Laparoscopic Pelvic Anatomy in Females

Shailesh Puntambekar • Sambit M. Nanda
Kajal Parikh

Laparoscopic Pelvic Anatomy in Females

Applied Surgical Principles

Springer

Shailesh Puntambekar
Galaxy Care Laparoscopy Institute Pvt. Ltd.
Pune
India

Kajal Parikh
Consultant Gynecologist and
Laparoscopic Surgeon
Thunga Hospital
Malad
Mumbai
India

Sambit M. Nanda
Consultant Gynecologist and
Laparoscopic Surgeon
Dr. Pattnaik's Hospital
Bandra
Mumbai
India

ISBN 978-981-13-8652-7 ISBN 978-981-13-8653-4 (eBook)
https://doi.org/10.1007/978-981-13-8653-4

This Springer imprint is published by the registered company Springer Nature Singapore Pte Ltd.
The registered company address is: 152 Beach Road, #21-01/04 Gateway East, Singapore 189721, Singapore

This book is dedicated to all the patients who allowed me to learn and relearn the concepts of anatomy. My sincere thanks also go to my colleagues who have tirelessly worked backstage, believing me as a leader for the last 25 years.

Dedicated to my parents, my wife and my children.

Preface

It has been my long dream to teach everything that I learnt and everything that I gained from my experiences to the world. I have always believed that there are anatomical planes that have been existing in the human body. For a surgeon to do a good surgery, it is the understanding of these planes that would make the difference between good and bad surgeons. I always thought that there is a reason why the anatomy exists in a particular way and how best its knowledge can be used for the betterment of dissection. That is the time I then realised that the entire surgery is based on the fascias which surround the various structures and spaces and, of course, the vessels. Where are these fascias? How do they cover the organs? Where are the spaces? How do we find them? Where are the vessels? How do we work not to damage them? These were the questions that always come to my mind. Some surgeons are God-gifted, while majority are not. But for any surgery to survive, it has to be duplicable and the steps reproducible. With this single-handed motto, I decided to embark on the journey of unravelling the mystery and the magic of anatomy. This was more relevant in the era of minimal access surgery where a 360-degree vision is not possible, and hence one has to predict the next structure before it arrives on the operative fields. Thus, we coined the term "predictive anatomy". Along with these words came a few sentences which are not in correct English but were accepted in the world like "fat belongs to the rectum", "fat belongs to the bladder" and "dissection should always be parallel to the tubular structures". I later realised, when I coined these phrases, a lot of surgeons do the dissection the same way. But we gave words in a way in which dissection is to be done. The understanding of anatomy was solely responsible for me to achieve my ultimate dream of live laparoscopic uterine transplant.

This book has been a compilation of 1200 images which were drawn and selected, reselected, rejected and then finalised after reviewing more than 10,000 images. This was done over a period of 2 years wherein even the camera systems changed and we could get better pictures every time that we changed the systems. This involved a huge team effort and hard work. A lot of nights and a lot of tempers were involved. I remain indebted to few people who have worked hard to make these images see the light of the day. I am especially thankful to Dr. Sambit Nanda, Dr. Kajal Parikh, Dr. Shruti Ugran and Mr. Nilesh Sonawane who have taken monumental efforts to scan and change the pictures at every point where I was not satisfied.

I also thank my wife, Dr. Seema, and my two daughters, Shreya and Dr. Aishwarya, for their continued support and excusing me from the daily courses of life. It would remain incomplete if I do not thank my team of surgeons and gynaecologists, Dr. Mangesh Panse, Dr. Ravindra Sathe, Dr. Manoj Manchekar, Dr. Mihir Chitale, Dr. Mehul Mehta, Dr. Advait Jathar, Dr. Raviraj Tiruke and Dr. Tejashree Bakre, who provided valuable inputs and helped me complete the book. Finally, I would like to thank the publishers and all my colleagues and staff at Galaxy Care Hospital who have stood behind me. I hope, you enjoy reading this book and learn anatomy in such a way as that of Shiv Khera's saying: "You can win too".

Pune, India Shailesh Puntambekar
Mumbai, India Sambit M. Nanda
Mumbai, India Kajal Parikh

Introduction

The pelvic anatomy is a constant anatomy with very few variations. Thus, it is easy to master the anatomy. A thorough knowledge of anatomy leads to better surgery. Surgery is an art of science, and anatomy is a network of fasciae and planes. Finding these planes would lead to bloodless surgery.

The art of surgery has been revolutionised due to the introduction of various technologies. There has been a long journey from open to minimal access surgery. The minimal access surgery has further evolved from multiport to single port to NOTES to robotic surgery. Though there has been advancement in the technology and modes of access, what has remained constant is the *anatomy*. The basic foundation of any ultramodern surgery was and will always remain anatomy. Thus, a deep understanding of this anatomy is needed to perform good surgery and not just the understanding of anatomy from the anatomy books.

The biggest disadvantage of minimal access surgery is a limited vision. Hence, one needs to predict the next structure, the next organ and the next fascia. This is what we call as "predictive anatomy". The entire book will give you an insight into the art and science of understanding the "predictive anatomy". The anatomy is beneficial to surgeons, gynaecologist, urologist and any other surgeons who wish to do pelvic surgery.

Contents

About the Authors

Shailesh Puntambekar is a cancer surgeon who specialised in laparoscopic cancer surgery. He is heading 'Galaxy Care Laparoscopy Institute', Centre for Advanced Laparoscopy and Robotic Surgery, in Pune. Considered as an expert in laparoscopic pelvic surgery and gynaecological cancer surgery in the world, he has developed laparoscopic radical hysterectomy for cervical cancer known to the world over as the "Pune technique". He has to his contribution the largest published series of laparoscopic exenteration for advanced pelvic cancers. His highest contribution comes in the form of laparoscopic live donor uterine transplant. This was done in May 2017 and remains the first in the world. The outcome of our transplant was with the delivery of a female child on 18th October 2018. He sincerely believes that every procedure in gynaecology from the simplest TLH to the uterine transplant is possible with an excellent understanding of the pelvic anatomy. He has coined the word "predictive anatomy", which is extremely helpful in anticipating the anatomical structures. He has developed applied surgical anatomy which means using the knowledge of anatomy to develop the surgical planes. Since the last few years, the annual congress of AAGL (American Association of Gynecologic Laparoscopy) has had him doing live cadaveric dissection at an inaugural event. He is also a regular faculty at the International School of Surgical Anatomy (ISSA) which rest the cadaveric courses at Tubingen, Germany. He has trained more than 150 international surgeons and gynaecologists and 300 Indian surgeons and gynaecologists who duplicate the anatomical steps devised by him. He has demonstrated live surgeries in 35 countries all around the world and in 200 national workshops. His teaching and concepts of pelvic anatomy have been widely acknowledged by surgeons and gynaecologists. He has authored four books, out of which the *Atlas of Laparoscopic Surgery in Gynecologic Oncology* is now in its third edition. He has had more than 100 publications in peer-reviewed journals.

Sambit M. Nanda is a consultant gynaecologist and laparoscopic surgeon from Mumbai and is associated with Galaxy Care Hospital (Pune) since 2016. He received his formal training in Advanced Gynaec Laparoscopic Surgery as a fellow to renowned Laparoscopic Oncosurgeon Dr. Shailesh Puntambekar (Pune). During his tenure as a FMAS-MUHS fellow at Galaxy Hospital, Pune, he was privileged to be a team member of India's first successful uterine transplant surgery and the ongoing uterine transplant project till the year 2018. He holds his special interests in gyne-oncology and was recommended and selected for the coveted UICC International Fellowship in Germany under Dr. Ivo Meinhold. He is forever indebted to Dr. Shailesh Puntambekar for giving him the opportunity to participate and contribute in all aspects of research and data analysis for studying the anatomy of the pelvis and further culminating in the making of this book.

Kajal Parikh is a consultant gynaecologist and laparoscopic surgeon from Mumbai and is associated with Galaxy Care Hospital (Pune). She has received her training in Advanced Gynaec Laparoscopic Surgery, Laparoscopic Gynaec-Oncosurgery from the renowned Dr. Shailesh Puntambekar (Pune) and Dr. Neeta Warty (Mumbai). During her tenure as a FMAS-MUHS fellow at Galaxy Care Hospital, Pune, she was privileged to be a team member of

India's first successful uterine transplant surgery and the ongoing uterine transplant project. She is forever indebted to Dr. Shailesh Puntambekar for giving her the opportunity to participate in the research and data analysis for studying the anatomy of the pelvis that was involved in the making of this book.

1 Pelvic Organs

The organs in the abdomen are classified as abdominal and pelvic organs (Figs. 1.1 and 1.2).

This classification is important to understand from the surgical point of view. All the organs of the pelvis lie in the midline (Fig. 1.3a, b).

Thus there is enough surgical space available for dissection on the lateral side for dissection. This is true even if the organ expands (myomas, bladder tumours) (Figs. 1.4, 1.5, 1.6, 1.7, 1.8, 1.9, 1.10, 1.11, and 1.12).

The organs have an external opening and thus all of them can be visualised through various scopies. Thus the intracavitary pathologies can be easily diagnosed and treated in the initial conditions (Figs. 1.13, 1.14, 1.15, and 1.16).

All the pelvic organs are supported by the fascias and muscles. Thus weakness of either the fascias or the pelvic muscles or both allows them to herniate either internally or externally (Figs. 1.17 and 1.18).

Understanding this concept is very important. Thus the organs are a victim of the weakness of the fascias and muscles and the pathology does not lie within them. The treatment therefore should be directed more towards the correction of the fascias rather than the resection of the organ except in the most advanced or serious cases. The tightening of the fascias can be done perineally or laparoscopically without removing any part of the organ (Fig. 1.19).

The pelvic organs are dynamic organs and hence are actively innervated with the nerves. The autonomic supply is distributed like a main pipeline with offshoots. Thus the main nerve can be preserved by cutting the offshoots of the nerve going to the organ. The nerve supply is always accompanied with a small vessel and hence it is called as neurovascular supply (Fig. 1.20).

These concepts are important to understand that just cutting the nerves going to the organ may lead to bleeding. Additionally the main nerve can always be preserved if we understand the neurovascular anatomy (Fig. 1.21).

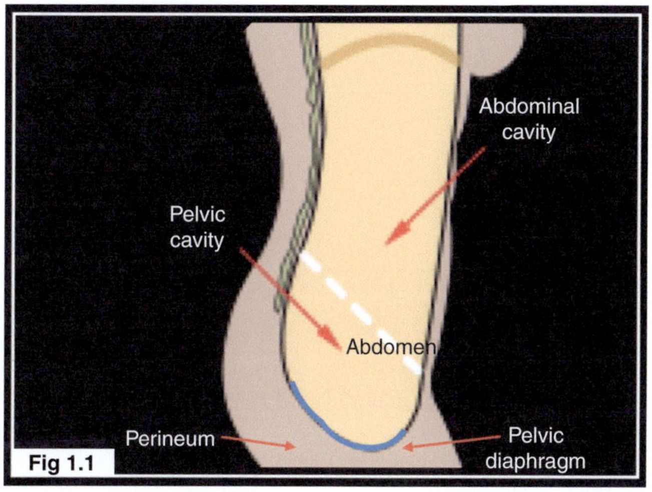

Fig. 1.1 Division of the abdomen into abdominal and pelvic cavity by an imaginary line from the sacral promontory to the pubic symphysis

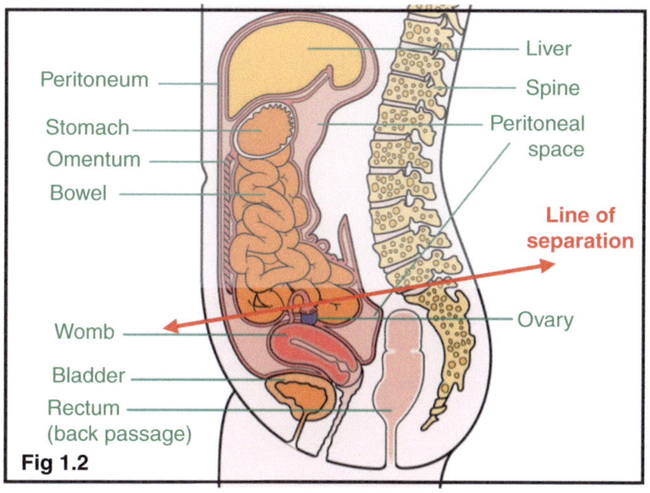

Fig. 1.2 Division of organs in the abdominal and the pelvic cavity

S. Puntambekar et al., *Laparoscopic Pelvic Anatomy in Females*, https://doi.org/10.1007/978-981-13-8653-4_1

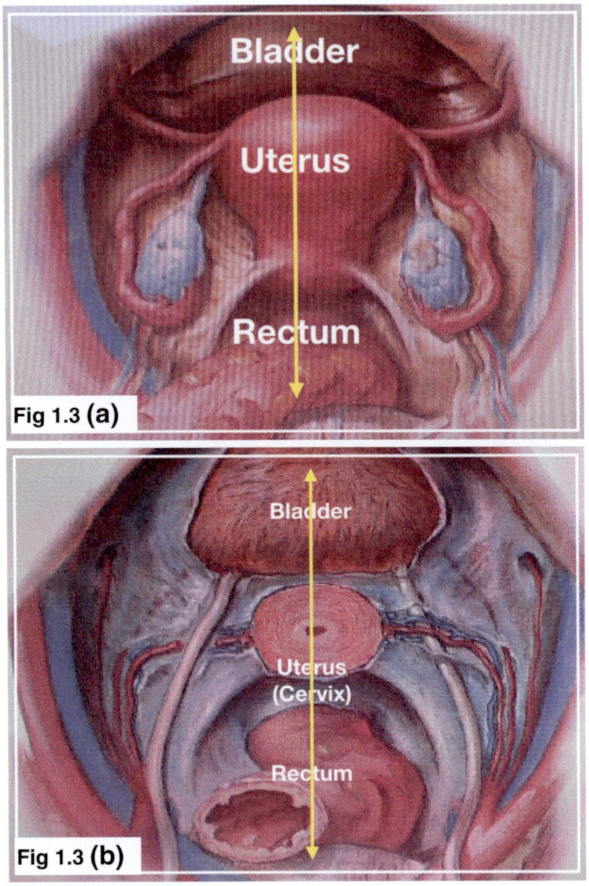

Fig. 1.3 (**a**) Surgical view point: Superior view of the pelvic cavity with normal anatomical position of organs. Uterus in the centre with the urinary bladder anteriorly and the rectum posteriorly. The organs are aligned in the centre. Image courtesy Parker-Macmillan Book of Pelvic Anatomy. (**b**) Surgical view point: Superior view of the pelvic cavity with the organs at the level of their vascular communications. Image courtesy Parker-Macmillan Book of Pelvic Anatomy

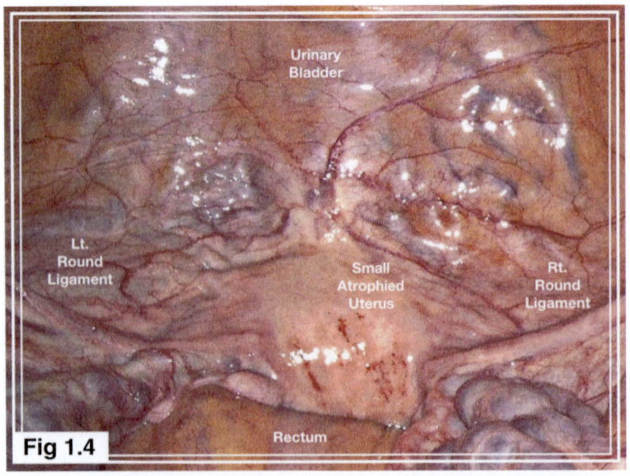

Fig. 1.4 Normal view on laparoscopy: Urinary bladder remains anterior, identification of the Foley can be appreciated. Small atrophic uterus with bilateral round ligaments retroverted and in midline, rectum identified along with the fat of appendices epiploicae identified posteriorly. Bilateral venous engorgement seen extending from near the cornua of uterus to the level of infundibulopelvic ligament

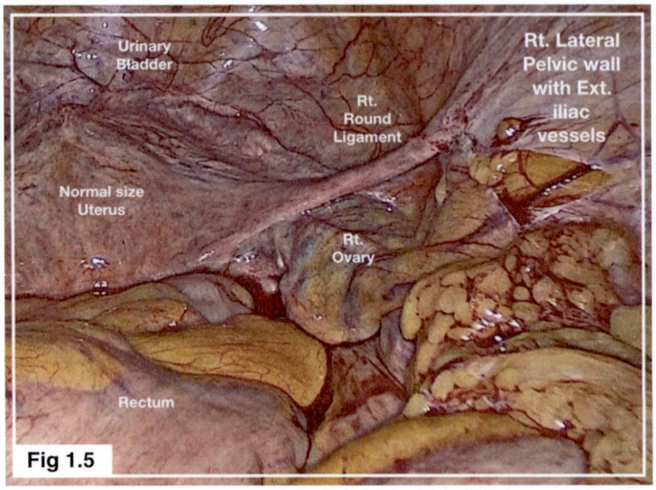

Fig. 1.5 Normal view on laparoscopy: Urinary bladder remains anterior; normal-size uterus retroverted and in midline position and the rectum lies posterior. The Right round ligament attached to the uterus can be used to trace up to the deep inguinal ring. The right lateral pelvic wall can be seen by the impressions of the Right external Iliac vessels and covered by retroperitoneal fat

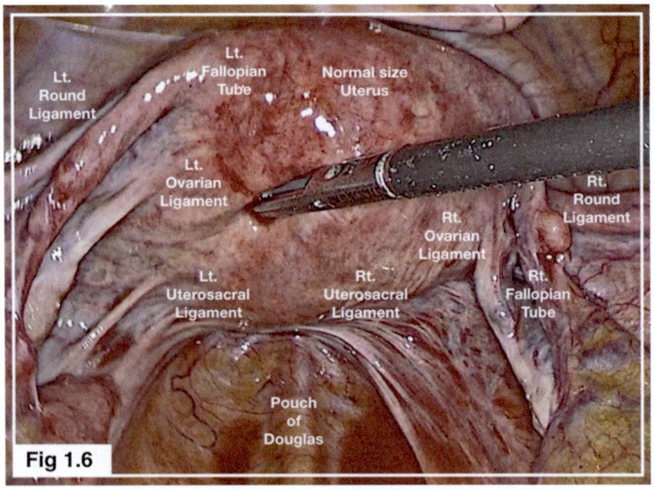

Fig. 1.6 Normal view on laparoscopy: Uterus in midline and mid-prone position with both round ligaments attached to the cornua. Both the fallopian tubes and the ovarian ligaments can be seen. The uterosacral ligaments can be identified inferiorly forming lateral boundaries for the pouch of Douglas which lies in the midline and inferior to the uterus. This patient had a history of tubal ligation which can be seen as the beaded appearance on the Right fallopian tube due to the silastic ring and engorgement of the mesosalpingeal vessels due to occlusion of the vessels with the silastic ring

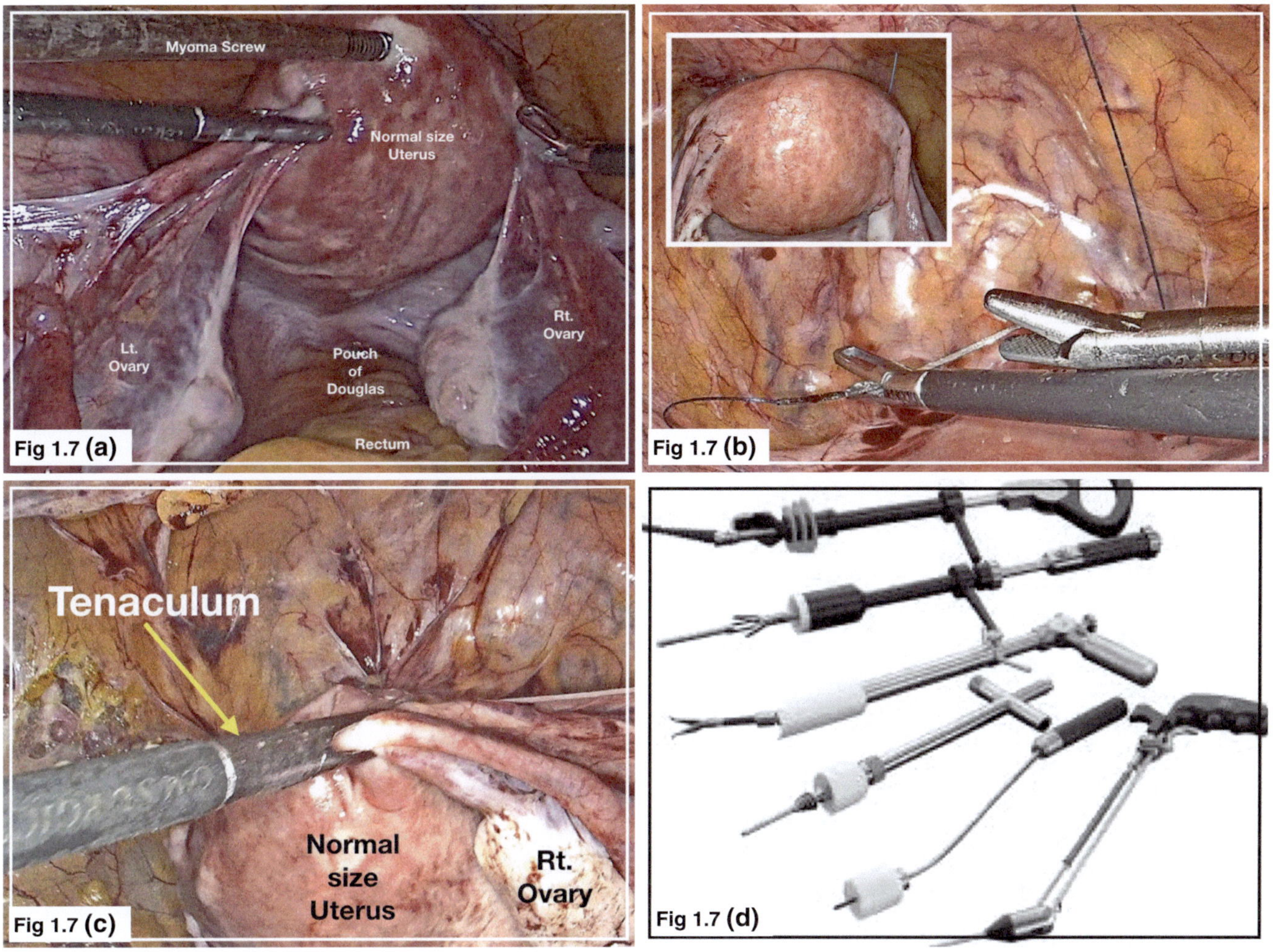

Fig. 1.7 (**a**) Uterine manipulation: Myoma screw inserted at the funds of the uterus used for manipulation and traction on the uterus. The myoma screw is a traumatic instrument and hence avoided in cases of fertility-preserving surgeries and cases of Ca endometrium. Both the ovaries are seen in their normal dependent positions, falling into the pouch of Douglas and towards the midline. The tubes appear ligated. (**b**) Tenaculum: In case of Ca endometrium or fertility-preserving surgery the uterus can be held and manipulated with the help of a tenaculum as well. (**c**) Hitch: Amongst the techniques of manipulation if the uterus is needed to be fixed upwards a uterine hitch can also be done to fix the uterus to the anterior abdominal in case of rectal surgeries as show here. Inset: The uterus is lifted to the anterior abdominal wall. (**d**) There are various vaginal manipulators available which are very popular amongst gynaecologists. Image courtesy: Karl Storz uterine manipulators

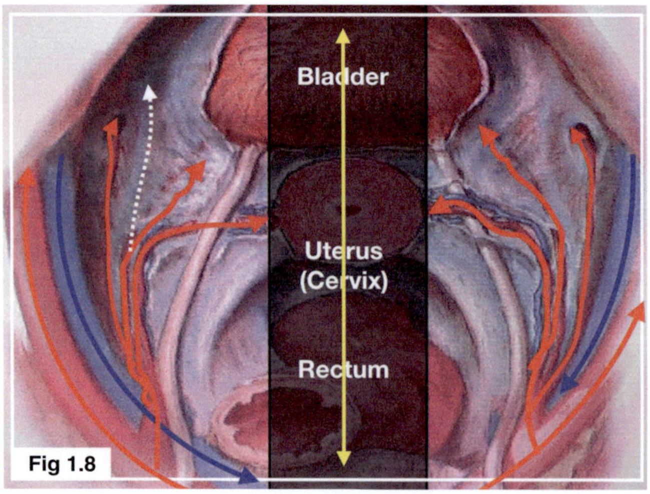

Fig. 1.8 Surgical view point: Organs of the pelvis receive the blood supply from the lateral side. The vessels flow from the lateral pelvic wall medially to drain into the organs. The chief vessel is the anterior division of the internal iliac artery which sends off branches travelling medially to the uterus as the uterine artery and the bladder as superior vesicle artery and then gets obliterated and travels to the anterior abdominal wall as the obliterated hypogastric ligament or the median umbilical ligament

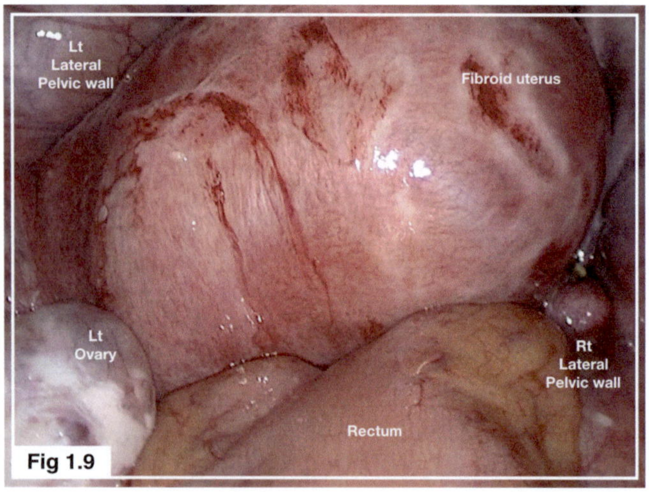

Fig. 1.9 Resilience of pelvic anatomy: Large-size myoma arising from the uterus, from the midline without involving or distorting the lateral pelvic wall anatomy

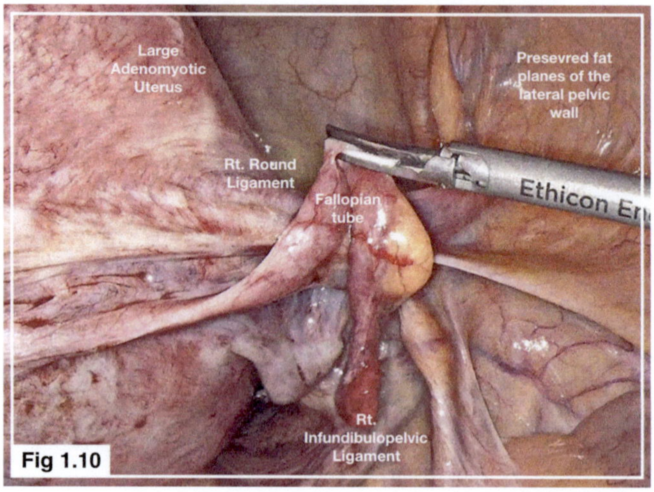

Fig. 1.10 Resilience of pelvic anatomy: Large adenomyotic uterus growing centrally and midline without distorting the anatomy of the lateral pelvic wall. Fat planes appear preserved. Right round ligament and fallopian tubes are intact and uninvolved

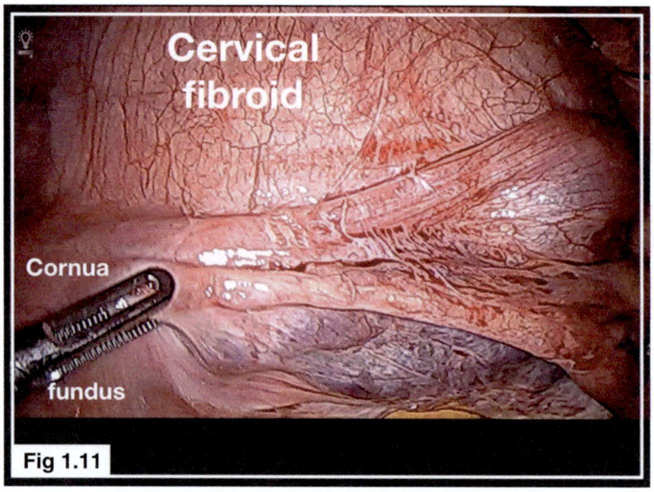

Fig. 1.11 A cervical fibroid can be seen in this image. The funds and the cornua can be easily identified

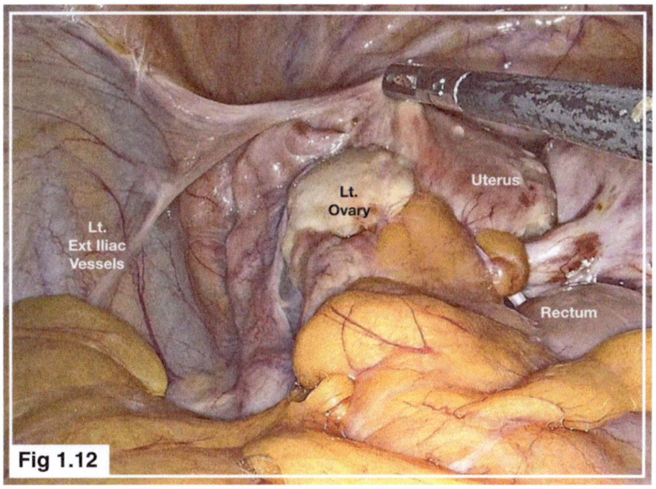

Fig. 1.12 A case of Grade IV endometriosis with uterus densely adherent on the posterior surface to the rectum with obliterated pouch of Douglas. Left external iliac vessels appear free and uninvolved. The left ovary has mixed components; the healthy solid component is seen on the surface anteriorly while the cystic component is embedded or wrapped or densely adherent to the lateral pelvic wall and rectum. The right structures, i.e. Right round ligament and possibly the Right ovary, are also engulfed in the adherent mass posterior to the uterus

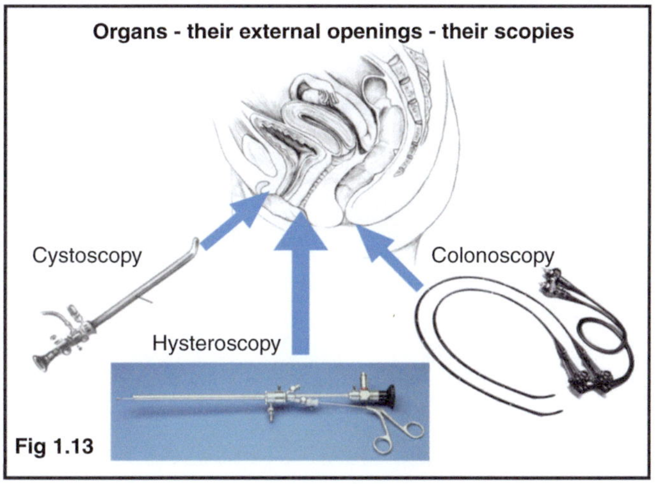

Fig. 1.13 Natural orifice endoscopy: Pelvic organs and their respective natural orifices and their related minimally invasive endoscopes and instruments

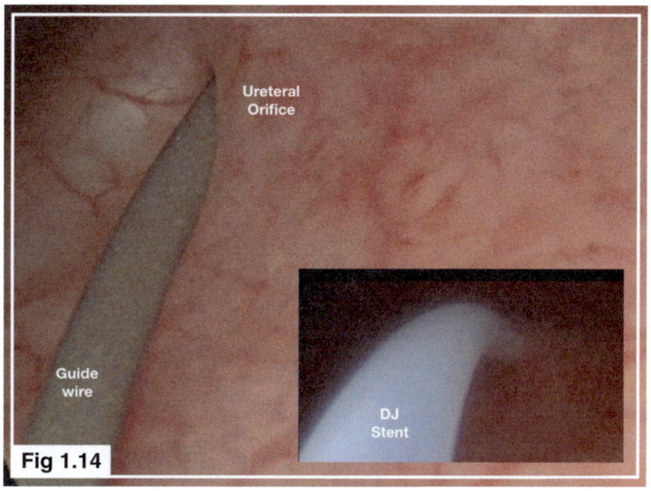

Fig. 1.14 Cystoscopy: A case of cervical cancer requiring cystoscopy-guided stenting post-operatively with a guide wire first followed by a DJ stent

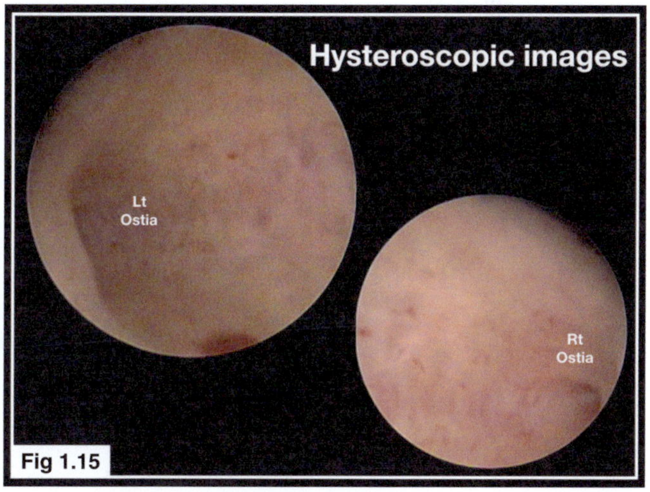

Fig. 1.15 Hysteroscopy: A case of postmenopausal bleeding being investigated by diagnostic hysteroscopy with biopsy. Bilateral ostia are visualised

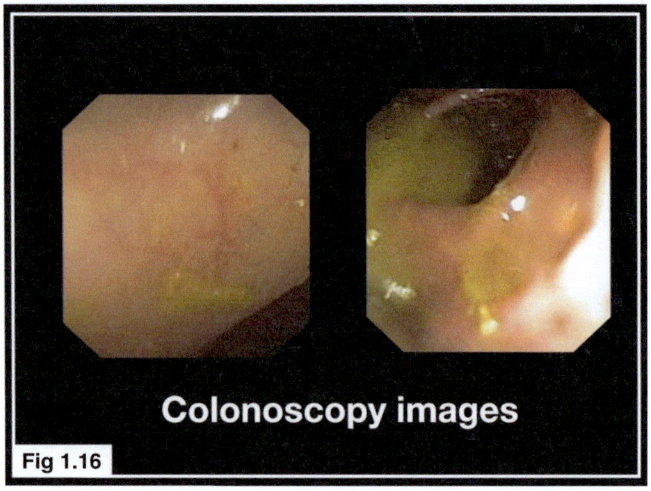

Fig. 1.16 Colonoscopy: Images of the sigmoid colon and the mucosal wall seen through colonoscopy

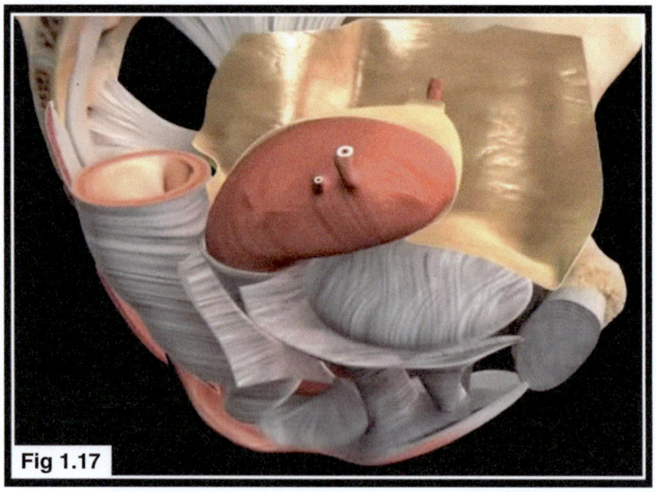

Fig. 1.17 All the fascias covering the organs of the pelvis

Fig. 1.18 All organs are lined by a sheet of fibrous connective tissue (fascia) and named as per their locations and organs covered

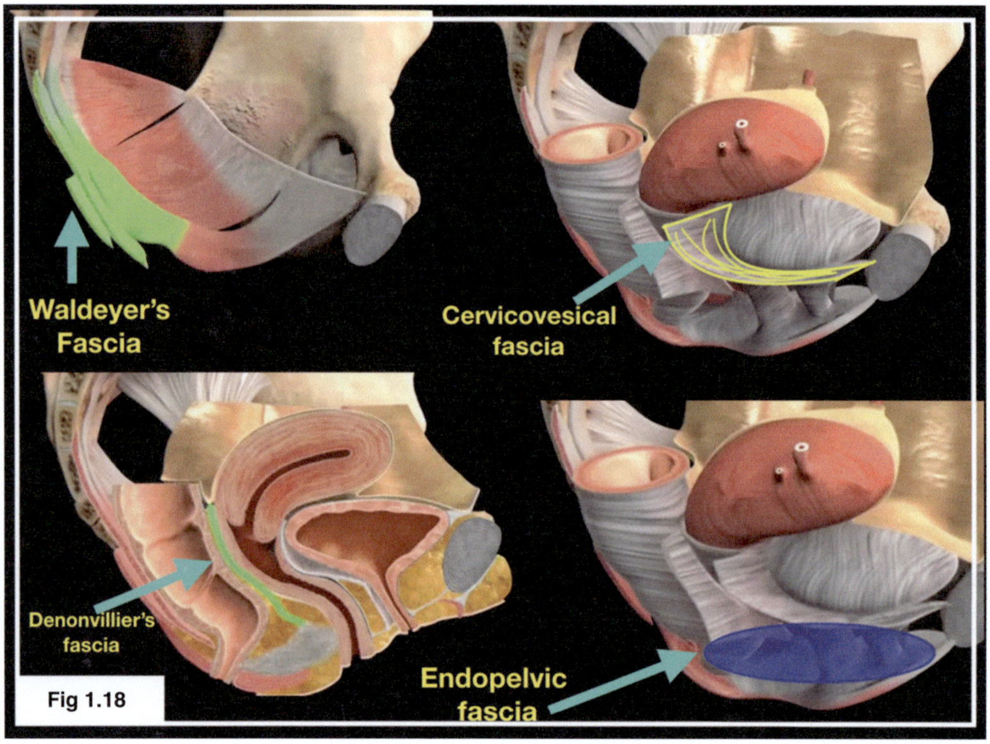

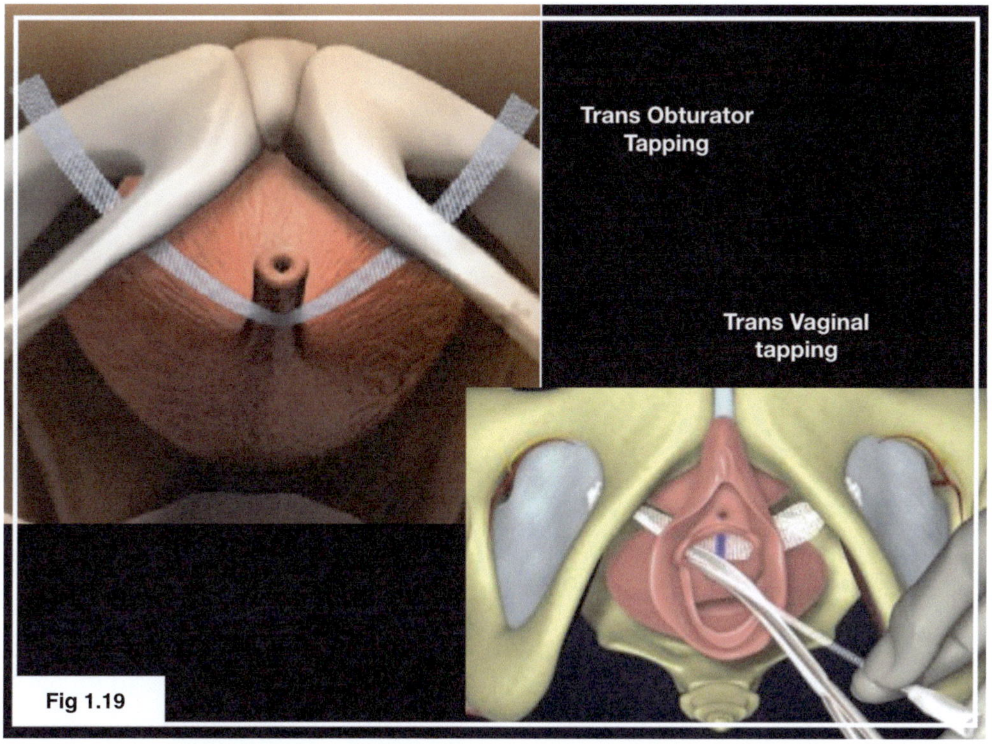

Fig. 1.19 Transobturator taping and transvaginal taping. Application of these principles of anatomy has helped develop slings for repairing fascial defects

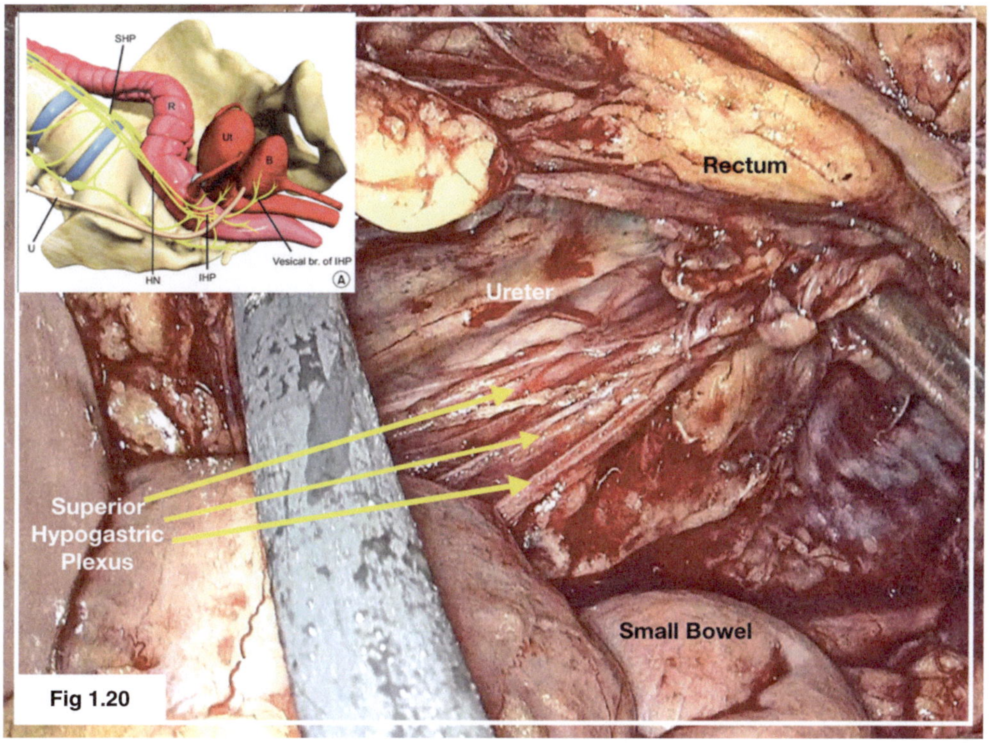

Fig. 1.20 Offshoots of hypogastric nerve plexus along the rectum travelling towards the uterus and supplying the bladder

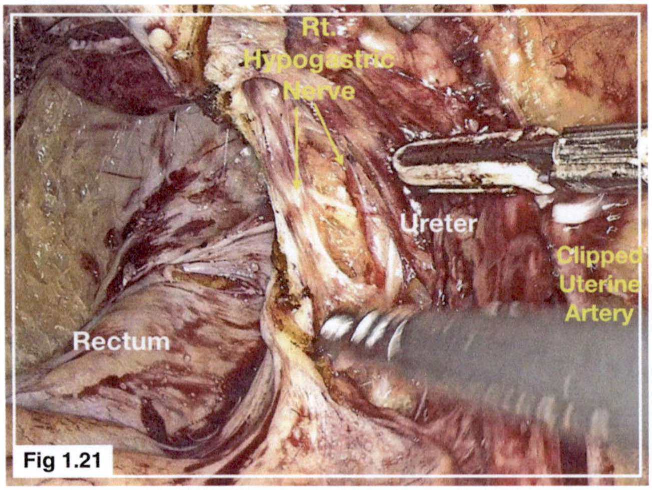

Fig. 1.21 A case of laparoscopic radical hysterectomy performing rectovaginal space dissection, demonstrating the significance of dissection in the correct avascular plane to prevent bleeding

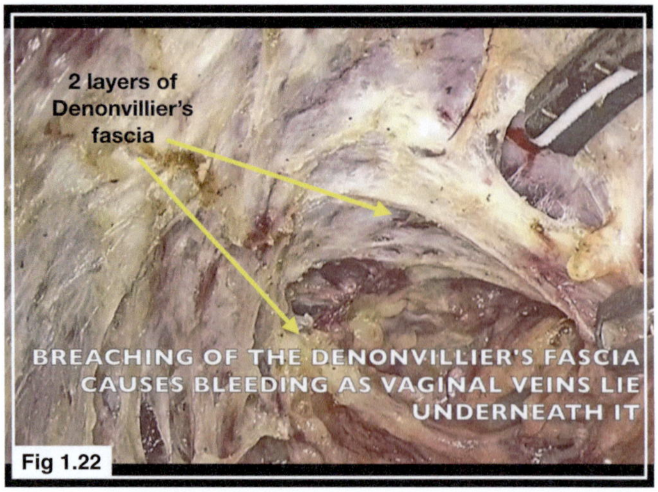

Fig. 1.22 A case of laparoscopic nerve-sparing radical hysterectomy showing the right hypogastric nerves and their dissection for nerve preservation

The main reason for this book is to make you understand why the anatomy exists in a particular way and how understanding this anatomy can help you strategise your surgical steps. The pelvis is unique not only due to the reasons mentioned above but also because the variations in the anatomy are extremely rare compared to the abdominal organs. Since the organs are dynamic care has to be taken during the surgical manoeuvres to preserve the integrity of the remaining organs (Figs. 1.22 and 1.23).

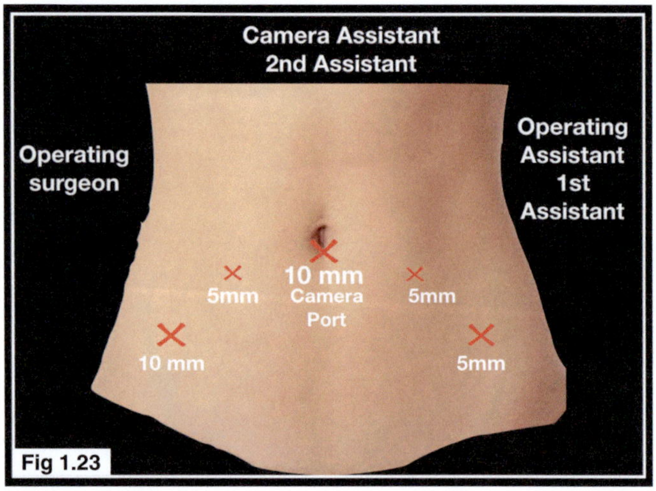

Fig. 1.23 Ports and surgeon position: All images in the atlas have been taken with these fixed positions of the ports and the surgeons as shown above. Pneumoperitoneum is achieved at the Palmer's point

2 Pelvis Boundaries

The pelvic cavity starts at the level of sacral promontory and is bounded by bony structures laterally. The caudal limit is pelvic floor (Figs. 2.1, 2.2, 2.3, 2.4, and 2.5).

The structures included are the uterus with adnexa, ureters, urinary bladder, rectum and prostate in males (Fig. 2.6).

The anatomy defers in males and females only in the region of prostate. The pelvic organs are the uterus, bladder and prostate. The rectum and ureters enter the pelvis from upper abdomen (Fig. 2.7).

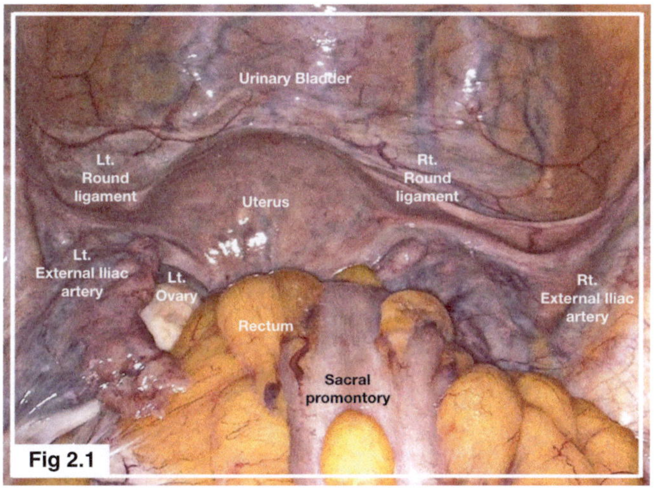

Fig. 2.1 View from the midline and above the level of sacral promontory: The sacral promontory at the centre covered by the rectum and sigmoid colon, flanked by the external iliac artery bilaterally. Anteriorly and below the level of sacral promontory, the uterus and the urinary bladder are well appreciated

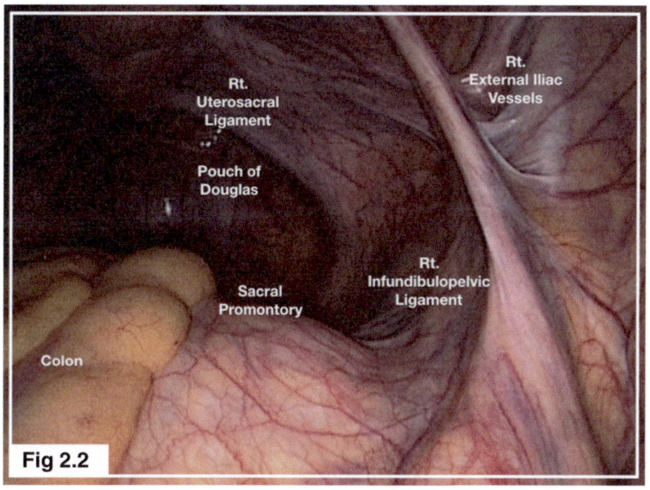

Fig. 2.2 Structures seen at the level of sacral promontory: A view from across the left side and above the level of sacral promontory with right infundibulopelvic ligament seen. The uterus is anteverted exposing the Right uterosacral ligament and the pouch of Douglas. The Right external iliac artery and vein can be seen lateral to the infundibulopelvic ligament

S. Puntambekar et al., *Laparoscopic Pelvic Anatomy in Females*, https://doi.org/10.1007/978-981-13-8653-4_2

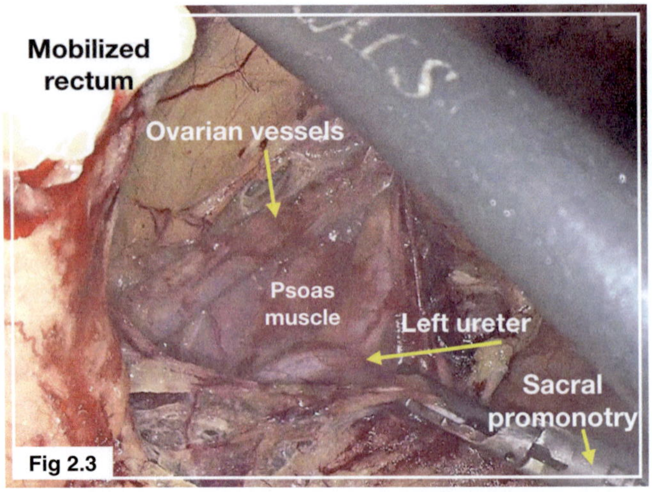

Fig. 2.3 Structure from right above sacral promontory: In a case of laparoscopic low anterior resection during mobilisation of the rectum the contralateral structures can be seen underneath the rectum. The left ureter and left ovarian vessel can be seen in this image. All these structures and their positions are visible at a level above the sacral promontory

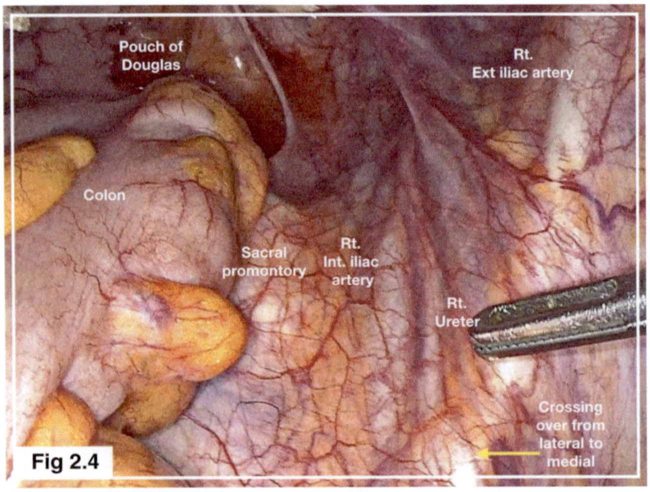

Fig. 2.4 Structures seen at the level of sacral promontory: The external iliac artery, the ureter tossing over to the medial side at the bifurcation of the common iliac artery and the internal iliac artery

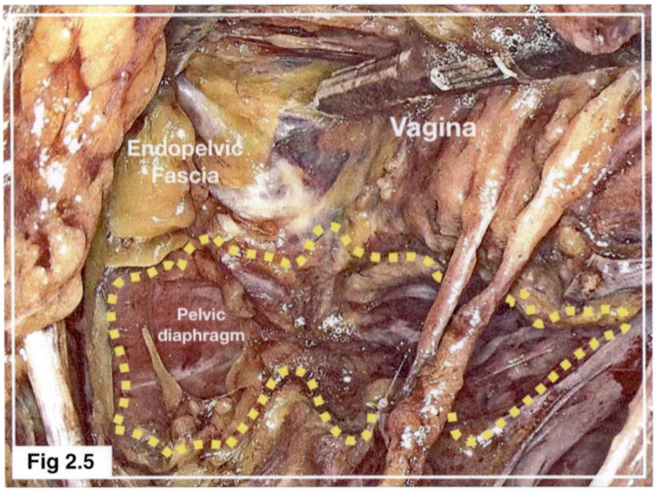

Fig. 2.5 Pelvic diaphragm: This dissection was done in a case of total pelvic exenteration for recurrent Ca ovary. The yellow dotted line represents the area of the pelvic diaphragm covered by the endopelvic fascia

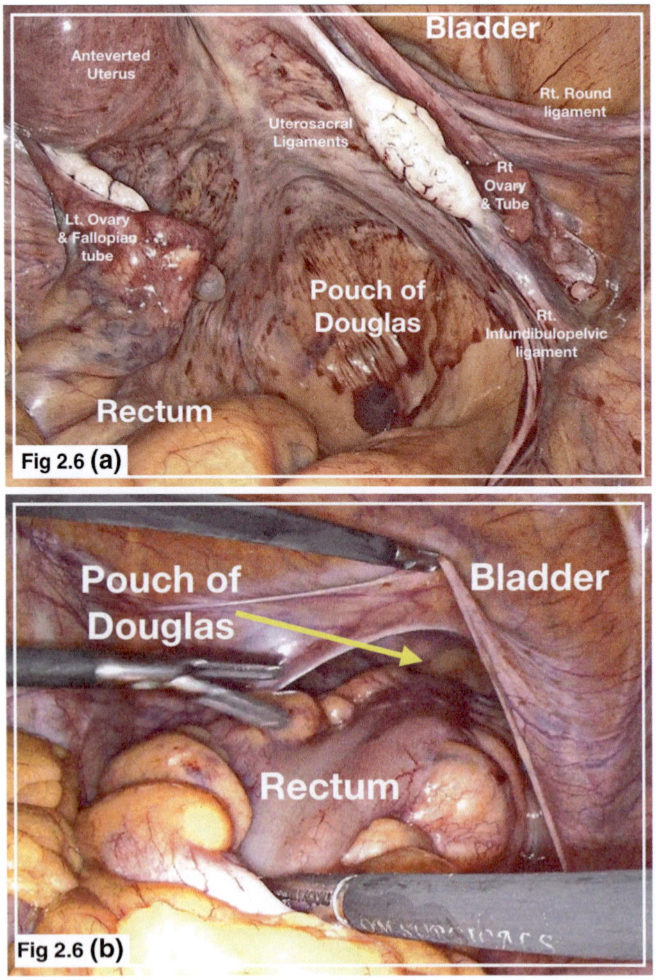

Fig. 2.6 (**a**) Structures with the female pelvic cavity: The rectum posteriorly, the uterus at the centre with Right ovary (adnexa), the urinary bladder (the fold of bladder peritoneum can be appreciated anteriorly). (**b**) Structures in the male pelvic cavity: The rectum posteriorly, the pouch of Douglas between the rectum and bladder. The bladder with prostate and ureters under the peritoneum

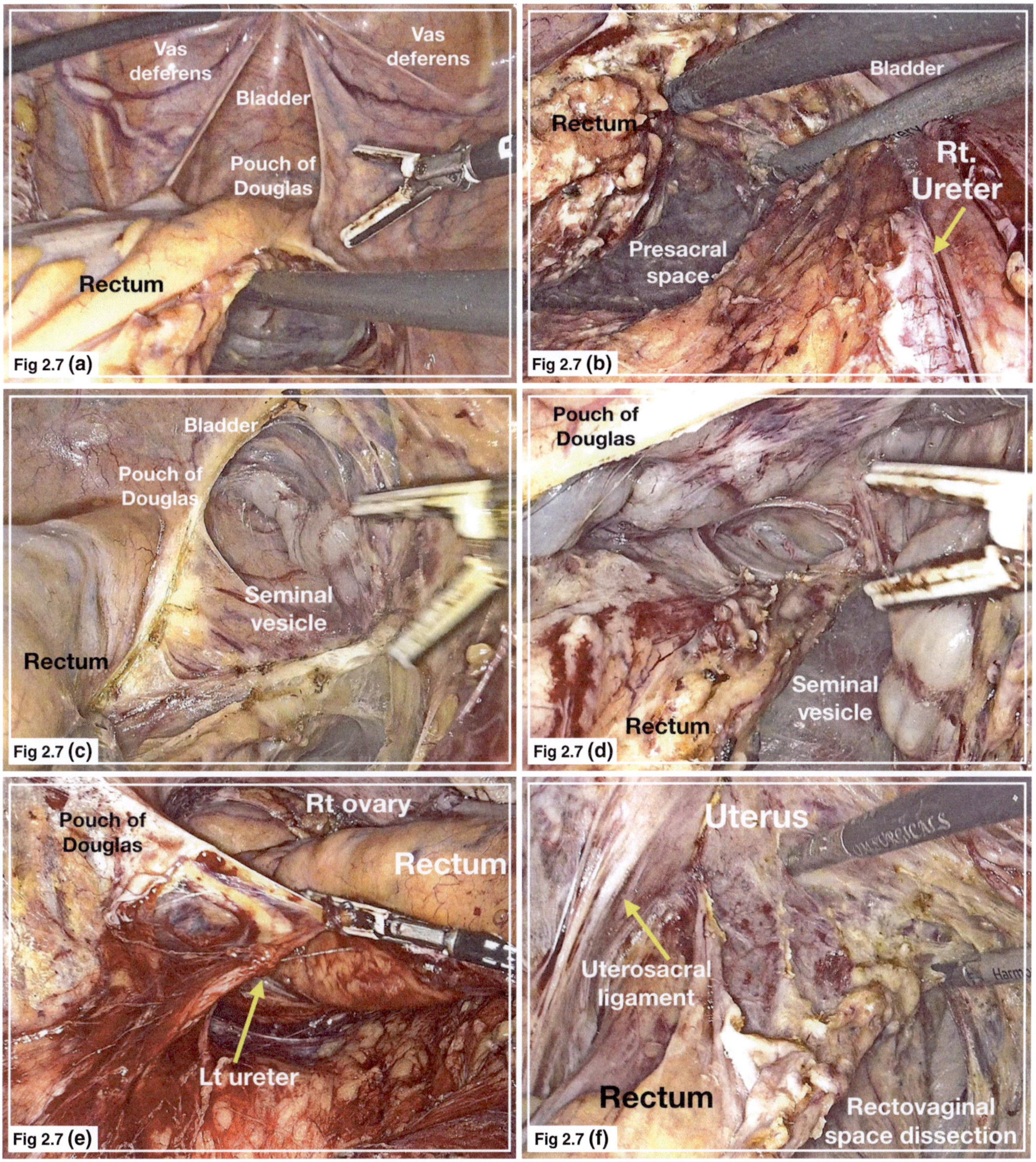

Fig. 2.7 (**a**) In a case of laparoscopic low anterior resection in male patient. The rectum is mobilised from the posterior surface. The pouch of Douglas is dissected exposing the seminal vesicles anteriorly along with the prostate. (**b**) The pouch of Douglas is dissected and the ureters are visualised in this image. The impressions of the vas deferens can be seen through the peritoneum travelling to the deep inguinal ring. (**c**) The seminal vesicles are visualised here in this case. The ureters are not visualised further ahead in the operating area as the bladder is not dissected any further and secondly the ureter goes deeper into its course and is inserted in the bladder. (**d**) The prostate appears as a vascular region between the spinal vesicles on either side. The pouch of Douglas has been completely dissected. (**e**) In a similar case of laparoscopic low anterior resection done in a female patient. The rectum is mobilised in a similar fashion but the pouch of Douglas leads to dissection of the rectovaginal space, thus exposing the ureters and the vagina on their posterior surface anteriorly. The right ovary can be seen in the upper right corner. The ureter is more frequently seen as it is closely associated with the uterus and due to a relative lack of space as compared to male pelvis. (**f**) Rectovaginal space dissection separates the rectum from the uterus. Dissection carried out between the two layers of Denonvilliers' fascia. (**g**) The rectum is completely from the uterus and uterosacral ligaments. Both the ovaries can be seen clearly

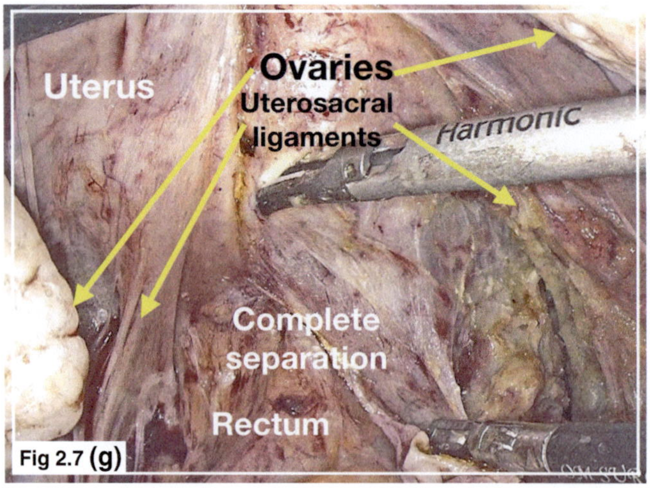

Fig. 2.7 (continued)

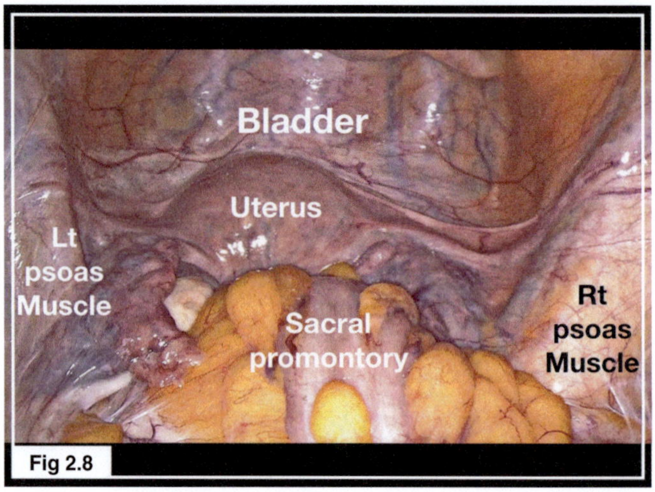

Fig. 2.8 The sacral promontory is the cranial boundary of the pelvis

2.1 Sacral Promontory (Fig. 2.8)

The view from sacral promontory showing the sacral promontory at the highest point on the pelvis. The uterus in midline and flanked by the psoas muscle on each side.

At this level the following anatomical things happen:

1. The common iliac divides into internal and external artery (Fig. 2.9).
2. The ureter crosses the common iliac artery from the lateral to the medial side and continues to remain as the most medial tubular structure. Thus remaining medial to the ureter during dissection will prevent damage to the major vascular structures (Fig. 2.10).
3. The superior hypogastric plexus lies at that level and the hypogastric nerves then travel on the posterolateral side of the organs. Care has to be taken during sacrocolpopexy as the suture at the level of sacral promontory can damage the superior hypogastric plexus. These nerves lie at a deeper plane than the ureter. Remaining at the level of ureter will prevent damage to the nerves; also the nerves are lateral and hence can be preserved during any of the pelvic organ removal (Figs. 2.11 and 2.12).
4. From the sacral promontory to the pelvic diaphragm there is Waldeyer's fascia which covers the presacral veins. During the surgical dissections this fascia should not be violated as there can be torrential bleeding. This fascia is seen during the dissection done for pelvic organ repair like sacrocolpopexy. The risk of damaging the fascia is when one takes suture to fix the mesh at the sacral promontory (Figs. 2.13 and 2.14).
5. None of the pathologies of the uterus reach the sacral promontory and hence in difficulty one can start the dissection at the level of sacral promontory (Figs. 2.15, 2.16, and 2.17).

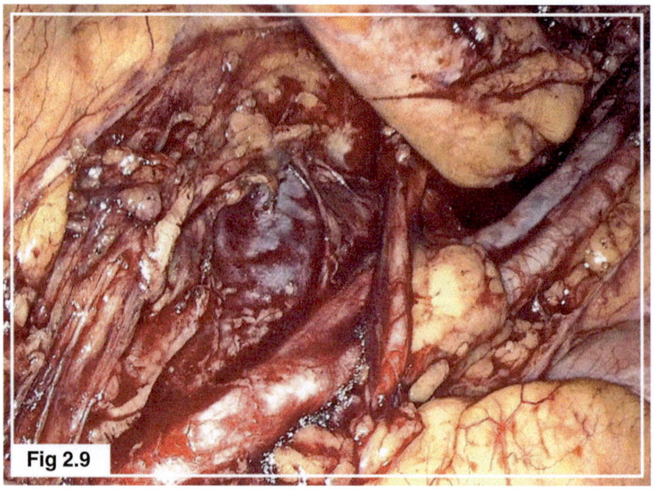

Fig. 2.9 At the level of sacral promontory the common iliac bifurcates into the external and internal iliac arteries and the ureter crosses over from lateral to medial over the bifurcation. This has been shown in the image

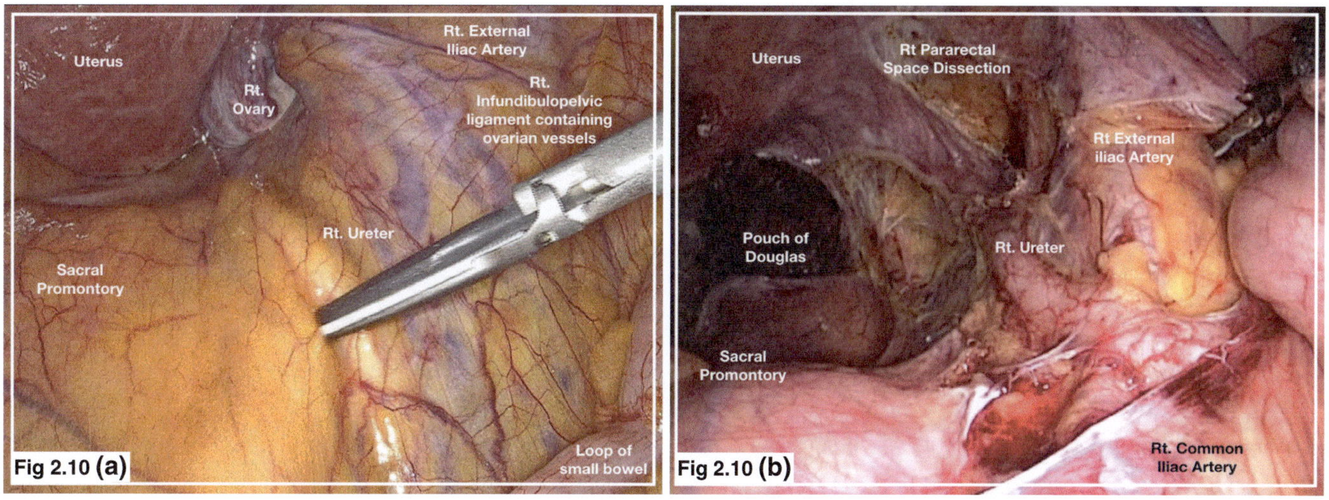

Fig. 2.10 (**a**) Structures seen on the right side of the sacral promontory: The sacral promontory, Right ureter, Right infundibulopelvic ligament and Right external iliac artery. The infundibulopelvic ligament contains ovarian vessels, and the veins can be seen more prominently as they are more superficial and appear engorged. (**b**) Structures seen on the right side of sacral promontory: The sacral promontory lies in the midline, and the Right ureter lies lateral to the sacral promontory. The Right ureter crosses over from the lateral to the medial side at the level of bifurcation of common iliac artery. Thus the common iliac artery can be appreciated when traced cranially from the ureter. The external iliac artery lies lateral to the ureter; it can be traced caudally from the ureter. The internal iliac artery lies at the level below the sacral promontory and medial to the ureter though its origin lies at the level of scrap promontory and just below the level of ureter

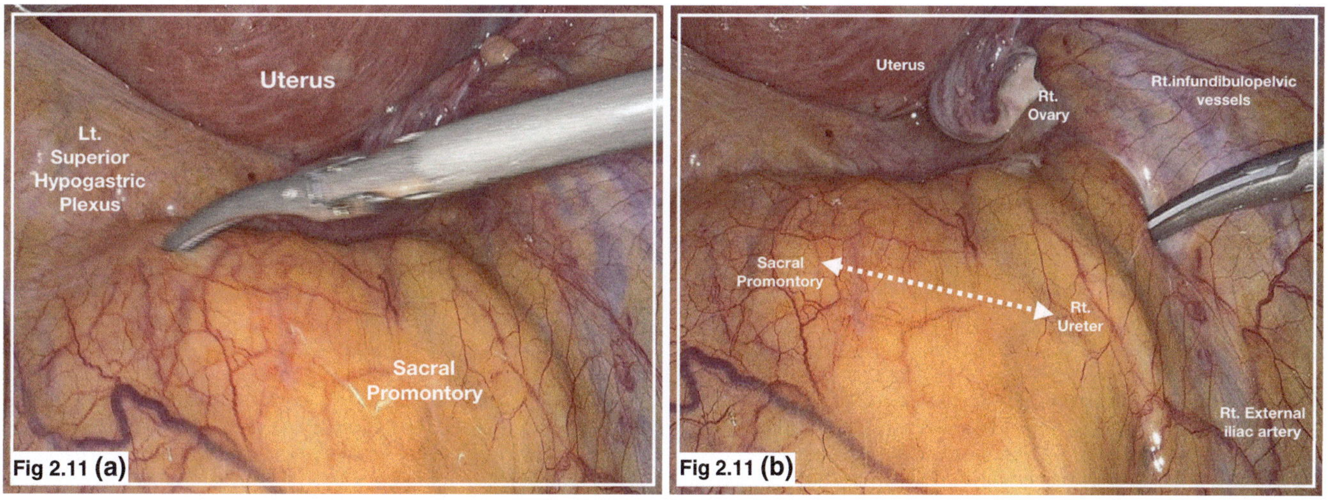

Fig. 2.11 (**a**) Structures seen at the level of sacral promontory when viewed from the right side: Sacral promontory on the left side (though midline) with the Right ureter crossing over from the lateral to medial side. There is a significant distance between them, and underneath the peritoneum is a tough fibrous relatively avascular tissue called anterior longitudinal ligament. This area is useful for suturing in cases of sacrocolpopexy and mesh repair. (**b**) The representative image of sacrocolpopexy. (**c**) Structures seen at the level of sacral promontory: The superior hypogastric plexus of the sympathetic nervous system is present under the peritoneum at the level of sacral promontory. They are pointed out by the grasper on the left side. Thus the sacral promontory is also an important landmark for nerve-sparing surgeries, i.e. nerve-sparing radical hysterectomy

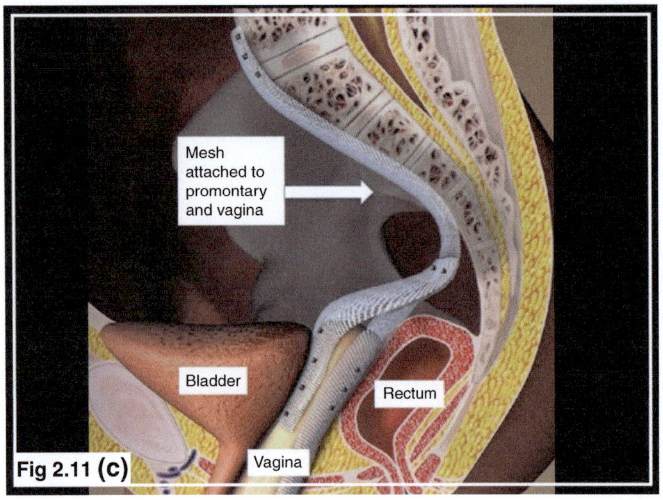

Fig. 2.11 (continued)

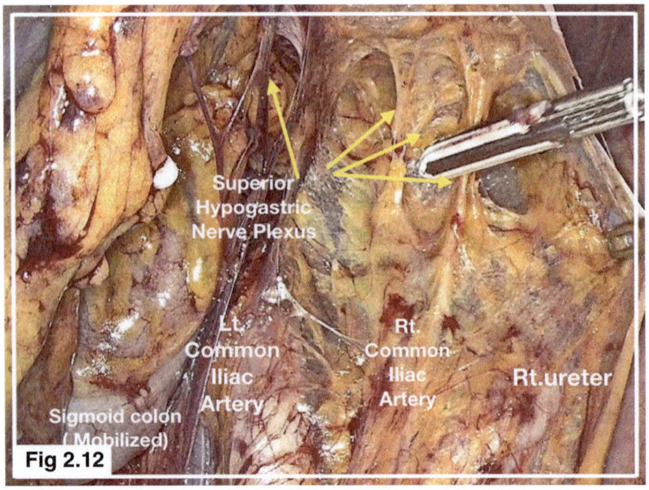

Fig. 2.12 Superior hypogastric plexus: In a case of posterior exenteration, dissection of the rectum from the presacral fascia at the level of the sacral promontory for mobilisation of the colon and the nerves is well appreciated. Fine dissection at this level reveals the nerves which are preserved to maintain the bladder function anteriorly

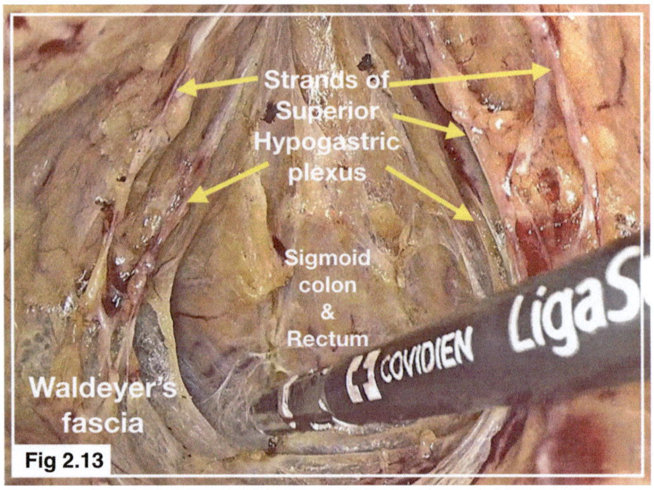

Fig. 2.13 Dissection of Waldeyer's fascia (presacral fascia): In a case of posterior exenteration mobilisation of the sigmoid colon and rectum is done by dissection of the Waldeyer's or presacral fascia. This completely exposes the superior hypogastric plexus of nerves as shown in the figure bilaterally

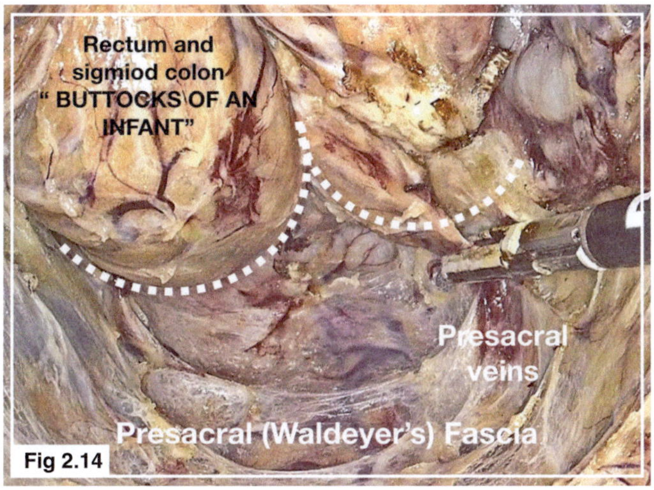

Fig. 2.14 Dissection of Waldeyer's fascia: In a case of posterior exenteration, mobilisation is done for the colon and the rectum. Dissection done in the correct plane is avascular and the classical appearance resembles the "buttocks of an infant"

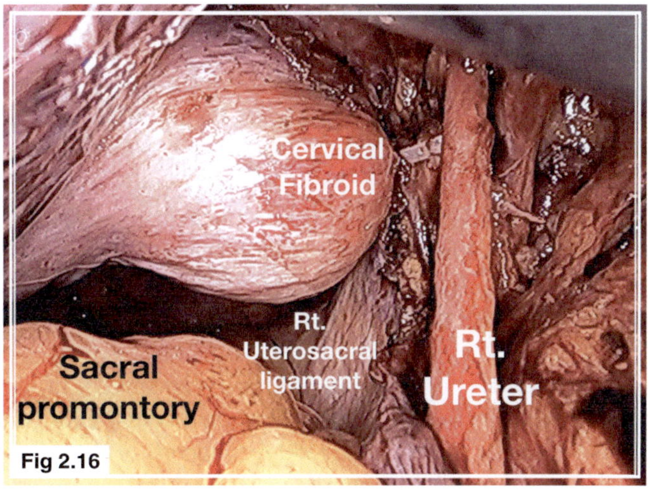

Fig. 2.16 Cervical fibroid: In a case of a 28-year-old secondary infertility with cervical fibroid was posted for myomectomy: As seen the sacral promontory lies above the pathology. The right ureter has been completely dissected along its entire pelvic course to help ease complete dissection of the cervical fibroid

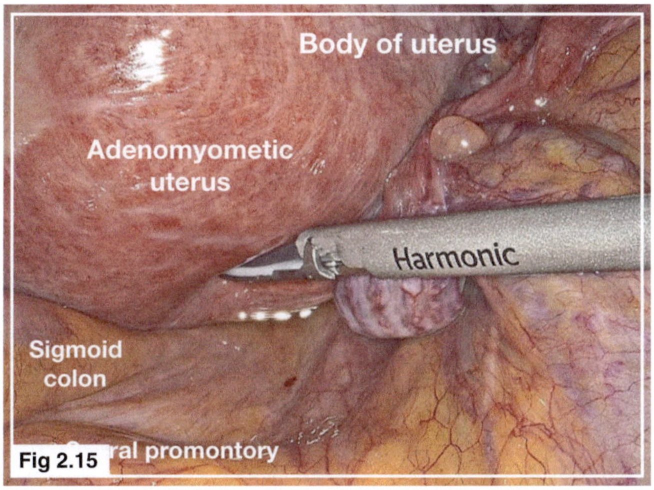

Fig. 2.15 Origin of pelvic pathologies: Pelvic pathologies do not arise from above the sacral promontory. The origin of the largest fibroid if traced is placed below the level of sacral promontory

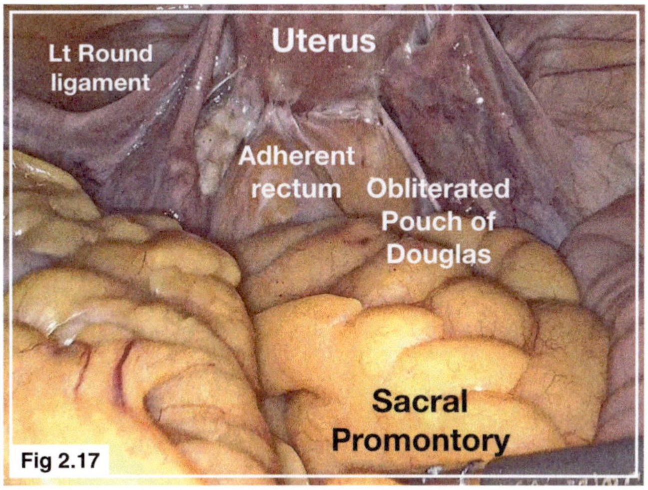

Fig. 2.17 Grade IV endometriosis: In this case of Grade IV endometriosis we can see obliterated pouch of Douglas due to adhesions between structures. This adhesiolysis can be initiated from a fixed bony point such as sacral promontory. Sacral promontory almost always/relatively remains free of adhesions in Grade IV endometriosis

2.2 Concepts of the Blood Supply

1. With the exception of rectum and ovaries all the other organs have their blood supply originating from the lateral pelvic wall of the pelvis (Figs. 2.18, 2.19, and 2.20).
2. The midline organs receive their blood supply from the lateral side. They have to travel a distance before they reach the organ. Surgically this concept allows you to clamp the vessel laterally. Also the fact that there is a long pedicle available for ligation helps in performing bloodless surgery (Fig. 2.21a–k).
3. The corollary to the above concept is the support of the uterus lying medial to the origin of the vessels. Thus one can modify or strengthen or cut the supports of the uterus without damaging the blood supply (Fig. 2.22a–c).
4. The ureter is always lateral to and at the base of uterosacral ligament. Thus remaining medial to and at the apex of the uterosacral ligament will prevent damage to the ureter (Fig. 2.23a–c).

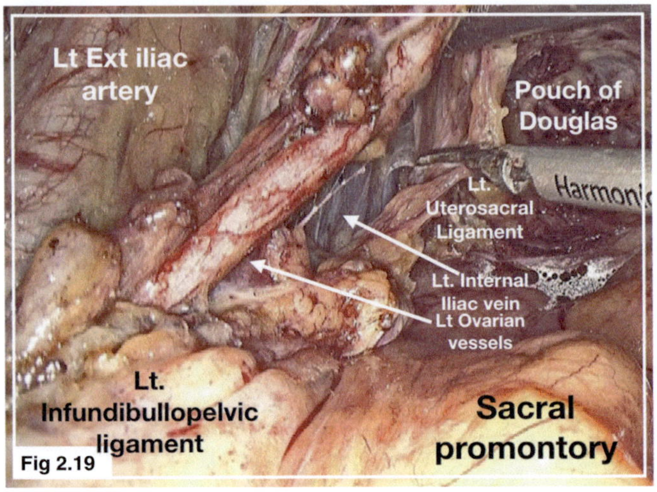

Fig. 2.19 Blood supply to the ovary: Careful dissection of the infundibulopelvic ligament exposes the ovarian artery and the vein. A shadowy figure of the internal iliac vein can be appreciated underneath. It follows the same course as the internal iliac artery and runs parallel to it. The left uterosacral ligament has been shown gripped between the harmonic blades

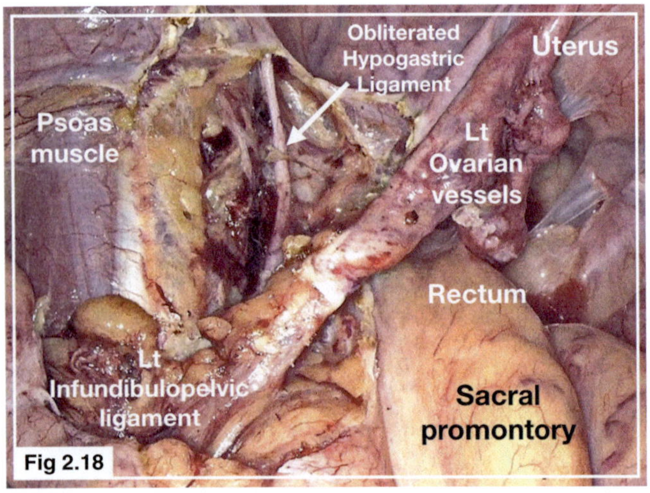

Fig. 2.18 Blood supply to the ovary: All organs of the pelvis except the ovaries and the rectum receive blood from the branches of internal iliac artery arising from the lateral pelvic wall. The ovarian vessels pass through the infundibulopelvic ligament to supply the ovaries. The rectum receives blood from the inferior mesenteric artery (superior rectal artery—primarily) above the sacral promontory and often from the middle rectal artery which is the branch of the internal iliac artery. The internal iliac artery can be seen at its terminal stage where it gets obliterated to form the obliterated hypogastric ligament or the median umbilical ligament

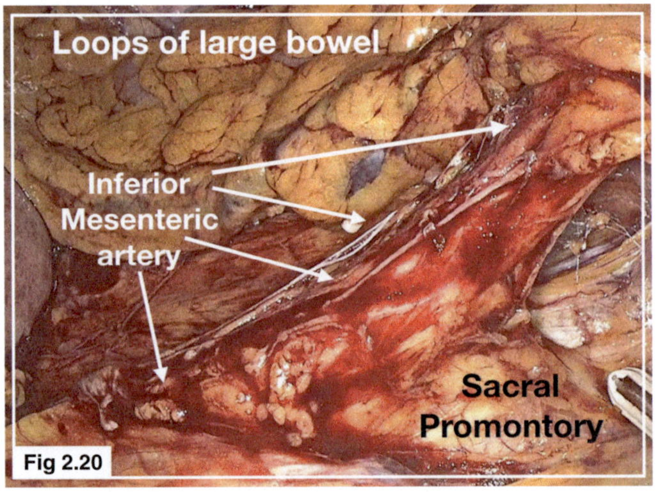

Fig. 2.20 Blood supply to the rectum: The inferior mesenteric artery seen as a thick band above the aural promontory. It is identified as the only vessel which crosses over across from the right to the left above the sacral promontory. This dissection was done for mobilisation of bowel up to the splenic flexure for resection and re-anastomosis of the large bowel

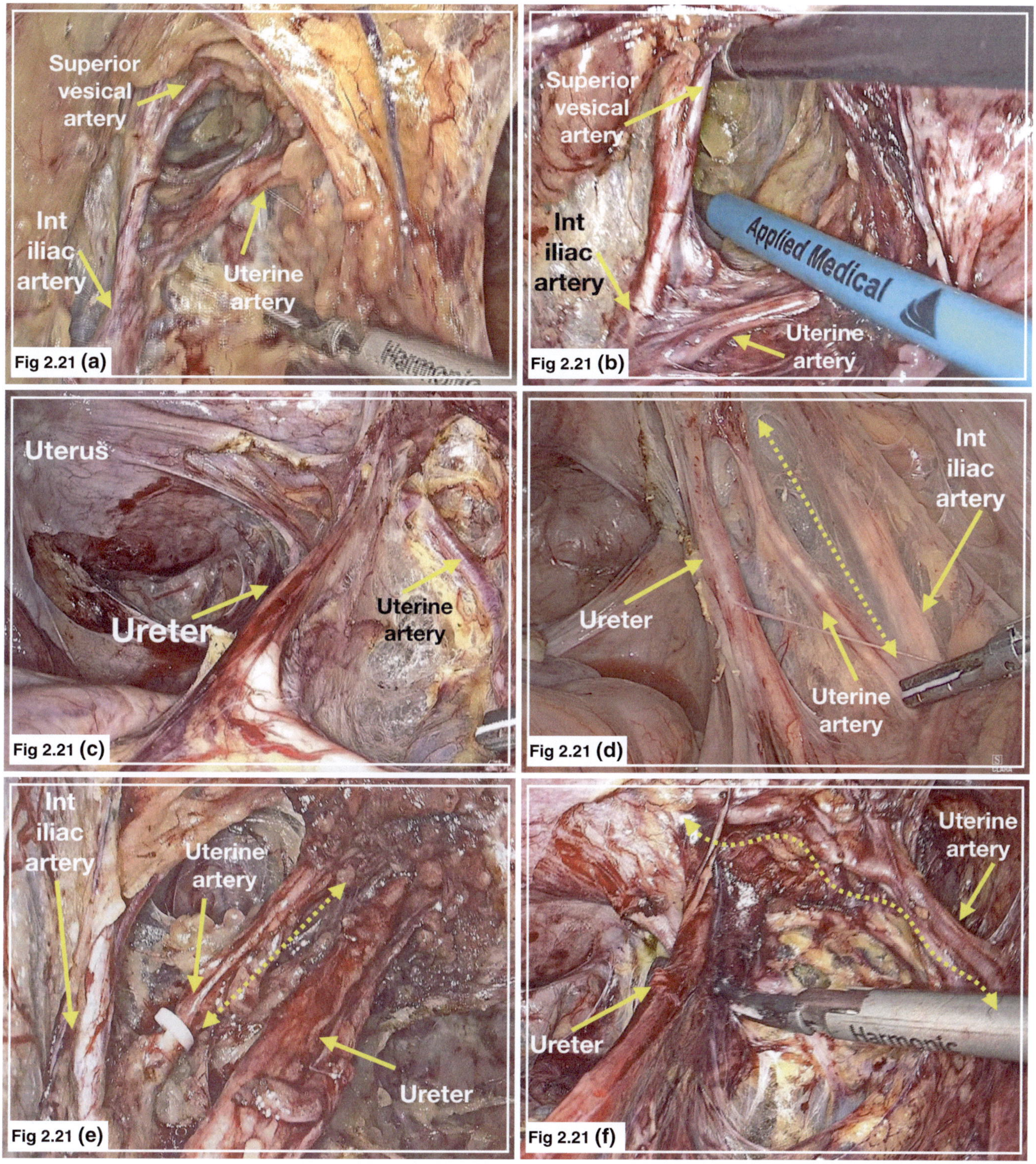

Fig. 2.21 (**a**) The uterine and the superior vesical artery can be seen travelling from the lateral pelvic wall to the medial side to supply the respective organs. (**b**) In case of paravesical space dissection the space is created by dissecting the uterine artery away from the superior vesical artery. This avascular space in between is called the paramedical space. (**c**) The relation between the ureter and the uterine artery can be seen here. The artery lies above the ureter at all times. (**d**) The relation of the ureter with the uterine artery can be seen in the pararectal space. Also the length of the uterine artery available for ligation can be seen with yellow dotted lines. (**e**) The uterine has already been clipped at its origin; however the entire length is available for ligation. The length of the uterine artery available for ligation can be seen with yellow dotted lines. The uterine artery often bleeds when clipped near the uterus. Thus it is best to clip it at its origin. (**f**) The entire tortuous course of the uterine artery can be seen here above the ureter. The length of the uterine artery available for ligation can be seen with yellow dotted lines. (**g**) The uterine artery and the ureter can be seen. The entire length of the uterine artery can be seen. The length of the uterine artery available for ligation can be seen with yellow dotted lines. (**h**) The uterine artery has been clipped at its origin. However there are higher chances of bleeding near the uterus as the uterine artery divides into the ascending branch and the descending cervical branch. In such conditions it is the descending cervical branch which bleeds in a retrograde fashion. (**i–k**) Similar uterine artery and ureter relation has been demonstrated

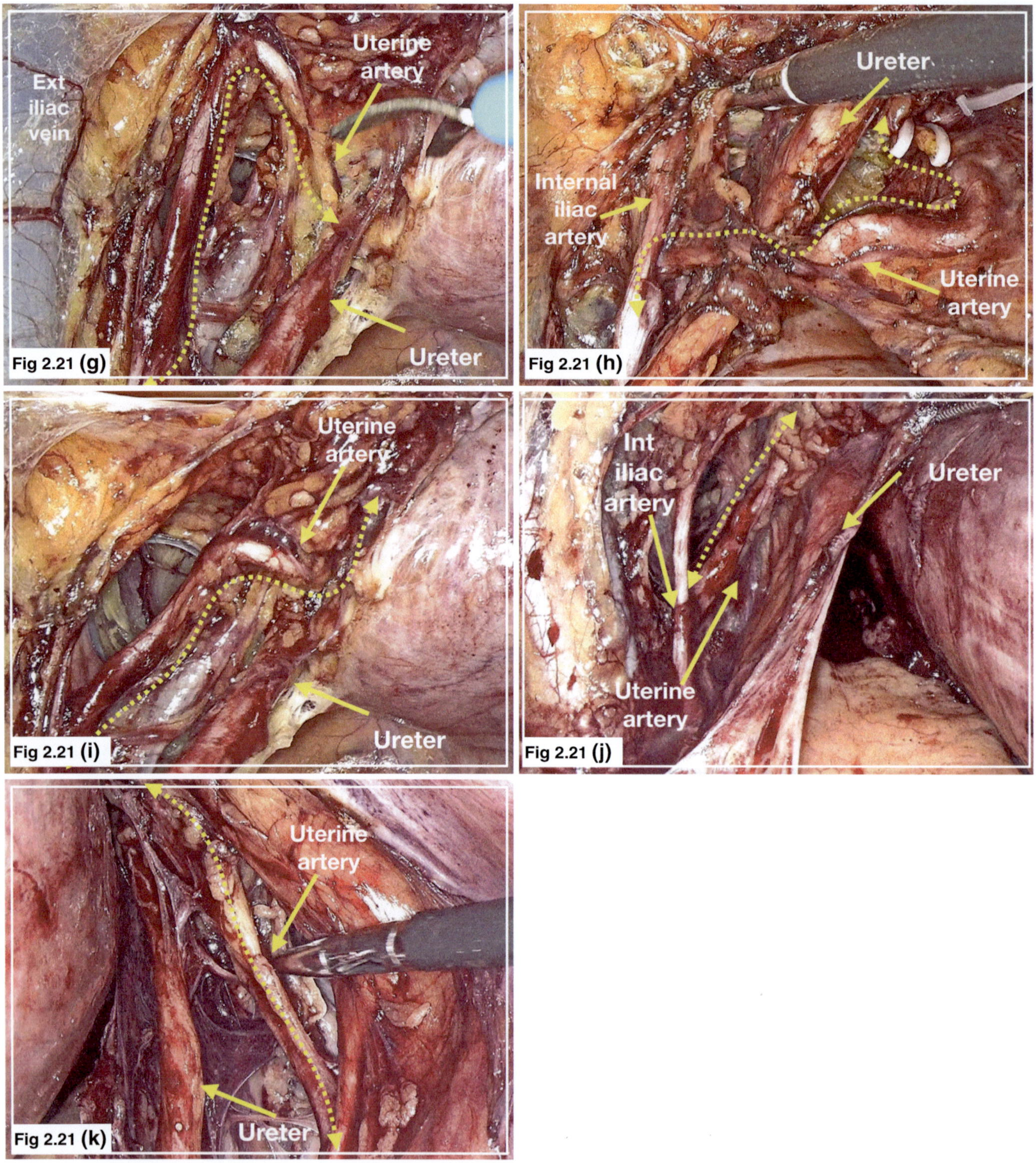

Fig. 2.21 (continued)

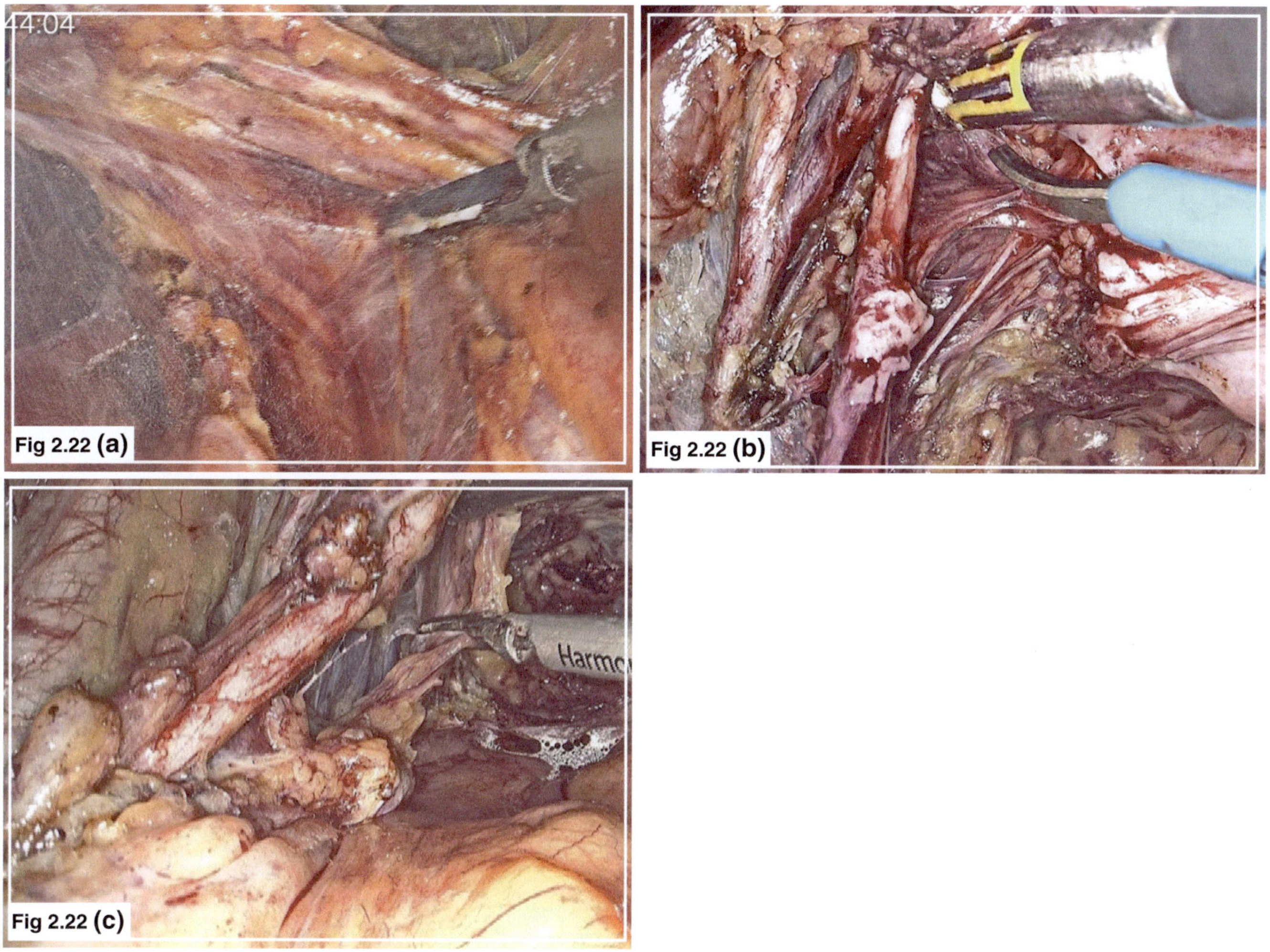

Fig. 2.22 (**a**–**c**) Supports of the uterus: Uterosacral and round ligaments can be easily appreciated. They lie medial to the major vital structure like the ureter and the uterine artery. Thus they can be intervened, cut, ligated, and plicated without disturbing the major vital structures

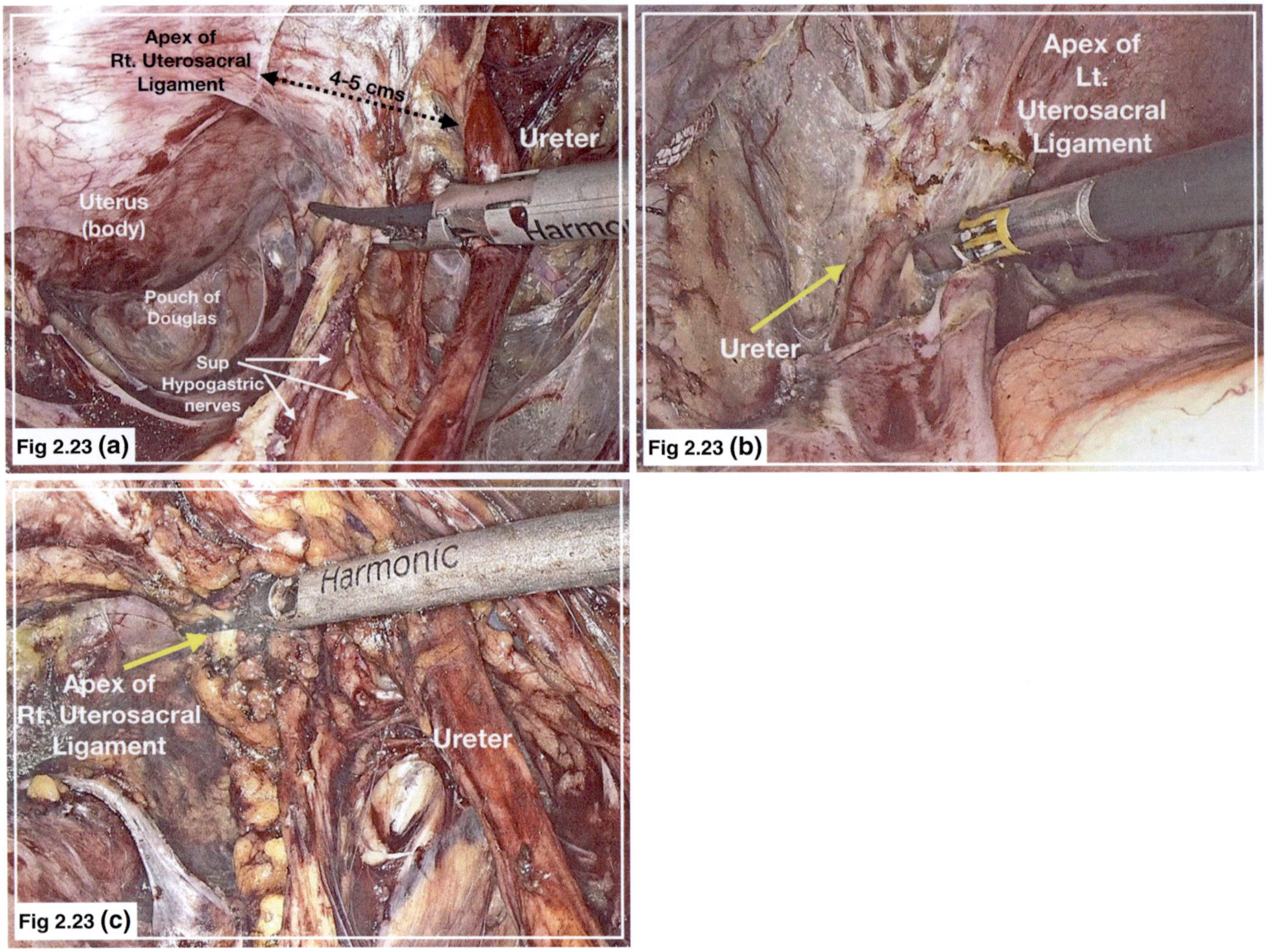

Fig. 2.23 (**a–c**) The ureter: In a case of nerve-sparing radical hysterectomy the orientation of the Right ureter has been demonstrated. It lies far and lateral to the apex of uterosacral ligament. The uterosacral ligament has been gripped by the harmonic blade near the apex. Finer superior hypogastric plexus of nerves can be appreciated

2.3 Lateral Boundary

The lateral boundary of the pelvic consists of muscles and bones (Fig. 2.24).

The availability of the space in the pelvis and the placement of the midline organs allow the pelvic pathologies to grow to a large size (Fig. 2.25).

The psoas muscle is the anatomical landmark on the lateral wall. The genitofemoral nerve along with the external iliac artery lies on the psoas muscle. The genitofemoral nerve is the lateral most limit for pelvic lymph nodal dissection (Fig. 2.26).

The ureteroneocystostomy is done with psoas hitch. The fundus of the urinary bladders stitched to the psoas muscle to avoid tension on the ureterobladder anastomosis (Fig. 2.27).

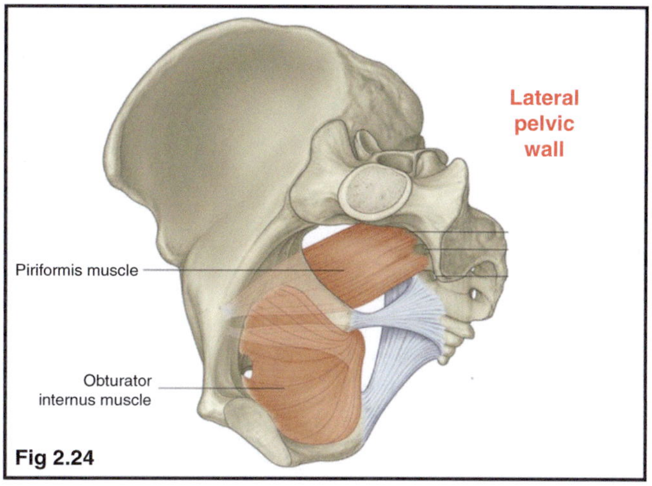

Fig. 2.24 Lateral pelvic wall: Diagrammatic representation of lateral pelvic wall demonstrating the levator ani and the obturator internus muscles

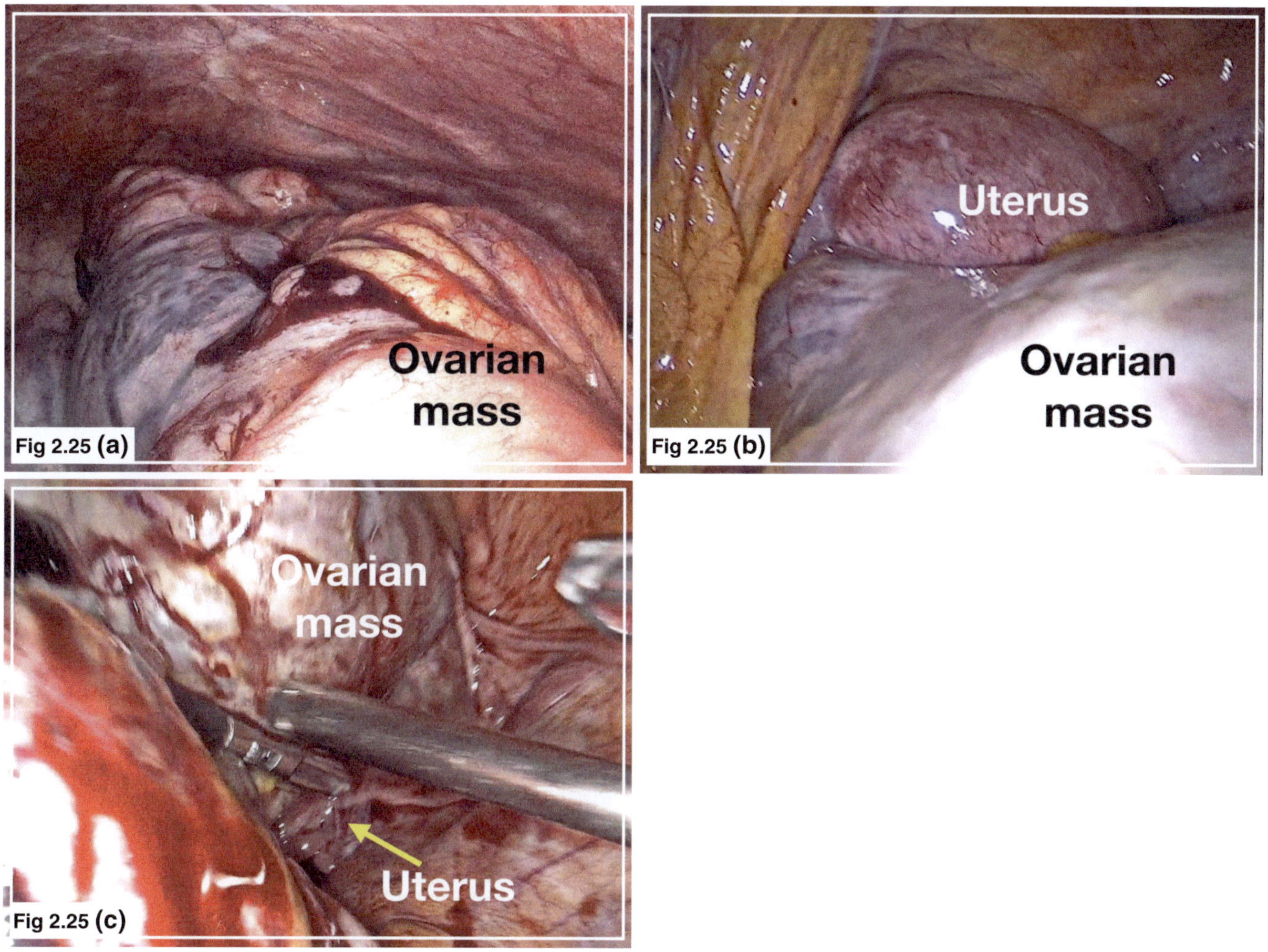

Fig. 2.25 (**a**, **b**) Large ovarian masses grow freely due to availability of space. Thus ovarian masses are diagnosed late as they become symptomatic after growing much larger and out of proportions

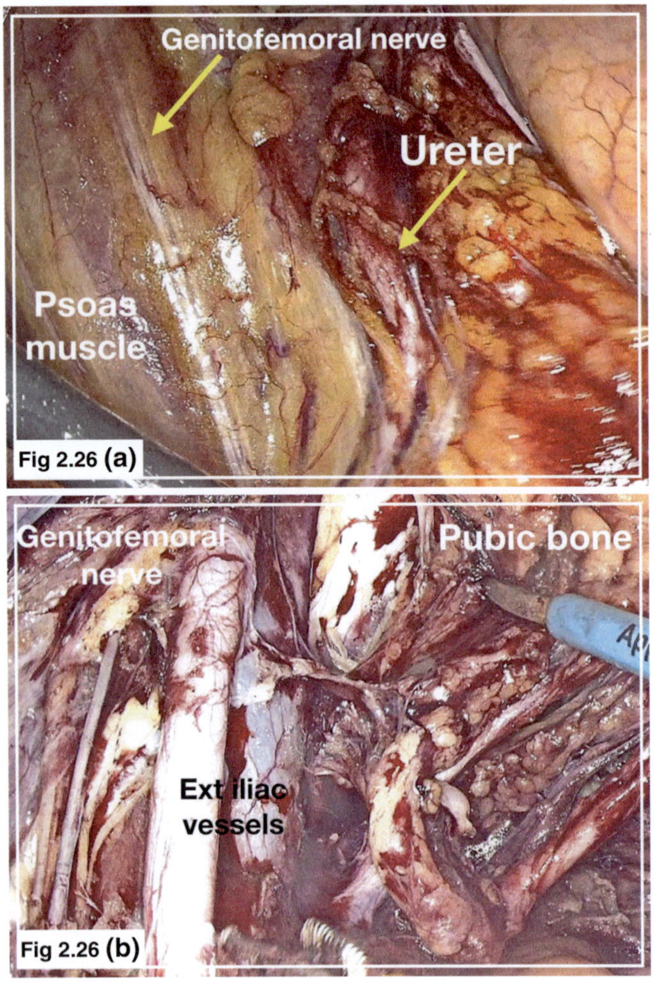

Fig. 2.26 (**a**) The psoas muscle on the left side can be even with the genitofemoral nerve on it running parallel. (**b**) The genitofemoral nerve and the pubic bone seen in one plane demonstrating that they are the lateral limit of the pelvic lymph node dissection

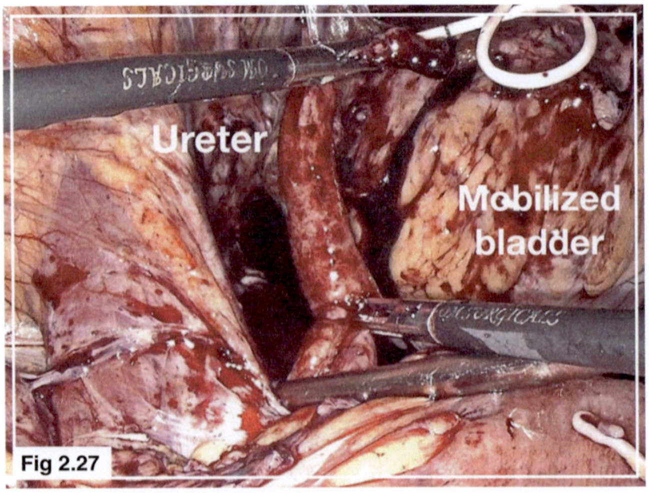

Fig. 2.27 In a case of ureterovaginal fistula (UVF) repair ureteroneocystostomy is done by mobilising the bladder anteriorly from the prevesical space and the ureter inserted into a newly made orifice on the anterior surface of bladder. To support the ureter the ureter is hitched to the psoas muscle

2.4 Caudal Boundary

The caudal boundary of the pelvis is formed by the pelvic muscles with its covering endopelvic fascias. The muscles of the pelvic diaphragm are the levator ani, obturator internus and coccygeus. These are responsible for keeping the pelvic organs in the midline. The pelvic sphincters are a part of the pelvic diaphragm. In a prolapse surgery the repairs are done by hitching the organs to these muscles (Figs. 2.28 and 2.29).

2.5 Anterior Boundary

Anteriorly is the pelvic peritoneum with the abdominal organs. This forms the roof of the pelvis. The inferior epigastric artery lies in the roof of the pelvis. Its location is important as this can be damaged during the later port entry (Fig. 2.30).

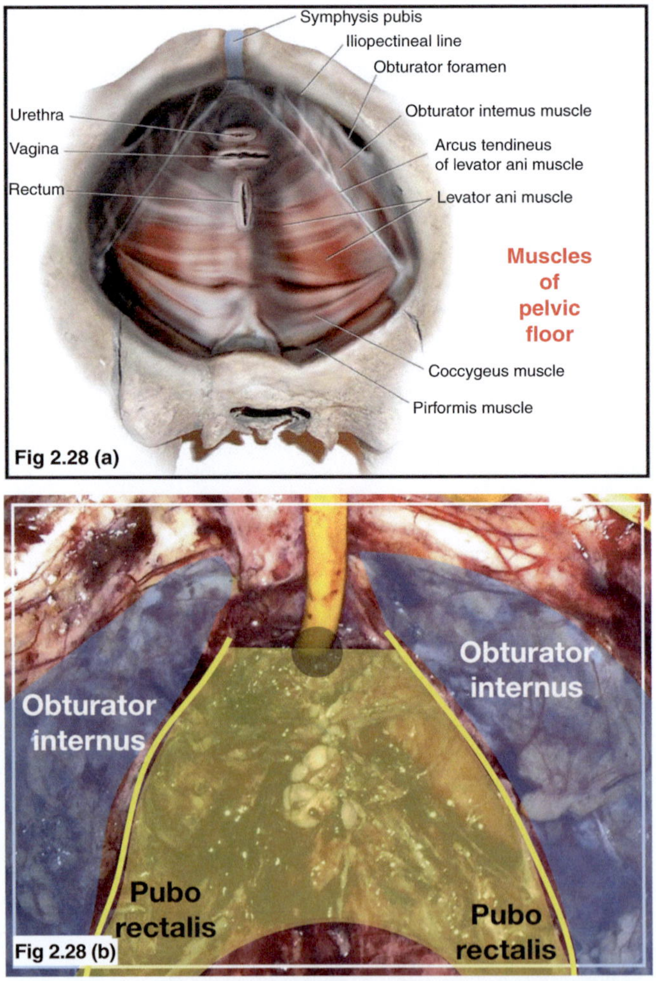

Fig. 2.28 (**a**) The pelvic floor diagrammatically represented. (**b**) The pelvic floor demonstrated in a case of laparoscopic anterior exenteration. The levator ani and the obturator internus have been labelled

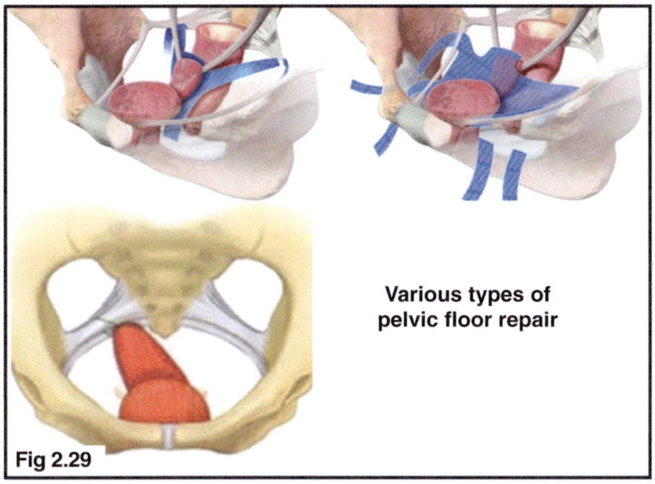

Fig. 2.29 Various types of pelvic floor surgeries where pelvic floor muscles are strengthened with the help of meshes

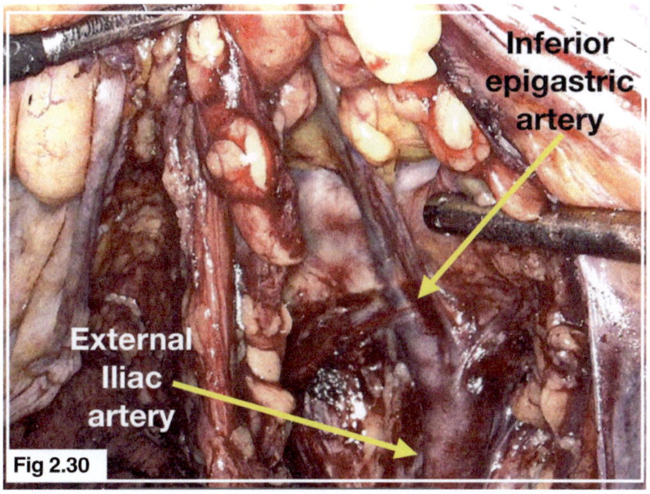

Fig. 2.30 The inferior epigastric artery can be seen reflected onto the anterior abdominal wall. It is a branch of the external iliac artery

3 Ligaments and Supports of the Uterus

The uterosacrals, cardinal ligaments and paracolpos form a continuous fan-shaped structure (Figs. 3.1 and 3.2).

Medially is the rectum, laterally is the internal iliac artery and caudally is the levator ani muscle. The ligaments go from the uterus to the sacrum. The pararectal and paravesical spaces are lateral to the uterine supports. Hence all the ligaments can be transected in oncology surgery (Fig. 3.3).

The ureter lies free lateral to the ligaments and hence has to be retracted laterally to go to the insertion of the ligament into the pelvic wall (Fig. 3.4).

The lymphatics and the veins traverse through these ligaments. Hence there is the necessity to transect them as laterally as possible in the oncology surgeries (Fig. 3.5).

The uterine artery traverses above the ureter and does not lie in the ligaments. Therefore the artery can be easily dissected off the ligaments (Figs. 3.6 and 3.7).

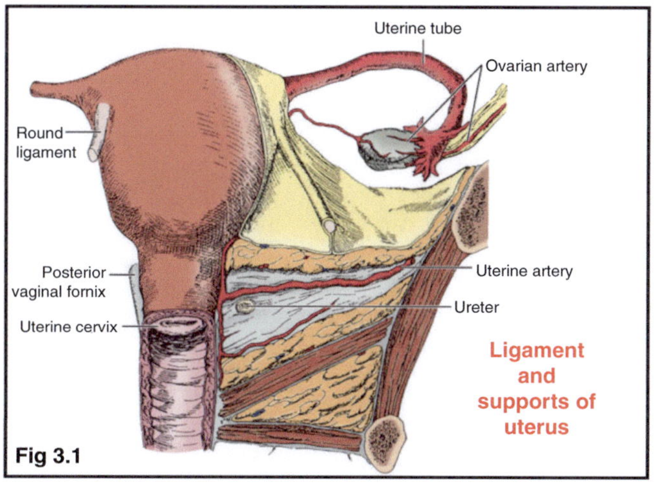

Fig. 3.1 Diagrammatic representations of ligaments of the uterus

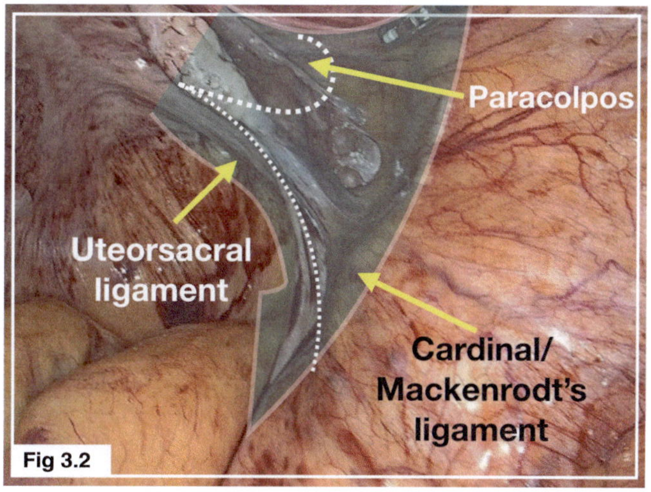

Fig. 3.2 The fan-shaped support of uterus comprises uterosacral ligament, paracolpos medially and Mackenrodt's or cardinal ligament laterally

S. Puntambekar et al., *Laparoscopic Pelvic Anatomy in Females*, https://doi.org/10.1007/978-981-13-8653-4_3

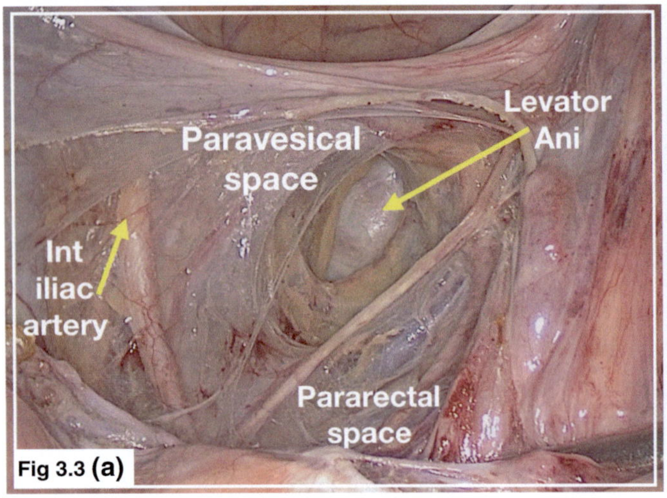

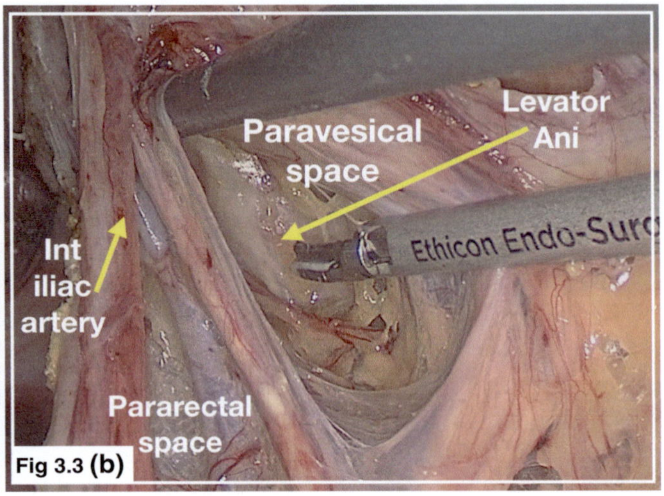

Fig. 3.3 (**a**, **b**) Images showing the levator ani (floor), the internal iliac artery laterally (lateral border), the pararectal and the paravesical space

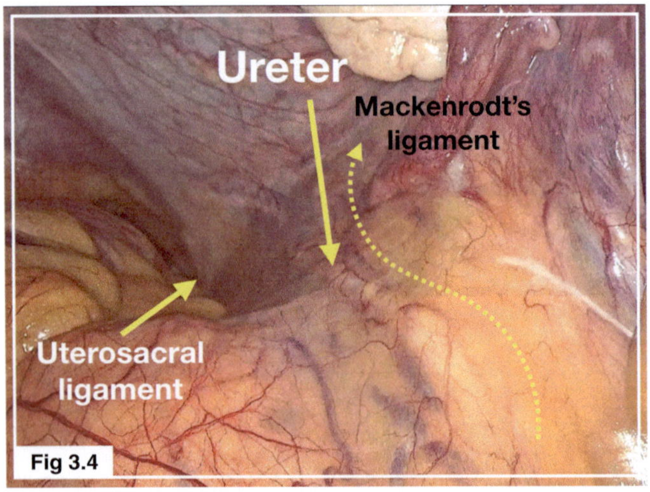

Fig. 3.4 The ureter though close to the uterosacral ligament always remains lateral to the uterosacral ligament. Thus it passes through the Mackenrodt's ligament to traverse under the uterine artery to reach the bladder

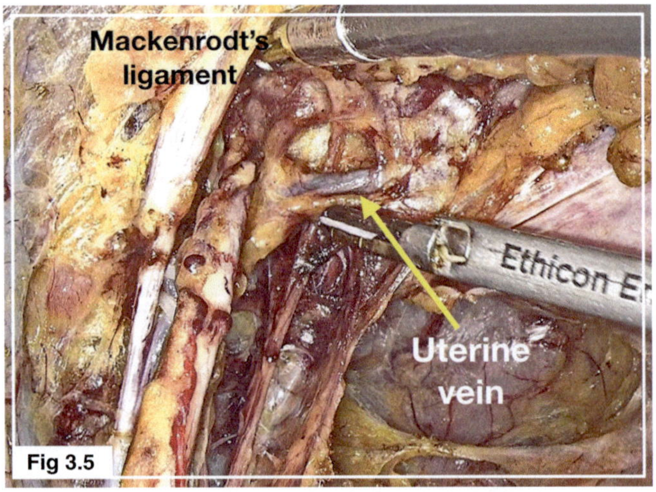

Fig. 3.5 The uterine artery and vein pass horizontally across the Mackenrodt's ligament from the uterus to the lateral pelvic wall

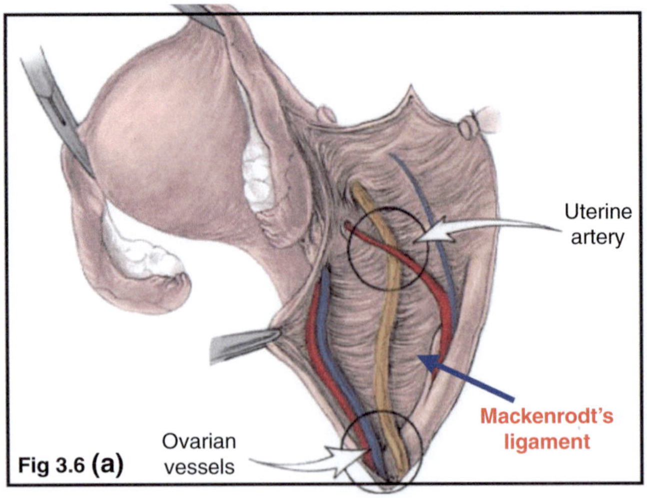

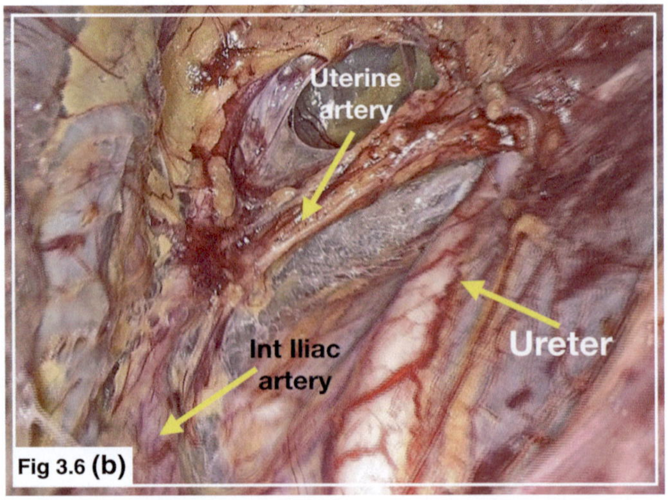

Fig. 3.6 (**a**) Diagrammatic image from the Mackenrodt's ligament exposing the uterine artery and vein underneath the peritoneum. (**b**) The image from a case of laparoscopic radical hysterectomy showing the uterine artery remaining above the ureter at all times. The origin of the uterine artery can be seen at the lateral pelvic wall. Thus the uterine artery can be ligated along its entire course

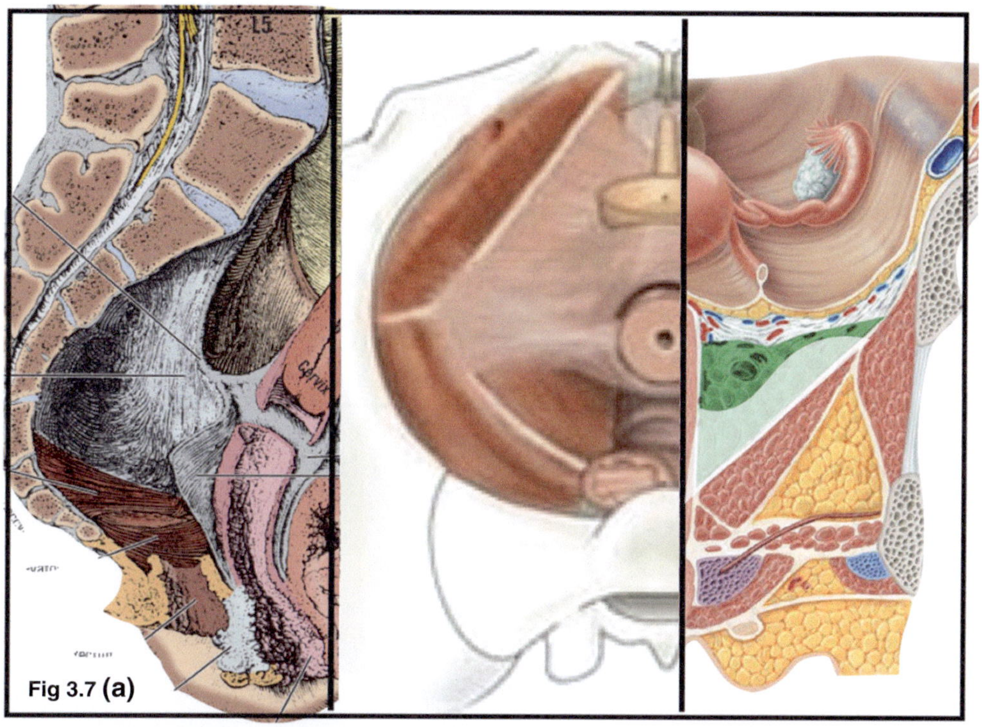

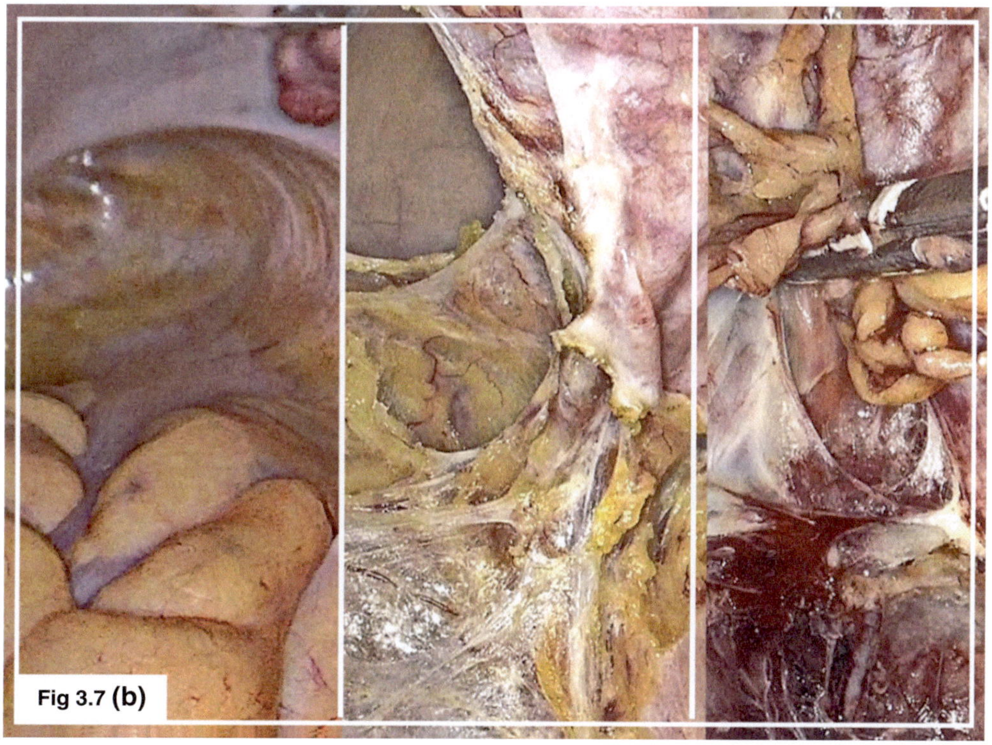

Fig. 3.7 (**a**, **b**) Collage of diagrammatic representations and real-time images of the ligaments to be discussed in the chapter

3.1 Uterosacral Ligaments (Fig. 3.8)

The uterosacral ligament is the fibromuscular support and is the true and the strongest support. The rectum lies between the uterosacral ligaments (Fig. 3.9a–d).

The ureter and all the vascular structure lie lateral to the uterosacral ligament. This anchors the uterus to the sacrum (Fig. 3.10a–c).

The uterosacral ligament is the medial boundary of the Okabayashi space (medial pararectal space) (Fig. 3.11a–e).

The uterosacral ligament is a strong support of the uterus and hence its laxity can lead to prolapse. Restoration of the uterosacral ligament is the most important step in the surgery of prolapse (Fig. 3.12).

The uterosacral ligament is fairly an avascular structure and hence can be cut without any fear of haemorrhage (Fig. 3.13).

In oncological surgery the uterosacral ligament can be cut right at the insertion without damage to the hypogastric nerves. This is the most important support as it is

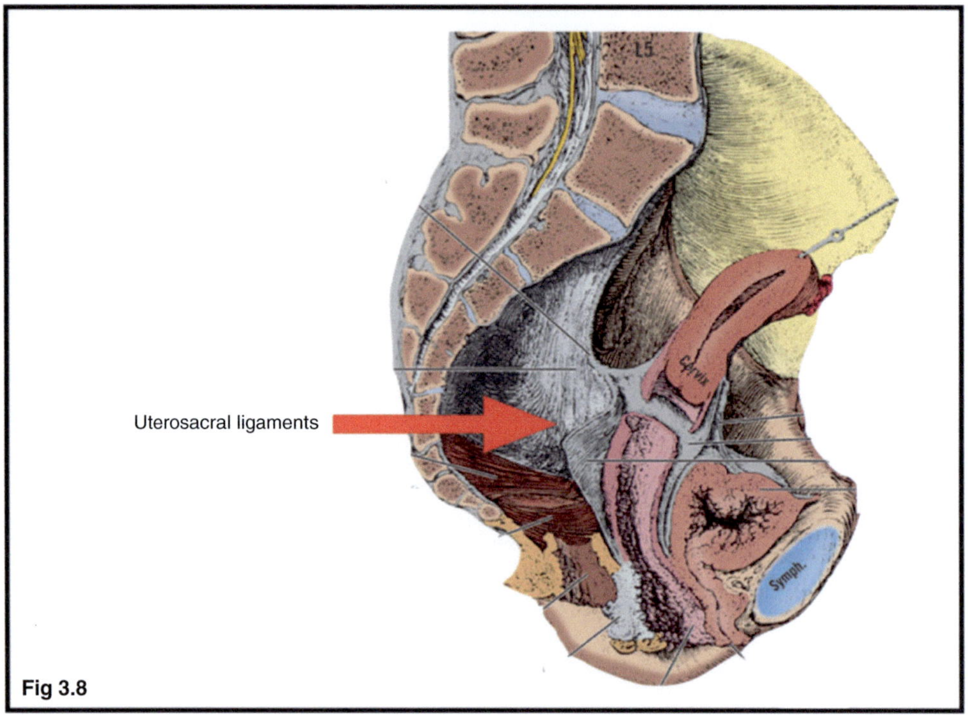

Fig. 3.8 Diagrammatic representation of the uterossacral ligaments

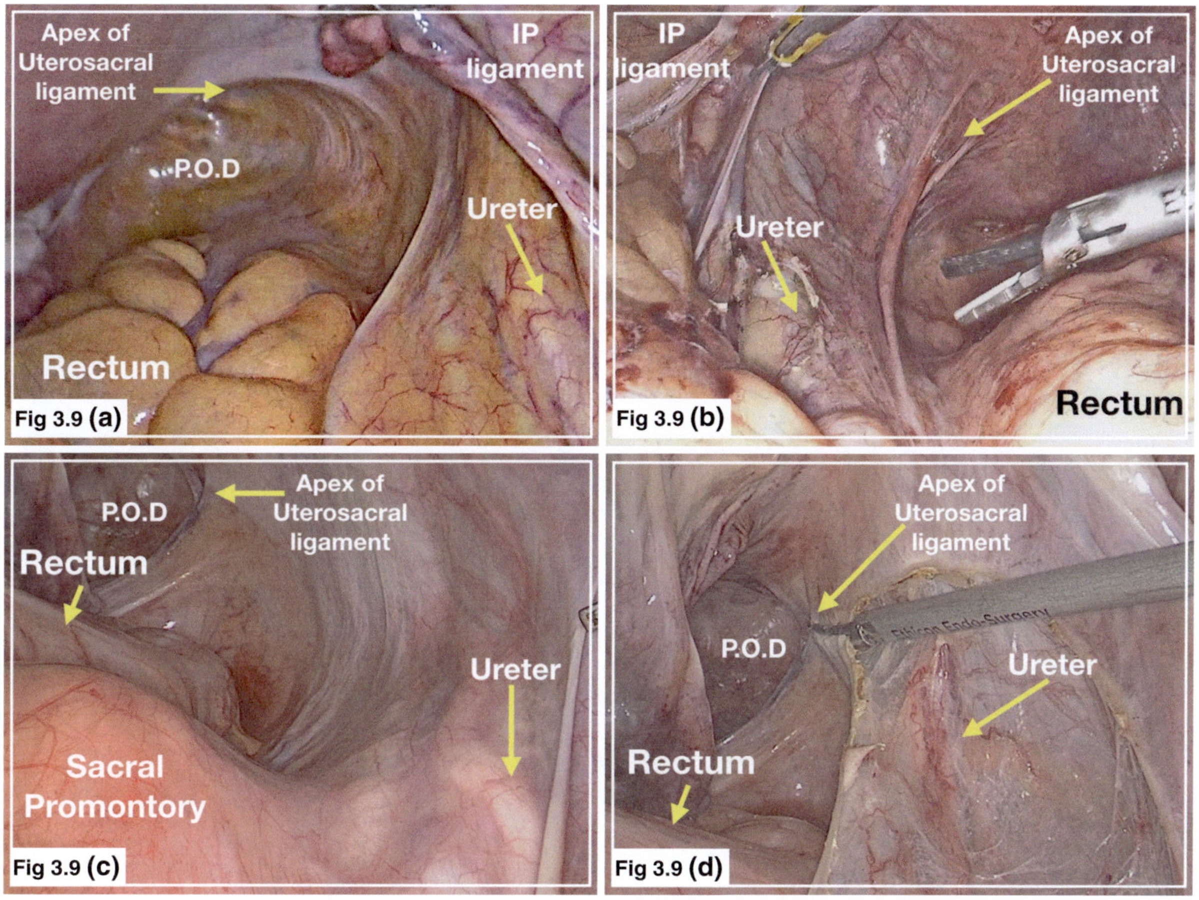

Fig. 3.9 (**a–d**) The series of images taken from a view from the infundibulopelvic ligament (IP ligament) shows the rectum as the media most structure bounded on both sides by the uterosacral ligaments. The ureter can be seen at the level of the pelvic bro after which it dips into the pelvis but remains lateral to the uterosacral ligament at all times

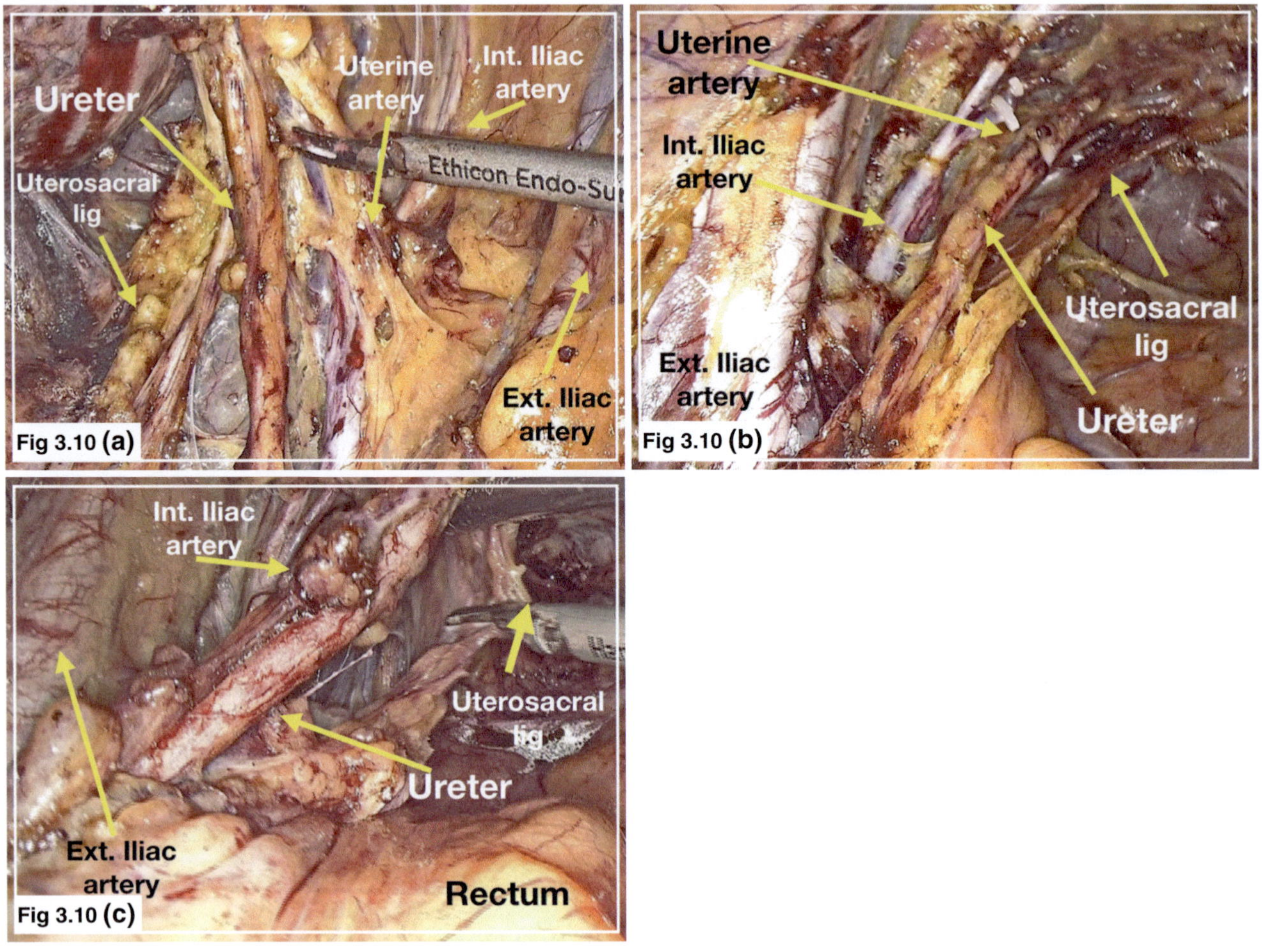

Fig. 3.10 (**a–c**) The lateral pelvic wall is dissected and the ureter and the vascular structures like uterine artery and internal and external iliac artery are seen. The uterosacral ligament has been shown as a separate entity from all the vital structures

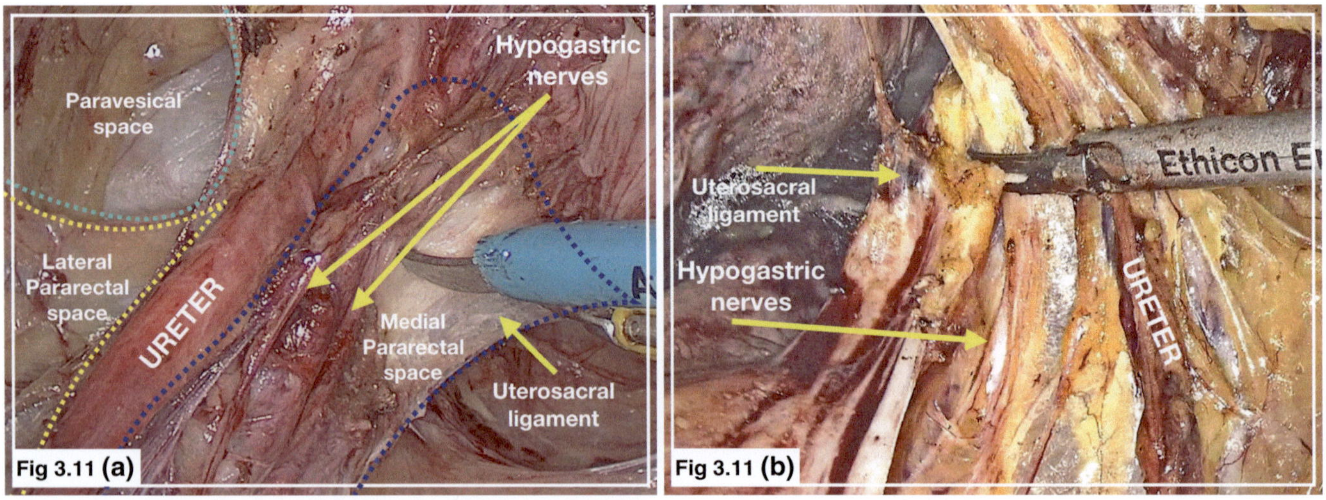

Fig. 3.11 (**a**) The medial pararectal space has been dissected at the apex of the uterosacral ligament. The slender, tubular structures seen close to the ureter are the hypogastric nerve fibres travelling along with the ureter and supplying the bladder and the uterus. This area is important in nerve radical hysterectomy. (**b**) Similar image seen on the right side as well. These images have been taken from cases of nerve-sparing laparoscopic radical hysterectomy. The ureter divides the pararectal space into medial and lateral pararectal space. (**c**) The superior hypogastric plexus converges as hypogastric nerves as they approach the apex of uterosacral ligament. Thus these nerves can be traced at the level of the sacral promontory and above as well. (**d**) The hypogastric nerves communicate with the parasympathetic nerves to form the inferior hypogastric plexus and from here the nerves further supply the bladder and the uterus. (**e**) The ureter can be seen dividing the pararectal space into medal and lateral pararectal space, though there is no firm structural partition in between

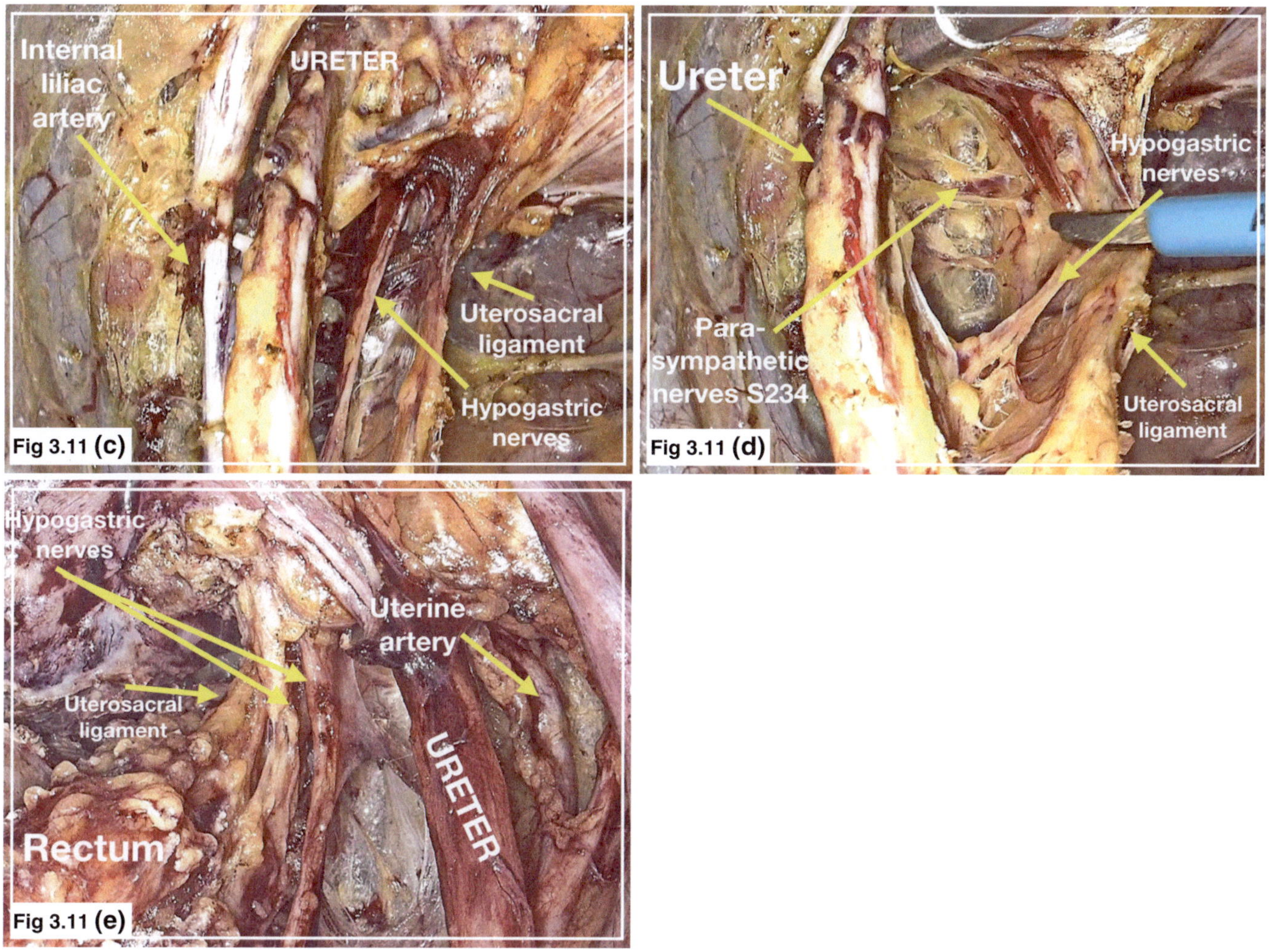

Fig. 3.11 (continued)

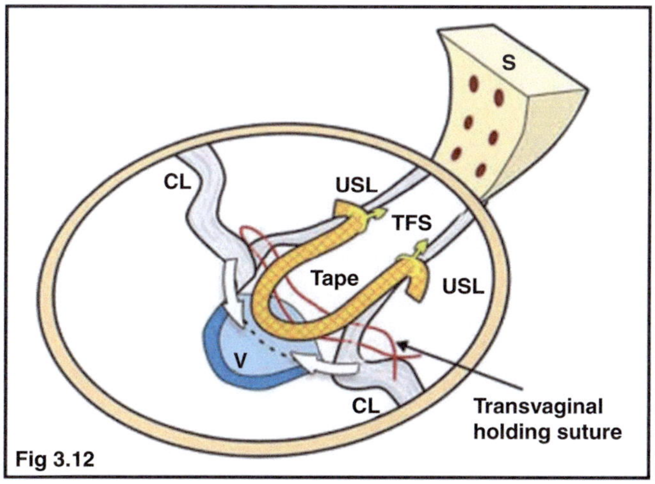

Fig. 3.12 Diagrammatic representation of uterovaginal prolapse and the possible repair surgeries

the border between the rectum and the ureter (Figs. 3.14 and 3.15).

The uterosacral ligament has been resected and the pararectal along with paravesical and rectovaginal space has been united to a common floor of the endopelvic fascia or the levator ani. The rectum and the ureter are close to the base/lower portion of the uterosacral (Fig. 3.16).

3.1.1 Concepts

1. Dissection at the apex of the uterosacral ligament will avoid damage to the uterus as well as the ureter (Fig. 3.17).
2. The restoration of the uterosacral ligament will allow better dissection when the pouch of Douglas is obliterated (Fig. 3.18).

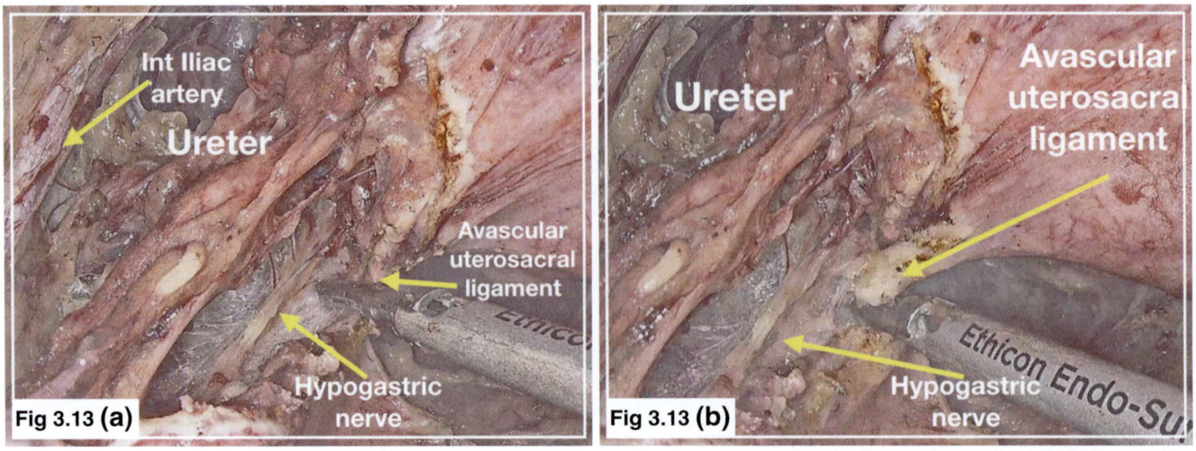

Fig. 3.13 (**a**) The uterosacral ligament is the fibromuscular support of the uterus. Lack of areolar tissue and presence of fibrous tissue make it more avascular. Thus it is easy to resect the tissue directly. (**b**) The various vascular structures lie lateral to the uterosacral ligaments. Hence it is easy to resect the alignment without a fear of injury to the structures as seen in the image

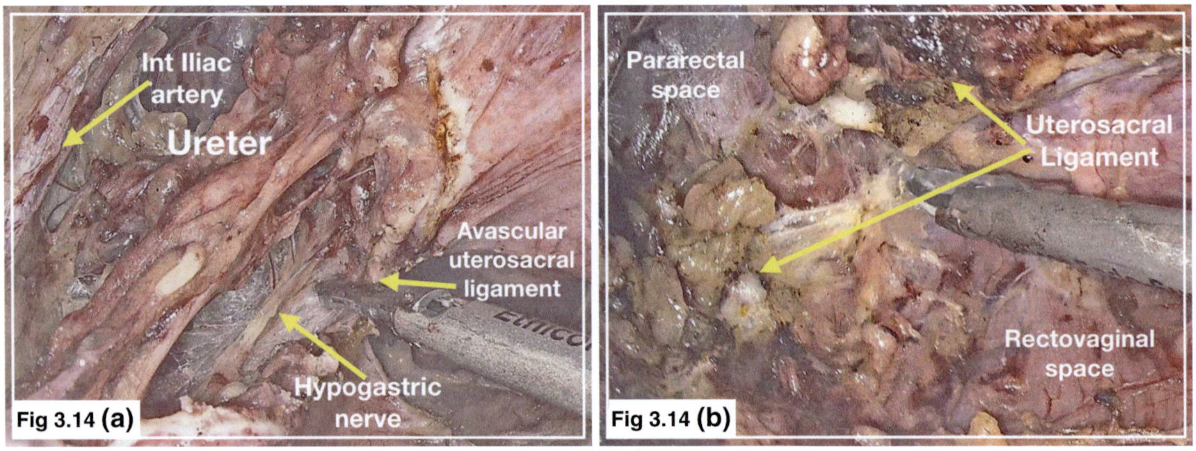

Fig. 3.14 (**a**) As previously seen in Fig. 3.13a the hypogastric nerve has been spared during resection of the uterosacral ligament. This image has been taken from a case of nerve-sparing laparoscopic radical hysterectomy. Thus resection has been done sparing the nerve. (**b**) The uterosacral ligament has been resected and the underneath endopelvic fascia is visible. There are still no signs of bleeding and the major support of the uterus has been resected

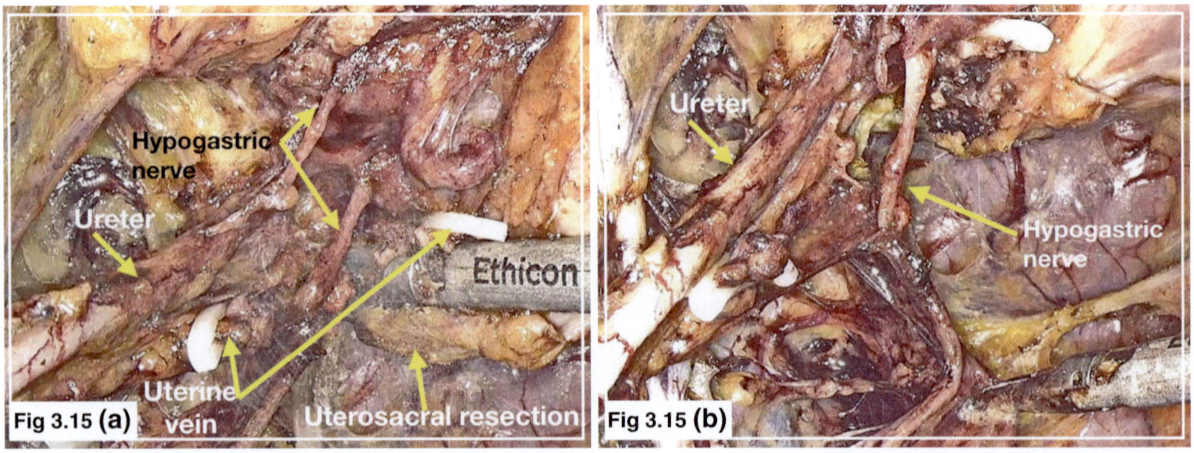

Fig. 3.15 (**a**) In another set of images the hypogastric nerve has been more clearly defined and the uterosacral ligament is being resected. The uterine vein has been clipped and cut medial to the ureter signifying that the parasympathetic nerve fibre to the bladder has been spared in this nerve-sparing laparoscopic radical hysterectomy. (**b**) Uterosacral ligament is being resected. The uterine vein has been clipped and cut medial to the ureter signifying that the parasympathetic nerve fibre to the bladder has been spared in this nerve-sparing laparoscopic radical hysterectomy

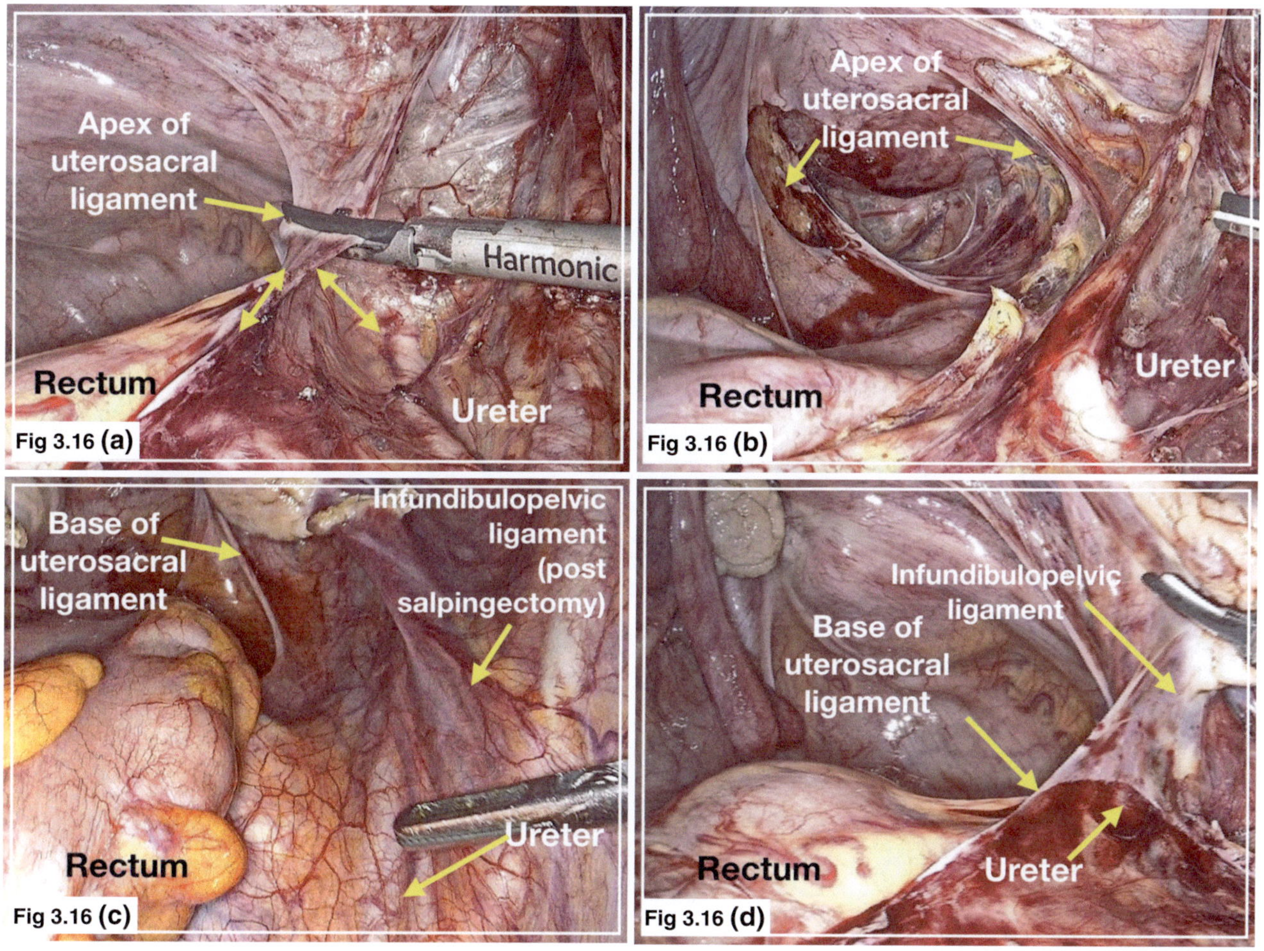

Fig. 3.16 (**a**, **b**) The pair of images show the close proximity of the rectum and the ureter to the base of the uterosacral ligament and at the apex. They however can be lateralised and kept away from the ligament during resection. (**c**, **d**) This pair of image has been taken at the level of sacral promontory where the base of the uterosacral ligament can be best explained an their proximity to the ureter and the rectum as well

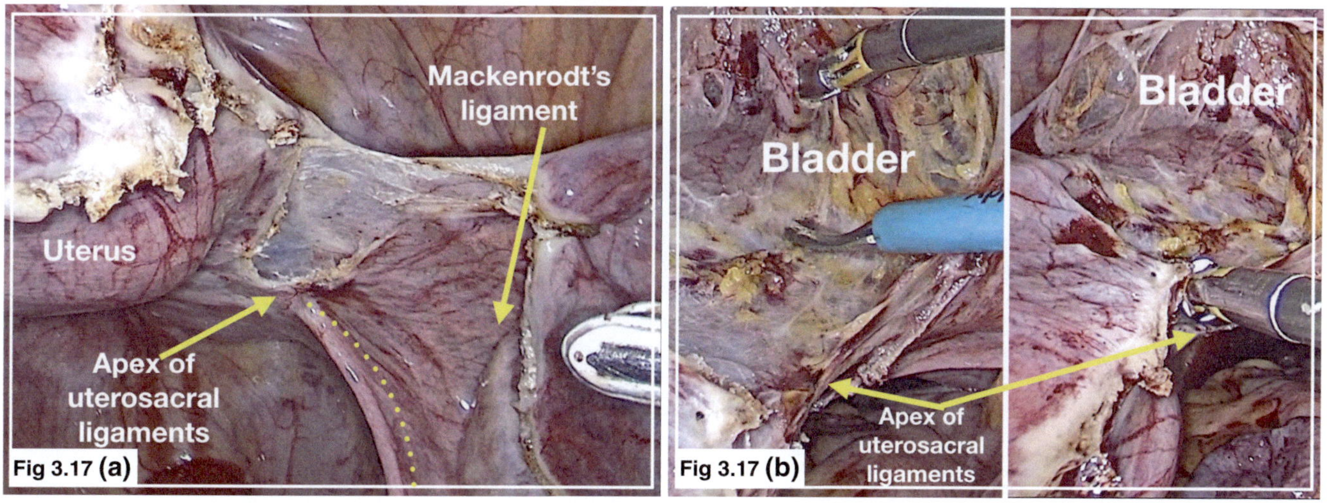

Fig. 3.17 (**a**) The image from a case of total laparoscopic hysterectomy for a case of AUB with failed medical management. The posterior leaf of broad ligament is exposed till the apex of uterosacral ligaments. The dissection in benign hysterectomy is done till the apex of uterosacral and the chief ligaments like uterosacrals and the Mackenrodt's ligament are not opened. (**b**) In this figure we can see the first half describing the dissection of the bladder and the apex of uterosacral ligaments explaining that anteriorly and posteriorly the broad ligament is opened till the apex of uterosacral ligament. The right half of the image shows the approach to colpotomy. The apex of uterosacral ligaments remains at the level of the uterovaginal junction. Thus colpotomy is best done at this level without loosing vagina length post-operatively

3. The hypogastric nerves always lie lateral to the uterosacral ligament. Thus remaining medial to the uterosacral ligament will avoid damage to the nerves (Figs. 3.14, 3.15, and 3.19).

The hypogastric nerves also lie lateral to the base of the uterosacral. The plane of the hypogastric nerve is close to the Waldeyer's fascia (lies at the deeper level) (Fig. 3.20).

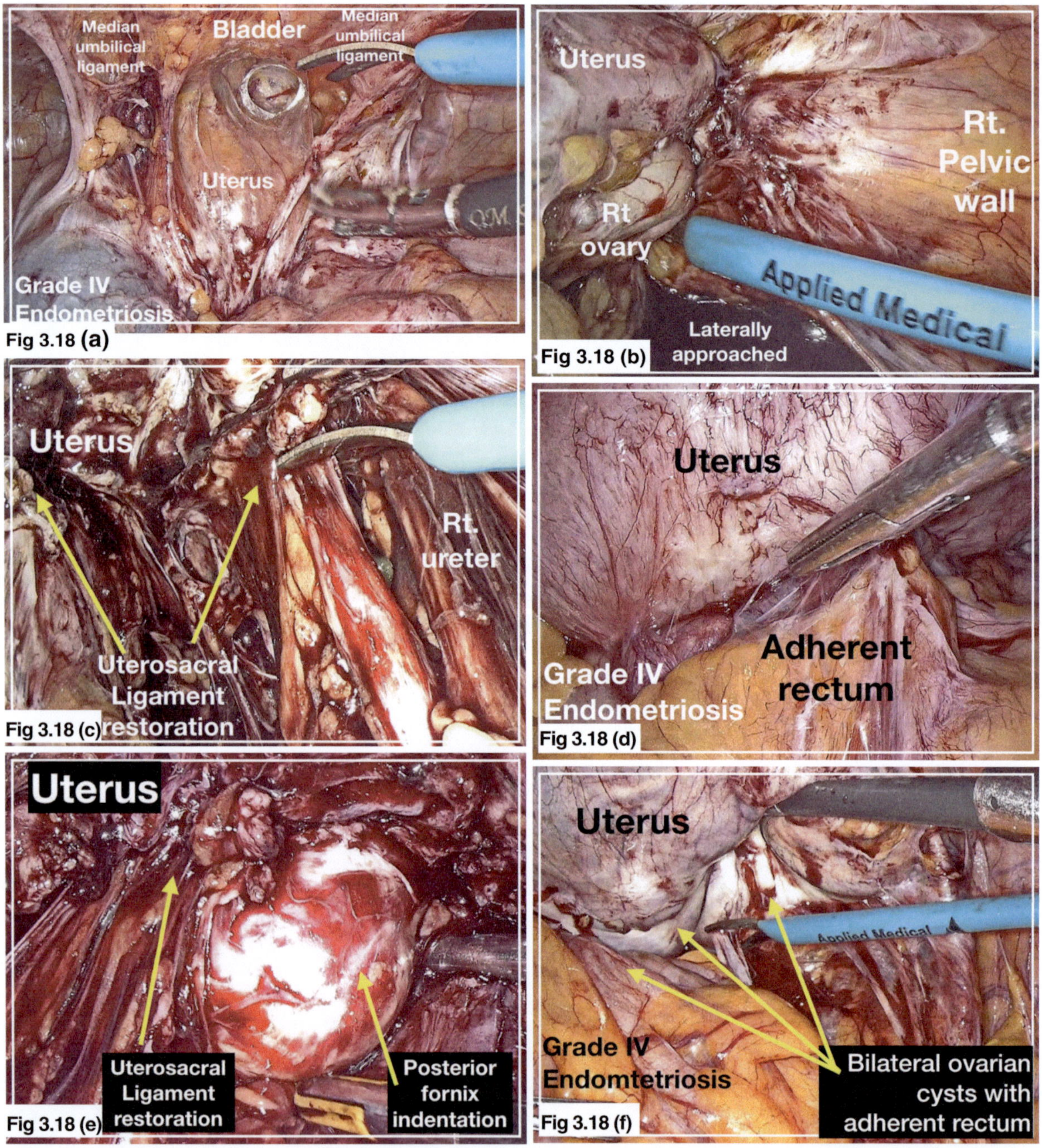

Fig. 3.18 Endometriosis. (**a–c**) This group of images show the dissection of the posterior region of the uterus in case of Grade IV endometriosis. The main purpose of dissection is restoration of the uterosacral ligament which helps in performing a hysterectomy as the surrounding structures become more well defined. Secondly restoration of the uterosacral ligaments recreates the pouch of Douglas which is helpful in ovum pickup for infertility. (**d**, **e**) Images of pelvis prior to intervention in a Grade IV endometriosis followed by uterosacral restoration. (**f**, **g**) Bilateral chocolate cysts in a patient seeking treatment from infertility. The uterosacral restoration here would help in forming a false pouch of Douglas meant for ovum pickup without injuring any other organs. (**h**, **i**) Similar pair of images showing restoration of the uterosacral ligaments in a case of Grade IV endometriosis

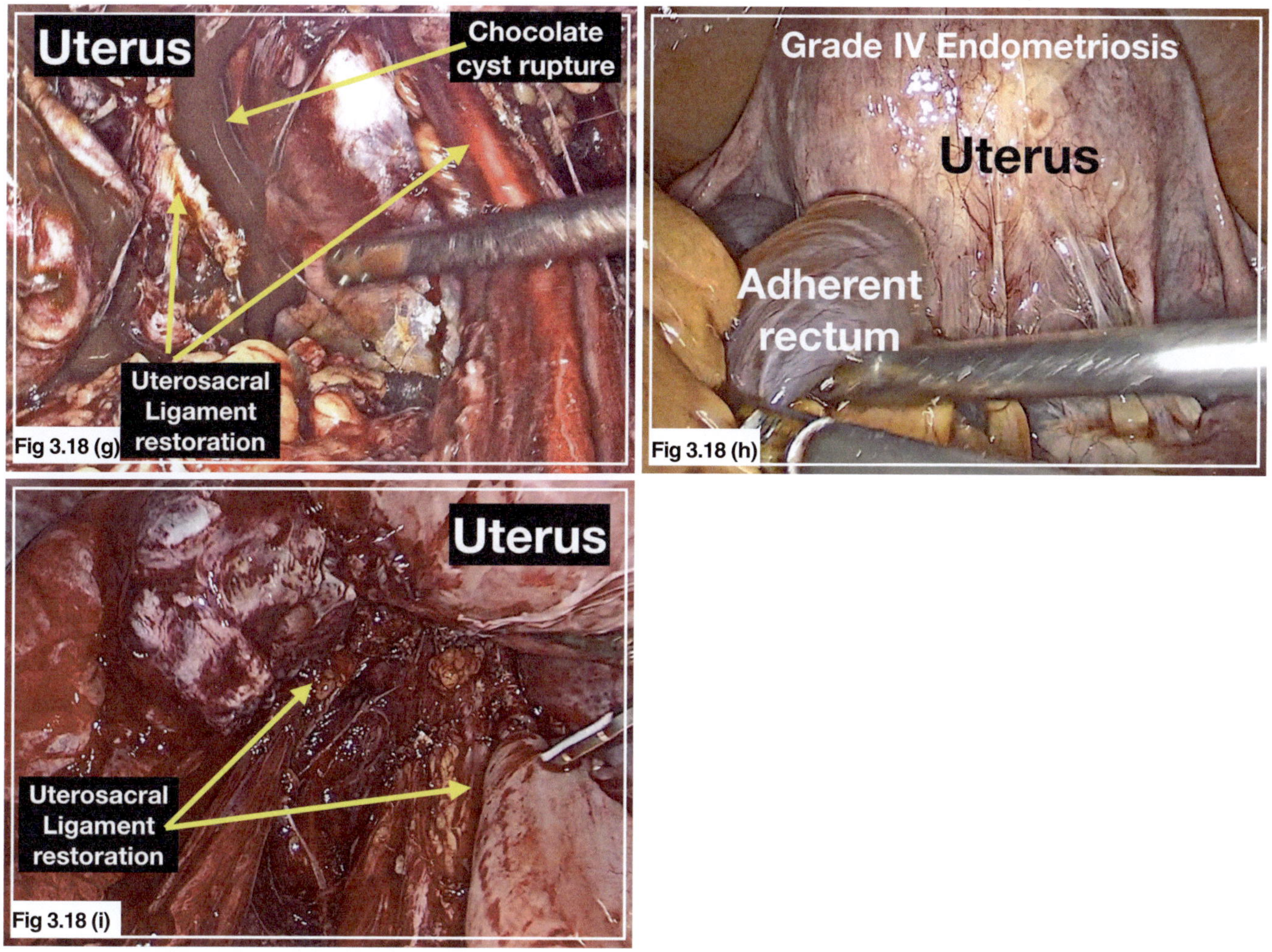

Fig. 3.18 (continued)

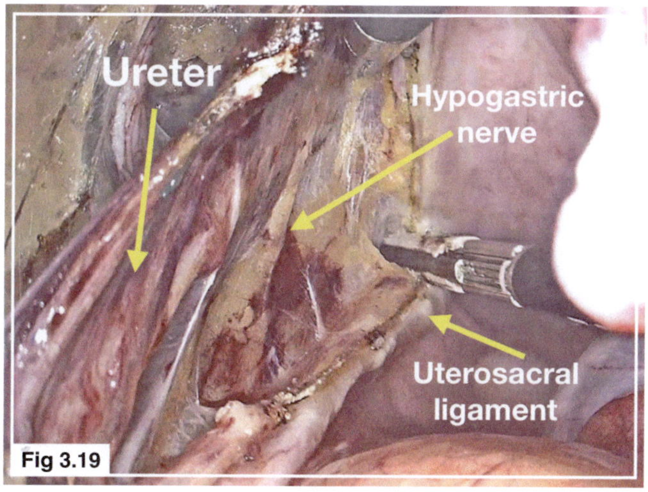

Fig. 3.19 The hypogastric nerve can be seen lying lateral to the uterosacral ligament. Thus dissection is being carried out on the medial side. Also refer to Figs. 3.14 and 3.15

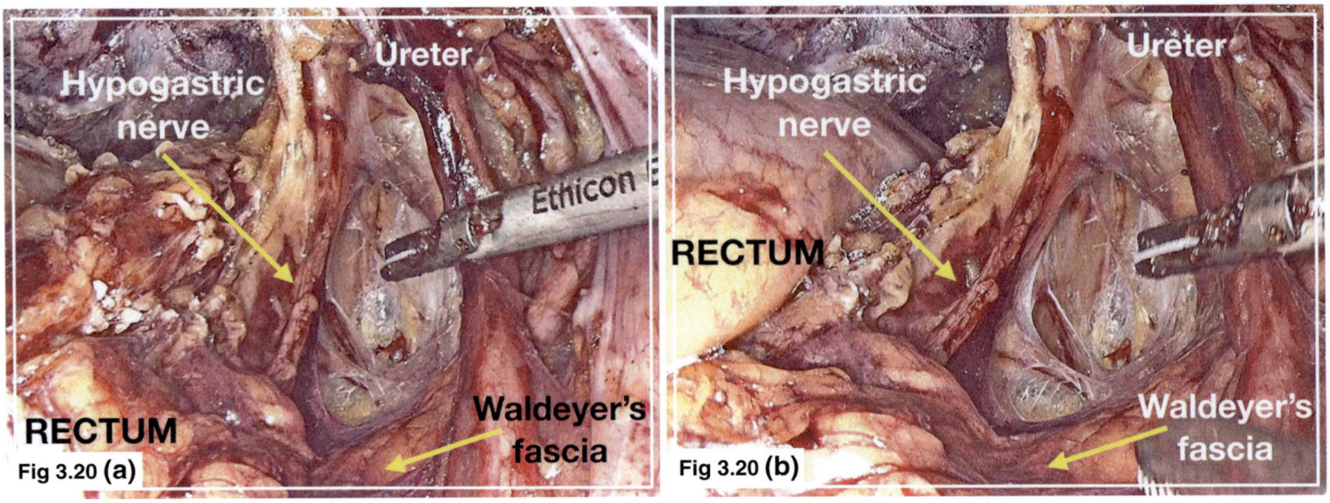

Fig. 3.20 (**a**, **b**) The pair of images show the hypogastric nerve lying closer and deeper to the rectum and thus closely associated with the Waldeyer's fascia as explained in the text. Thus the nerve lies deep to the base of the uterosacral ligament

Fig. 3.21 Uterosacral ligaments can be used for plication to strengthen the support of prolapsed uterus

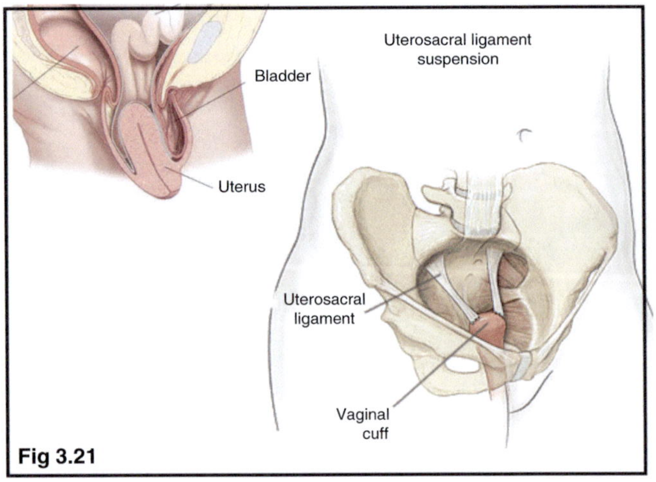

3.1.2 Rules

1. Remaining at the apex of the uterosacral avoids damage to the rectum, ureter and nerves.
2. The uterosacrals can be transacted at the base (even in NSLRH). Thus the lateral transaction limit is the same as that in the LRH.
3. The uterosacral plication/strengthening is the most important step in the uterine suspension (Fig. 3.21).

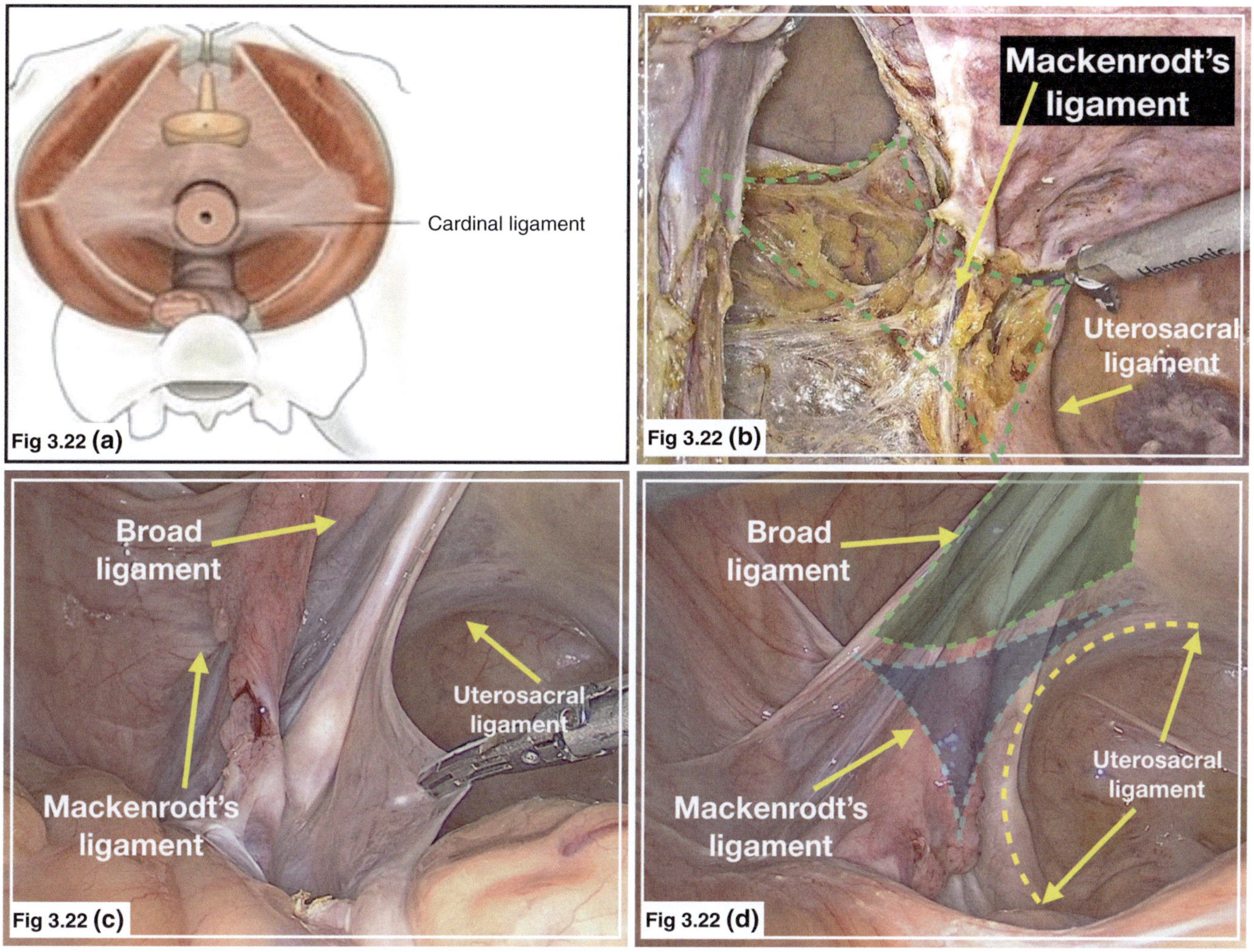

Fig. 3.22 (**a**) Diagrammatic representation of the cardinal or Mackenrodt's ligament. (**b**) The image shows the isolated Mackenrodt's ligament without the broad ligament and only a fragment of the uterosacral ligament can be seen as the common borders to the Mackenrodt's ligament. The dissection of the broad ligament has been done for explaining the purpose to the viewers so that the Mackenrodt's ligament can be solely focussed here. (**c**) The image shows the uterosacral ligament medially as the border of the Mackenrodt's ligament and the broad ligament on top. (**d**) This image shows the boundaries of all three ligaments mentioned previously. The brand ligament lies on top as a canopy over the Mackenrodt's ligament contains the round ligament and the tubes while the Mackenrodt's ligament consists of the substance of the lateral support of the uterus. The fibroareolar tissue underneath communicating with the teal pelvic wall and the uterus at the level of the lower half of uterus and cervix with the lateral pelvic wall. The uterosacral ligaments form a type of medial border of the Mackenrodt's ligament

3.2 Mackenrodt's Ligaments (Fig. 3.22a–c)

These are the fibroareolar support of the uterus. The vessels, nerves and lymphatics travel through the ligaments. The uterus is suspended to the lateral pelvic wall by the cardinal ligaments (Fig. 3.23a–d).

Since these are not the true supports of the uterus these are not strengthened during the prolapse surgery. The significance of the ligaments lies in the lymphatic drainage and the vascular supply (Fig. 3.24).

The basic rule is that the lymphatics follow the venous drainage, since uterine vein lies in the cardinal ligaments and thus the lymphatics drain into the internal iliac/obturator nodes (Fig. 3.25a, b).

3.2.1 Rules

1. Cervical cancer drains into obturator/internal iliac nodes. Thus the sentinel node is found here (Fig. 3.26).
2. In pelvic inflammatory disease, the vessels and the ureter get adherent due to the surrounding inflammation (Fig. 3.27a, b).
3. The hypogastric nerves and the parasympathetic fibres are in relation to the lateral part of the ligament. Hence in nerve-sparing surgery the ligament length transacted is less as compared to the non-nerve-sparing (Fig. 3.28).
4. The cardinal ligament strengthening is not done in prolapse surgery since this is a weak support of the uterus (Fig. 3.29).

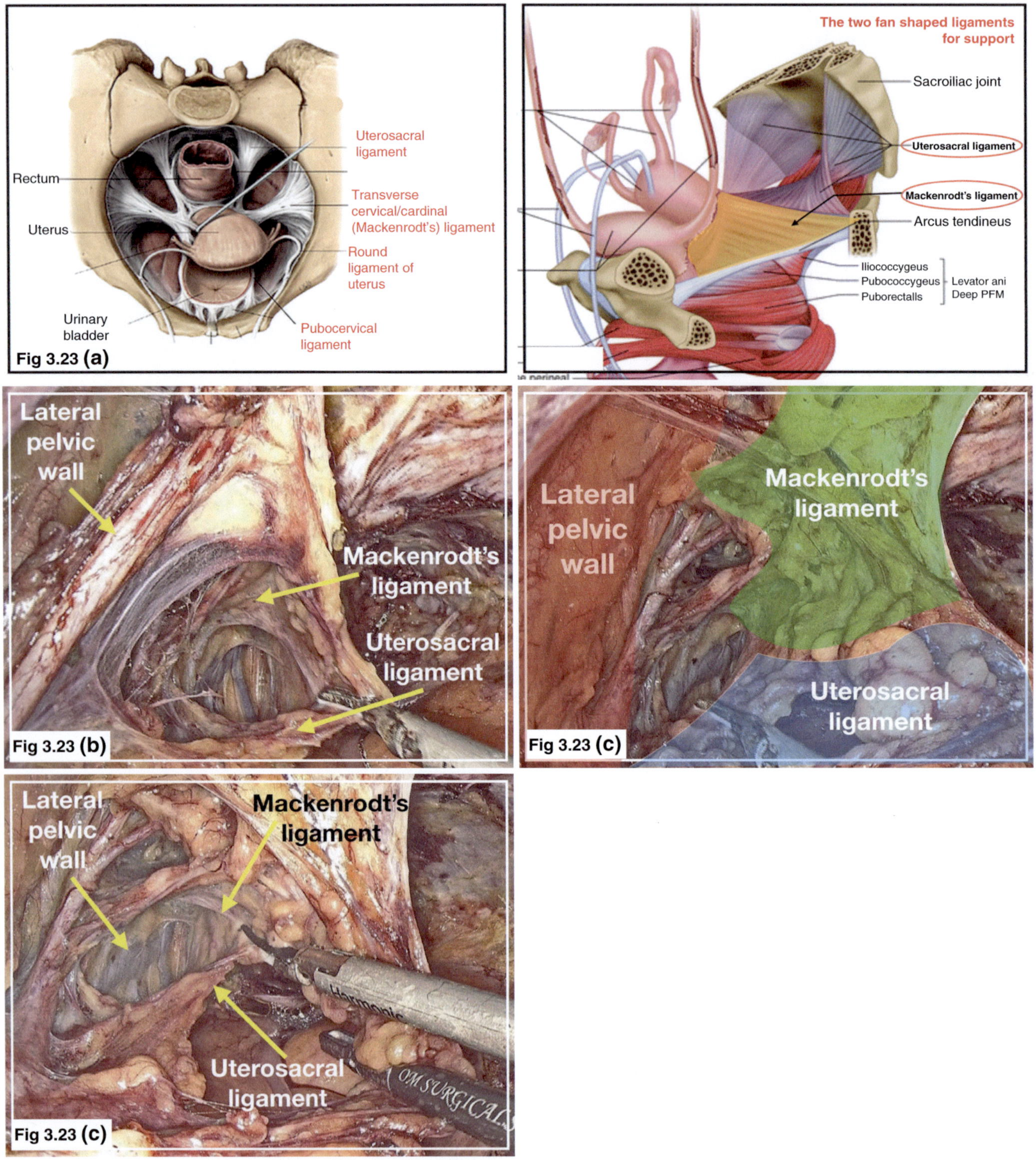

Fig. 3.23 (**a**) Characteristic image of the Mackenrodt's ligament seen in the pelvis. (**b**) The extent of the Mackenrodt's ligament lies from the bladder to the uterosacral ligament, thus forming a fan-like structure as explained universally. The Mackenrodt's ligament is a fan-shaped structure in a superior view of the pelvis spanning from the outside of the bladder to the outside of the sacrum, while the uterosacral ligament is a fan-shaped ligament in the sagittal section of the pelvis spanning along the entire lateral border of the sacral region. (**c**) In a case of nerve-sparing laparoscopic radical hysterectomy the Mackenrodt's and the uterosacral ligament have been dissected and demonstrated. The relation previously explained with graphs and images has been demonstrated in real-time images here. (**d**) The territory of the lateral pelvic wall, uterosacral ligaments and Mackenrodt's ligament has been defined for the purpose of understanding. Each structure mentioned has been shaded and labelled with a different colour. (**e**) As mentioned previously in the text the length of uterosacral resection remains the same for both the nerve-sparing and non-nerve-sparing radical hysterectomy. Thus the uterosacral ligament has been resected near to its base at the sacral region

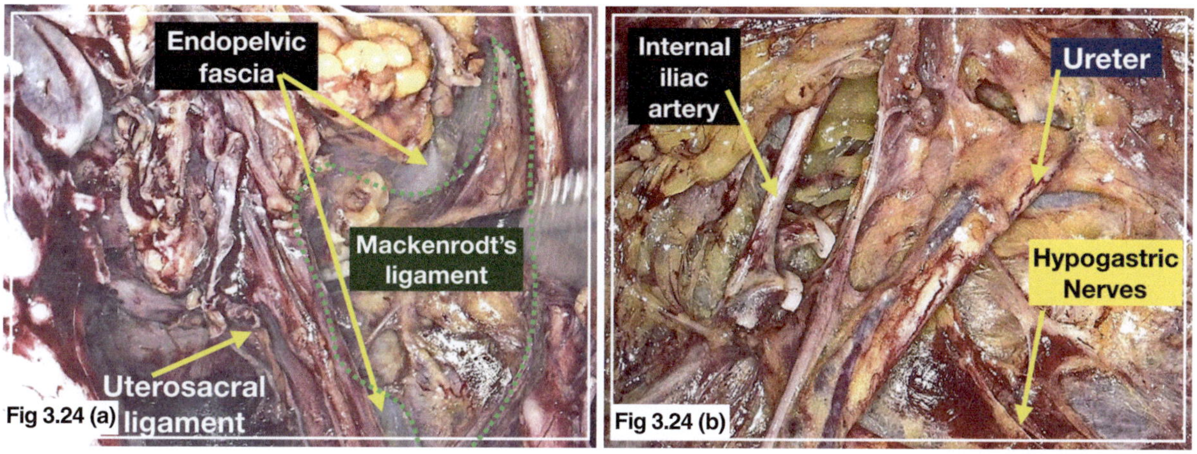

Fig. 3.24 (**a**) The image from a case of anterior exenteration demonstrates the uterosacral ligament and the Mackenrodt's ligament individually along with the endopelvic fascia seen glistening underneath from both sides of the Mackenrodt's ligament. The Mackenrodt's ligament can be seen laden with fibre areolar tissue containing vessels and lymphatics. (**b**) Even if both the uterosacral ligaments and the Mackenrodt's ligament share a common floor for levator ani muscle, the contents are very different. While the uterosacral ligament contains fibromuscular tissue it actually anchors the uterus in the pelvis and thus it is mainly plicated in prolapse surgeries. The Mackenrodt's ligament as seen in the image contains frail delicate structures like the ureter and blood vessel and nerves. They do not provide any mechanical support and have no role to play in UV descent. Thus they are not intervened in prolapse surgeries

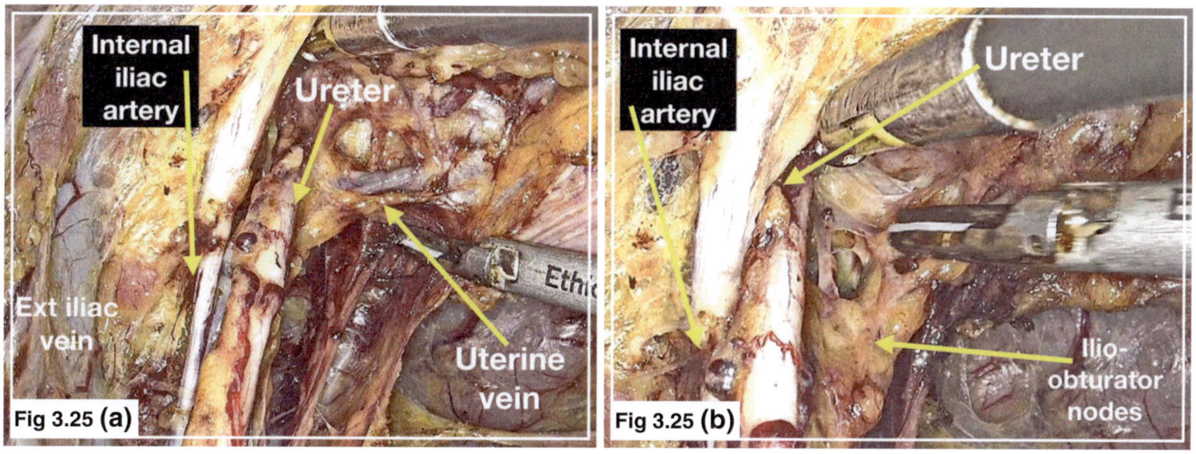

Fig. 3.25 (**a**) Lymphatics follow veins. In this image the uterine vein is seen travelling through the Mackenrodt's ligament. The uterine vein lies under the ureter and it carries parasympathetic nerve fibres and ilio-obturator nodes travel along the uterine vein as well. (**b**) The ilio-obturator lymph nodes can be seen along the way of uterine vein. The ilio-obturator lymph nodes drain into the internal iliac nodes. These are dissected off during pelvic lymph node dissection

Fig. 3.26 This series of images show the lymph nodes draining from the cervix. The ilio-obturator node is the sentinel lymph node that drains from the cervix

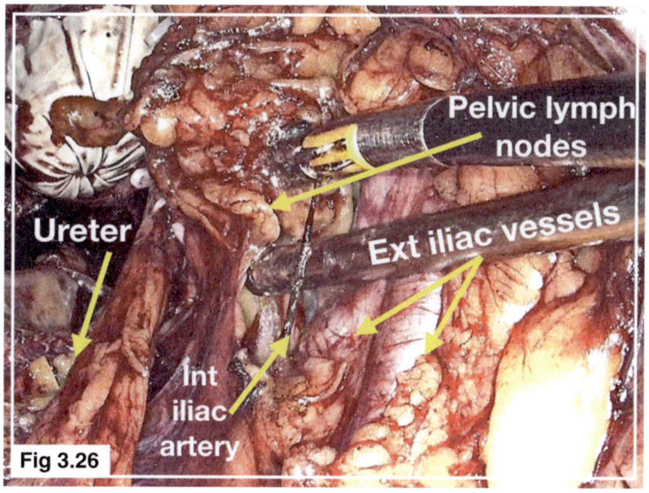

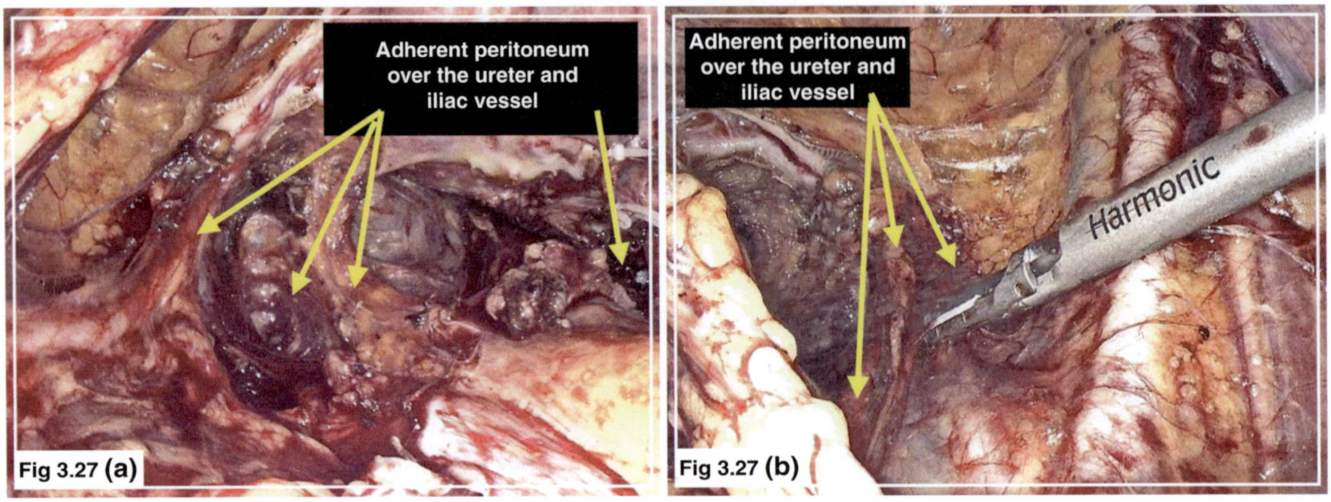

Fig. 3.27 (**a**, **b**) These images show adherent peritoneum over the ureter and the major vascular structures. Dissection in these cases leads to minor amount of haemorrhage as shown in the image

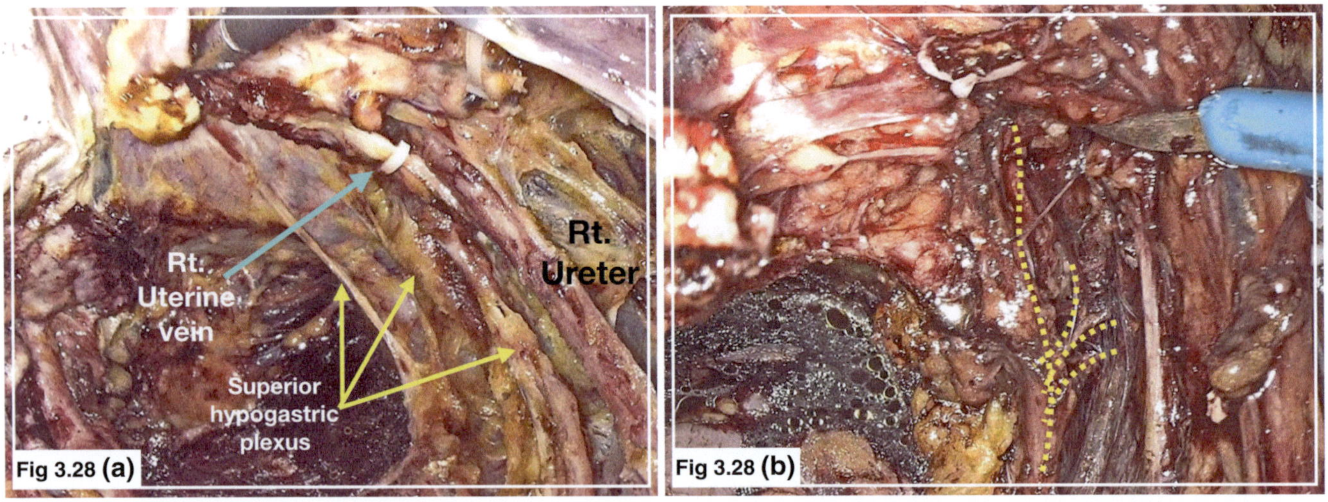

Fig. 3.28 (**a**, **b**) These images taken from a case of nerve-sparing laparoscopic radical hysterectomy show the dissection of the uterine vein medial to the ureter to spare the nerves which supply the bladder. The details of nerve-sparing radical hysterectomy have been explained further in the chapters of nerves of pelvis and the application of anatomy

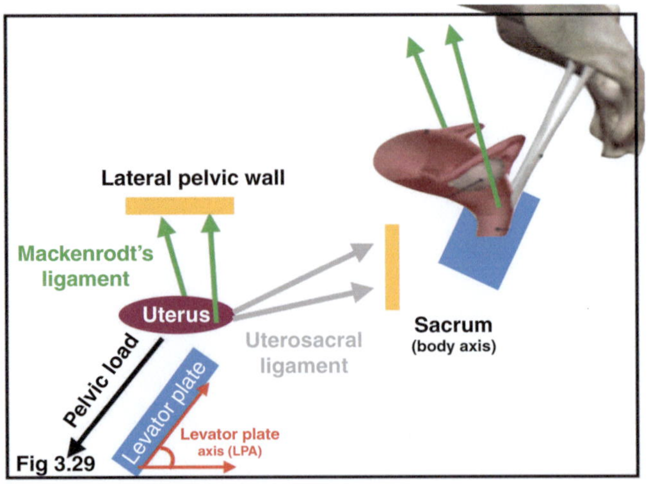

Fig. 3.29 The basis of Slings and their mechanical advantage have been explained in this image. The uterosacral ligaments are strengthened in most cases in posterior descent. The Mackenrodt's ligament has minimal role in providing support

3.3 **Paravaginal/Paracolpos** (Fig. 3.30)

These support the lower portion of the cervix and the upper part of the vagina to the lateral pelvic wall (Fig. 3.31).

The paracolpos is covered by the endopelvic fascia. The fascia extends laterally and continues as the fascia covering the levator ani/obturator internus muscle (Fig. 3.32).

The veins lie underneath the endopelvic fascia and hence staying above the fascia will avoid damage to the veins (Fig. 3.33).

This is the most vascular support of the uterus. The vaginal and the vesicle vein travels in this ligament to join the pudendal vein (Fig. 3.34).

The arborisation of these veins near the vagina gives high vascularity to the vagina (Fig. 3.35).

The ureter travels on the floor of this ligament (Fig. 3.36).

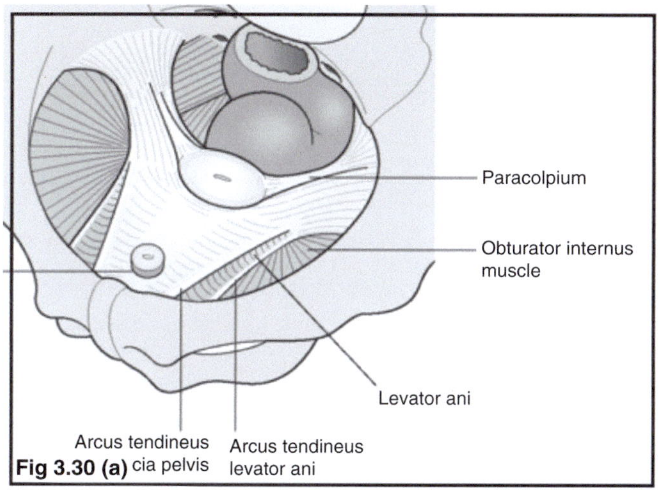

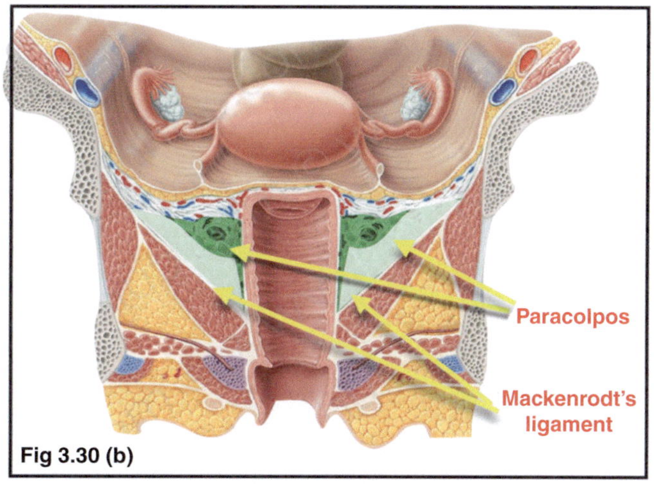

Fig. 3.30 (**a**) Diagrammatic representation of the paracolpos. The paracolpos is the postero medial aspect of the Mackenrodt's ligament, while the anterolateral part is the Mackenrodt's ligament proper. (**b**) Diagrammatic representation of the paracolpium/paracolpos in a cross-sectional image of the pelvis

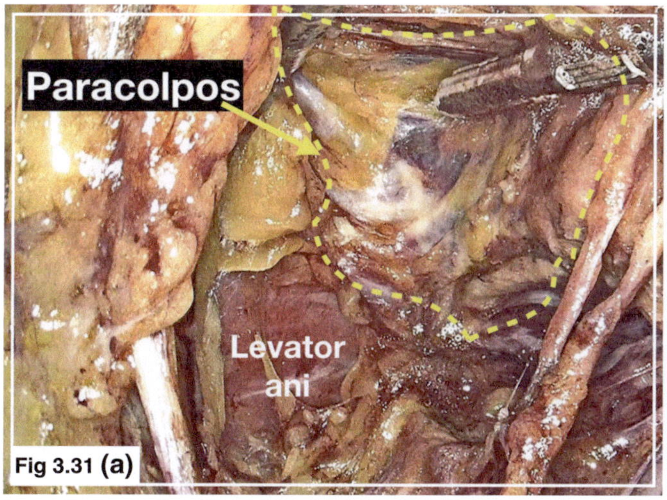

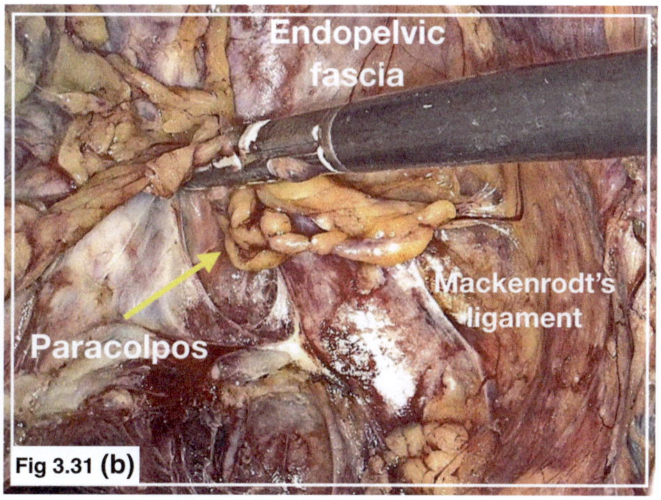

Fig. 3.31 (**a**) The image has been taken from a case of radical hysterectomy type IV where the endopelvic fascia has been dissected and the levator ani muscle can be seen. The thin white fascial tissue covered on the vaginal region is the paracolpos. By definition the paracolpos comprises the lower part of Mackenrodt's ligament covering the lower part of cervix and upper vagina. (**b**) The paracolpos extends only below the level of endopelvic fascia. It covers the vascular venous plexus of Santorini around the vagina. It is dissected in case of radical hysterectomy along with vaginectomy as shown here. The Mackenrodt's ligament can be seen separately from the paracolpos here

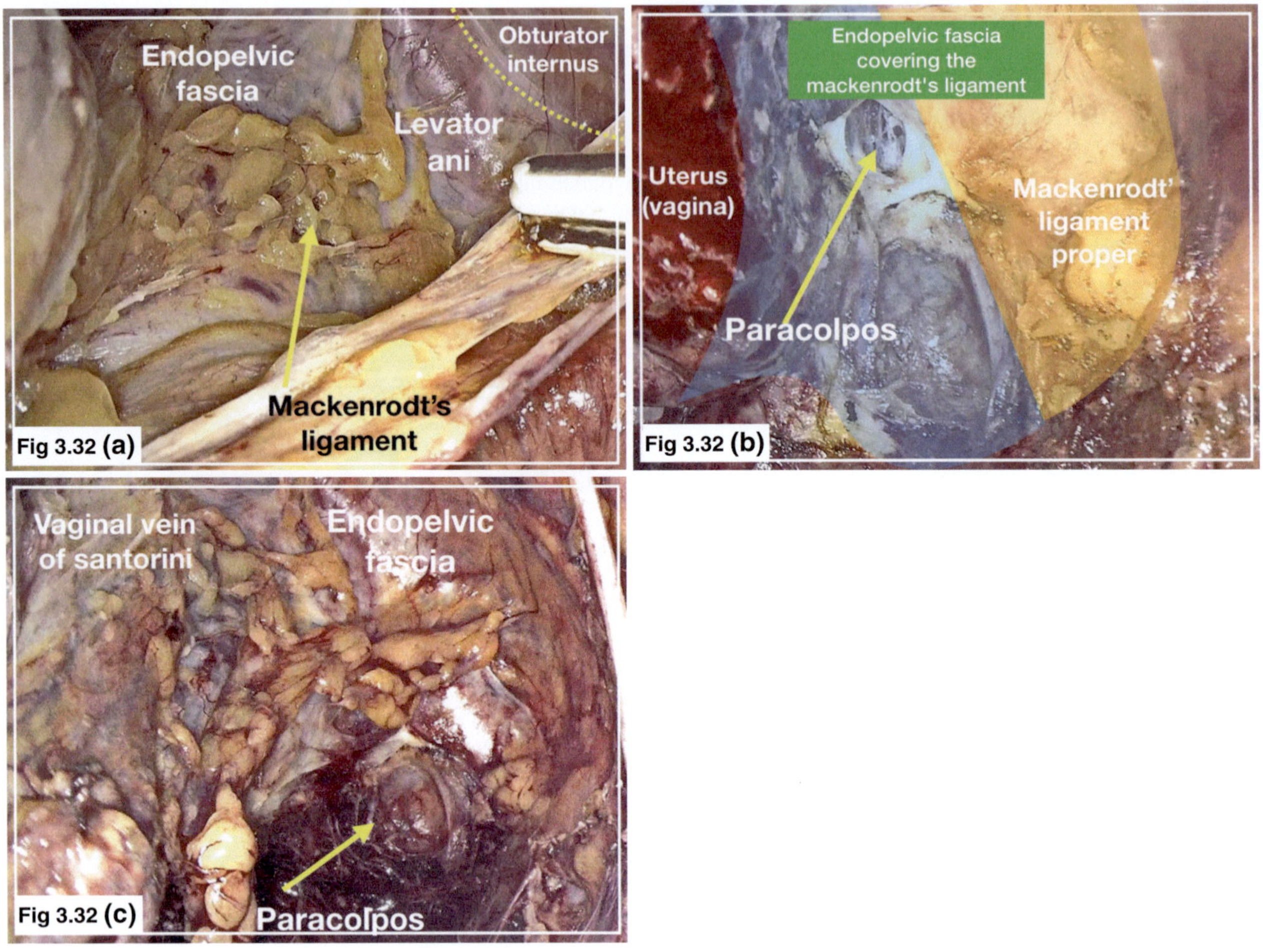

Fig. 3.32 (**a**) The yellow fibroareolar tissue seen over the endopelvic fascia belongs to the Mackenrodt's ligament while the endopelvic fascia can be seen extending and covering the levator and the obturator internus muscle. (**b**) In a case of radical hysterectomy along with vaginectomy the endopelvic fascia has been breached away from the vagina as they contain vessels of Santorini which bleed profusely. This helps in taking longer margins of the vagina for better oncological clearance. (**c**) The breach on the endopelvic fascia is extended around the vagina and thus longer length of the vagina is made resectable providing superior ontological clearance. The vaginal veins of Santorini can also be seen. These veins drain the vagina and the bladder and coalesce to form uterine veins high above

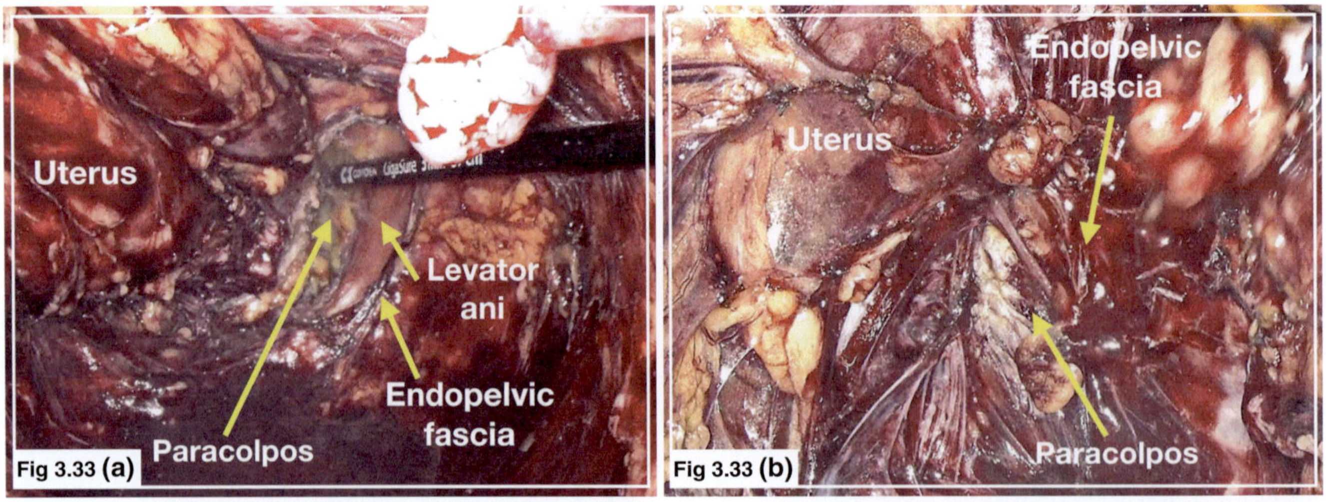

Fig. 3.33 (**a–d**) The series of images show breach in the endopelvic fascia near the vagina to direct the paracolpos leading to bleeding from the vaginal veins, thus also demonstrating the concept of veins lying underneath the fascia. This concept has been explained later in the subsequent chapters. The yellow fibroareolar tissue underneath the endopelvic fascia is called as the paracolpos. It provides support to the vagina and lower cervix

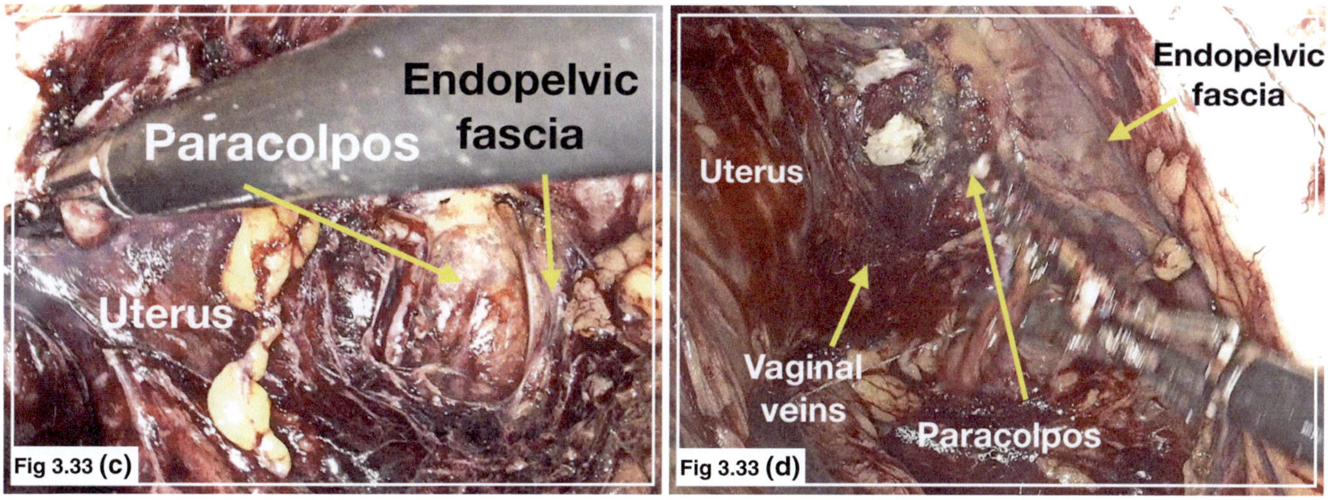

Fig. 3.33 (continued)

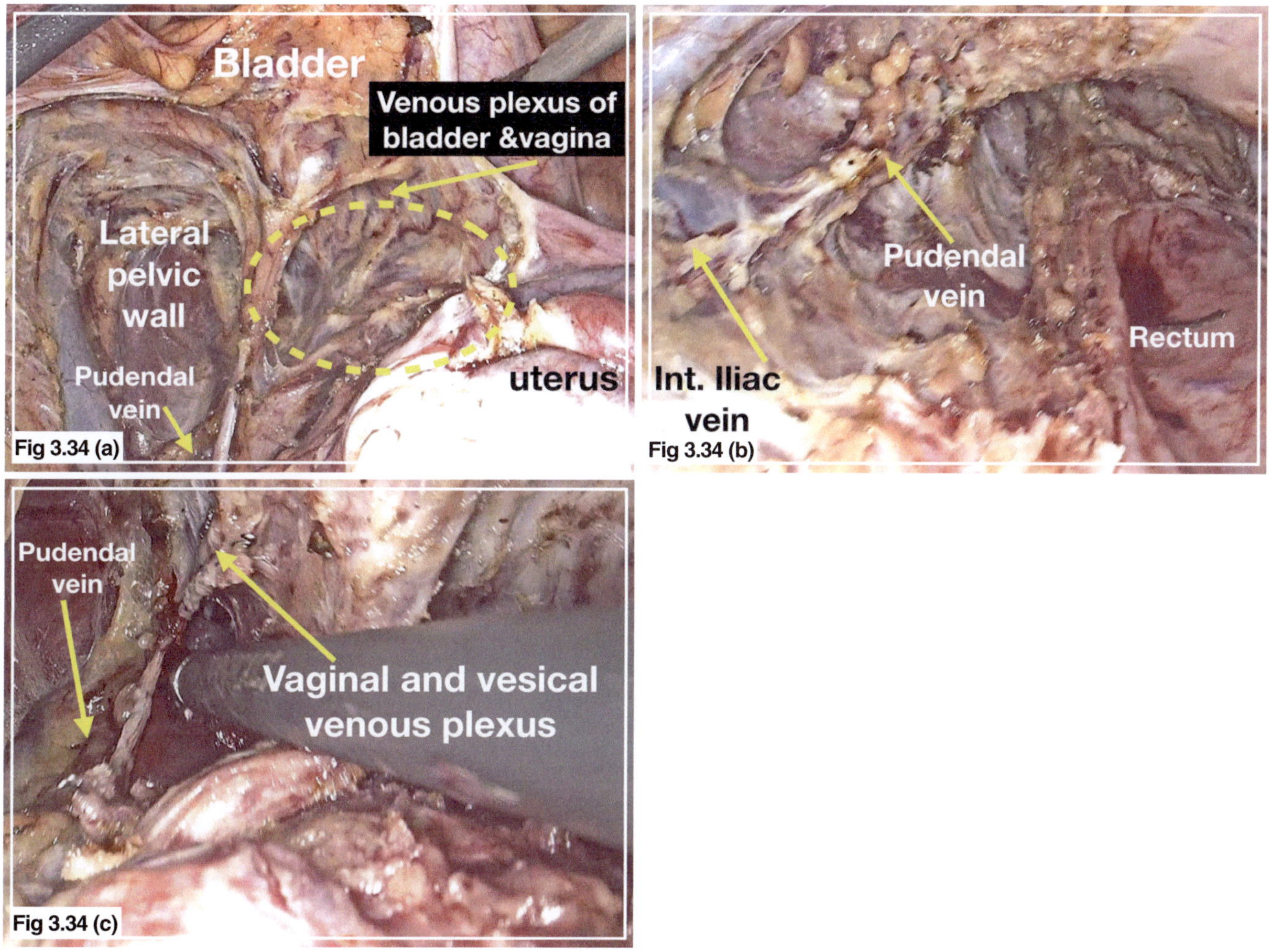

Fig. 3.34 (**a**) The venous plexus of the vagina and the bladder (vesical) is also called as the Santorini's plexus or the vesicovaginal plexus. They do not have a fixed drainage pattern. Commonly seen to drain into the pudendal vein as seen in this image taken from a case of dissection of uterine transplant. (**b**) In the same patient the pudendal vein travels below the uterosacral ligament to drain into the internal iliac vein as seen in the image. (**c**) In the case of dissection of donor for uterine transplant, the entire internal lilac vein has been harvested. Thus the vessels have been cut up to the pudendal vein. Plexuses are detrimental for the graft during re-anastomosis due to leakage

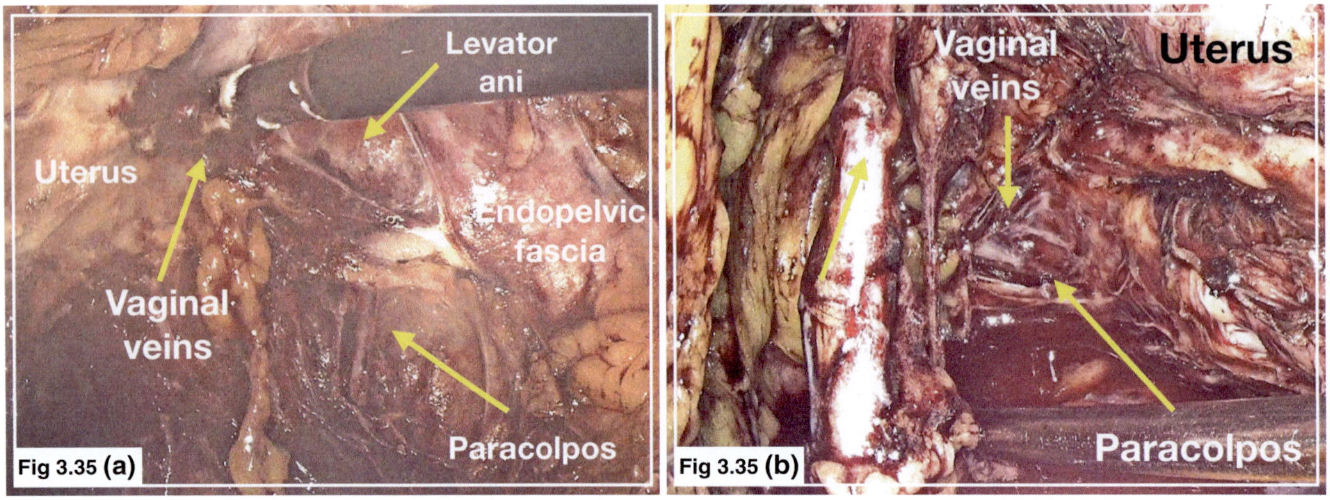

Fig. 3.35 (**a**, **b**) The images show the network of venous blood vessels around the vagina, thus called as arborisation. They are also called as the veins of Santorini and often bleed when breached into the endopelvic fascia

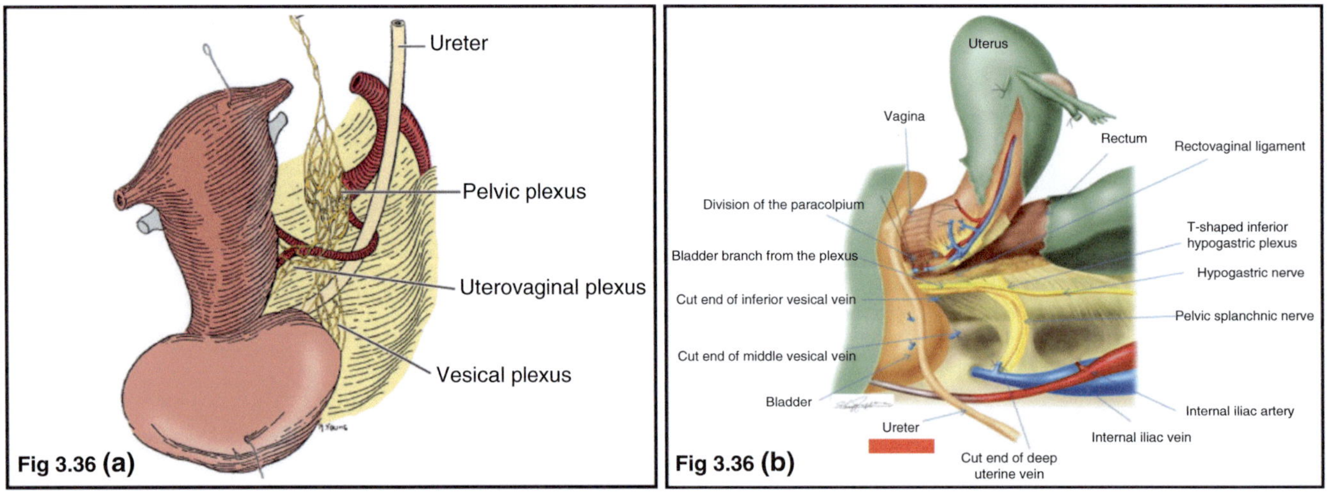

Fig. 3.36 (**a**, **b**) Ureter passes through the floor of the ligament. Below the ureter lies the uterine vein, which is a component of the Mackenrodt's ligament

3.3.1 Rules

1. Separation/lateralisation of the ureter at this level has to be done carefully due to underlying veins.
2. Since the vein lies underneath the fascia the ureter can be lateralised without damaging the vein (Fig. 3.37).
3. During LRH, the paracolpos has to be transacted laterally to get good lateral margin. The transaction has to be done carefully; otherwise haemorrhage is common (Fig. 3.38).

3.4 Round Ligaments (Fig. 3.39)

They are the true supports of the uterus and suspend the uterus anteriorly. The round ligament supports the uterus anterolaterally (Fig. 3.40).

It originates at the uterine horn, in the parametrium. The round ligament enters the pelvis via the deep inguinal ring, passes through the inguinal canal and continues on the labia majora where its fibres spread and mix with the tissue of the mons pubis (Fig. 3.41).

There is an artery which always accompanies the round ligament, called the Sampson's artery (Fig. 3.42).

3.4.1 Rules

1. The round ligament cannot be cut with cold scissors.
2. Lateral clearance of the round ligament has nothing to do with the oncological clearance.
3. Round ligament plication is done for correcting acutely retroverted uterus (Fig. 3.43).

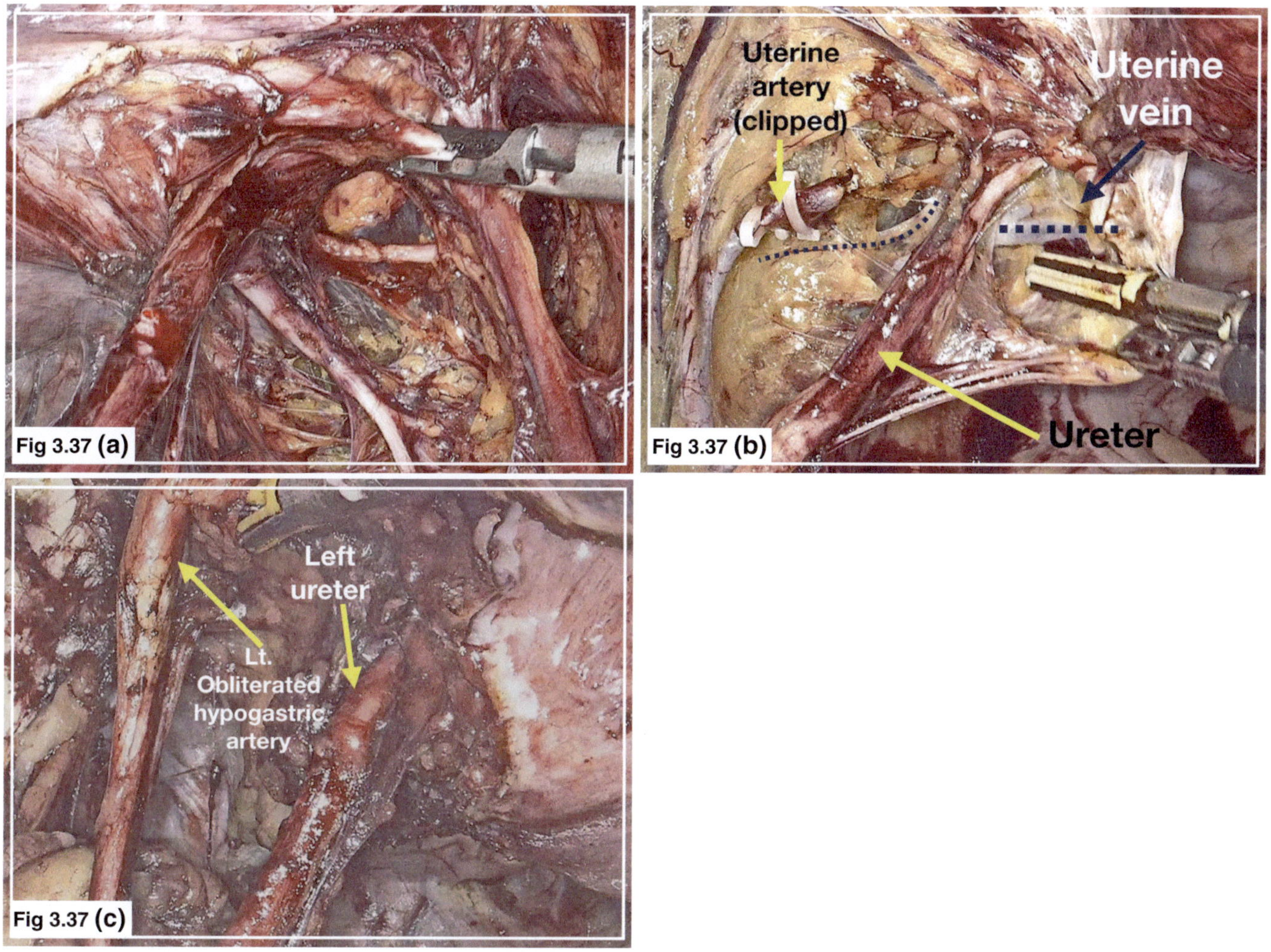

Fig. 3.37 (**a**–**c**) Mobilisation of the ureter does not cause any blood loss as the ureter lies above the endopelvic fascia and the veins lie below the fascia

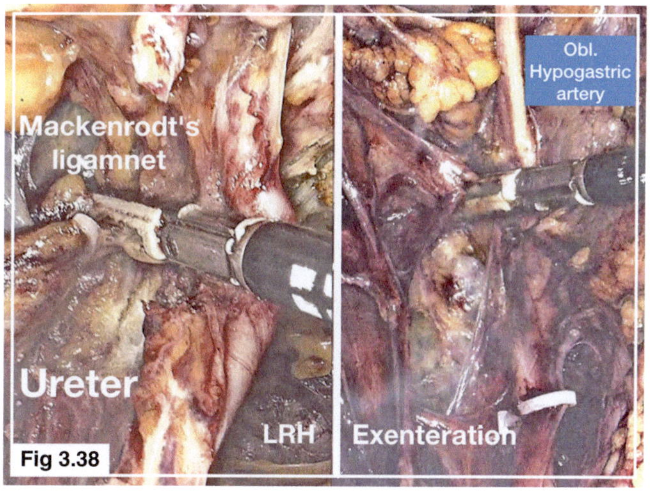

Fig. 3.38 The left-half image shows the paracolpos being resected lateral to the ureter in a case of laparoscopic radical hysterectomy and the right-half image shows the paracolpos resected further lateral near the internal iliac artery for better oncological clearance and good lateral margin

Fig. 3.39 Round ligament in its entire course from the uterus to the pubic symphysis anteriorly has been shown here

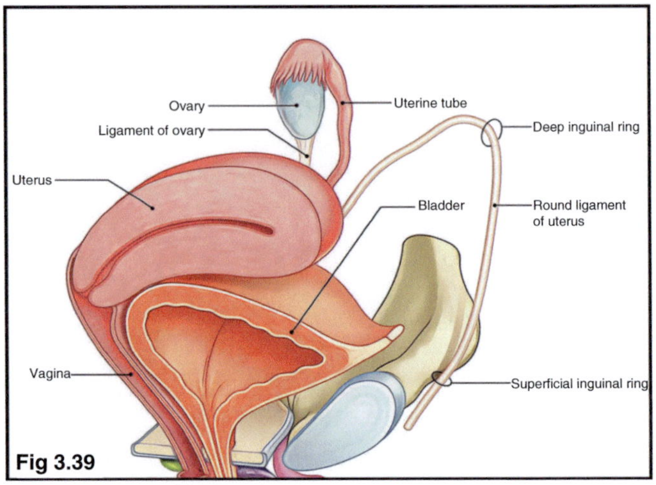

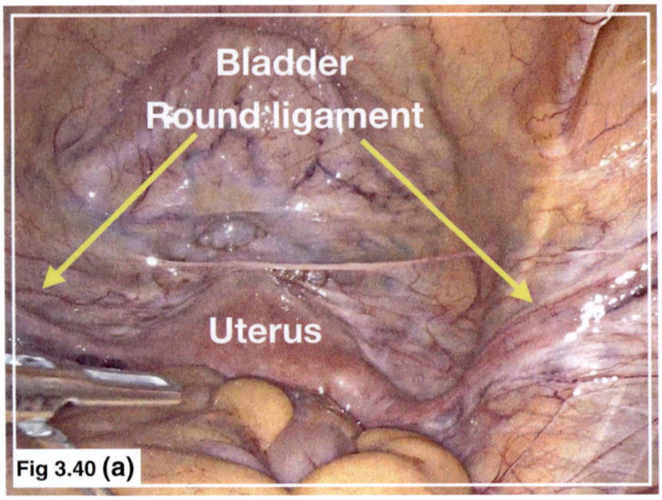

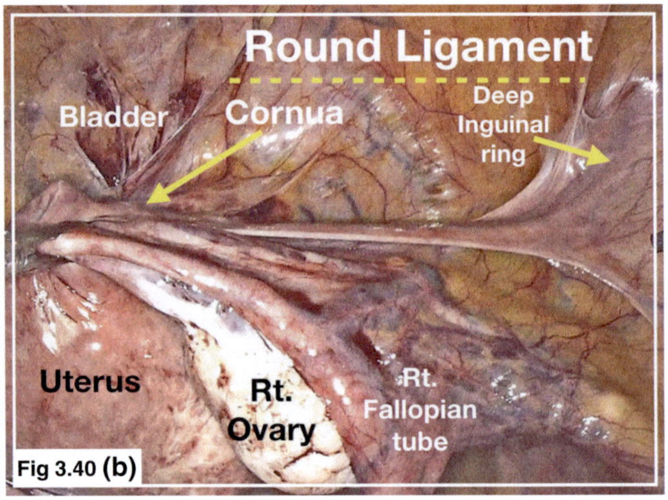

Fig. 3.40 (**a**) The first view in the pelvis often shows the following structures distinctly in a normal pelvis after retracting the loops of intestine. The bladder and rectum anteriorly and posteriorly and fundus of the uterus supported by the round ligaments on each side supporting the uterus form the sides onto the lateral pelvic wall. (**b**) The uterus has been retracted to the left side and the right round ligament can be seen taut from its origin on the cornua to its passage into the anterior abdominal wall at the level of the deep inguinal ring. The round ligament is the true support for the uterus

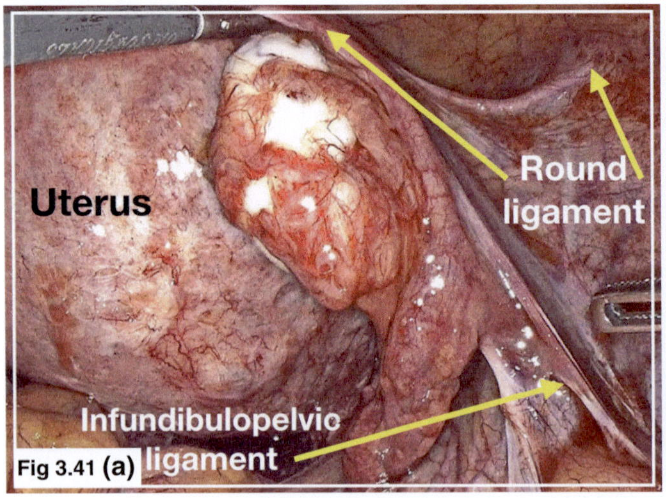

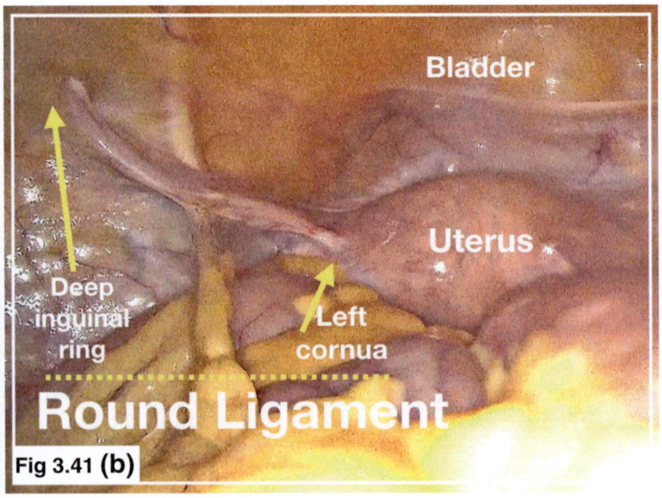

Fig. 3.41 (**a**) The round ligament here can be seen from its origin at the level of the cornua. The ligament further disappears after it reaches the lateral pelvic wall. But on dissection of the peritoneal layer it is seen entering the deep inguinal ring. (**b**) The entire course of the round ligament has been shown in this image. From the cornua to just before its entry into the deep inguinal ring

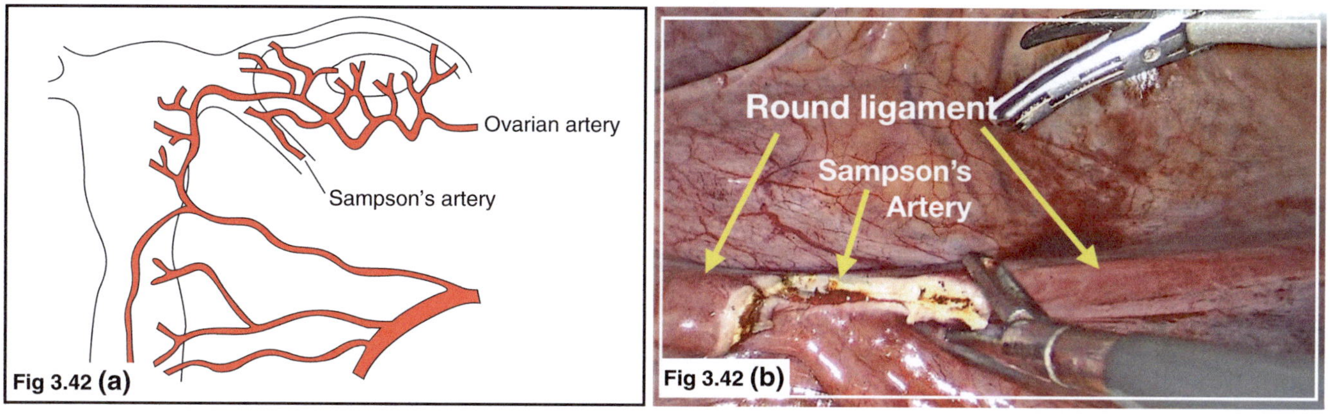

Fig. 3.42 (**a**) The diagrammatic representation of Sampson's artery which travels with the round ligament. (**b**) Bleeding from round ligament is commonly seen due to the Sampson's artery. Hence cold scissors are discouraged to use while cutting the round ligament

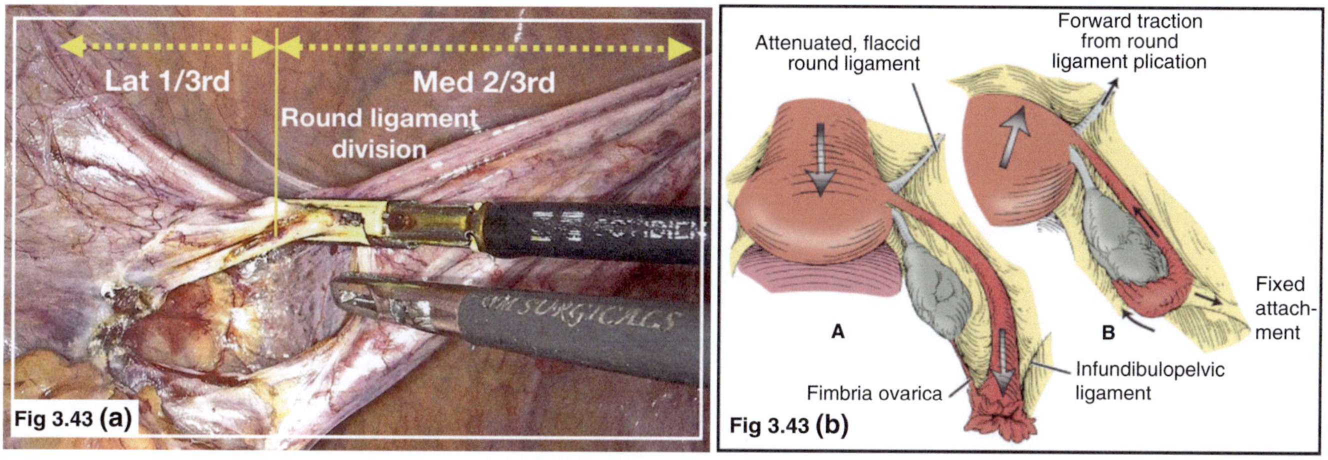

Fig. 3.43 (**a**) Round ligament is best cut with energy sources so as to coagulate the season's vessel as we cut the ligament from the outside. For a case of radical hysterectomy the round lateral resection of round ligament does not provide any oncological clearance. However it helps in easy exposure of the retroperitoneum and thus helps in dissection of the blood vessels and the pelvic lymph nodes. Hence in cases of radical hysterectomy it is advised to cut the round ligament at least beyond the medial 2/3rd and lateral 1/3rd junction. In case of hysterectomy, they can be cut near the uterus. (**b**) Round plication done to provide additional support to the uterus

3.5 Broad Ligament (Fig. 3.44)

It consists of two layers of peritoneum (photo). This connects the sides of the uterus to the lateral and posterior parts of the pelvis (photo).

The uterine vessels lie between the two layers of broad ligament (photo) (Fig. 3.45).

The access to the retroperitoneum can be done by cutting the anterior or posterior leaf of the broad ligament (Fig. 3.46).

Since the broad ligament consists of loose areolar tissue, the only pathology which can arise is the fibroid. A broad ligament fibroid always displaces the ureter and so a careful dissection should be done (photo) (Fig. 3.47).

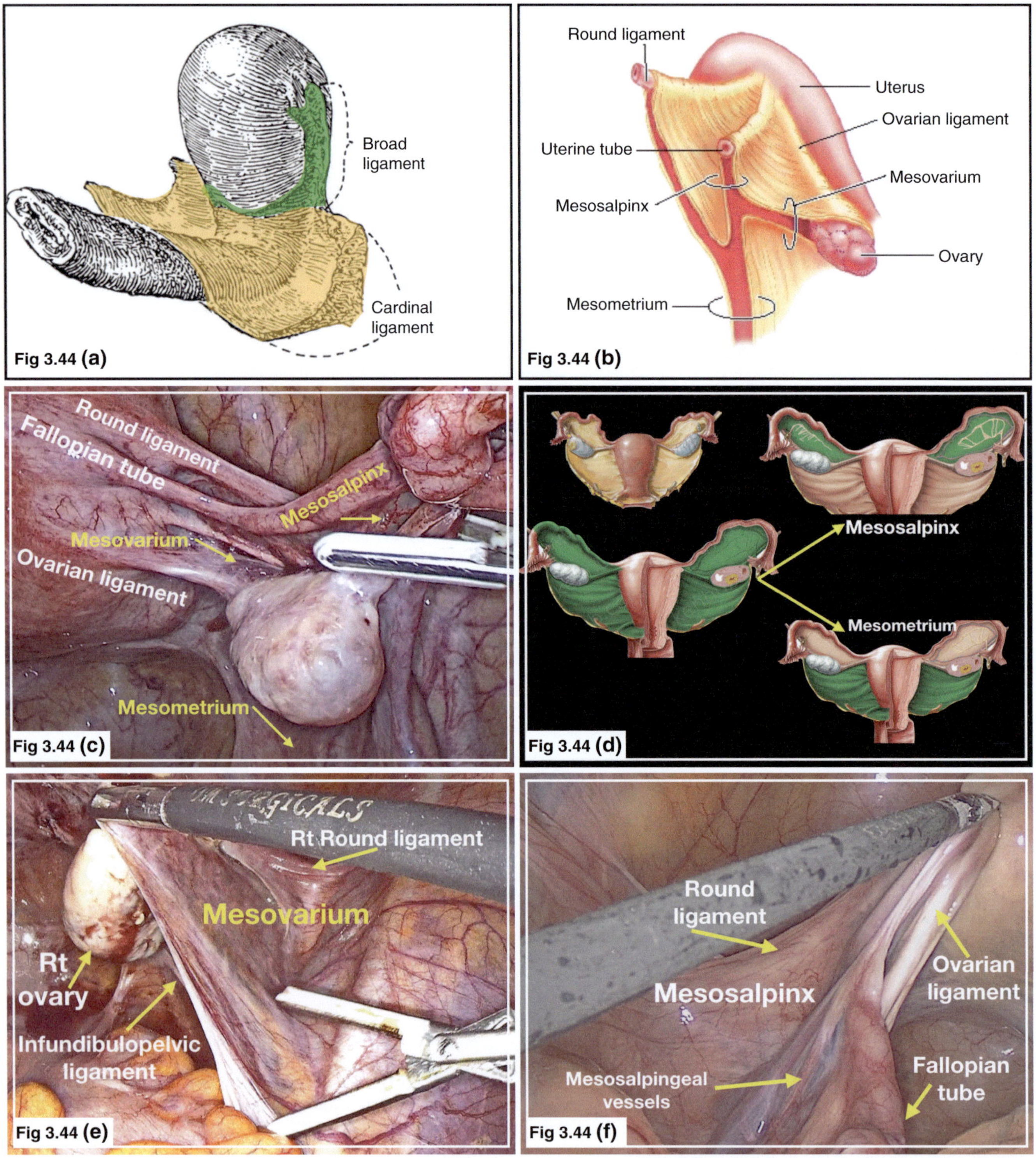

Fig. 3.44 (**a**) The broad ligament has been shaded in green while the Mackenrodt's ligament is shaded in yellow. Often the Mackenrodt's ligament is misrepresented by showing both ligaments in the same colour. Hence this differentiation is essential to understand the concept of Mackenrodt's ligament as well as the broad ligament. The broad ligament is a canopy over the uterus; thus it exists till the lower uterine segment, before the level goes to the internal os of the cervix. Below that point is the Mackenrodt's ligament. (**b**) The broad ligament is divided into the mesovarium, mesometrium and mesosalpinx by the ovarian ligament, uterus and fallopian tubes, respectively. (**c**) Real-time image supporting the previous diagrammatic image explaining the parts of the broad ligament. (**d**) The diagrammatic representation of the mesosalpinx and the mesovarium has been shown in the image. (**e**) The mesovarium has been demonstrated on this image more clearly than previous images. (**f**) The mesosalpinx with the blood vessel has been demonstrated in this image. It is advised to coagulate the mesosalpingeal vessel prior to salpingectomy. (**g**) The mesometrium is both the leaves of broad ligament together. Thus it can be seen easily. Here the posterior leaf of road ligament has been cut as a manner of approaching the retroperitoneum

Fig. 3.44 (continued)

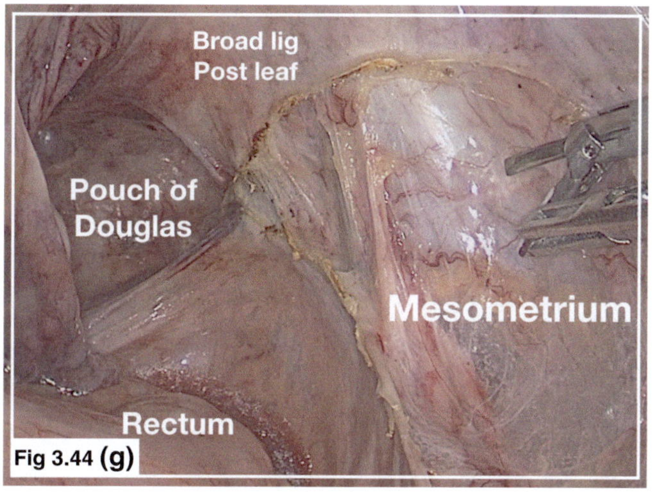

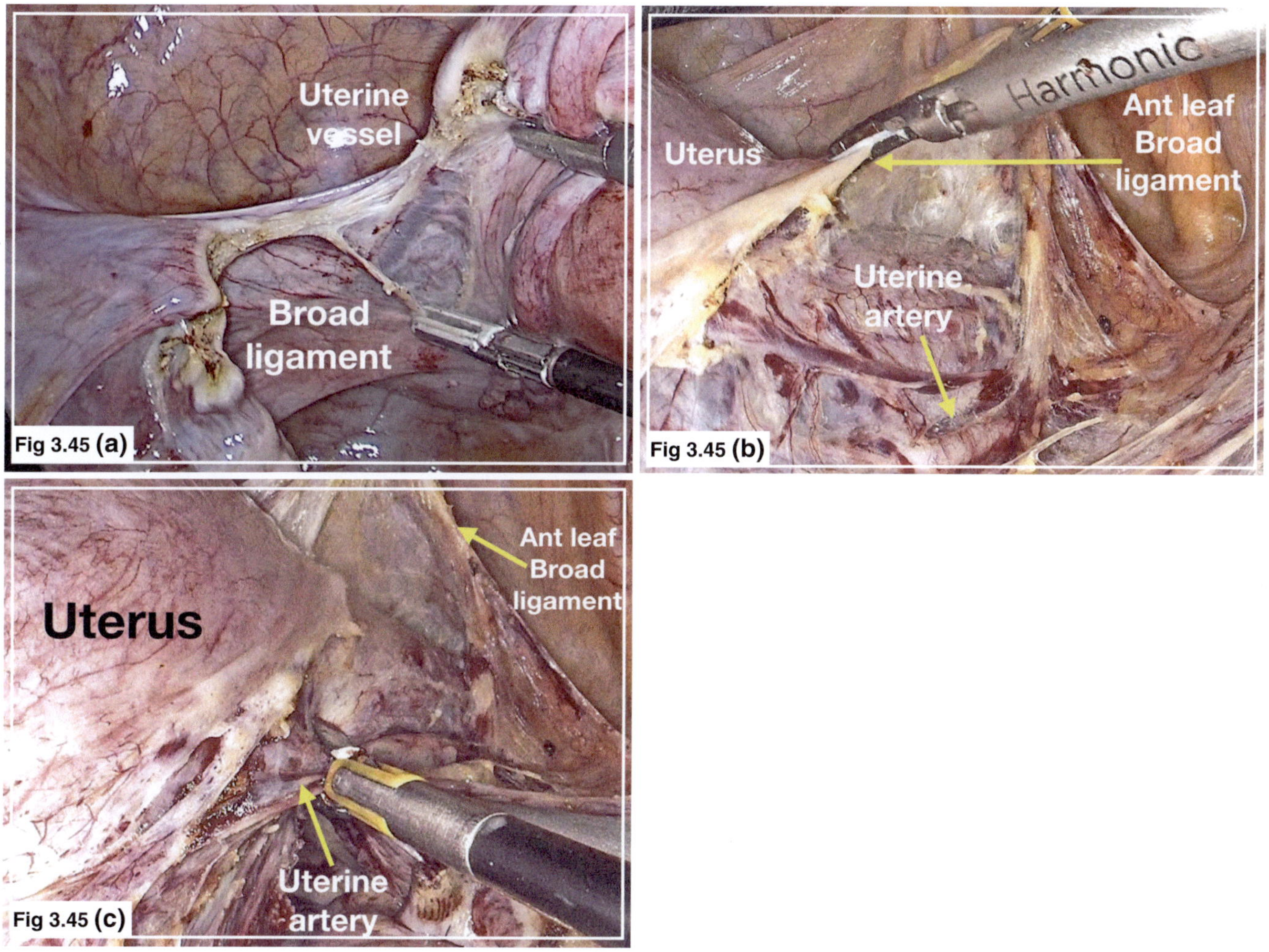

Fig. 3.45 (**a**) The left uterine vessels, artery and vein can be seen travelling along the contour of the uterus in between the leaves of broad ligament. (**b**) The right uterine artery can be seen travelling along the side of the uterus. The anterior leaf of broad ligament has been lifted upward to separate the bladder. (**c**) The uterine artery has been grasped by a bipolar cautery for coagulation in this case of benign hysterectomy

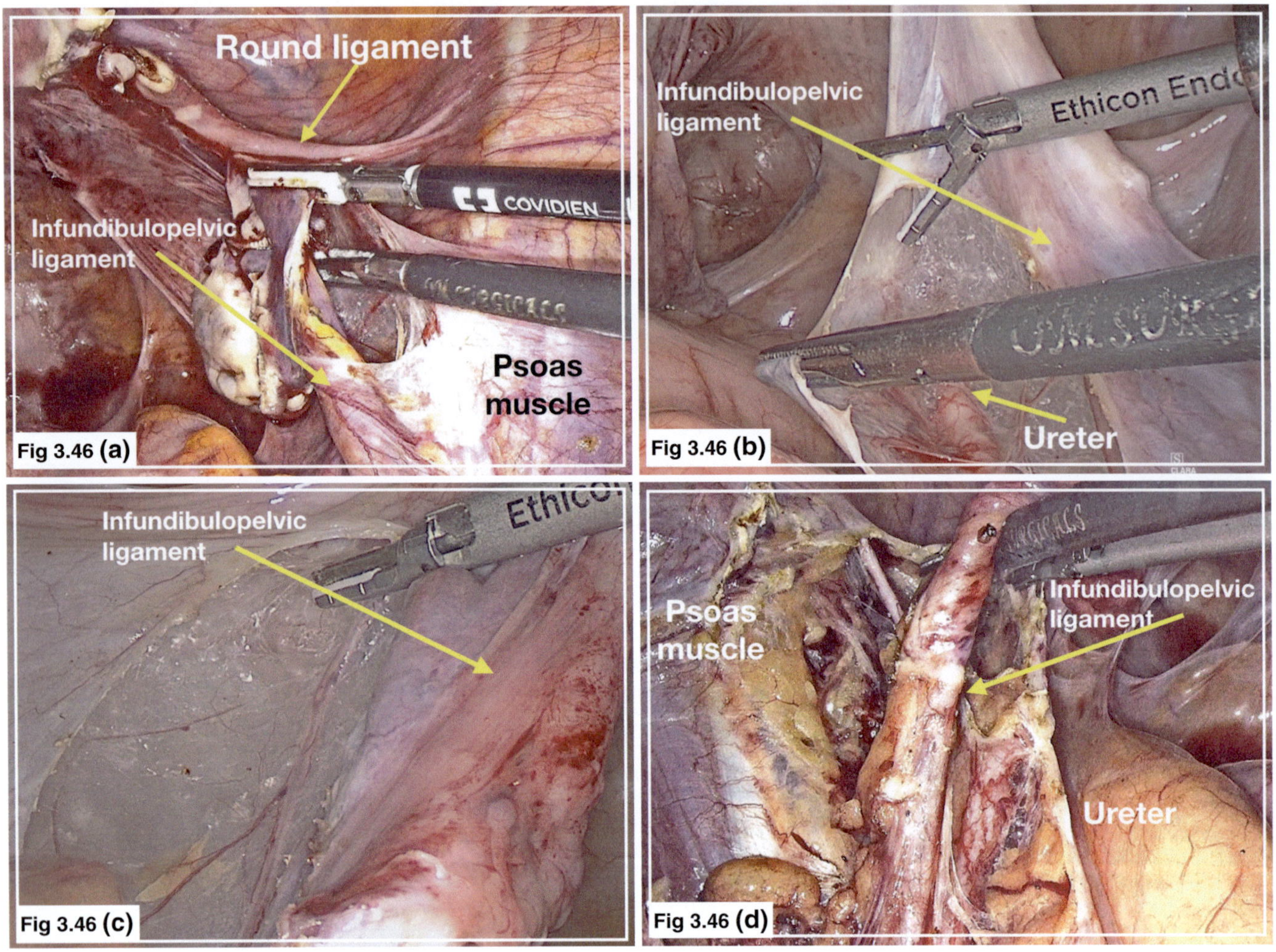

Fig. 3.46 (**a**) Lateral approach of retroperitoneum has been demonstrated. The broad ligament is cut lateral to the infundibulopelvic ligament. The psoas muscle is visible. (**b**) Medial approach has been demonstrated in this image. The ureter is visible. (**c**) Lateral approach has been demonstrated on the opposite side for approaching the retroperitoneum. (**d**) Both the medial and the lateral approaches done for this case to dissect the ovarian vessels. The ureter and the psoas muscle both are visible

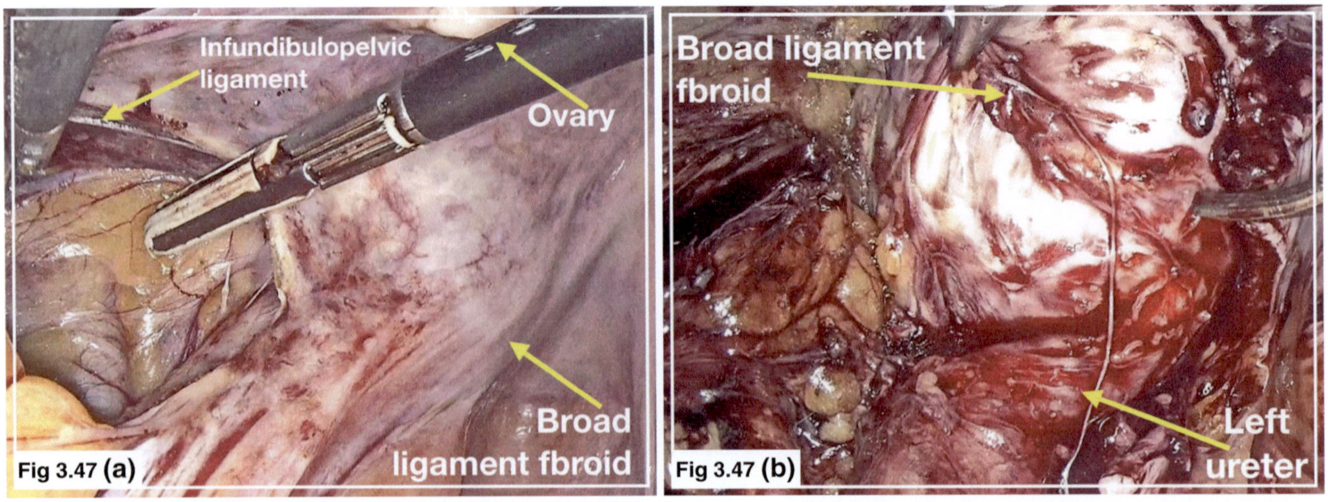

Fig. 3.47 (**a**) Broad ligament fibroid identified and its relations identified with the infundibulopelvic ligament, and ovary and posterior leaf of broad ligament itself. (**b**) The broad ligament dissects retroperitoneally, and is adherent to the ureter underneath leading to hydroureter proximal to the fibroid

4 Bones and Muscles

Levator ani is formed of three muscles, namely, pubococcygeus, puborectalis and iliococcygeus (Figs. 4.1 and 4.2a–g).

4.1 Coccyges (Fig. 4.3)

The levator ani and the obturator internus muscle form the base of the pararectal space and they are covered by the endopelvic fascia. This is a tough fascia. This fascia forms an important landmark for all pelvic floor repairs (Fig. 4.4).

4.2 Psoas Muscle

The psoas muscle is the lateral-most structure in the pelvis. The external iliac artery rests on the muscle (Figs. 4.5 and 4.6).

The pubic bone is exposed as the lateral-most boundary during the ilio-obturator lymphadenectomy. The circumflex iliac vein is in close proximity to this bone. This vein forms the distal limit of the lymphadenectomy (Fig. 4.7).

Anteriorly the pubic symphysis is visualised during the exenteration and pelvic floor repairs (Fig. 4.8).

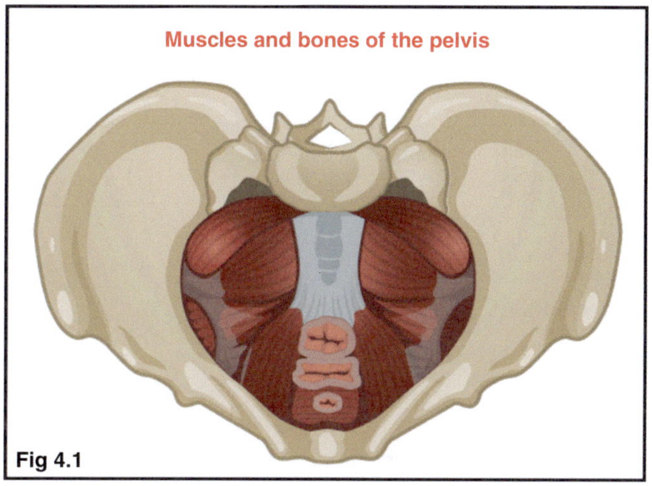

Fig. 4.1 Pelvic diaphragm

S. Puntambekar et al., *Laparoscopic Pelvic Anatomy in Females*, https://doi.org/10.1007/978-981-13-8653-4_4

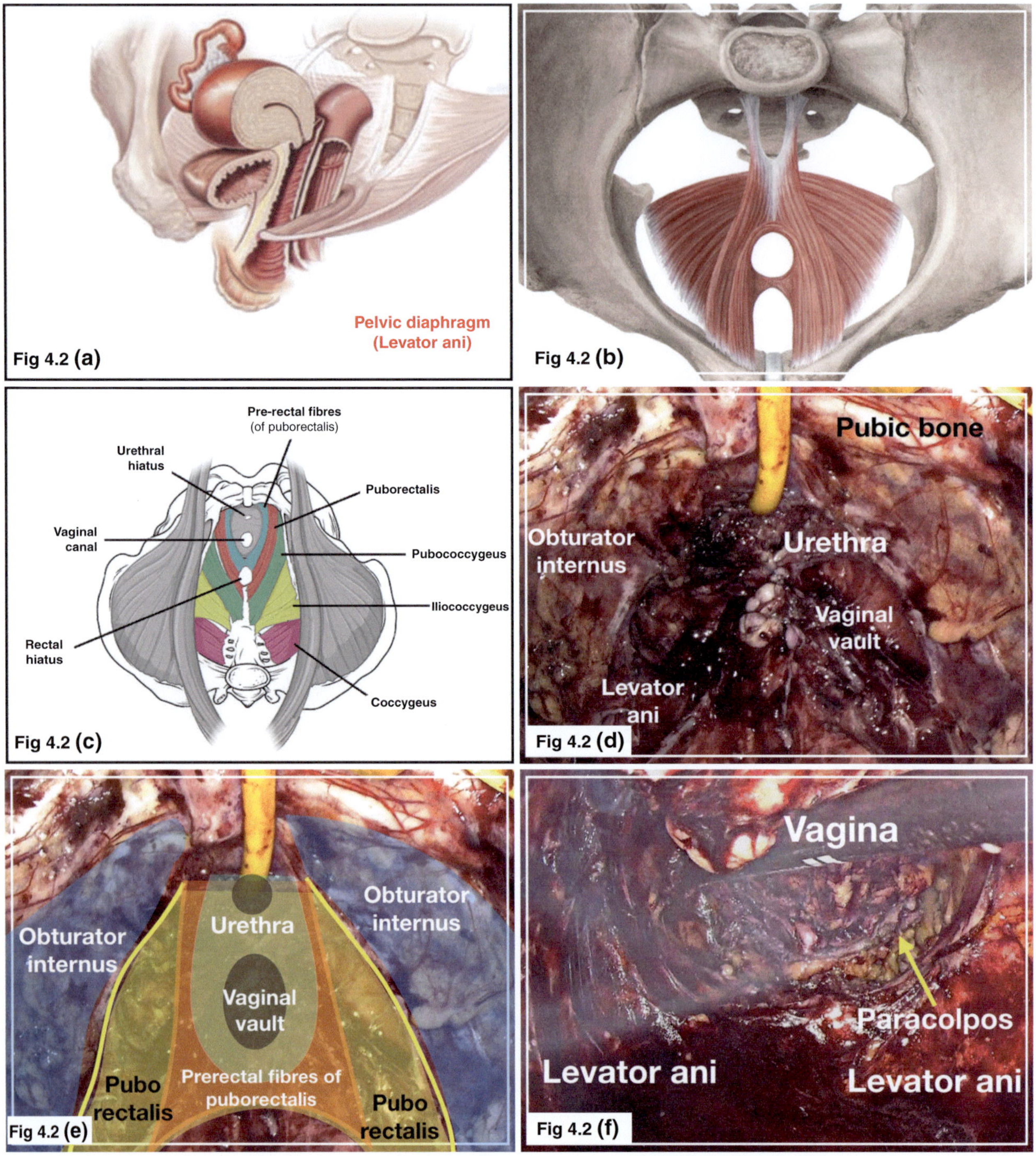

Fig. 4.2 (**a**) Three-dimensional diagrammatic representation of the pelvic diaphragm (levator ani). (**b**) Only the levator ani has been shown in this image. The puborectalis, pubococcygeus and iliococcygeus muscle form the levator ani. The pelvic diaphragm comprises coccygeus, pyriformis and obturator internus along with the levator ani muscle. The obturator internus on the anterolateral side and the coccyges and pyriformis muscle on the posterior aspect have not been shown. (**c**) The view of pelvic floor from the perineal region has been shown. Each muscle shown here in different colour has been shown in the real-time images in subsequent images. (**d**) The image from a case of anterior exenteration shows the final image of the pelvic floor after the uterus and bladder have been removed. The stump of vagina (vault) and the urethra (Foley's catheter) can be seen. The levator ani muscle and the obturator interns muscle can also be seen covered by the endopelvic fascia. (**e**) The same image has been used as graphic representation of all the various structures visualised. The green-shaded region is the urogenital diaphragm, the orange-shaded region shows the prerectal fibres of puborectalis and the yellow-shaded region is the puborectalis muscle proper. The pubococcygeus and the ischiococcygeus cannot be visualised in this region as they have no direct correlation to the anal canal or the vagina. These three muscles do not have clear distinction amongst themselves and thus in real-time images they together form the levator ani. The blue-shaded region is the obturator internus. (**f**) The dissection of the paracolpos has been demonstrated. The breach in endopelvic fascia at the level of paracolpos and the region behind it forms the levator ani muscle. Here too, the prerectal fibres of puborectalis and the puborectalis proper can be seen. The pubococcygeus and the iliococcygeus remain behind the rectum. (**g**) Diagrammatic representation of prerectal fibres and the puborectalis muscle has been shown here

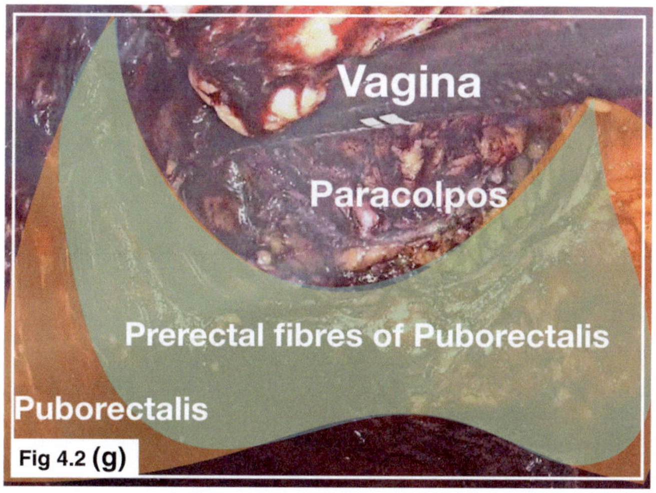

Fig. 4.2 (continued)

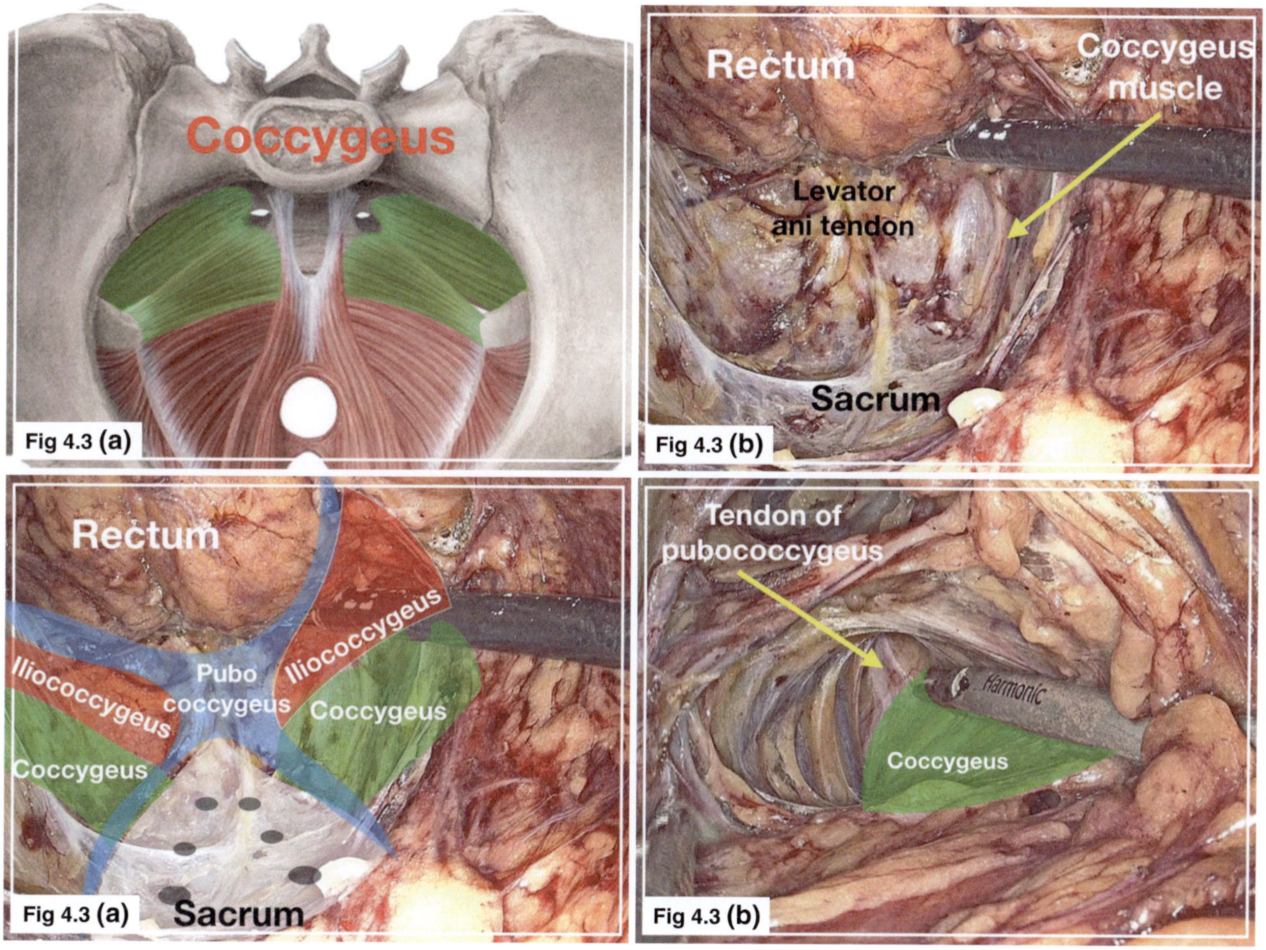

Fig. 4.3 (**a**) The coccyges muscle forms a part of the pelvic diaphragm. It has been shaded separately in green. (**b**) In a case of mobilisation of rectum for low anterior resection or posterior exenteration the interior aspects of the rectum are dissected which exposes the endopelvic and the Waldeyer's fascia and the underneath muscle is the levator ani and the coccyges muscle. (**c**) The diagrammatic representation. The blue-shaded region is the tendon of pubococcygeus muscle, and the red-shaded region is the iliococcygeus muscle. These two muscles are a part of the levator ani group of muscles. The coccyges which is free from the group lies more posterior and higher up on the sacrum. The coccyges has been shaded in green. (**d**) In a case of radical hysterectomy during dissection of the internal iliac vein the Waldeyer's fascia can be exposed high up above the endopelvic fascia. The muscle underneath this fascia is the coccyges muscle. The tendon of the pubococcygeus can be seen clearly

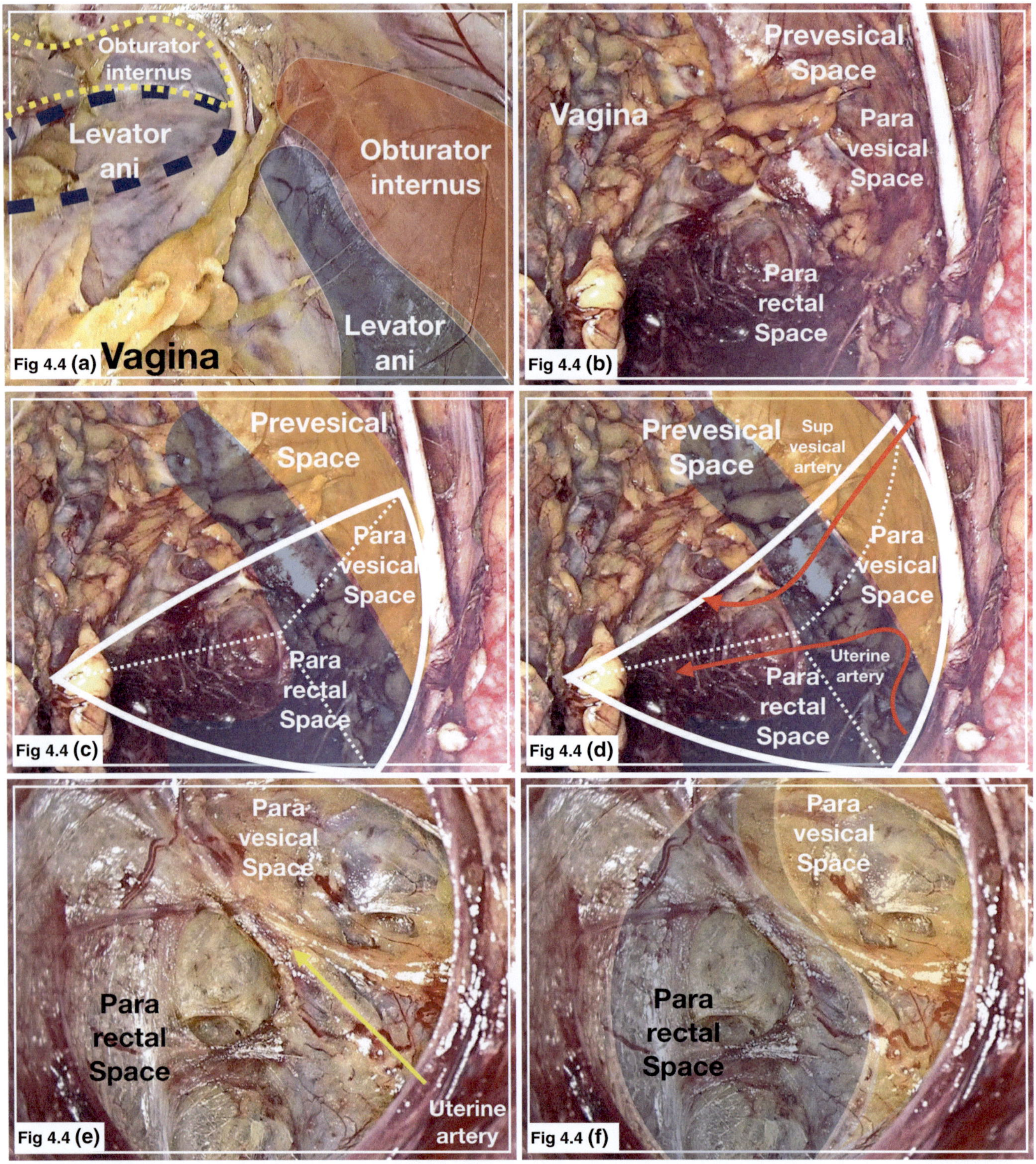

Fig. 4.4 (**a**) The image from a case of anterior exenteration showing the levator ani muscle along with the obturator internus muscle. The blue-shaded region on the right and the encircled region on the left both represent levator ani. Similarly the yellow-shaded region and the encircled region both represent the obturator internus muscle region. (**b**) Lower down where the prevesical, the pararectal and the paravesical space have been dissected from a common floor can be seen. The endopelvic fascia can be seen covering the obturator internus and the levator ani muscle. (**c**) Diagrammatic representation of the previous image with the individual muscle has been demonstrated. The white pyramidal structure represents the pararectal and the paravesical space. Both spaces share a common floor (levator ani muscle). (**d**) The same image from previous except the uterine artery and the superior vesical artery has been introduced in a schematic fashion to explain the division into the pararectal, the paravesical space and the prevesical space. (**e**) In a case of radical hysterectomy the pararectal space dissection has been done to expose the uterine artery closely. The uterine artery is divided into the pararectal and the paravesical space. Both have been dissected till the endopelvic fascia (levator ani floor). (**f**) The diagrammatic representation of the previous image showing the division of the endopelvic fascia by underneath levator ani and obturator internus muscle

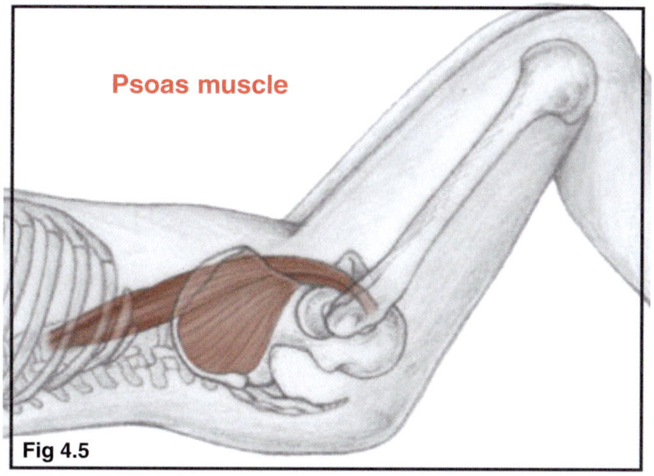

Fig. 4.5 Diagrammatic representation of psoas muscle

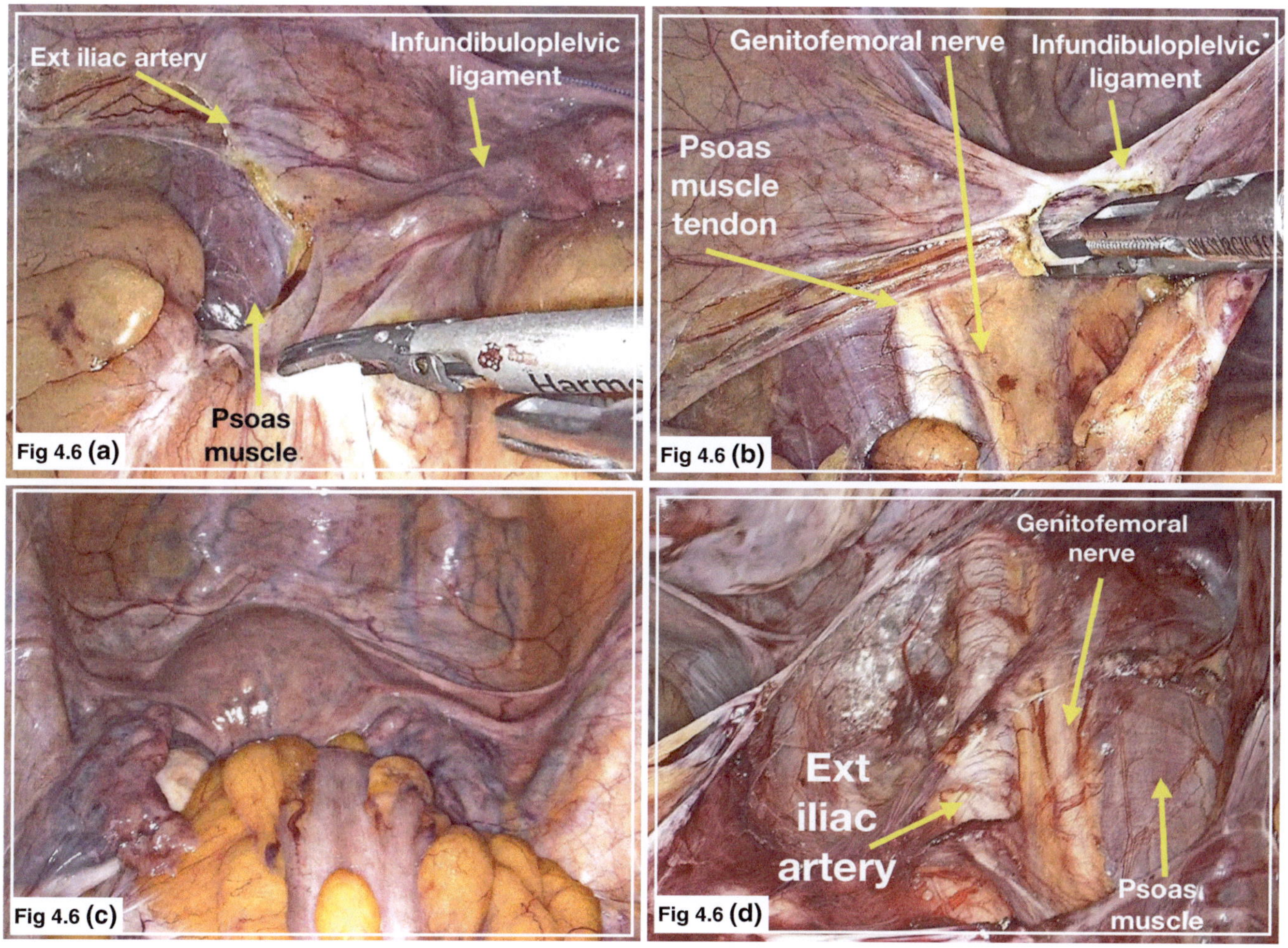

Fig. 4.6 (**a**) In a case of radical hysterectomy the retroperitoneum can be opened from lateral to the infundibulopelvic ligament. This exposes the psoas muscle easily as shown in the image. (**b**) The psoas muscle tendon and the genitofemoral nerve can be seen in this image. (**c**) Bilateral psoas muscle can be seen in this image. (**d**) Right-sided psoas muscle with the genitofemoral nerve can be seen

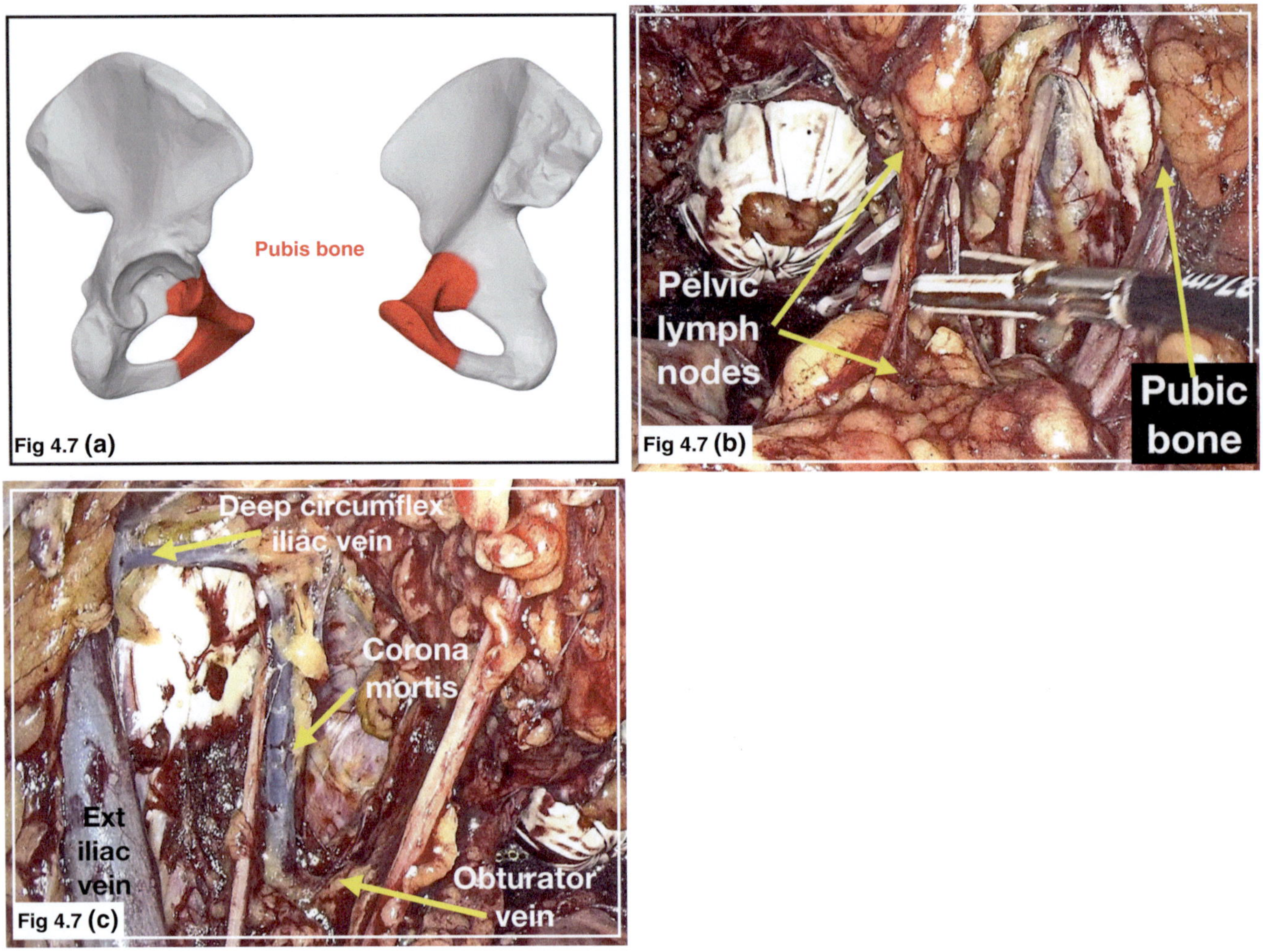

Fig. 4.7 (**a**) Pubis bones on the medial and lateral surfaces. (**b**) In a case of right pelvic lymph node dissection the lateral limit of dissection is the pubis bone as shown in the image. (**c**) The deep circumflex iliac vein is a branch of the external iliac vein which communicates with the obturator veni (branch of the internal iliac vein); this communication is called as corona mortis. This is the only communication between the external and the internal iliac veins

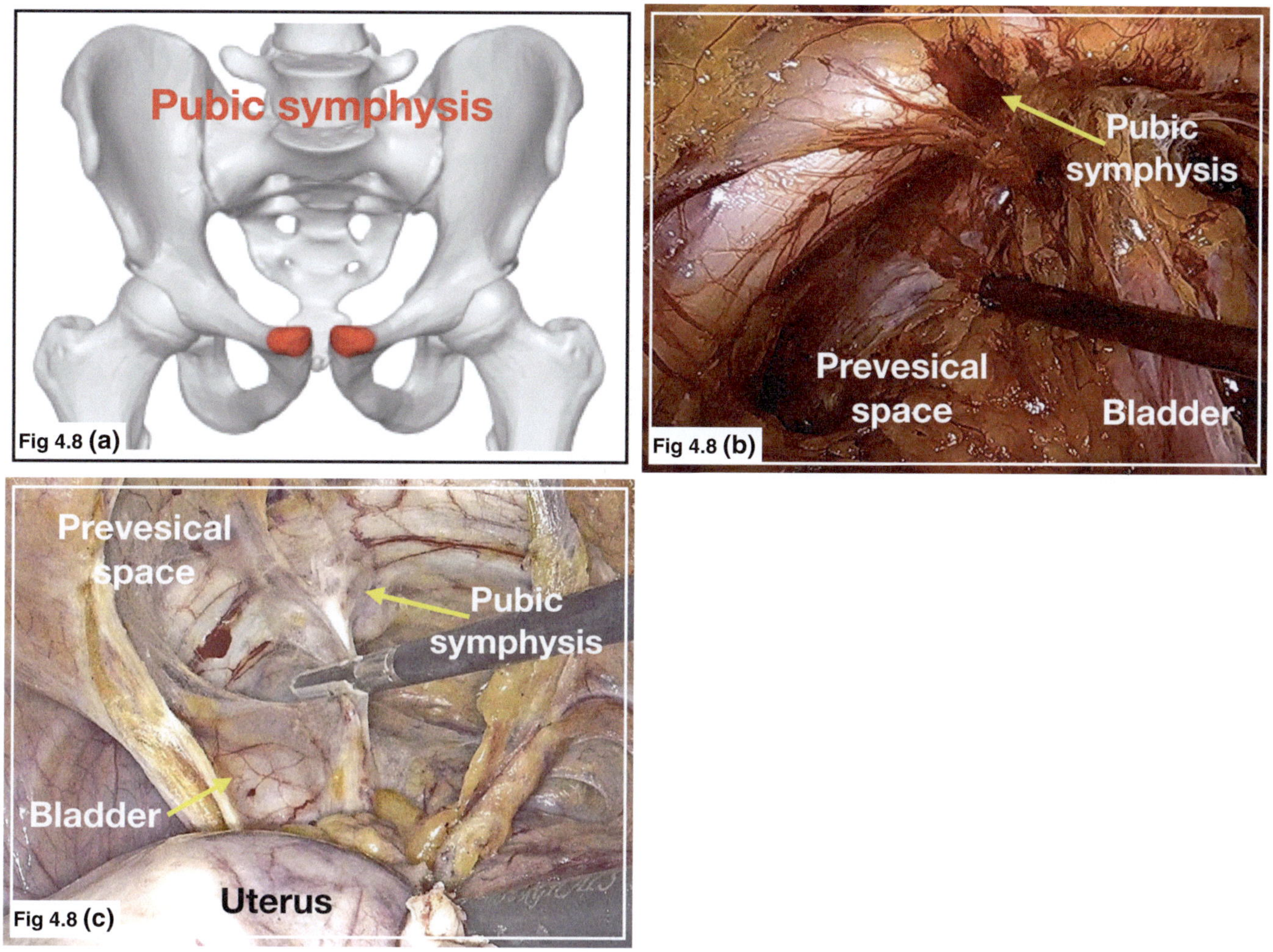

Fig. 4.8 (**a**) Diagrammatic representation of the pubic symphysis. (**b**) Image from a case of anterior mobilisation bladder in a case of burch colposuspension. The bladder is mobilised till the level of urethra. Thus the pubis bones are easily visualised. (**c**) The pubic symphysis appreciated in a case of anterior exenteration

4.3 Bones

Thus, the bony boundaries of the pelvic cavity are:

- Superiorly sacral promontory
- Laterally the ala of the pelvic bone
- Posteriorly sacrum

4.4 Inferiorly Pubic Symphysis (Figs. 4.9 and 4.10)

The importance of the pelvic floor, pelvic floor repair, SUI sling surgery like transobturator tape (TOT) and tension-free vaginal tape (TVT) procedures (Fig. 4.11).

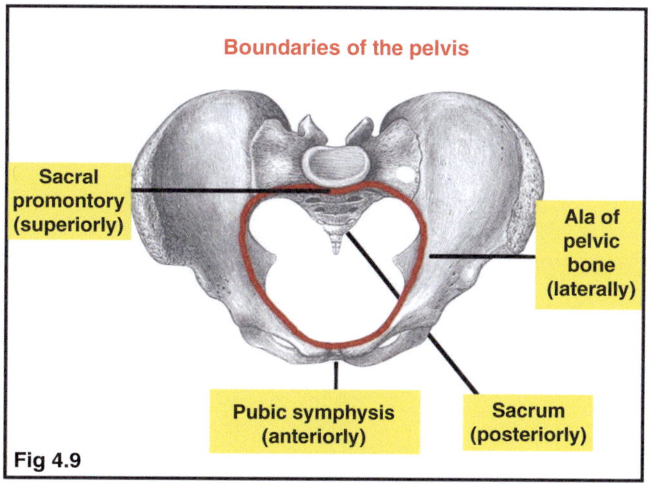

Fig. 4.9 Diagrammatic representation of the boundaries of pelvis

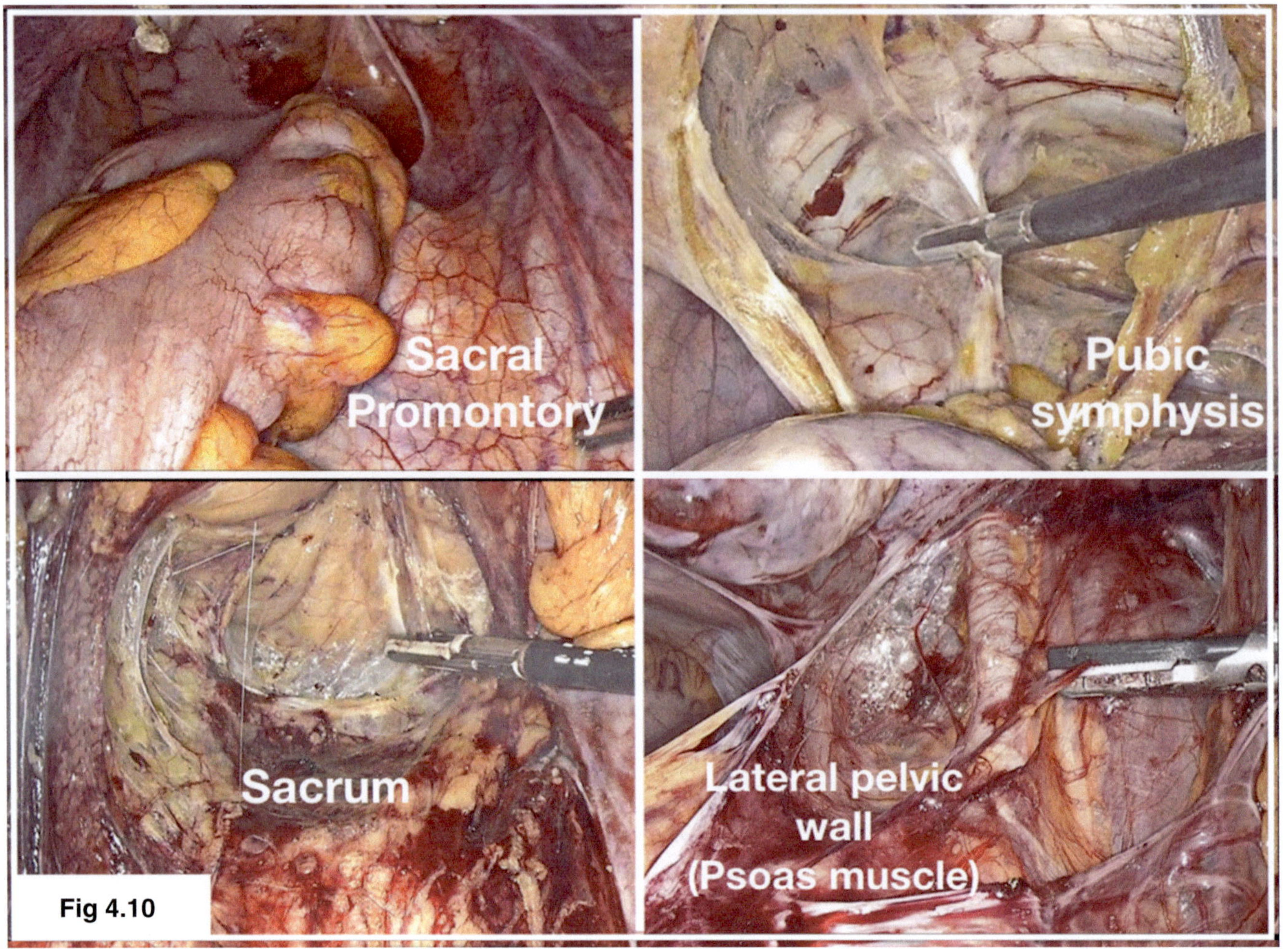

Fig. 4.10 Real-time collage of the boundaries of pelvis starting from top left in clockwise manner—sacral promontory, pubic symphysis, lateral pelvic wall and sacrum

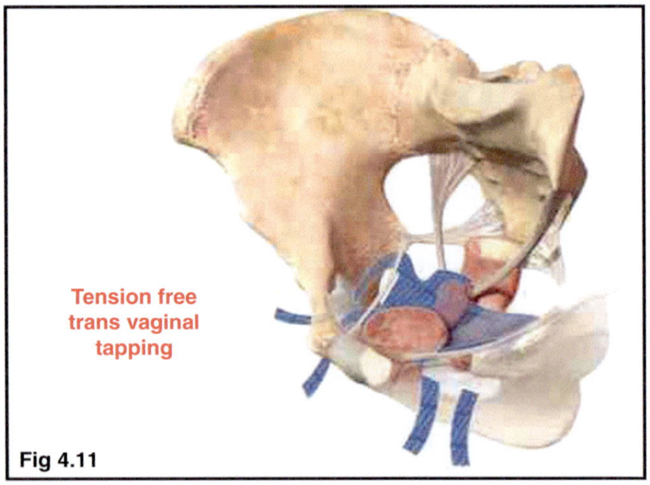

Fig. 4.11 Tension-free transvaginal taping shown in the image

5 Vascular Anatomy

The vascular anatomy will be described from the bifurcation of the aorta. *The bifurcation of the common iliac is at the level of sacral promontory* (Figs. 5.1 and 5.2c).

This is an important anatomical landmark. The line of small bowel mesentery crosses at the level of sacral promontory on its way to the right sacroiliac joint (Fig. 5.3a–c).

Thus the pelvic organs can be separated at this level from the upper abdominal organs. *Thus the organs anterior to the bifurcation can be easily separated from the great vessels* (Fig. 5.4a–d).

There are no vessels (branches) arising from the major vessels at this level anteriorly (Fig. 5.5a, b).

It is important to recognise these fascial planes. Unless there is inflammation, the loose areolar planes can be easily dissected (Fig. 5.6a, b).

In the presence of any branches of aorta or vena cava this would not have been possible. These planes are essential in the surgeries of the rectum and the vault suspension in females (Fig. 5.7a, b).

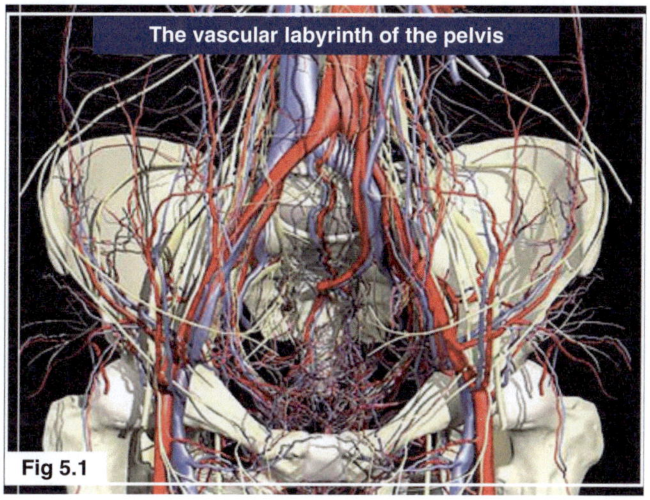

Fig. 5.1 The chaotic vascular labyrinth of the pelvis. Our goal is to bring order to this chaos and help understand better

S. Puntambekar et al., *Laparoscopic Pelvic Anatomy in Females*, https://doi.org/10.1007/978-981-13-8653-4_5

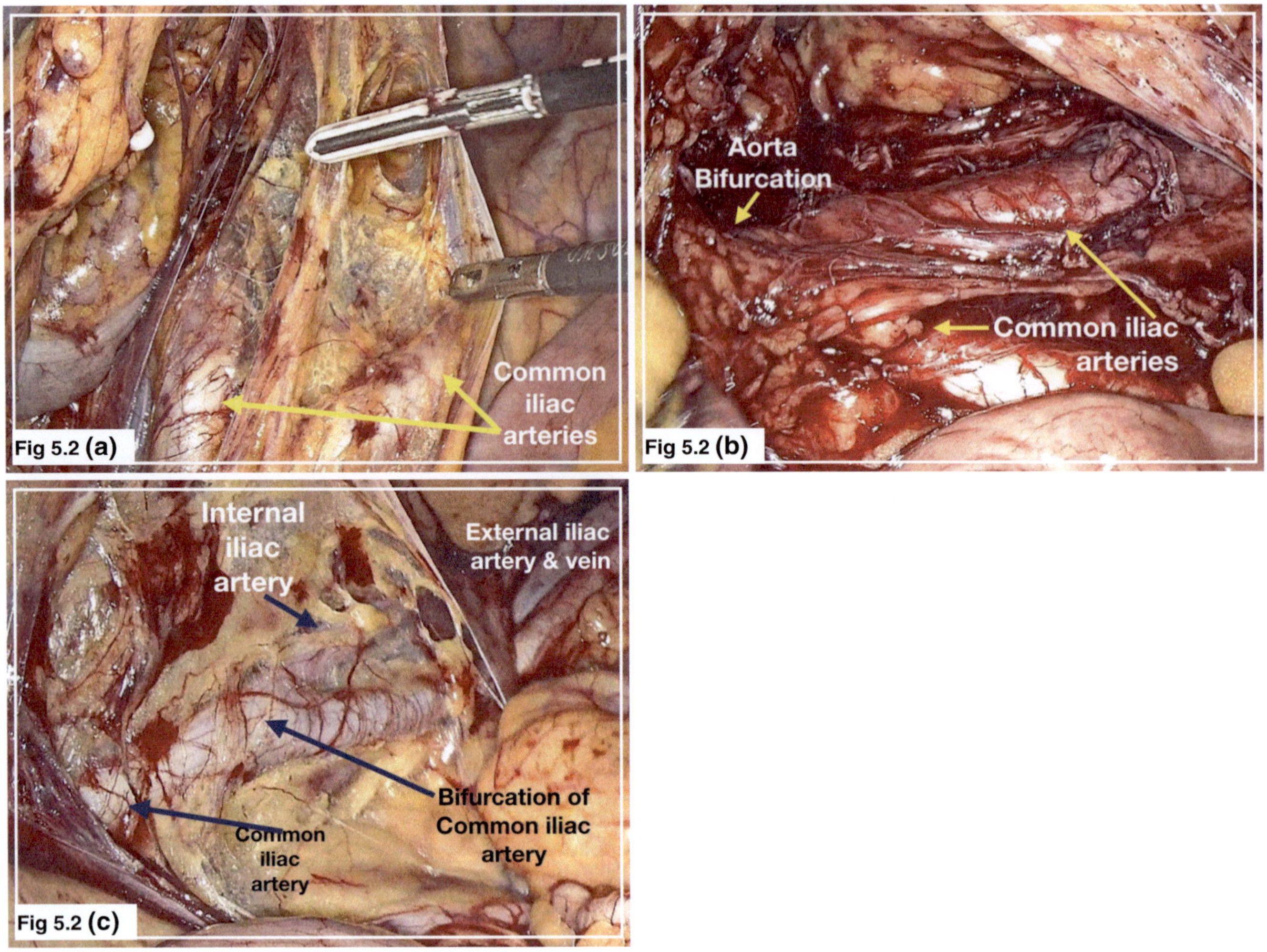

Fig. 5.2 (**a**) In a case of transperitoneal para-aortic lymph node dissection the bifurcation of the aorta is exposed and both the common iliac arteries can be clearly visualised. The discussion of the vascular anatomy of a gynaecological pelvis begins at the level of the bifurcation of the aorta and the common iliac arteries. (**b**) The bifurcation of aorta occurs at the level of L4 vertebrae where it gives rise to common iliac arteries. (**c**) The common iliac artery further bifurcates into the external and internal iliac artery at the level of sacral promontory. The sacral promontory is the summit of the pelvis. Hence all discussion of the vascular anatomy of the pelvis begins at this level or a level above at the level of bifurcation of the aorta. The inferior vena cava (IVC) labelled in the image lies below and towards the right of the aorta and thus is easily visible at the level of the common iliac artery

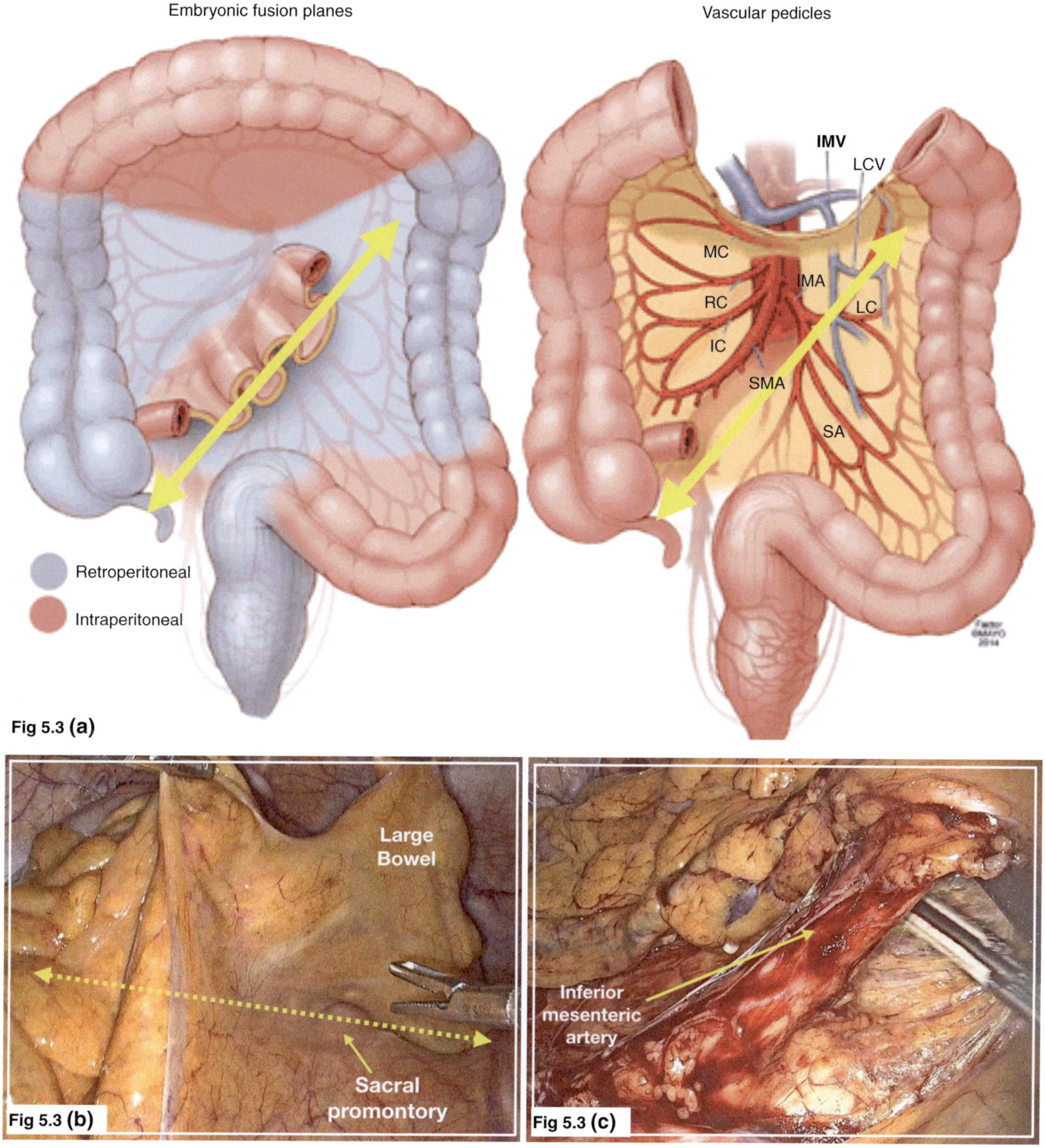

Fig. 5.3 (**a**) The line of mesentery as explained in the image is marked in yellow line. It crosses the sacral promontory on its way to the sacro-iliac joint. This becomes the line along which the small bowel can be reflected backwards to prevent it from entering the pelvis frequently. (**b**) Real-time image of the large bowel held with forceps. The sacral promontory has been identified. The small bowel has already been reflected to show the sacral promontory. Line of mesentery is an imaginary line for conceptual purposes only. (**c**) The inferior mesenteric artery is the chief vessel of the mesentery concerned with the pelvic area. It supplies the sigmoid and rectum. The origin of the inferior mesentery artery lies above the bifurcation of aorta at L3. It is often encountered during posterior exenteration surgery

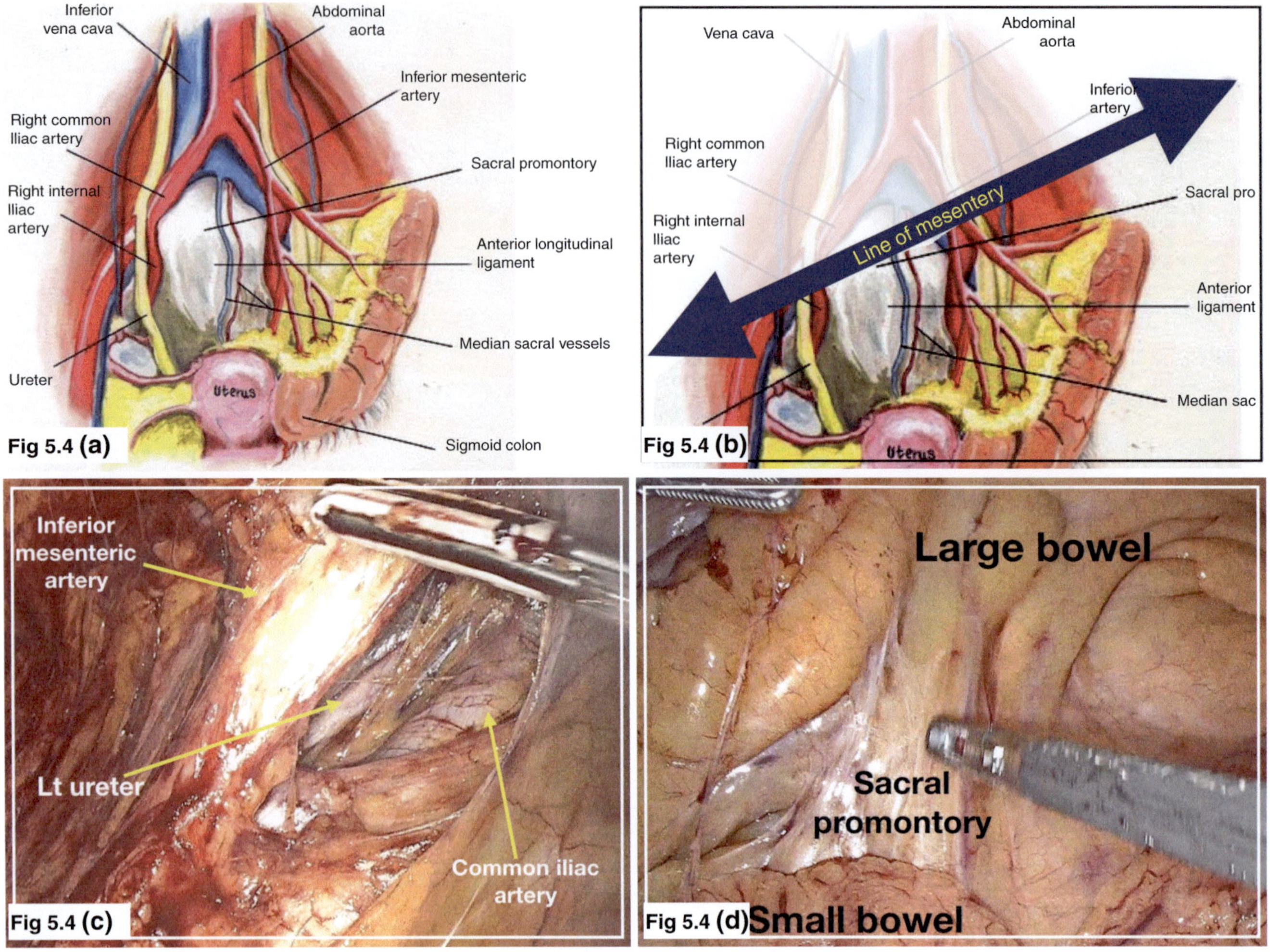

Fig. 5.4 (**a**) Schematic diagram showing the pelvic organs and their blood supply being separated from the abdominal organs and their mesentery by an imaginary line. Pelvic organs receive their blood supply at level below the line of mesentery while abdominal organs receive above the line of mesentery. (**b**) An imaginary line of mesentery has been shown in dark blue line. The bowels may remain below the line of mesentery but their blood supply (inferior mesenteric artery) can be traced above the line of mesentery. Thus abdominal organs can be separated from the pelvic runs based on other blood supply. The abdominal organs and their blood supply lying above the line of mesentery have been shaded lighter to highlight the focus of discussion, the pelvic organs and their blood supply lying below the line of mesentery. (**c**) Real-time image taken from a case of posterior exenteration where the inferior mesenteric artery has been dissected. The common iliac artery is the chief vessel of pelvic organs and has been shown separately and below the origin of the inferior mesenteric artery. The left ureter can also be seen lateral to the common iliac artery. The ureter will cross over to the medial side of the vessel at the level of bifurcation of common iliac at the level of sacral promontory. (**d**) The large bowel can be seen separated from the small bowel based on the line of mesentery. The sacral promontory is in the centre and pointed out by the forceps

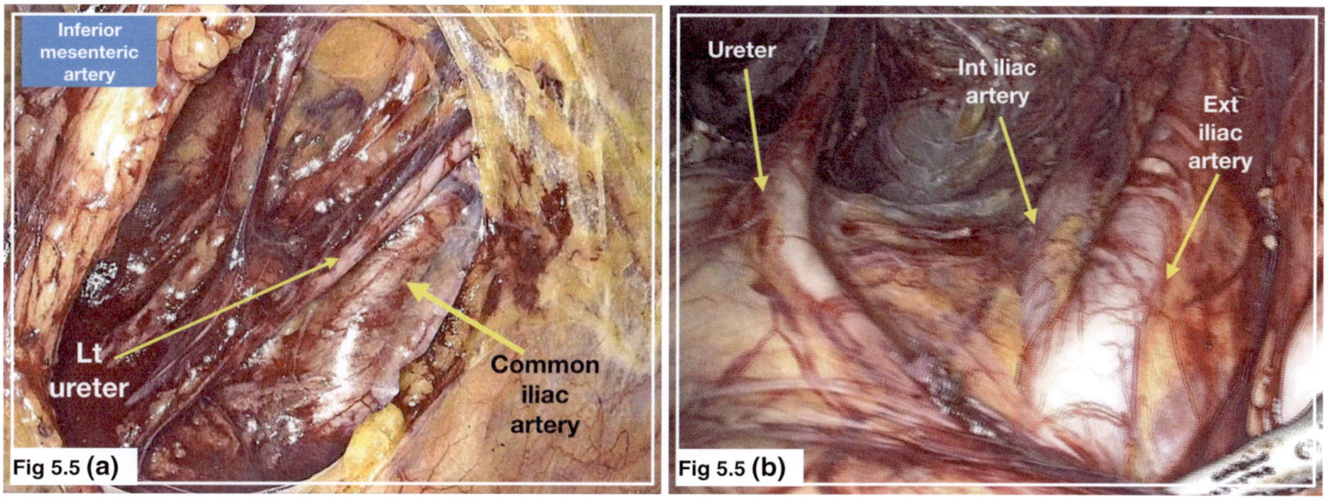

Fig. 5.5 (**a**) There are no major vessels of the pelvis arising from the anterior surface of the aorta. The inferior mesenteric artery supplies the large bowel arising at L3 vertebrae, and the aorta bifurcates into the common iliac arteries at L4 vertebrae. The common iliac arteries lie in the lateral sides. The aorta bifurcates onto its sides instead of anterior-posterior. This also reinstates the rule of laterality of blood supply in the pelvis. The ureter is seen crossing over on to the medial side. (**b**) The common iliac artery divides into the external and internal iliac artery. The internal iliac artery lies medial to the external iliac artery. The external artery also does not have any branches arising from its anterior surface making the lymph node dissection much easier

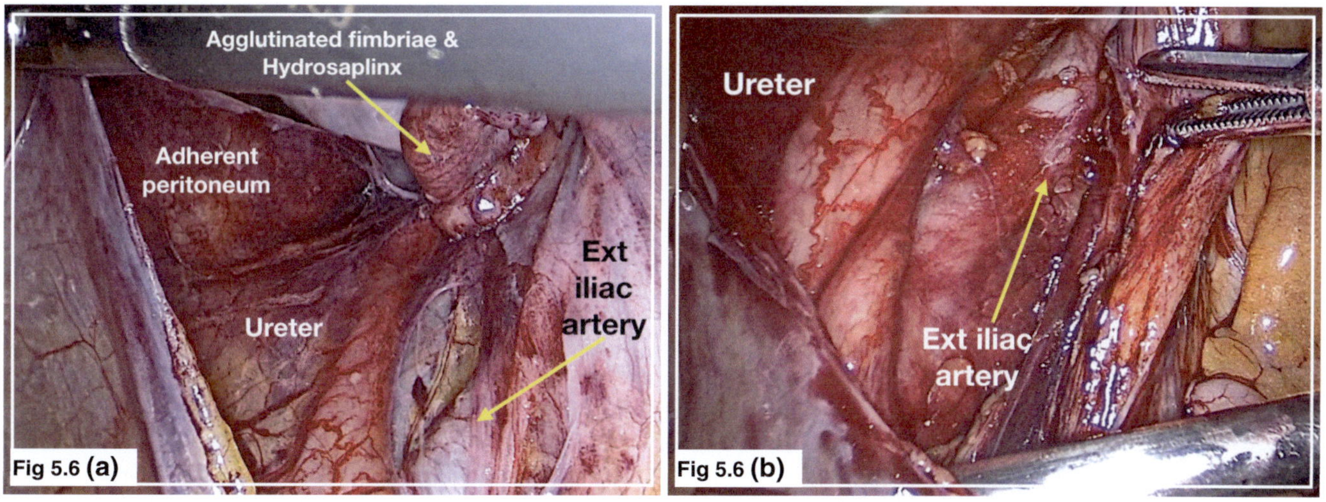

Fig. 5.6 (**a**) Inflammation in the loose areolar tissue causes more haemorrhage. The ureter can be seen crossing over the external iliac artery underneath in inflammatory conditions. This image has been taken from a case of pelvic inflammatory disease (PID) for total laparoscopic hysterectomy. The agglutinated fimbriae end and the hydrosalpinx can be seen. The peritoneum appears adherent and haemorrhagic. (**b**) Closer image of the ureter crossing over the iliac vessels. The adhesive peritoneum makes it difficult to identify structures and thus difficult to dissect as it also leads to significant haemorrhage obscuring the operative field

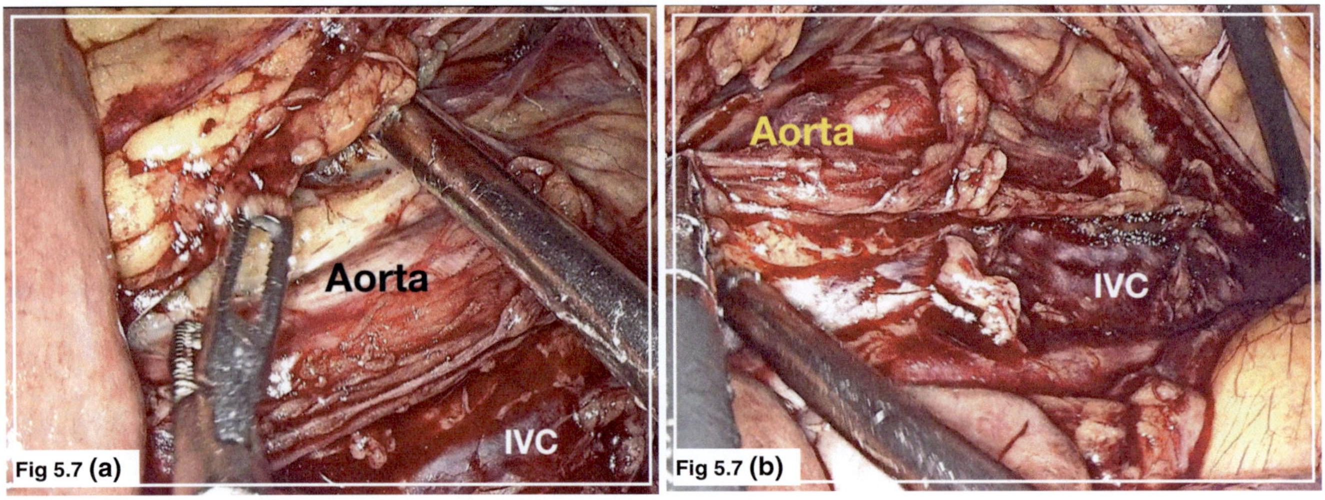

Fig. 5.7 (**a**) Image from para-aortic lymph node dissection showing no branches of the aorta anteriorly making it easy to dissect planes for lymph nodes. The inferior vena cava can be seen underneath the aorta. (**b**) The inferior vena cava is given better exposure. No branches drain anteriorly into the inferior vena cava as discussed in text

5.1 Aorta/Vena Cava

The bifurcation of aorta is always at the level above the sacral promontory and it can be considered as the upper boundary of the pelvis (Fig. 5.8a–c).

The only structure of importance is the hypogastric plexus which is formed at this level. This will be described in details later. The aorta divides into the common iliac vessels on either side. The inferior vena cava divides caudal to the bifurcation of aorta (Fig. 5.9a–e).

The veins are in close proximity to the arteries. The lymphatic clearance anterior to the arteries can be easily achieved without the fear of damaging the veins (Fig. 5.10a–c).

The common iliac and the external artery and vein have no branches or tributaries arising from the anterior or lateral surface (Fig. 5.11a–c).

This is important to understand as this is the reason why the lymph node dissection can be performed by sweeping on the anterior aspect remaining parallel to these vessels (Fig. 5.12a–c).

Any branch would have prevented this from happening. These fibrofatty tissues are outside the fascial covering of the vessels. Hence the fibrofatty tissues with lymph nodes can be easily removed en bloc. Knowledge of this plane is important for the lymph nodal dissection (Fig. 5.13a–e).

There are small vasa vasorum on the external iliac vessels. They lie below the fascial covering and if one remains in the correct plane these do not get damaged (Fig. 5.14a–e).

The ureter crosses the common iliac artery from the lateral to the medial side at this level. The ureter thus continues to remain medial to the internal iliac artery in the pelvis (Fig. 5.15a–e).

This should take out the misconception that the ureter has segmental supply. There is a direct branch of internal iliac supplying the ureter which can be preserved in radical hysterectomy. The ureter can be completely separated from the major vascular structures caudal to this artery, thus enabling major cancer surgery to be performed (Fig. 5.16a–c).

The common iliac artery then divides into the external and internal iliac arteries (Fig. 5.17a–d).

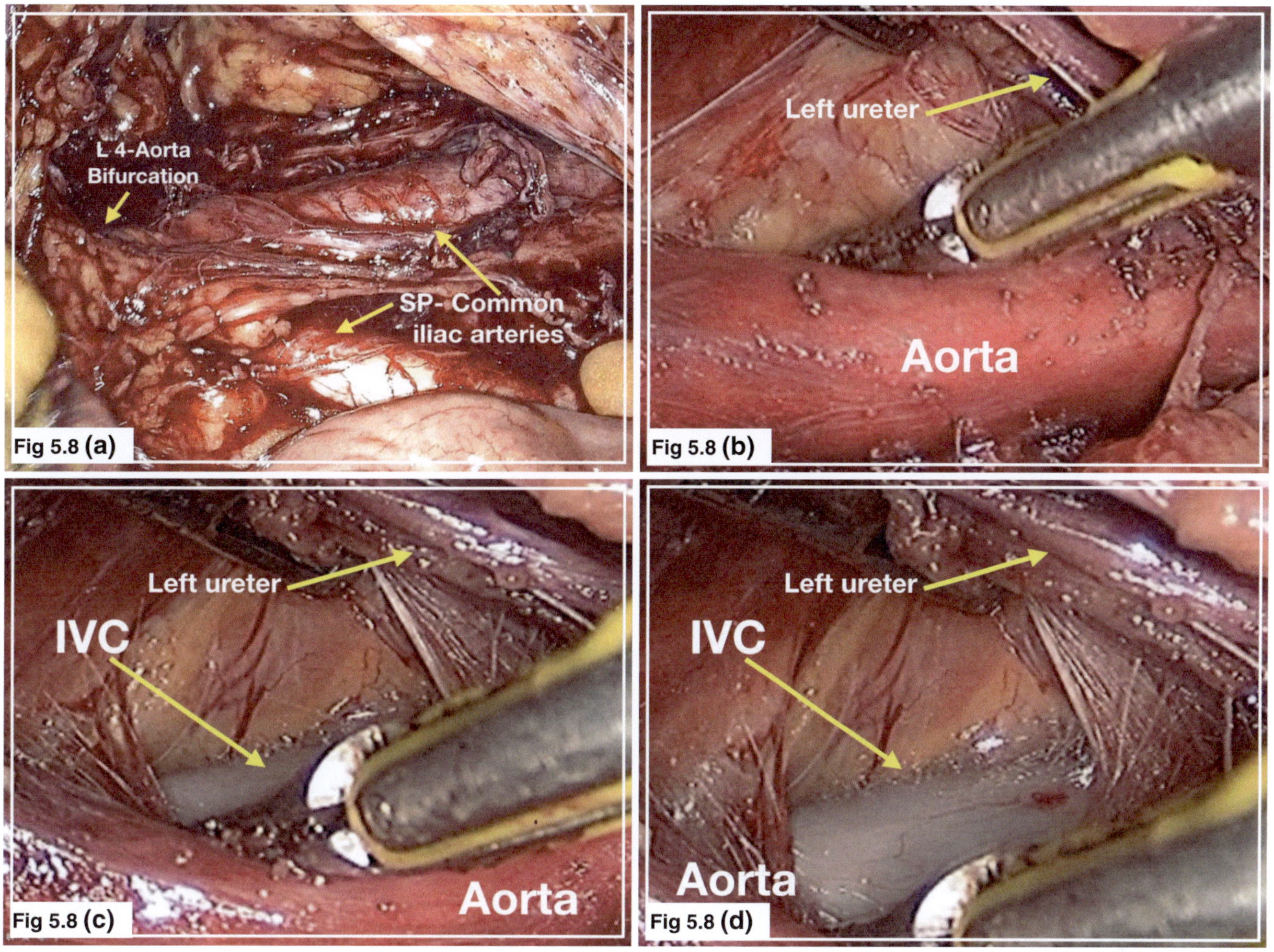

Fig. 5.8 (**a**) As discussed previously the image shows the aorta bifurcation at L3 and common iliac arteries at sacral promontory (SP) from a case of transperitoneal para-aortic lymph node dissection. (**b**–**d**) These series of images are taken from a case of extraperitoneal para-aortic lymph node dissection. All vascular structures here appear horizontal and parallel to each other in different planes. The aorta can be seen as a singular unbranched vascular structure. The IVC can be seen by retracting the aorta down slightly. Both aorta and IVC are unbranched structures seen; hence their dissection is easier than most other vessels

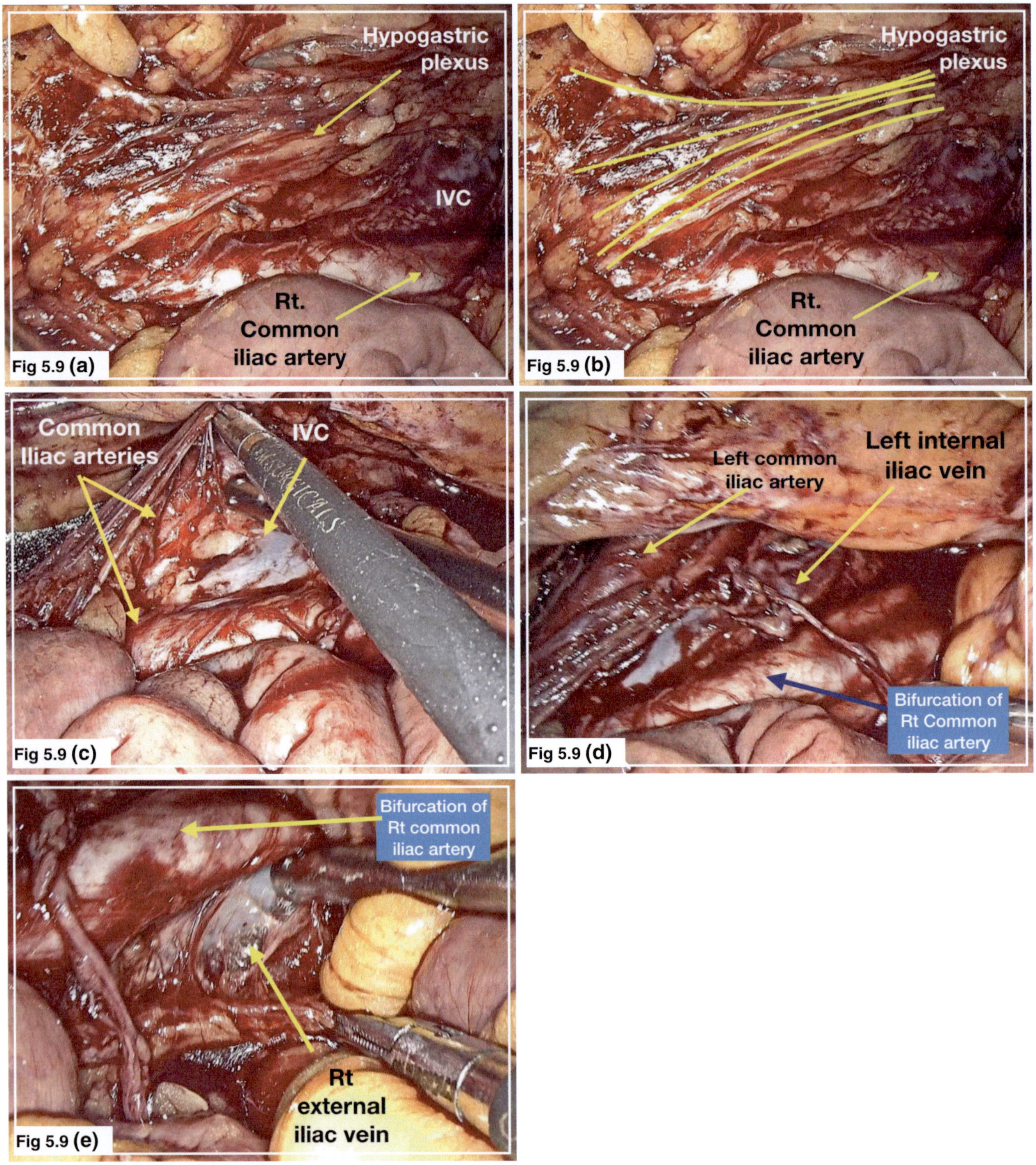

Fig. 5.9 (**a**) The superior hypogastric plexus can be seen as a layer of nerve fibres covering the aorta. They lie on the lateral side of the aorta and are commonly encountered during transperitoneal [para-aortic lymph node dissection]. (**b**) The superior hypogastric plexus nerve fibres have been highlighted in this image for a better understanding of the viewers. (**c**) The inferior vena cava (IVC) lies lower and to the right of the aorta. Hence the communication of the common iliac veins or the bifurcation of the IVC lies below the bifurcation of the aorta. They can be seen by dissecting gently between the common iliac vessels. (**d**) The Inferior venae cava and common iliac veins remian inferior and to the right of the aorta and the common iliac arteries respectively. The left internal iliac even lies closer yet lower to the right internal iliac artery as seen in the image. The internal iliac vein shortly dips steeply into the pelvic cavity and remains under the Waldeyer's fascia. (**e**) The right external iliac vein can be seen by retracting the external iliac artery medially. It originates lateral to the external iliac artery but soon travels parallel and exactly under it

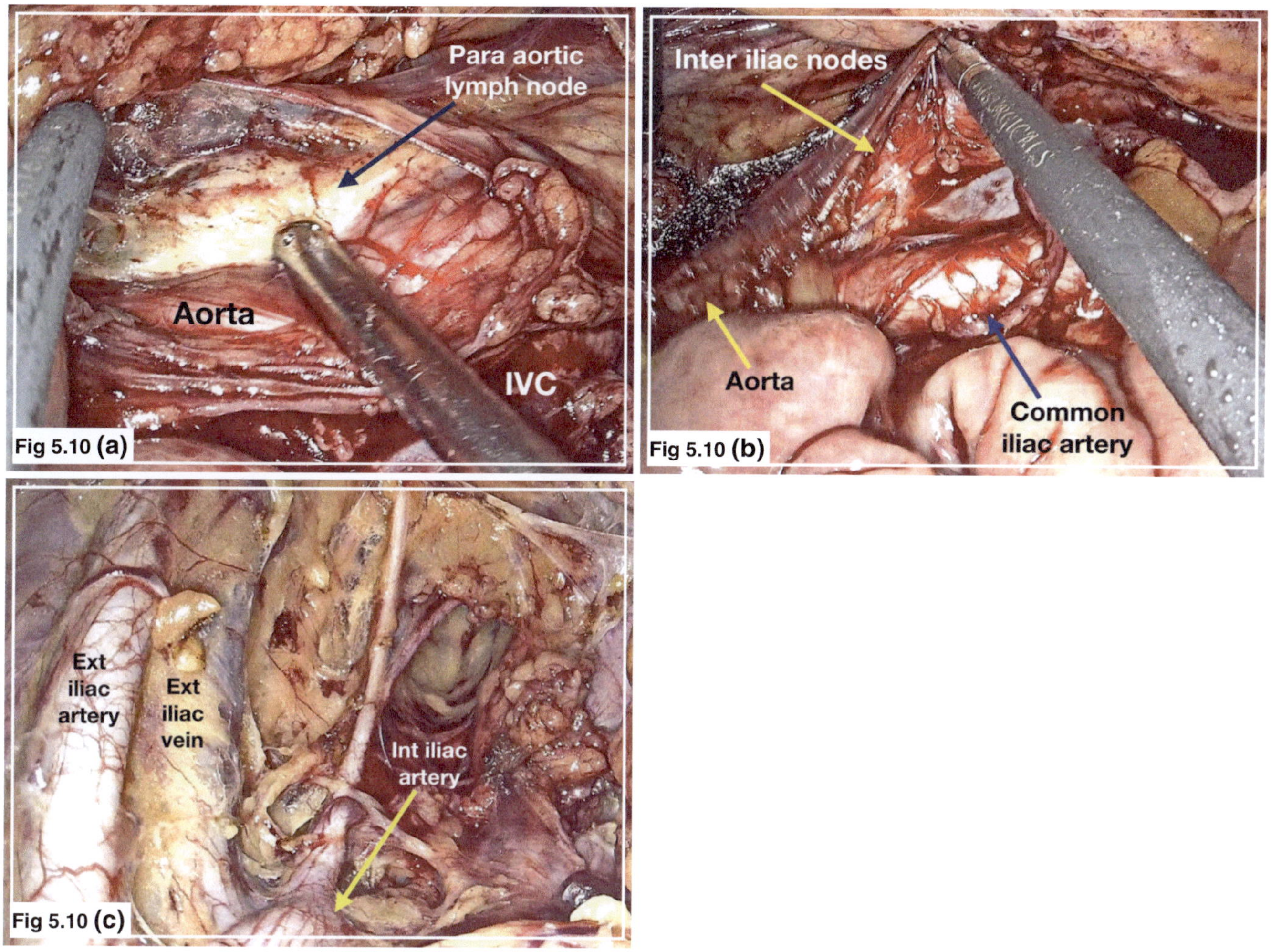

Fig. 5.10 (**a**) The aorta lies anterior to the IVC and the para-aortic lymph nodes lie anterior to the aorta. Even though lymphatics follow the veins by principle, they are located close to the arteries. Thus dissection of lymph nodes rarely injures the veins. (**b**) Similarly here the inter iliac nodes are dissected from the bifurcation of aorta and the IVC lies underneath the junction. The IVC remains more guarded here during lymph node dissection. (**c**) The external iliac vein lies inferior and medial to the eternal iliac artery. The lymph node dissection of the ilio-obturator nodes begins at the level of the external iliac artery and the psoas muscle. Similarly here too the external iliac vein lies deeply seated by the external iliac artery

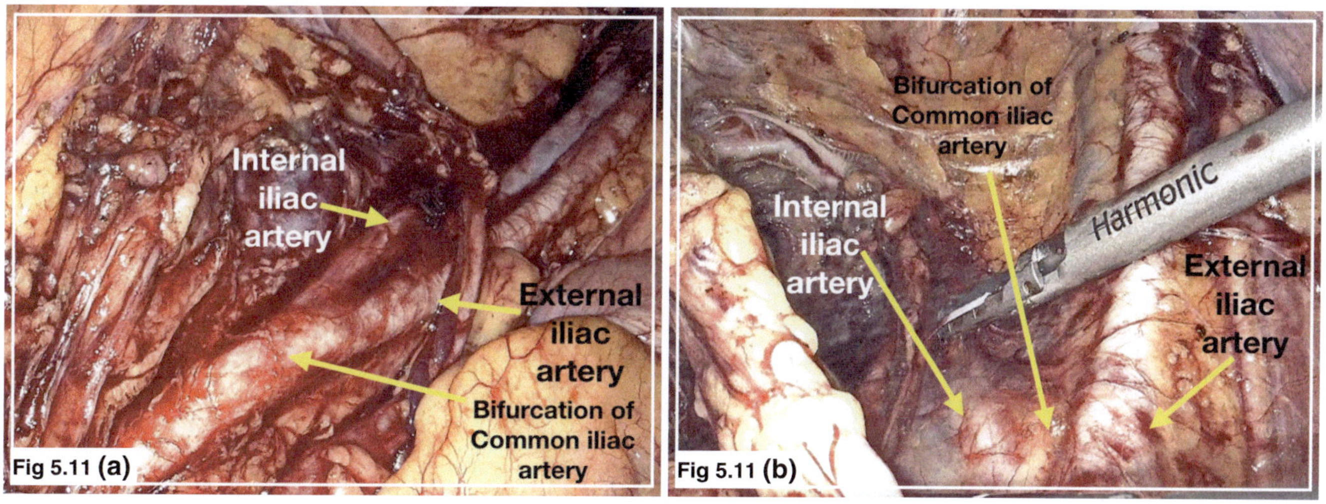

Fig. 5.11 (**a–c**) Show the bifurcation of the common iliac artery into the external and internal iliac artery. Neither common iliac artery nor the external iliac artery has anterior and lateral branches

Fig. 5.11 (continued)

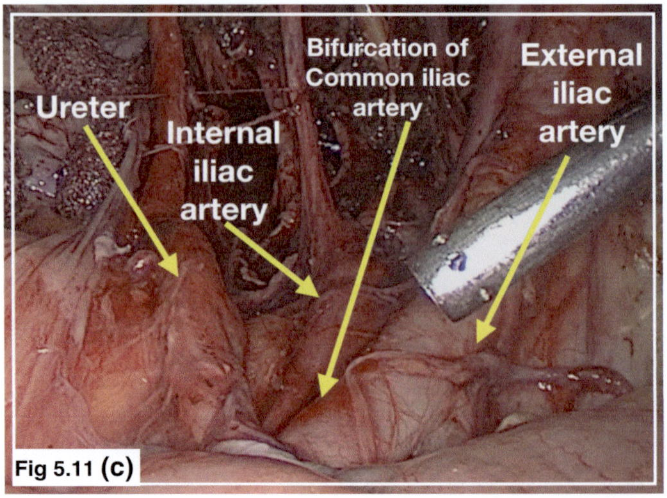

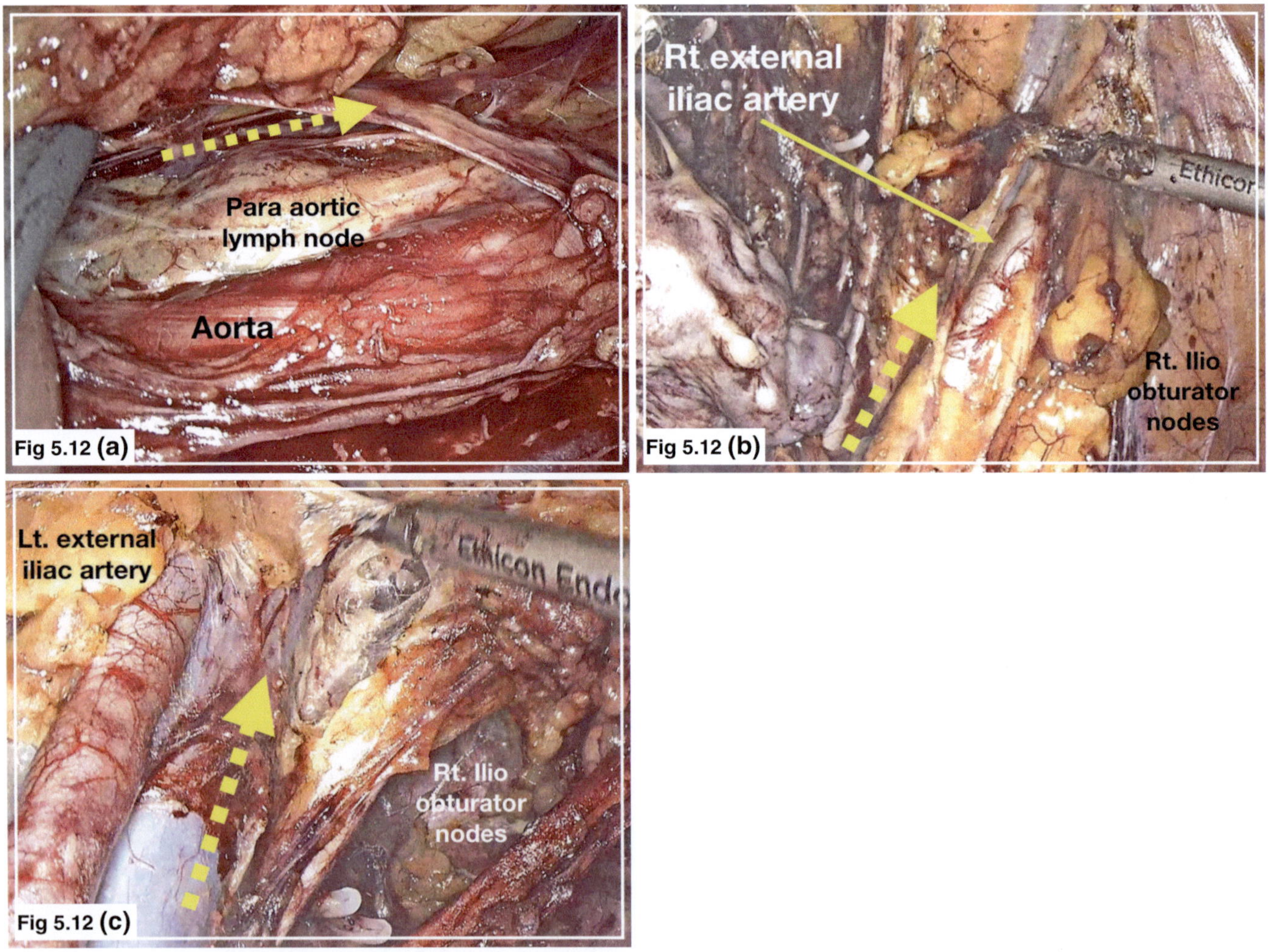

Fig. 5.12 (**a**) In this image the yellow dotted line denotes the direction of dissection during lymph node dissection. The para-aortic lymph nodes are dissected from the anterolateral aspect of the aorta in a cranial to caudal direction. (**b**) The right external iliac artery lies in close approximation to the right ilio-obturator lymph nodes. Here too the lymph nodes are dissected anteriorly and in a cranial to caudal direction. (**c**) Similar dissection of ilio-obturator lymph nodes is done on the left side as well

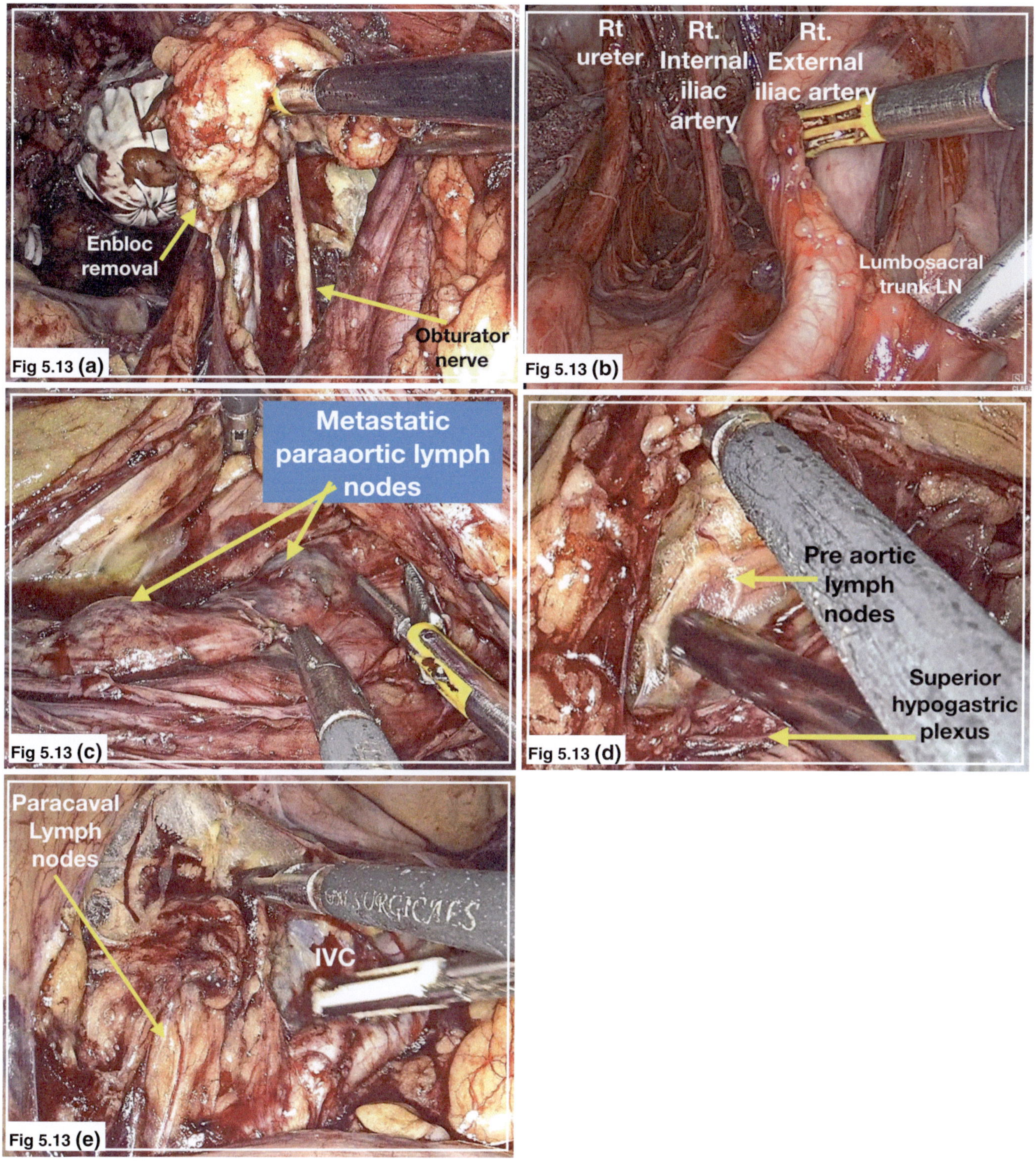

Fig. 5.13 (**a**–**e**) Various different types of lymph node dissection have been demonstrated explaining the lack of intervening fascia which aids in smoother and bloodless dissection

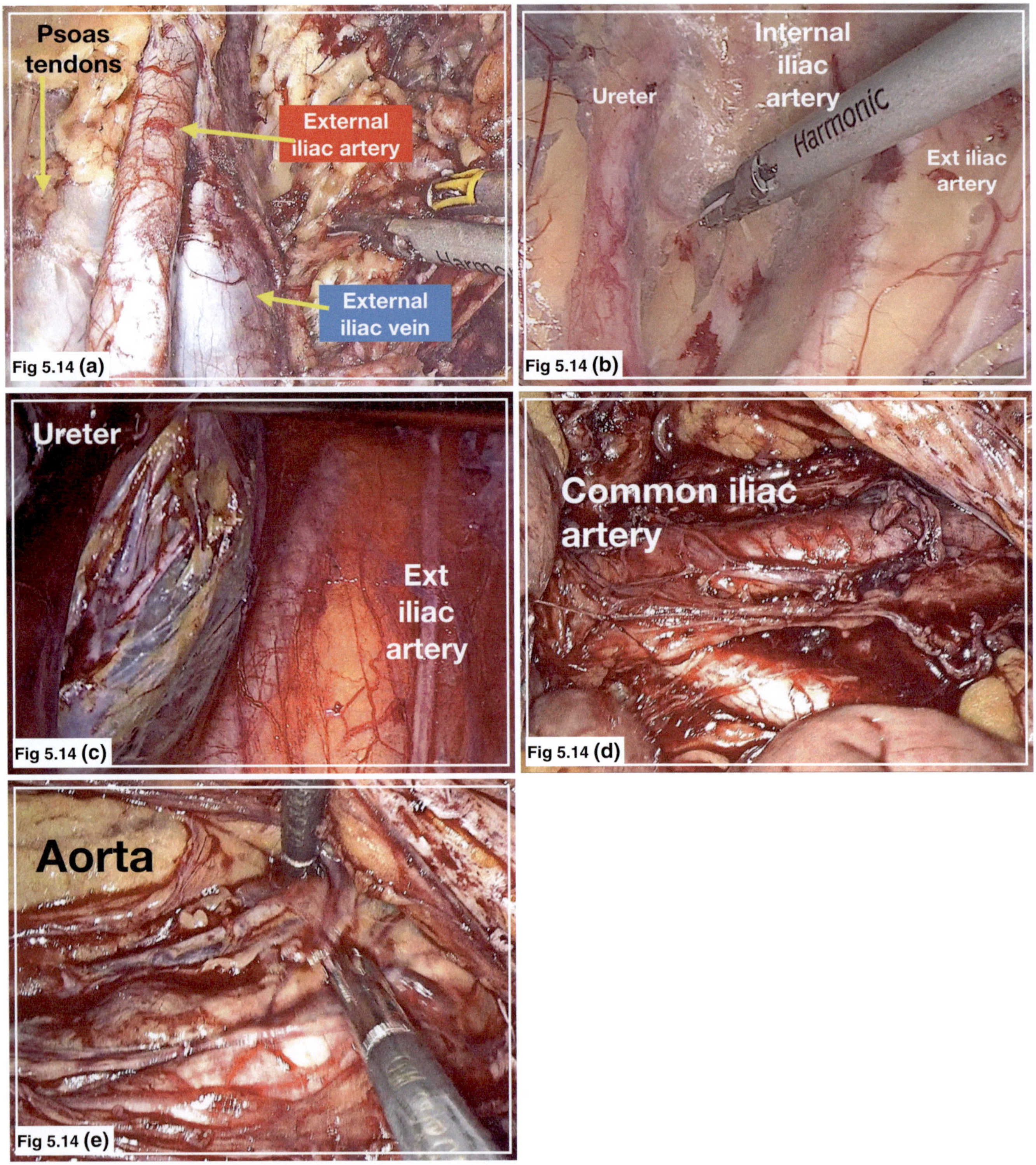

Fig. 5.14 (**a**) The image shows the left external iliac artery between the psoas muscle tendon and the external iliac vein. However a fine meshwork of capillary-sized vessels feeds the vessels itself called vasa vasorum and is seen across the entire length of the artery. It is not seen on tendons and seldom seen on veins. (**b**) In this image we can see the right external iliac artery with its vasa vasorum on the right side of the image and the ureter appears on the medial side. The internal iliac artery lies between the ureter and the external iliac artery. The patchy areas of haemorrhage are due to injury to the vasa vasorum of the internal iliac artery, injured during dissection. The second important finding to appreciate is a similar network of vessels seen on the ureter. It must be noted that the ureter has its own mesentery, the vessels are thicker than vasa vasorum, they are more tortuous and they are surrounded by their own layer of fat which is not seen on the vasa vasorum. (**c**) In case of inflammation of the loose areolar tissue the peritoneum is adherent to the vessels. Here in a case of laparoscopic radical hysterectomy the dissection of the pararectal space leads to injury of the capillaries over and then external iliac artery leading to haemorrhage as shown in the image. (**d**) Vasa vasorum can be appreciated over the bifurcation of the aorta and the common iliac arteries. (**e**) The vasa vasorum appreciated over the aorta as well

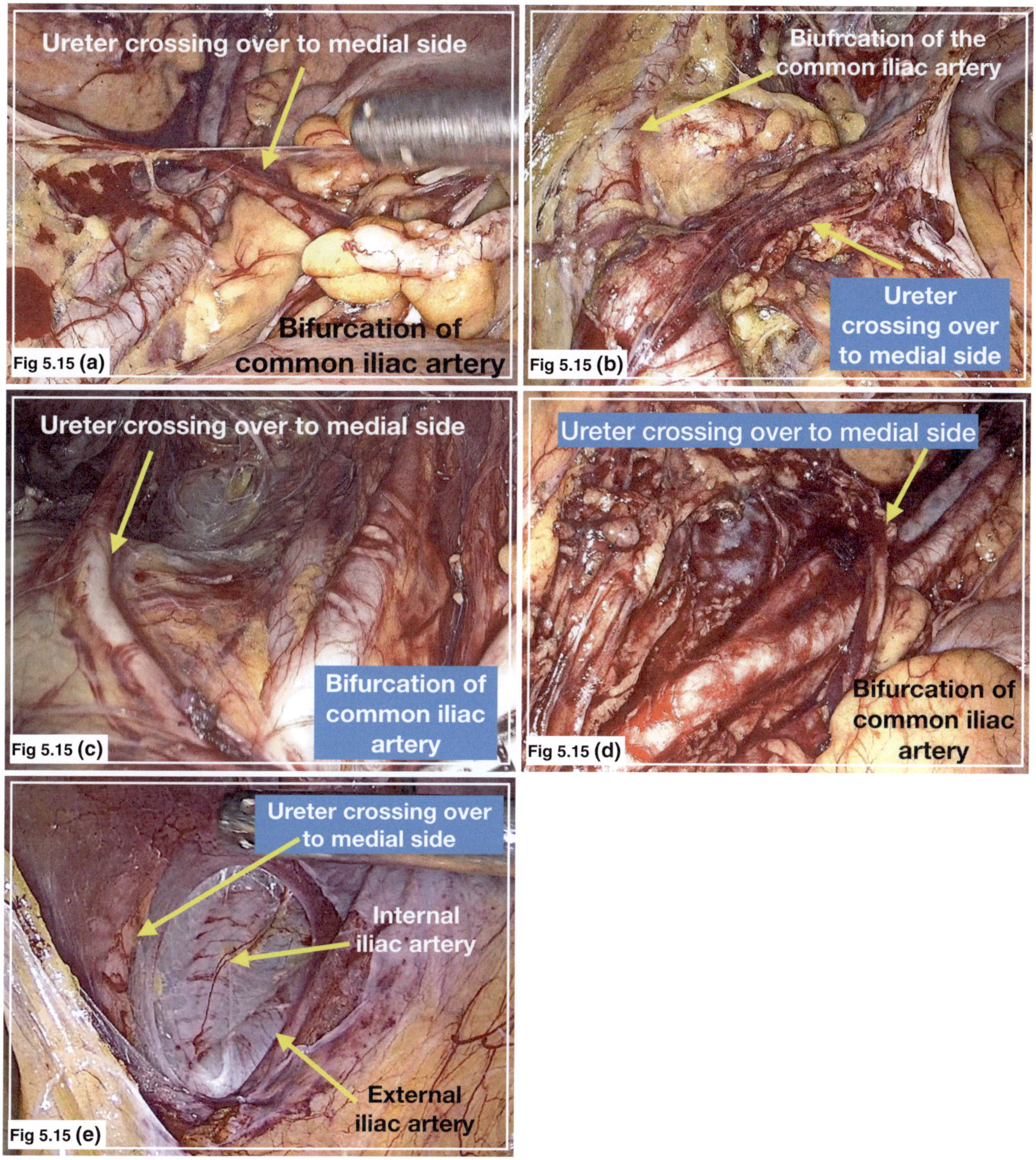

Fig. 5.15 (a–e) Series of images showing that the ureter crosses over the iliac vessels near the bifurcation of the common iliac artery. The ureter has been retracted medially and laterally to expose the exact bifurcation but left to its natural state prior to dissection the ureter crosses over exactly above the bifurcation of the common iliac artery

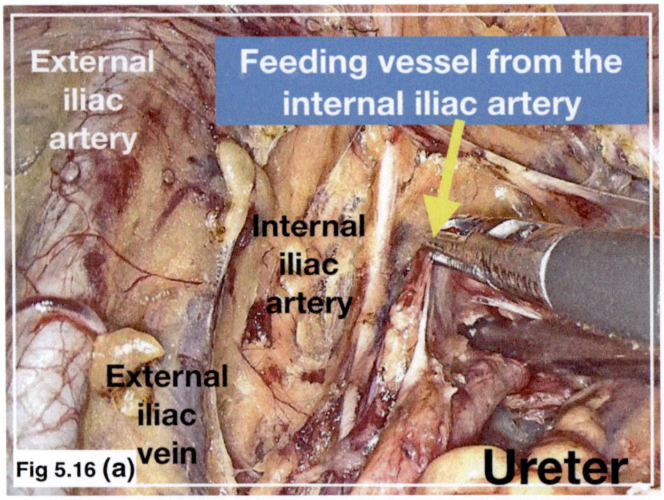

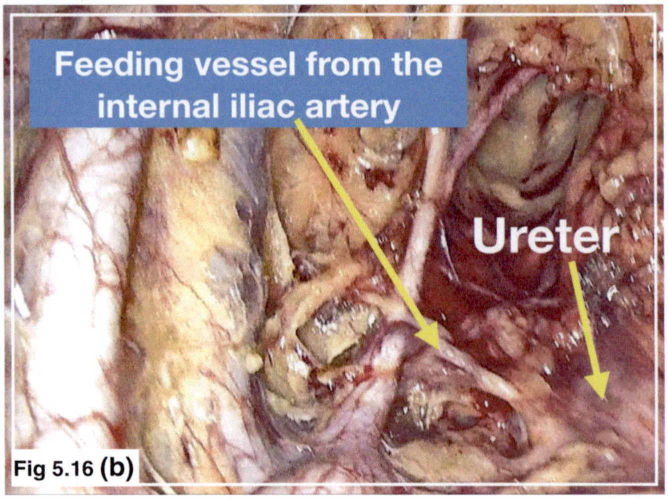

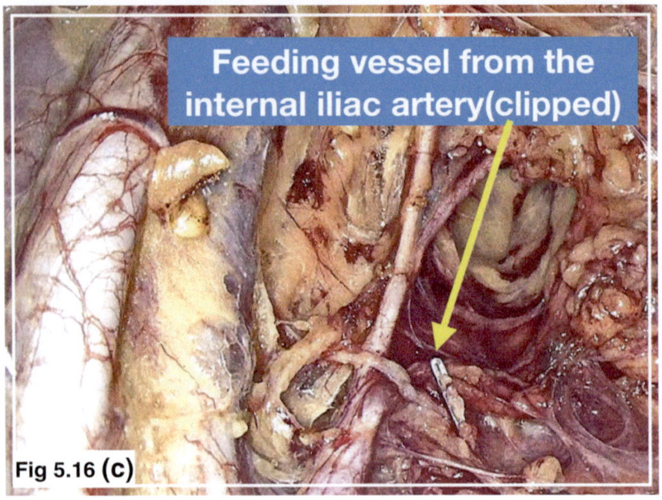

Fig. 5.16 (**a**) The feeding vessel directly from the internal iliac artery can be seen held by the forceps. The fibrofatty tissue around it is dissected and the vessel itself is clipped and cut. These series of images have been taken from a case of uterine transpose where each such vessel is important to identify as later they cause reperfusion bleeding as leaking vessels. (**b**) The vessel has been dissected from its fibrofatty tissue covering exposing its entire course and inserted into the ureter. (**c**) The feeding vessel has been clipped and dissected off from the ureter

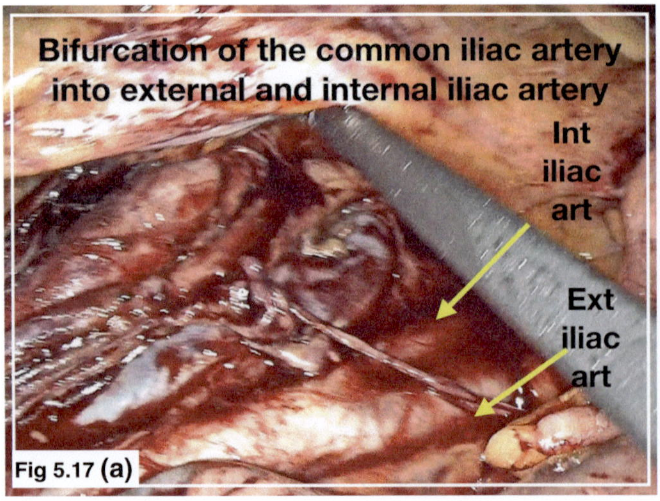

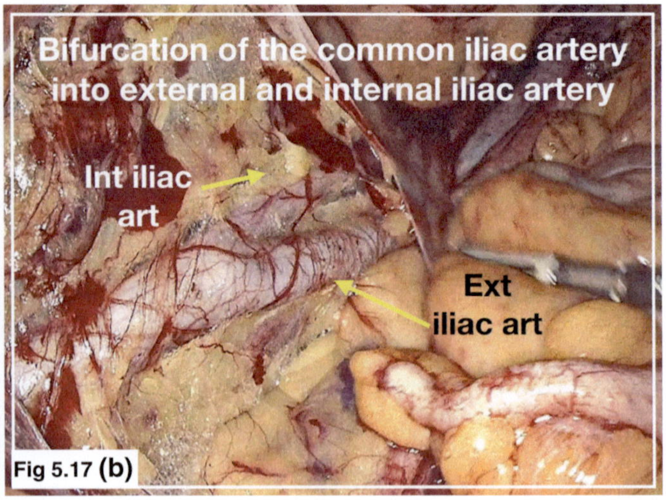

Fig. 5.17 (**a–d**) The series of images show the common iliac artery bifurcating into the internal and external iliac artery. The internal iliac artery lies medially and the external iliac artery laterally

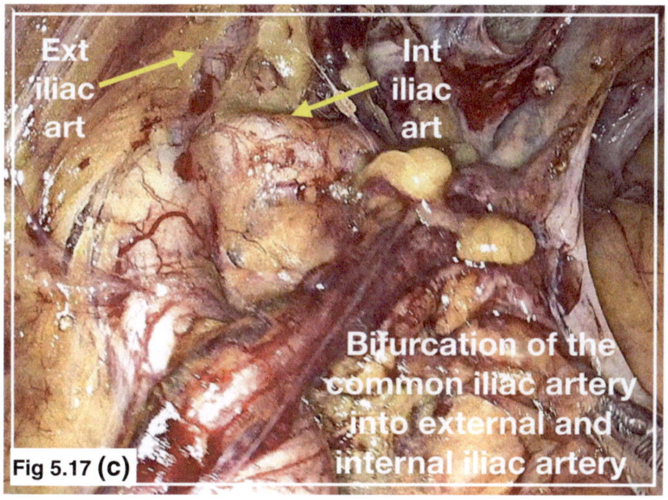

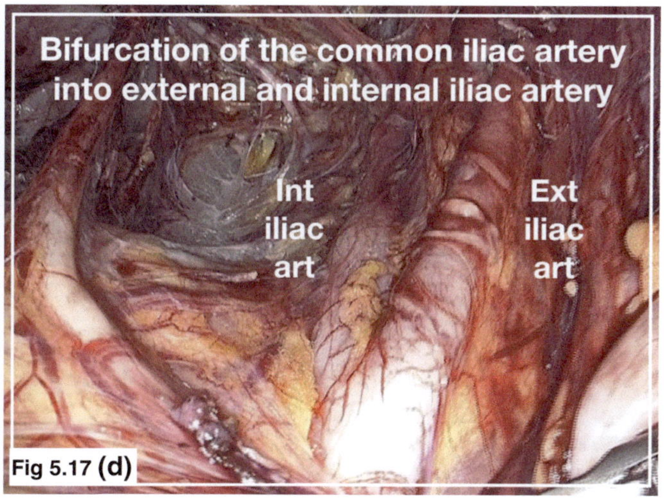

Fig. 5.17 (continued)

5.2 External Iliac Artery and Vein

The external iliac artery travels along the ilio-psoas muscle on its way to the lower limbs. The external iliac vein lies posteromedial to the artery (Fig. 5.18a–d).

Both the external iliac artery and vein are devoid of any branches till they reach the inguinal ligament. At this level the inferior epigastric artery arises from the anteromedial aspect of the external iliac artery (Fig. 5.19a–f).

This artery then ascends on the posterior aspect of the transversalis fascia extraperitoneally and goes cranially to supply the lower abdominal muscles (Fig. 5.20a–e).

The position of the inferior epigastric artery is important to prevent damage during secondary port insertion. The origin of inferior epigastric artery is the distal limit of ilio-obturator nodal dissection (Figs. 5.21 and 5.22).

There are three tributaries of the external iliac vein, namely, inferior epigastric vein, deep circumflex iliac vein and the femoral vein (Fig. 5.23).

The deep circumflex iliac vein remains closely applied to the pubic bone and is the caudal limit of lymph node dissection. This vein joins the obturator vein. This area is called as the corona mortis (Fig. 5.24).

Medial to the external iliac vein is the femoral canal which harbours the sentinel node of Cabana (Fig. 5.25a–e).

5.2.1 Important Aspects of Inferior Epigastric Artery and Vein

The inferior epigastric vein also drains into the external iliac vein on the anteromedial aspect. Both the vein and artery are closely approximated and are on the medial side of internal inguinal ring. *The inferior epigastric artery is close to the position of inferior ports and has to be visualised before the port insertion as it is likely to be damaged.* These vessels are the dividing line of direct and indirect inguinal hernias (Fig. 5.26a–e).

(a) Inferior epigastric artery runs extraperitoneally after its origin (Fig. 5.26f, g).
(b) They are the only branches of external iliac artery and vein in the pelvis (Fig. 5.27a, b).
(c) They lie on the medial aspect of deep inguinal ring and form the boundaries for classifying hernias into either direct or indirect hernias (Fig. 5.28a–c).

The only tributary of external iliac vein is the deep circumflex iliac vein and it hugs the pelvic bone (Fig. 5.29a–d).

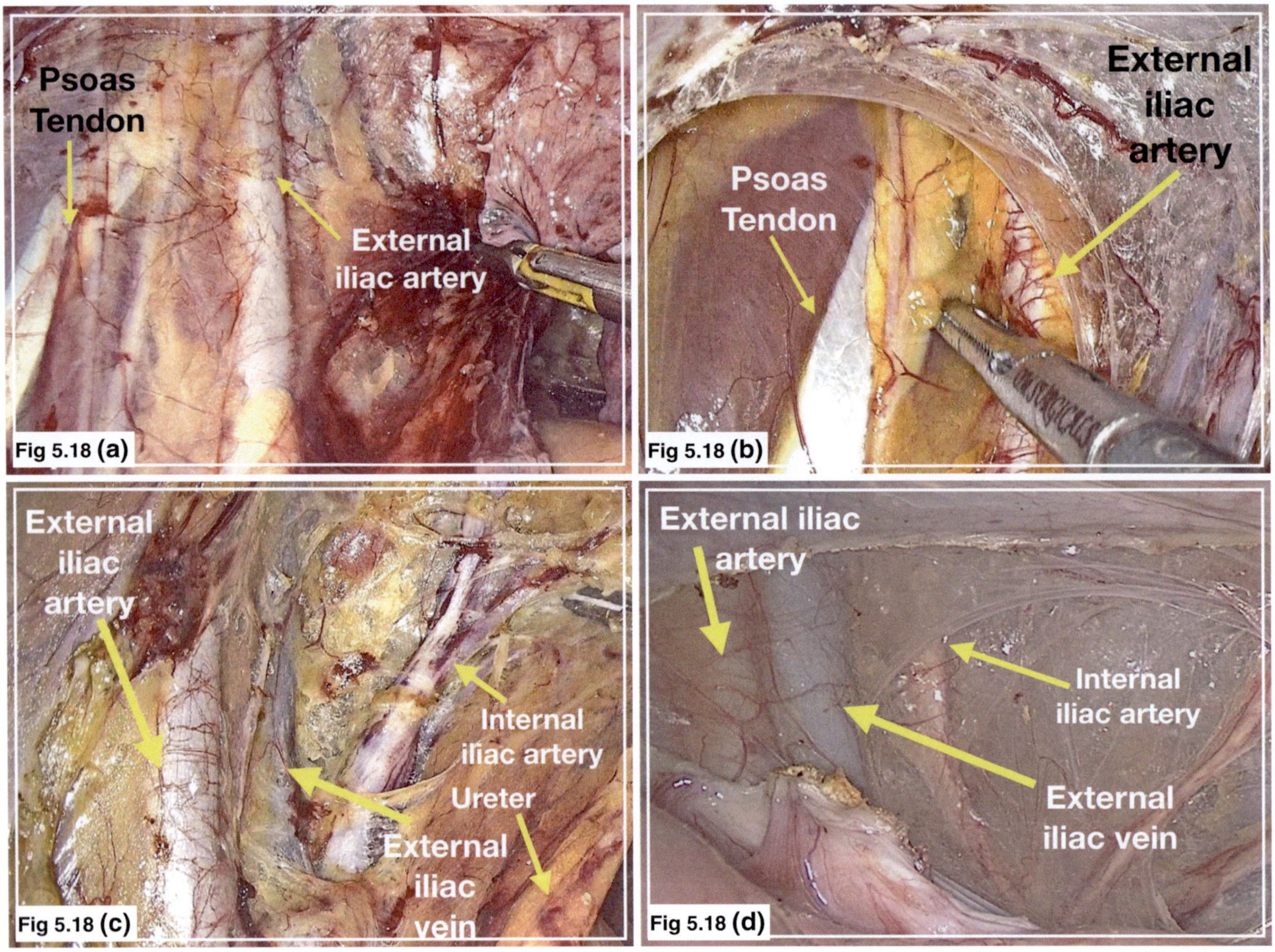

Fig. 5.18 External iliac artery. (**a**) Psoas tendon lies lateral to the external lilac artery. (**b**) Psoas tendon lies lateral to the external lilac artery. The genitofemoral nerve lies on the psoas muscle. (**c**) The external lilac artery and vein seen later in the internal iliac artery. (**d**) The sequence of vessels from lateral to medial is external iliac artery > external iliac vein > internal iliac artery

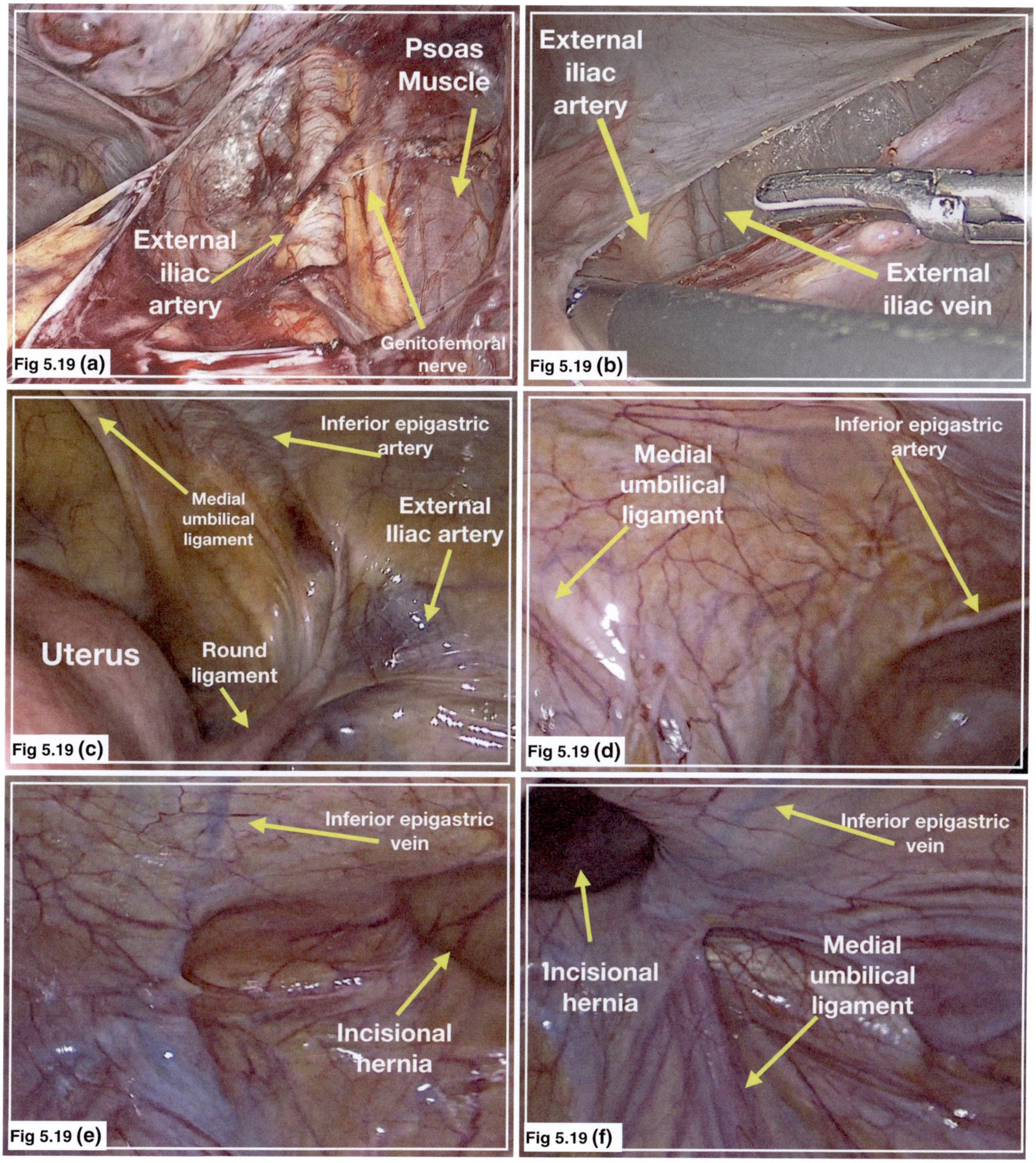

Fig. 5.19 (**a**) The external iliac rate and vein seen on the lateral pelvic wall are devoid of any branches in the initial 6 in. of the vessel length on their anterior or lateral surface. (**b**) The external lilac vessels are covered by the peritoneum and their impressions are often seen throughout it. They travel parallel and towards the anterior abdominal wall without giving out any branches along its course. (**c**) In this picture of a large-sized fibroid uterus, the impression of the external iliac vessels can be seen along with the impression of the inferior epigastric vessels travelling along the posterior surface of the anterior abdominal wall. (**d**) In this image the relation of the obliterated hypogastric artery or the medial umbilical ligament has been explained with the inferior epigastric artery. The medial umbilical ligament always remains medial to the inferior epigastric artery. The inferior epigastric artery lies near the deep inguinal ring. (**e, f**) These pair of images have been taken from a case of incisional hernia for meshplasty. The impressions of inferior digastric veins can be seen clearly on the lateral edges of the hernial site. In the images to follow, meshplasty has been demonstrated which exposes the inferior epigastric vessel more clearly

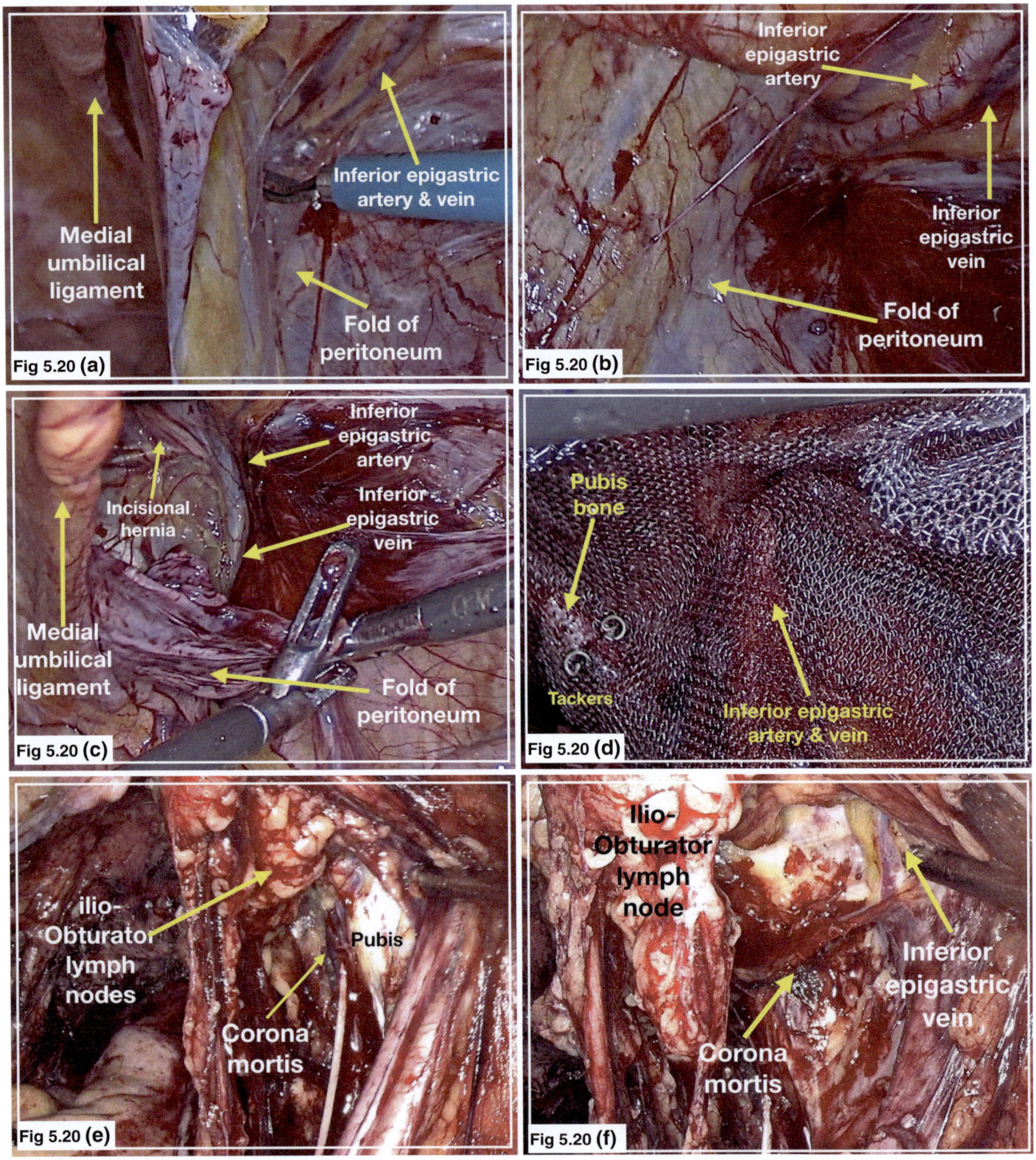

Fig. 5.20 Hernia meshplasty. (**a**) The series of images are taken from a case of incisional hernia explained in the previous message. The peritoneum covering the hernia is extricated and the inferior epigastric vessels are exposed. The medial umbilical ligament can also be seen under the peritoneum. The inferior epigastric artery is identified by the vasa vasorum seen over arteries. (**b**) A better view of the inferior epigastric artery and the vein can be seen in this image. (**c**) Final image taken after dissection of the peritoneum dissected off and before application of the mesh for meshplasty. The major vessels seen along with important landmarks like the pubis bone for application of tackers and the medial umbilical ligament. (**d**) Mesh applied for meshplasty. Tackers applied on the pubic bone. The vessel protected from any injury. (**e**) In a series of images showing the extent of ilio-obturator lymph node dissection, the image shows the corona mortis and the initial inferior epigastric vein tributary draining into the external iliac vein. (**f**) The dissection is further continued towards the posterior surface of the anterior abdominal wall. The inferior epigastric vein is exposed along with its course. (**g**) A closer view of the inferior epigastric veins can be appreciated from this image. (**h**) Final view of the inferior epigastric vein dissection can be seen from this image. The vein travels along the posterior surface of the anterior abdominal wall

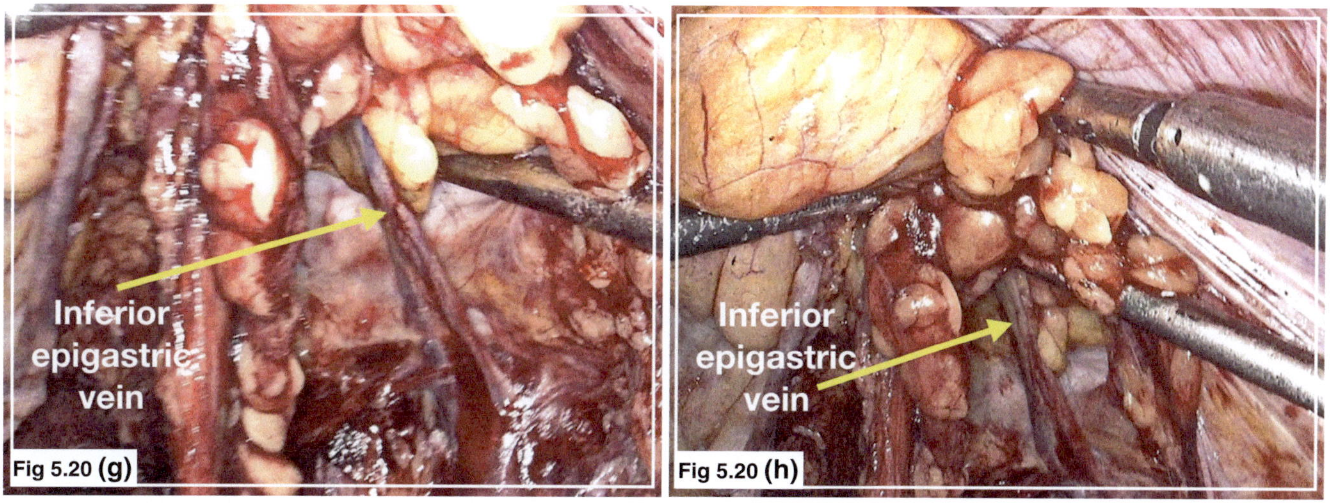

Fig. 5.20 (continued)

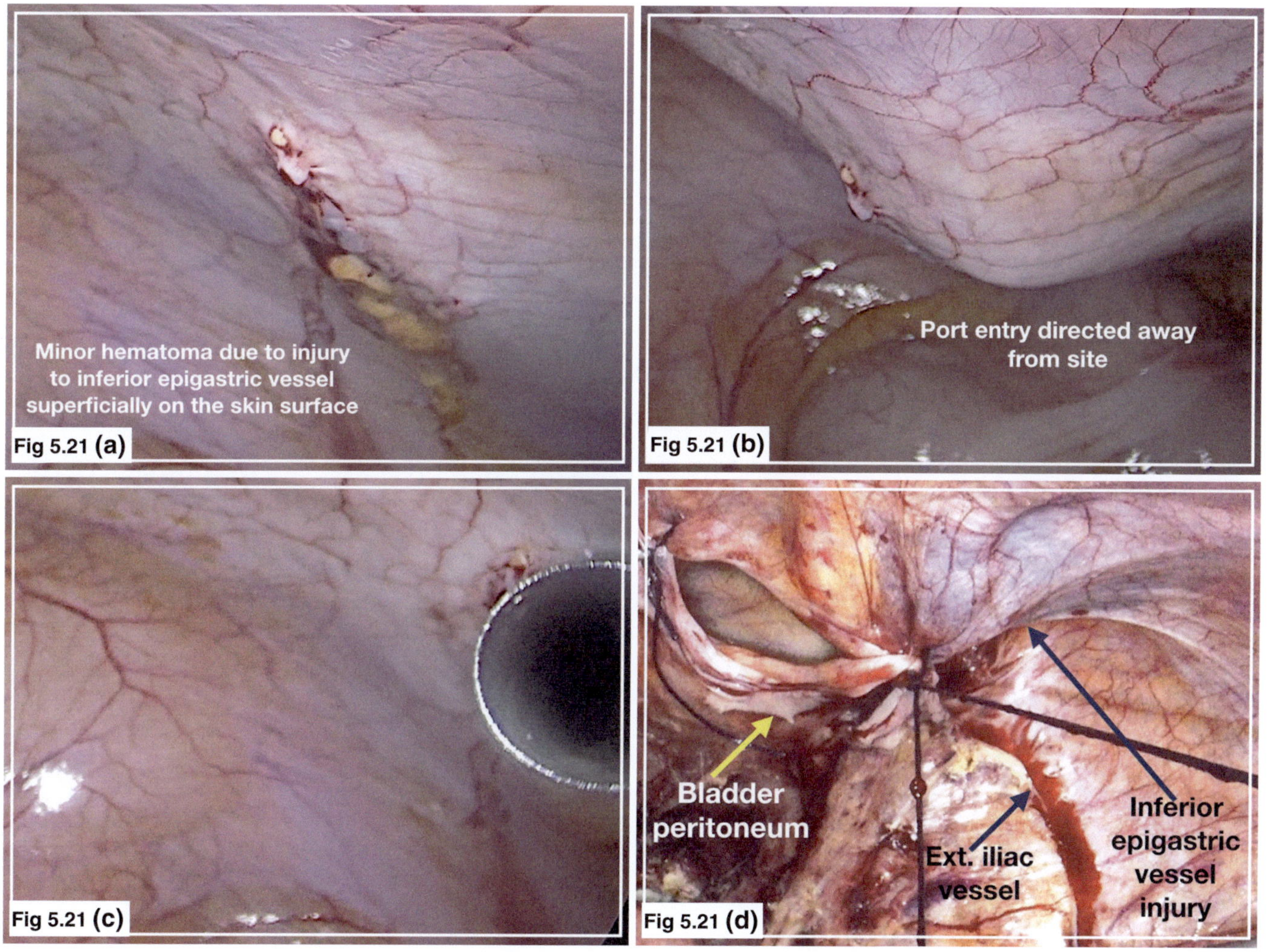

Fig. 5.21 Port insertion. (**a**) Small haematoma formed seen on the peritoneal surface due to injury to the inferior epigastric vessel on the skin surface. (**b**) Port inserted directed away from the possible site of the inferior epigastric vessels and away from its course. (**c**) Port enters the peritoneum at a site closer but away from the site of inferior epigastric artery without injuring the vessel in its course. (**d**) The image is taken from a case of dissection of donor for uterine transplant. The bladder peritoneum is etched to the anterior abdominal wall to keep it in fixed position and during the process injury to the inferior epigastric vessels leads to formation of a significant haematoma. The external iliac vessels can be traced underneath and the site of haematoma lies nearly at the plane corresponding to the origin of the inferior epigastric artery. (**e**) The most common condition of inferior epigastric injury is during secondary port insertions. These images have been taken from such a condition

Fig. 5.21 (continued)

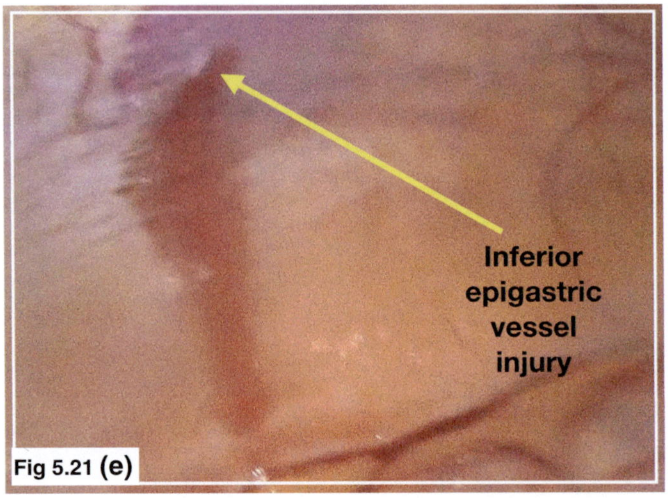

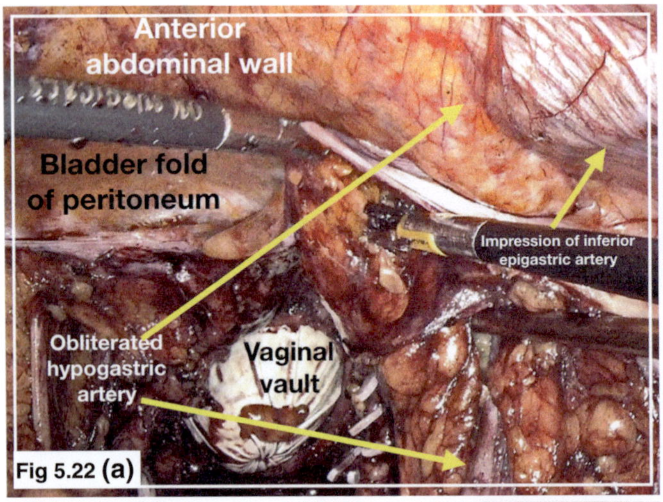

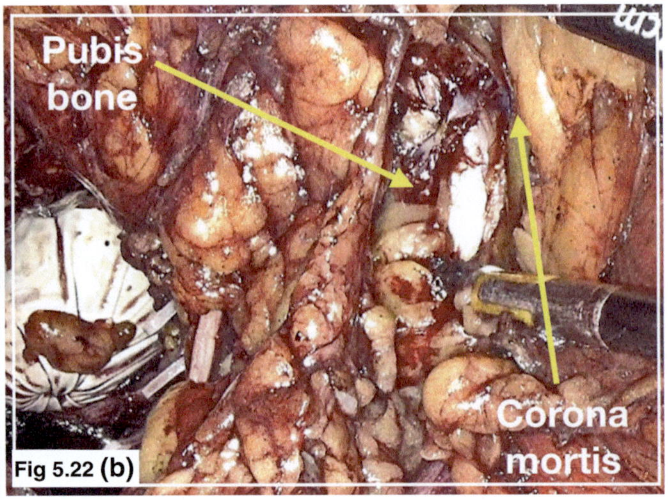

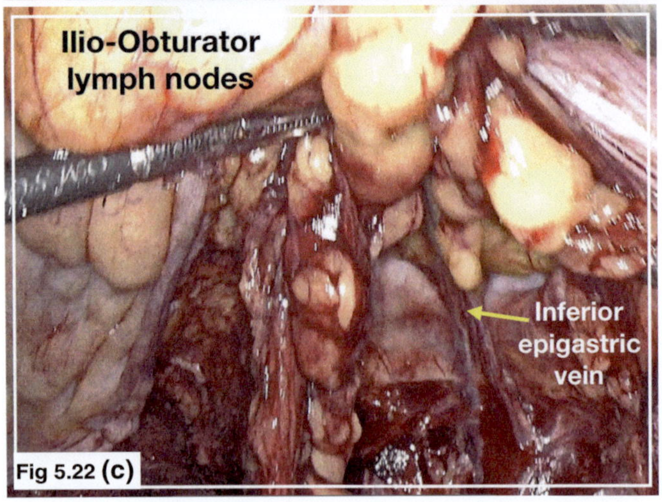

Fig. 5.22 (**a**) The limit of ilio-obturator lymph node dissection can be seen in the image. The user limit can be seen, the limit being medial to the origin of inferior epigastric artery along the obliterated hypogastric artery. (**b**) The pubis bone can be seen. The corona mortis (the deep circumflex vein) is also visible. Thus the inferior epigastric vein arises at the same place as the deep circumflex vein but perpendicular and along the abdominal wall. Hence it forms the limit of lymph node dissection. (**c**) The origin of the inferior epigastric vein has been demonstrated in this image. This is the anterior limit of ilio-obturator lymph node dissection

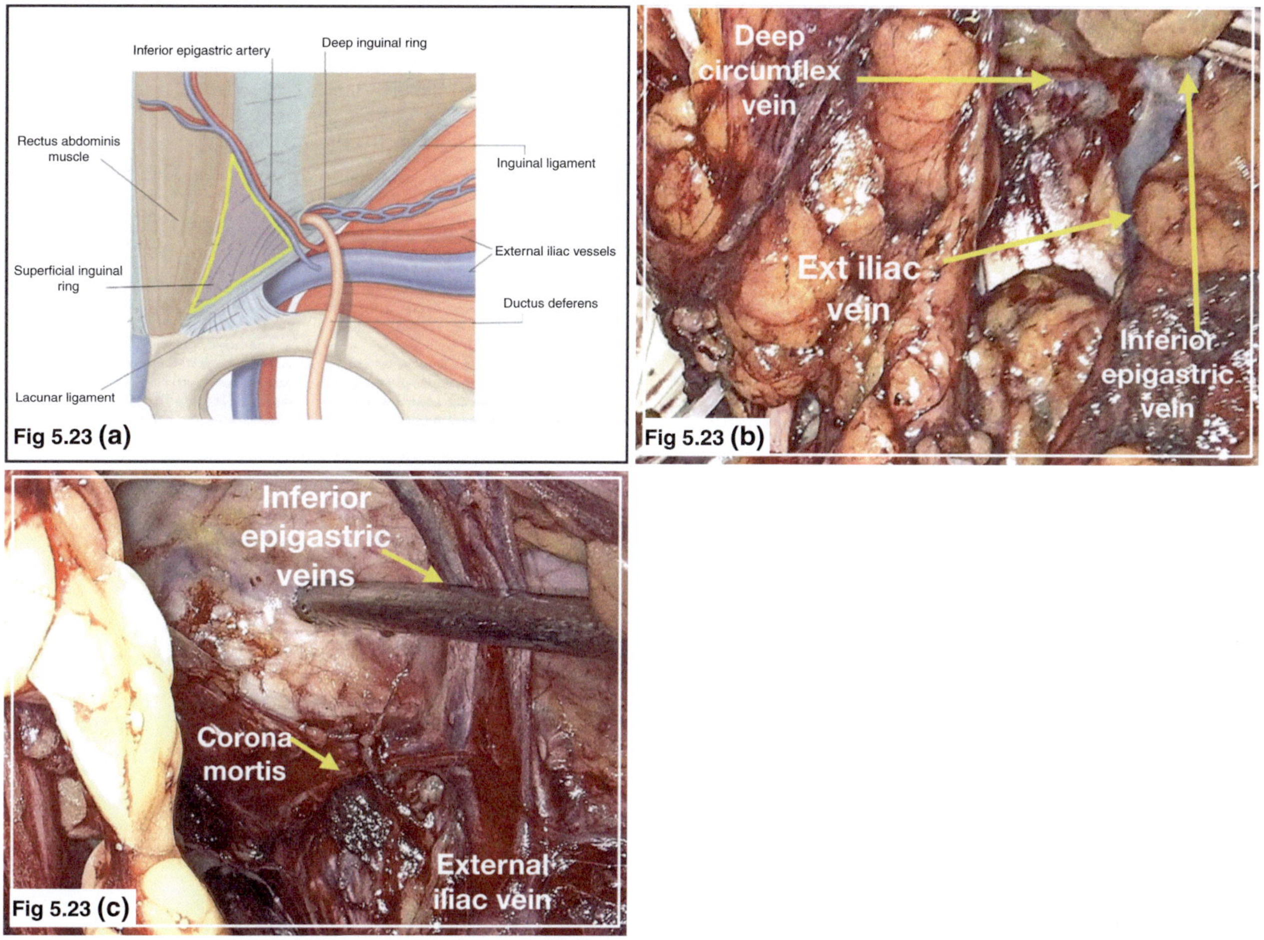

Fig. 5.23 (**a**) Diagrammatic anatomical representation of the inferior epigastric artery. (**b**) The inferior epigastric vein can be seen travelling to the anterior abdominal wall during lymph node dissection and the deep circumflex vein can also be seen travelling medially. The external iliac vein continues further as the femoral vein after crossing under the inguinal ligament. (**c**) The three tributaries of the external iliac vein have been demonstrated in the inferior epigastric vein, the deep circumflex iliac vein and the external artery continuing as the femoral vein

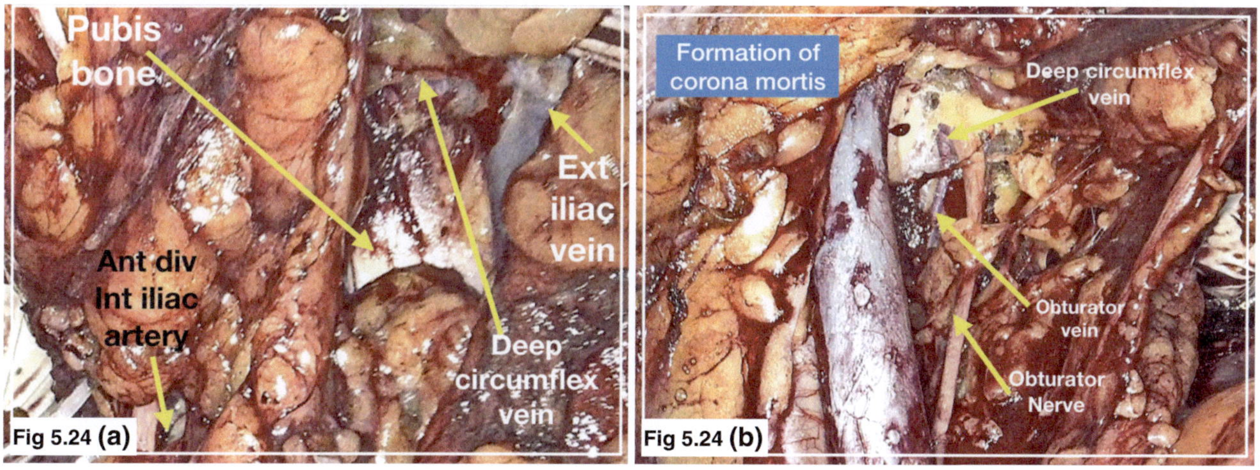

Fig. 5.24 (**a**) The deep circumflex vein, a tributary of the external iliac vein, has been seen travelling medially into the pelvis along the pubis bone. (**b**) The deep circumflex vein can be seen travelling down to communicate with the obturator vein. The communication is called as the corona mortis. (**c**) The deep circumflex vein travels through the fibre fatty tissue containing lymph nodes which is why the vein is often injured during lymph node dissection. (**d**) The corona mortis can be seen clearly along its entire course intact. The corona mortis thus can be seen as the only communication between the internal and the external iliac veins. (**e**) The deep circumflex vein is seen as thin tributary of the external iliac vein passing through the fibrofatty tissue (ilio-obturator lymph nodes). (**f–i**) These series of images show the corona mortis dissected in various cases of laparoscopic radical hysterectomy with ilio-obturator lymph node dissection

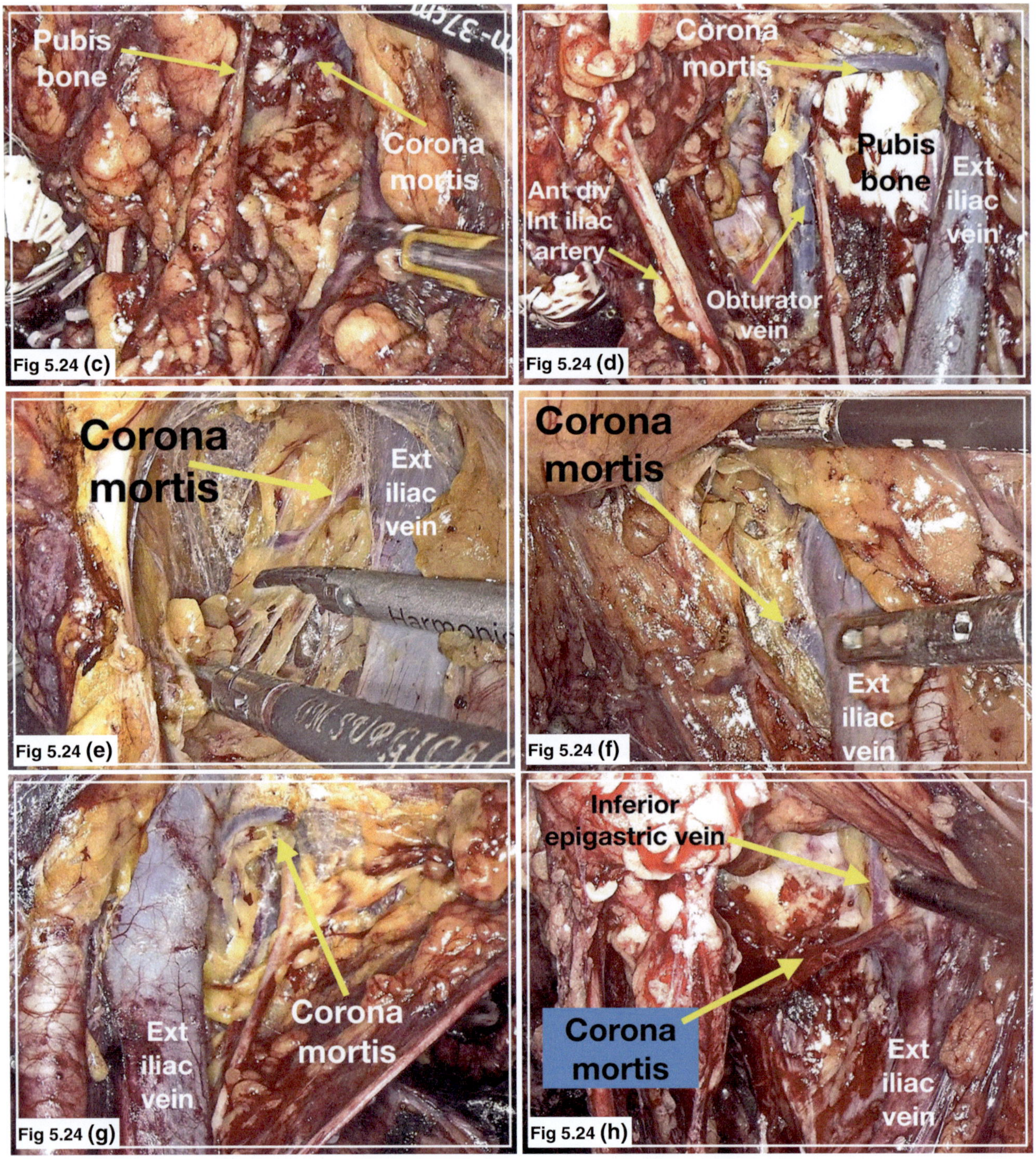

Fig. 5.24 (continued)

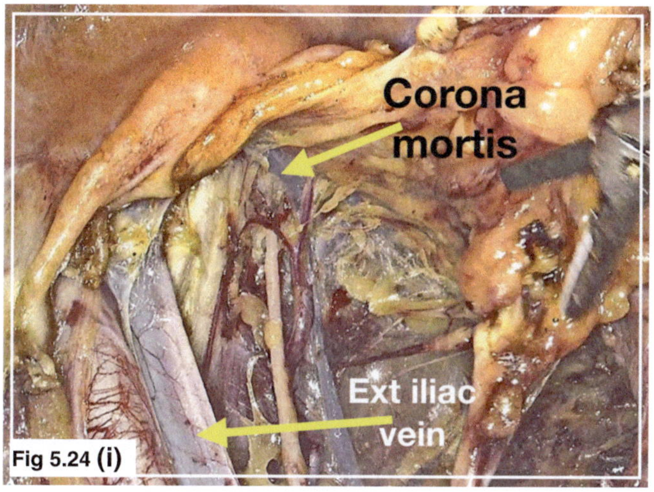

Fig. 5.24 (continued)

5.2.2 Internal Iliac Artery

The internal iliac artery arises from the common iliac artery at the level of sacral promontory (Fig. 5.30a–f).

It courses downwards and medially and divides into two divisions—the anterior and the posterior. This division takes place about 2–3 cm distal to the division of common iliac (Fig. 5.31a–c).

The anterior division continues to give branches on the medial and lateral sides and then continues to the anterior abdominal wall to end as obliterated hypogastric artery or also known as the medial umbilical ligament (Fig. 5.32a–i).

The anterior division continues downwards towards the iliac bone and is the main source of supply to the pelvic organs. The first branch arises about 5–6 cm distal to the origin of the posterior division (Fig. 5.33a–c).

Thus, enough length of the anterior division of internal iliac artery is available for ligation before the origin of its first branch (Fig. 5.34a, b).

This is the most important anatomical landmark. *The internal iliac vein closely hugs the artery posteriorly and hence care should be taken while ligating the artery as during emergency situations the vein can be damaged* (Fig. 5.35a–d).

Just 1–2 cm proximal to the first branch (uterine artery) there is a natural separation between the internal iliac artery and internal iliac vein which makes the distal ligation of the anterior division of internal iliac artery easy. A window posterior to the artery can be created without the fear of damage to the vein (Fig. 5.36a–c).

The first branch of the anterior division of internal iliac is the uterine artery in females and the superior vesical artery in males (Fig. 5.37a–c).

Both the uterine and the superior vesicle traverse a long distance through the pararectal space before they supply the organs (Fig. 5.38a–c).

This makes the ligation of these arteries easy laterally (Fig. 5.39a–c).

Both the vessels cross the ureter anteriorly and supply the ureter through a small branch (Fig. 5.40a–f).

Thus, there is enough length of these vessels available for the surgeon from its origin to its insertion. In case of bleeding from the organ, one can go laterally and be sure that there is enough length of artery available for ligation (Fig. 5.41a–c).

Also, one has to differentiate between the arterial and venous bleeding. If it is arterial bleeding, then one should depress the ureter posteriorly and go lateral to the ureter while if it venous bleeding one should retract the ureter upwards and go lateral because the vein comes from below the ureter (Fig. 5.42a, b).

The posterior division dips into the presacral fascia to supply the gluteal vessels. The anterior division of internal iliac artery should be ligated distal to the posterior division; otherwise there is claudication in the gluteal region (Fig. 5.43a–c).

Lateral vascular control can be easily achieved once this anatomy is understood. The easiest way of achieving this lateral control is to open the peritoneum at the level of sacral promontory and identify the ureter as it crosses the common iliac from lateral to medial and then open the plane parallel to the ureter in the direction from cranial to caudal. This opens the pararectal space and the first structure which crosses transversally is the artery which can be ligated. *The main trick is remaining lateral and parallel to the ureter* (Fig. 5.44a–d).

After giving the first branch the anterior division continues caudally and gives two branches in females and one branch in males and then continues as obliterated hypogastric artery and ends. The two branches in females are superior and inferior vesicle while in males it is the inferior vesicle (Fig. 5.45a–c).

Since the bladder lies anterior to the uterus the superior vesicle also arises at a plane higher than the uterine artery. *This allows the preservation of superior vesicle during radical surgeries of the uterus* (Fig. 5.46a–d).

The middle rectal artery on its way to the rectum crosses anteriorly the two deep uterine veins before their insertion into the internal iliac vein. This anatomy is important for the harvest of the internal iliac vein during the transplant of the uterus (Fig. 5.47a–d).

The only lateral branch of the internal iliac is the obturator artery. This artery is always posterior to the obturator nerve (Fig. 5.48a–c).

Thus, during the rectal surgery for cancer, this artery may not be visualised. The area lateral to the obliterated artery is vascular and harbours the lymph nodes (Fig. 5.49a, b).

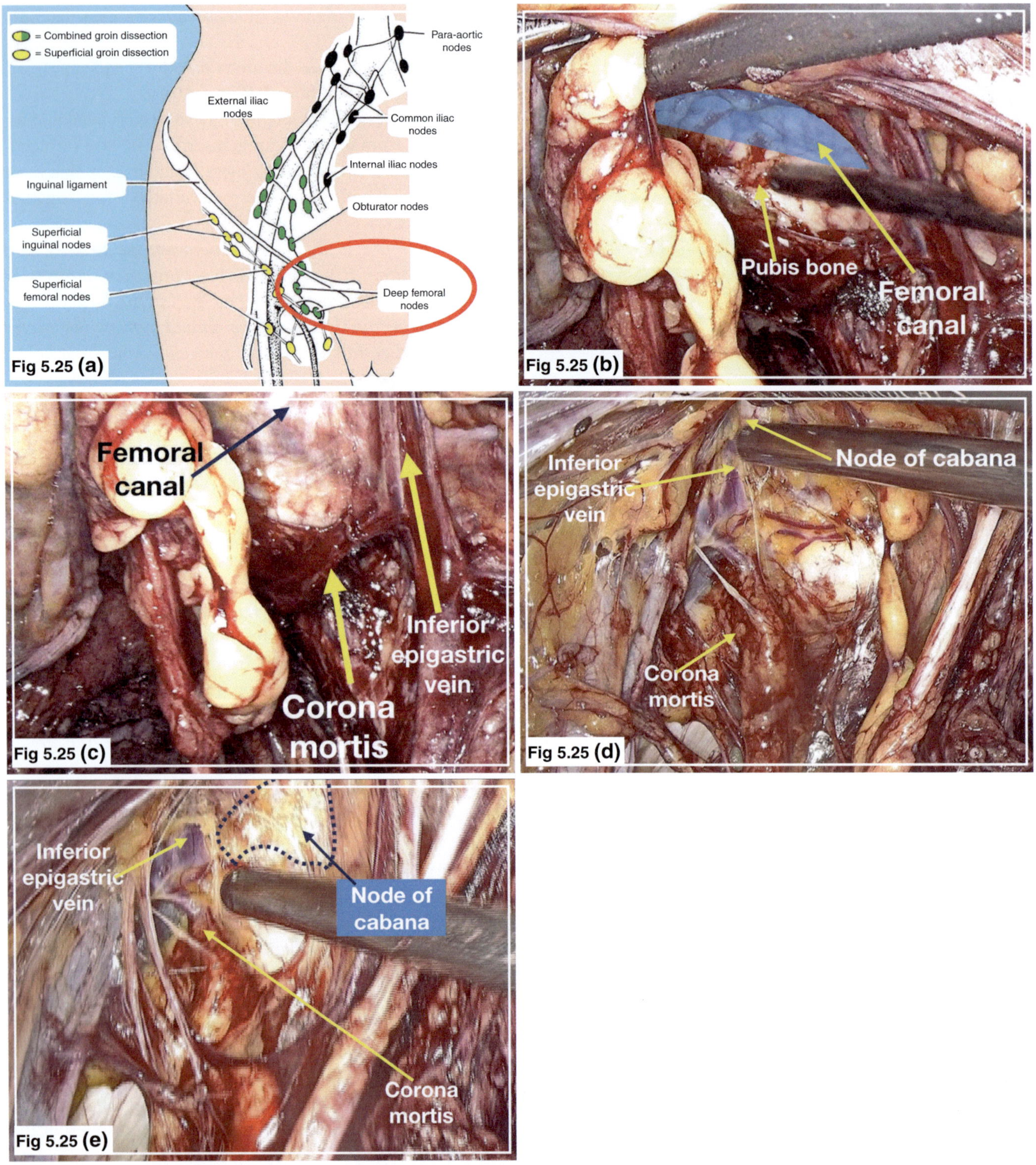

Fig. 5.25 (**a**) Graphic image of the sentinel node of Cabana or the femoral lymph nodes. (**b**) The area shaded in blue is the femoral canal which lies medial to the inferior epigastric veins. The fibrofatty tissue contains lymph nodes of cloquet/cabana. They are of clinical significance in case of carcinoma of the vulva. (**c**–**e**) The panoramic view of the femoral canal that can be seen in this image along with its relation to the inferior epigastric and the deep circumflex iliac veins

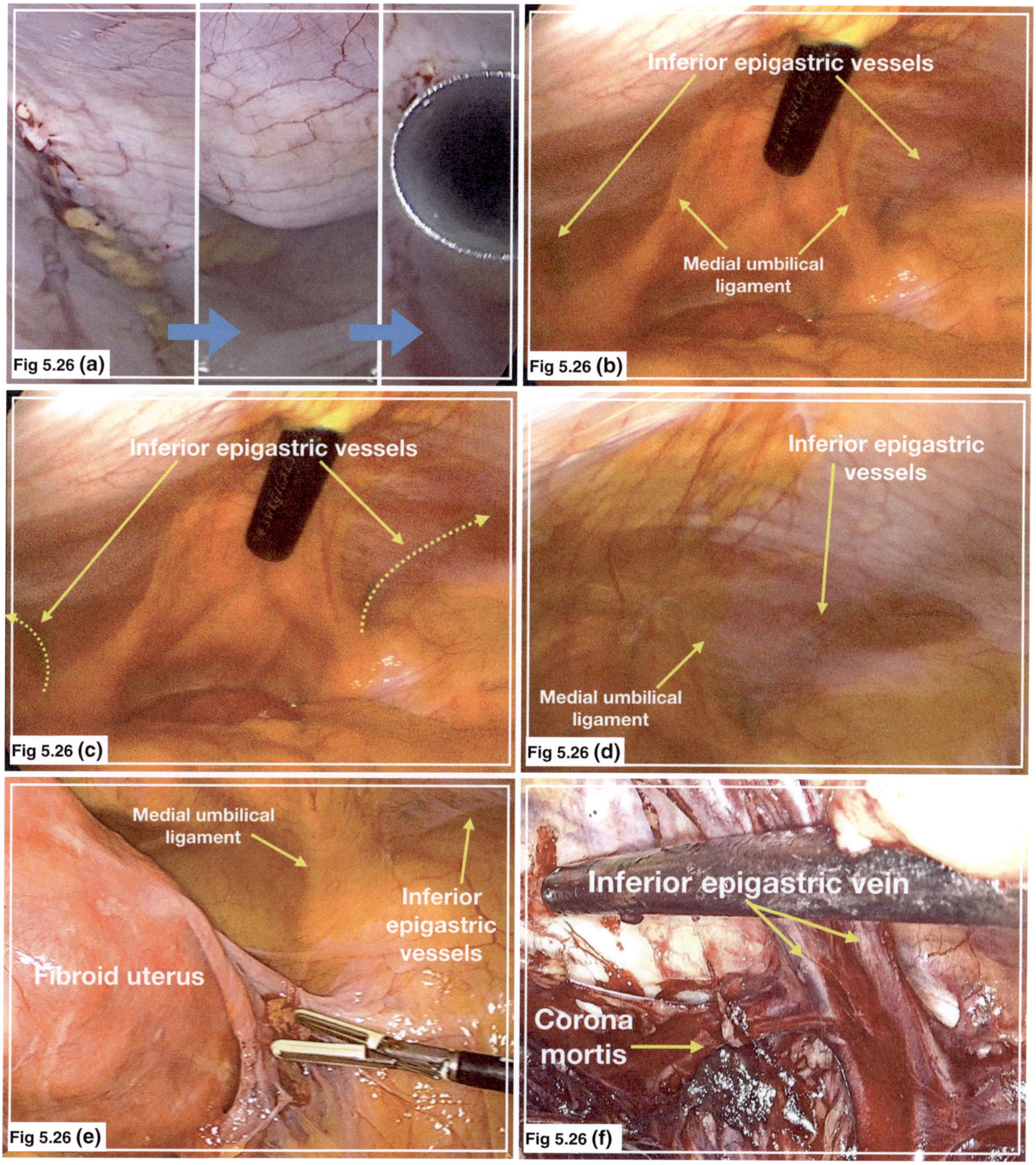

Fig. 5.26 (**a**) As previously explained how the position of the port with respect to inferior hypogastric vessel plays an important role. (**b**) The inferior epigastric vessels are clinically important in laparoscopy in terms of the port positions primarily and in condition of hernia surgeries. Thus they are seldom exposed in gynaecological procedures. The inferior epigastric vessel impressions can be seen on the anterior abdominal wall but seldom intervened in gynaecology. The vessels are seen bilaterally arising lateral to the medial umbilical ligament and travelling away from the ligament as well. (**c**) A diagrammatic representation of the inferior epigastric vessel has been shown with yellow arrows indicating the court of the inferior epigastric vessels. (**d**) Impression of inferior epigastric vessels can be seen on the peritoneal surface of the anterior abdominal wall. (**e**) The inferior epigastric vein is dissected during the case of ilio-obturator lymph node dissection. The corona mortis can also be seen travelling medially and into the pelvis. (**f**) The inferior epigastric vein shown in the previous image can be seen in a more panoramic view. When traced anteriorly along the posterior surface of the abdominal wall the vessels coincide with the impressions seen on the anterior abdominal wall. (**g**) The inferior epigastric vein shown in the previous image can be seen in a more panoramic view. When traced anteriorly along the posterior surface of the abdominal wall the vessels coincide with the impressions seen on the anterior abdominal wall

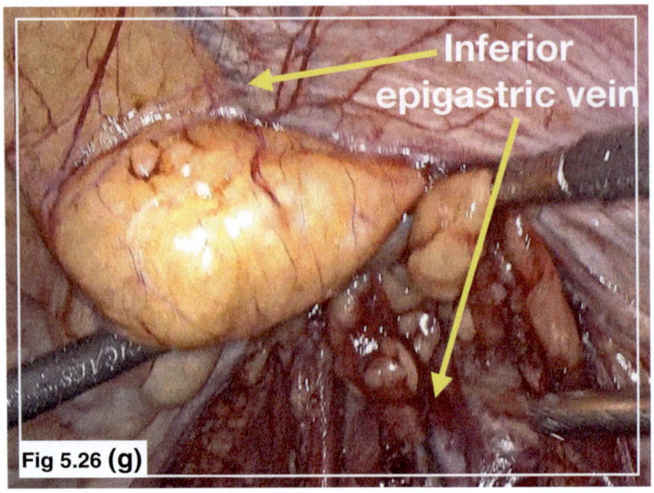

Fig. 5.26 (continued)

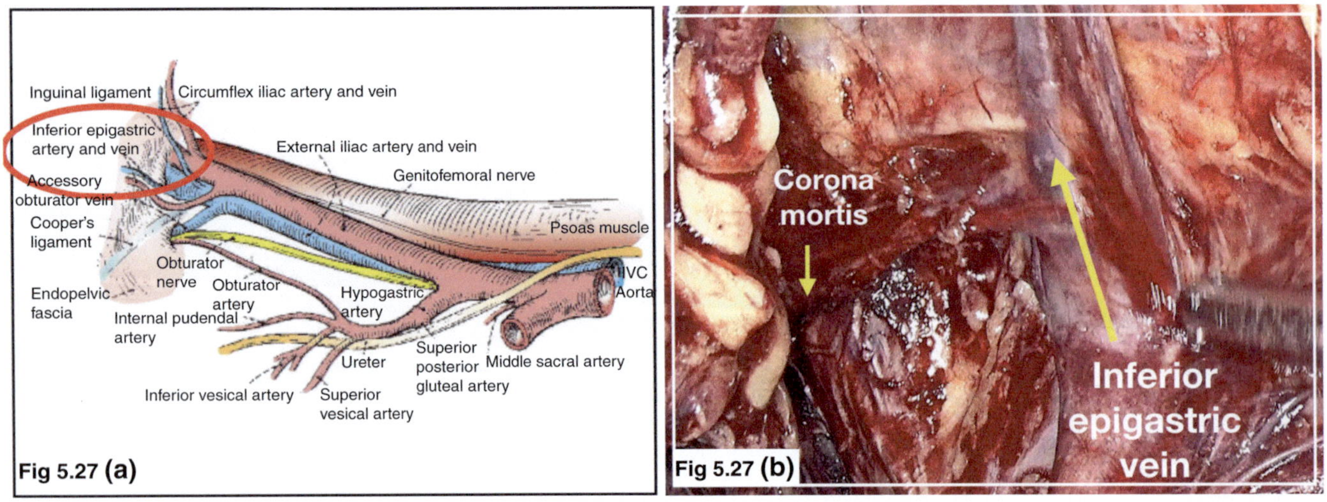

Fig. 5.27 (**a**) Diagrammatic representation of the external iliac artery with its branches. (**b**) There are no arterial counterparts of the corona mortis. Thus the inferior epigastric vessels are the only true branches of the external iliac vessels

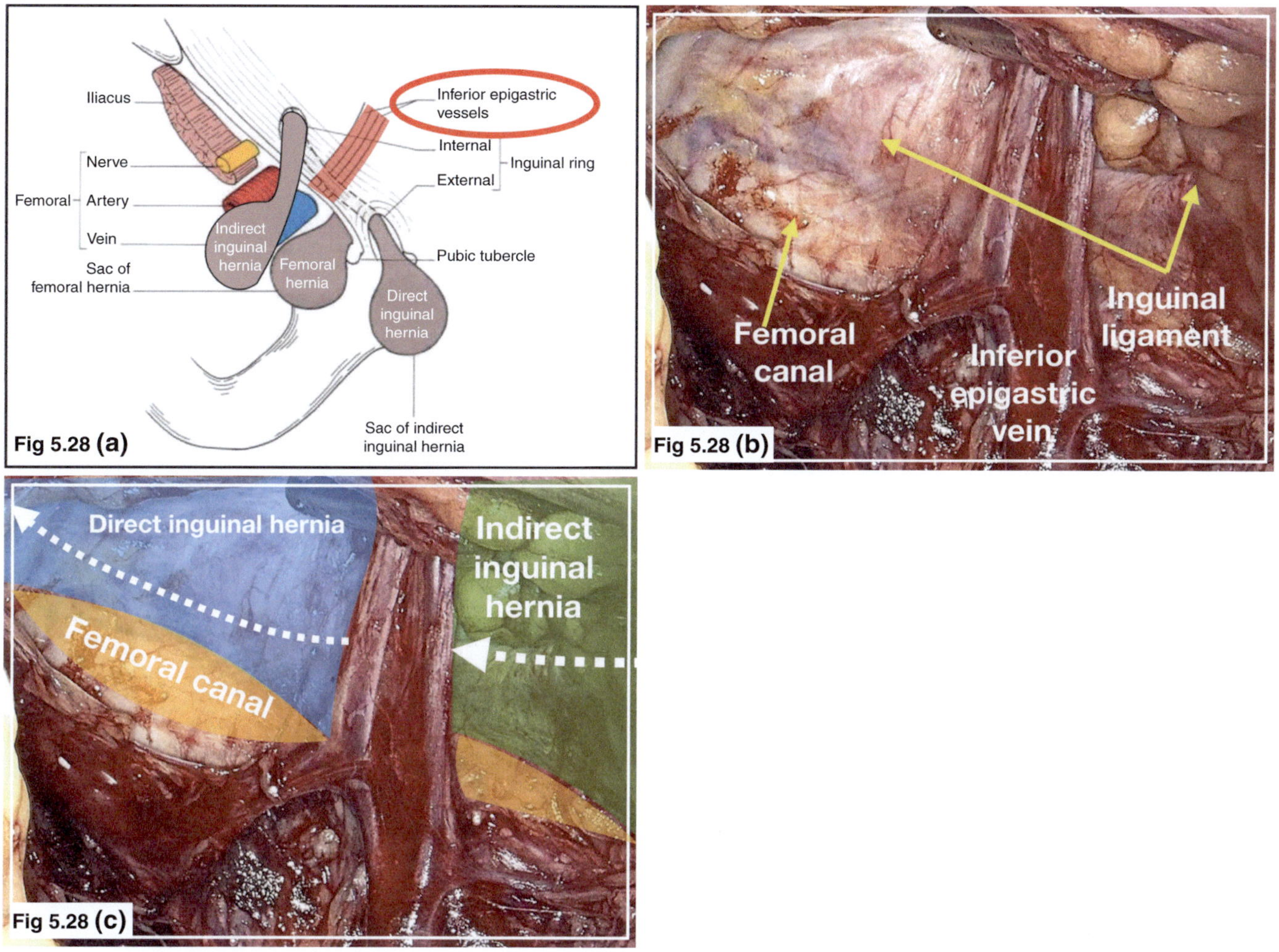

Fig. 5.28 (**a**) Diagrammatic representation of how inferior epigastric artery differentiates hernias; if the origin is medial to the vessels, it is direct inguinal hernia, and if lateral to the vessel it is indirect inguinal hernia. If it is below the inguinal ligament then it is femoral hernia. (**b**) The inguinal ligament can be seen more clearly lateral to the inferior epigastric vein as compared to the medial side of the abdominal wall. The location of hernia with respect to the inferior epigastric vessels decides whether the hernia is direct or indirect. (**c**) Diagrammatic representation of the previous image. The white dotted line represents the inguinal ligament. The area shaded in blue is for the direct inguinal hernia while the area in green is for indirect inguinal hernia. The area shaded in yellow represents the area of femoral canal covered with fibrofatty tissue of Cloquet lymph nodes

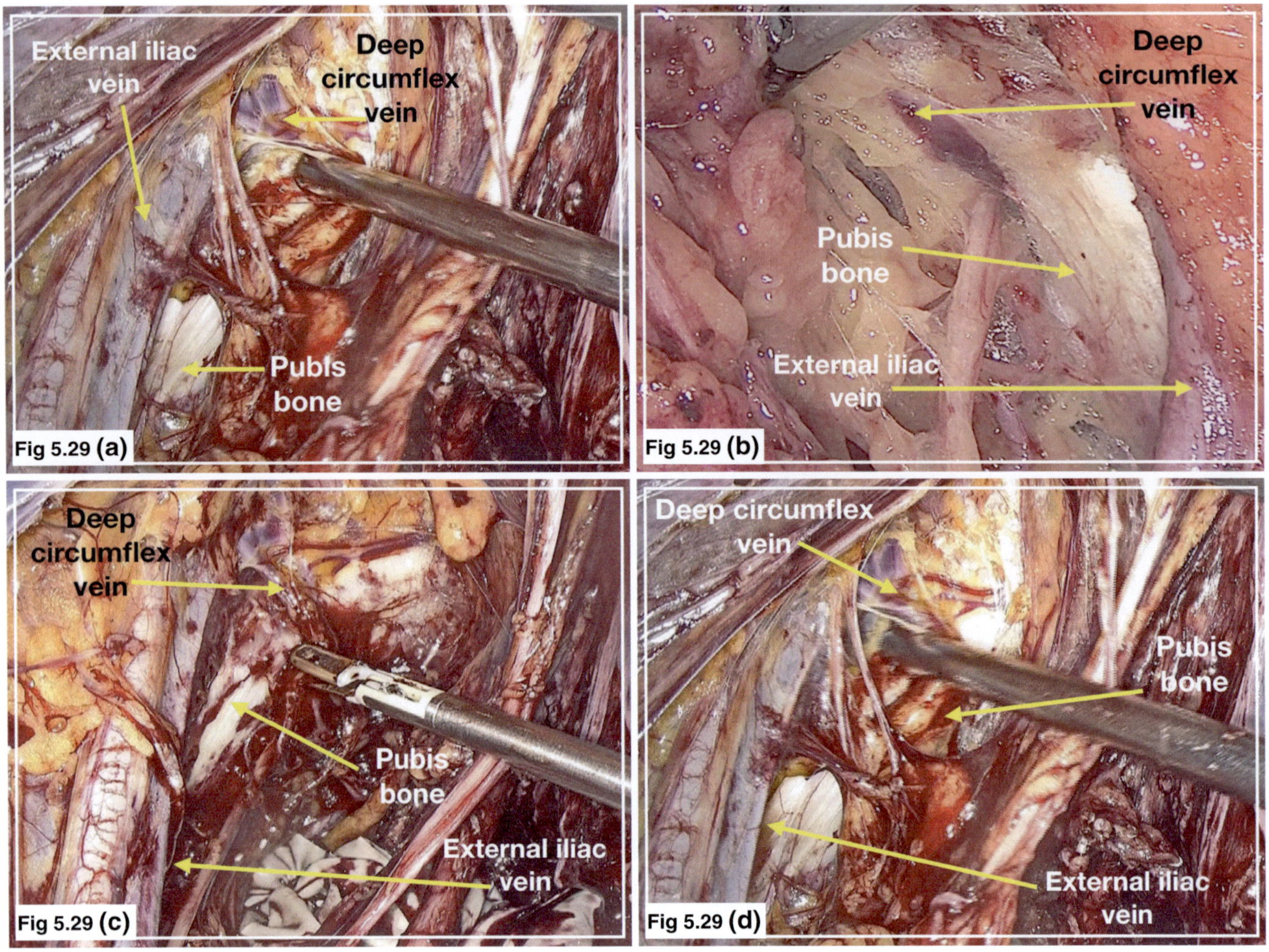

Fig. 5.29 (**a**–**d**) Series of images showing the corona mortis in various different cases of laparoscopic radical hysterectomy with pelvic lymph node dissection. The appearances may vary though the anatomy remains constant

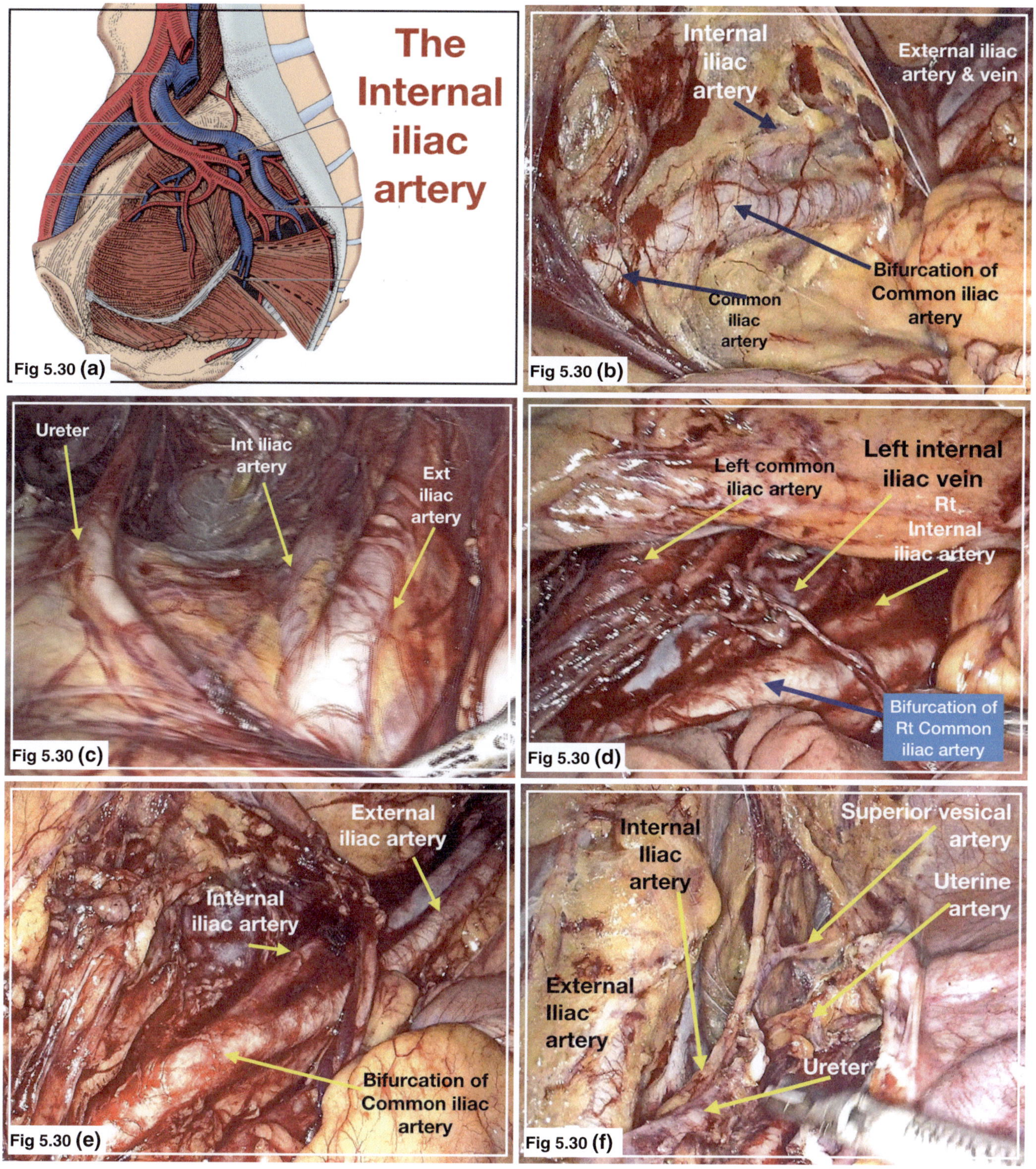

Fig. 5.30 (**a**) Diagrammatic representation of the internal iliac artery and its course in the pelvis. Also check Figs. 5.2c, 5.5b, 5.9d, and 5.11a. (**b**) Previously viewed images with internal iliac artery as one of the important structures (Fig. 5.2c). (**c**) Previously viewed images with internal iliac artery as one of the important structures (Fig. 5.5b). (**d**) Previously viewed images with internal iliac artery as one of the important structures (Fig. 5.9d). (**e**) Previously viewed images with internal iliac artery as one of the important structures (Fig. 5.11a). (**f**) The image has been taken from a case of dissection of donor for uterine transplant. The internal iliac artery can be seen along its entire length along with its medial branches, the uterine and the superior vesical artery

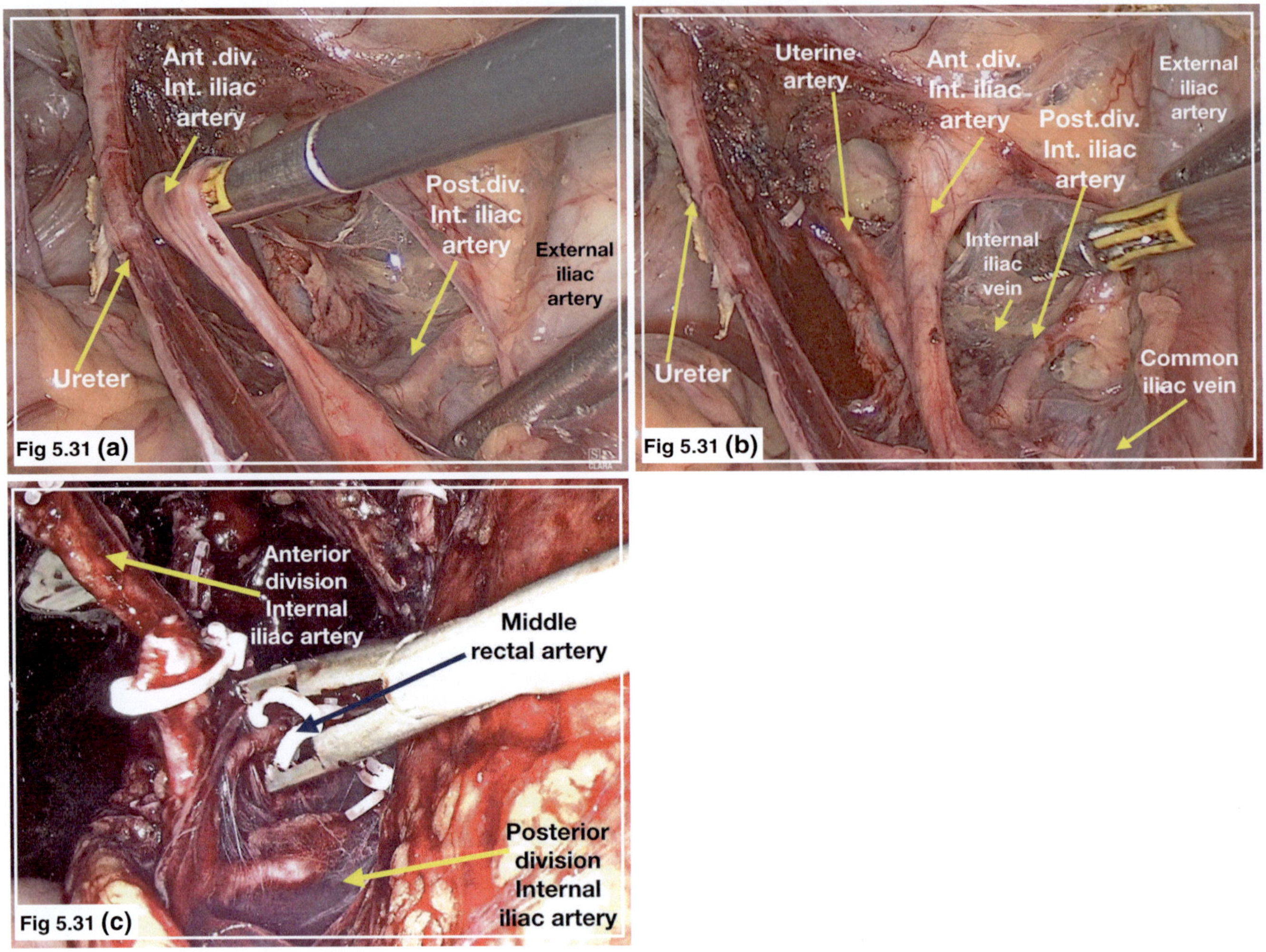

Fig. 5.31 (**a**) The image shows a stretched and retracted anterior division of the internal iliac artery. The anterior division is retracted so as to dissect the fibre fatty tissue underneath and expose the posterior division of the internal iliac artery. The posterior division has a short course in the pelvis. It turns backwards to supply the gluteal region as soon as it branches out from the main trunk of the internal iliac artery. (**b**) The image shows the anterior and posterior division of the internal iliac artery. The identity of anterior division can be reconfirmed by the uterine artery seen arising from the division and crossing over to reach across the ureter. Underneath the anterior division a pale image of the internal iliac vein can be seen. It can be seen terminating as the common iliac vein underneath the external iliac artery as it communicates with the external iliac vein to form the common iliac vein. (**c**) The image has been taken from a case of dissection of donor for uterine transplant. The posterior division of the internal iliac artery can be seen clearly along the side of the middle rectal artery which is an inconsistent branch in the anterior division of the internal iliac artery. The clip is being applied to the middle rectal artery in this image

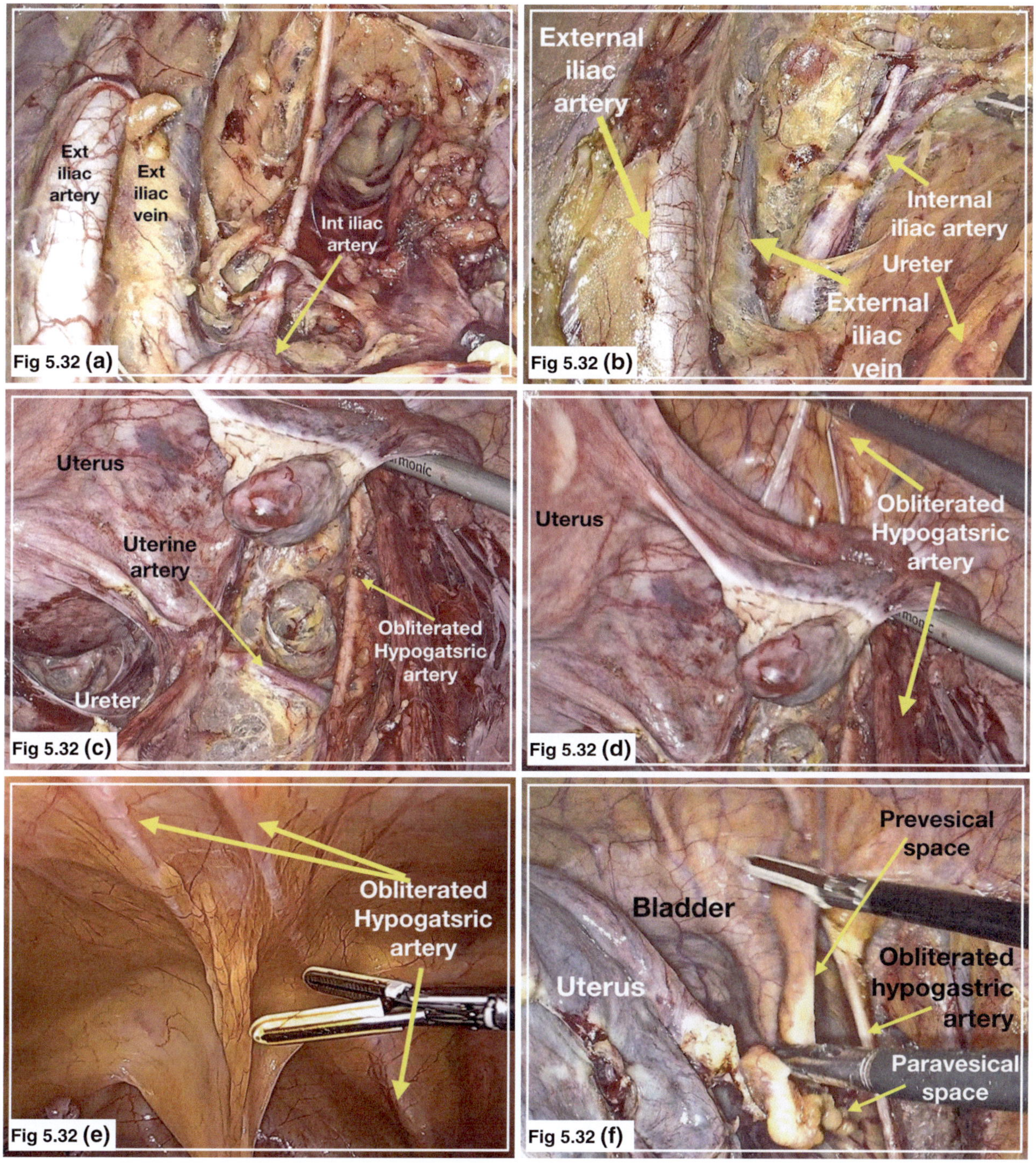

Fig. 5.32 (**a**) Previously viewed images with internal iliac artery as one of the important structures (Fig. 5.10c). (**b**) Previously viewed images with internal iliac artery as one of the important structures (Fig. 5.18c). (**c**) In a case of laparoscopic radical hysterectomy the internal iliac artery is dissected leaving medial branches of uterine artery shown in the image and then further dissected till the termination of the obliterated hypogastric artery. (**d**) The obliterated hypogastric artery continues on the anterior abdominal wall as the medial umbilical ligament. The medial umbilical ligament and the obliterated hypogastric artery can be seen in continuity. (**e**) The image is of a case of Burch's colposuspension showing anterior mobilisation of the bladder into the prevesical space. The traction on the bladder midline brings the medial umbilical ligament closer and the medial umbilical ligament can be seen continuing as the obliterated hypogastric artery at the level below the pubis where the anterior abdominal wall continues as uterovesical fold of peritoneum of the bladder. (**f**) The image is from a case of anterior exenteration where the bladder dissection of the prevesical space is approached from the paravesical space by remaining medial to the obliterated hypogastric artery. It is seen that the obliterated hypogastric artery continues as the medial umbilical ligament on the posterior surface of the anterior abdominal wall. (**g**) The mage is taken from the final view after a complete laparoscopic radical hysterectomy showing the vault in the centre, the obliterated hypogastric artery, the obturator nerve and the external iliac artery in the medial to lateral order. (**h**) Both the obliterated hypogastric artery shown as medial umbilical ligament and the urachus forming the median umbilical ligament. (**i**) In this image the medial umbilical ligament is tugged on the anterior abdominal wall and the movement is appreciated on the obliterated hypogastric artery in the retroperitoneal spaces in the pelvis

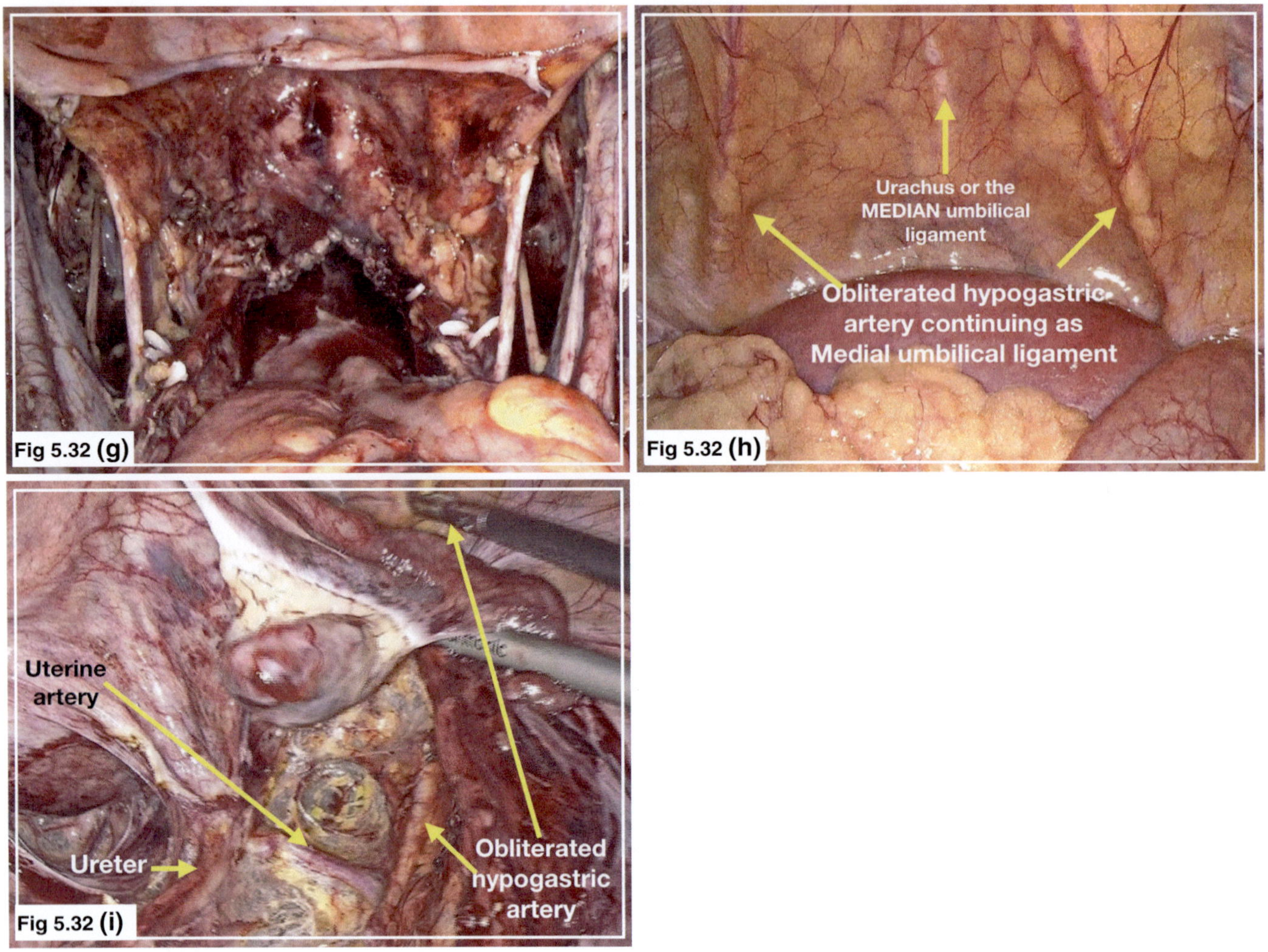

Fig. 5.32 (continued)

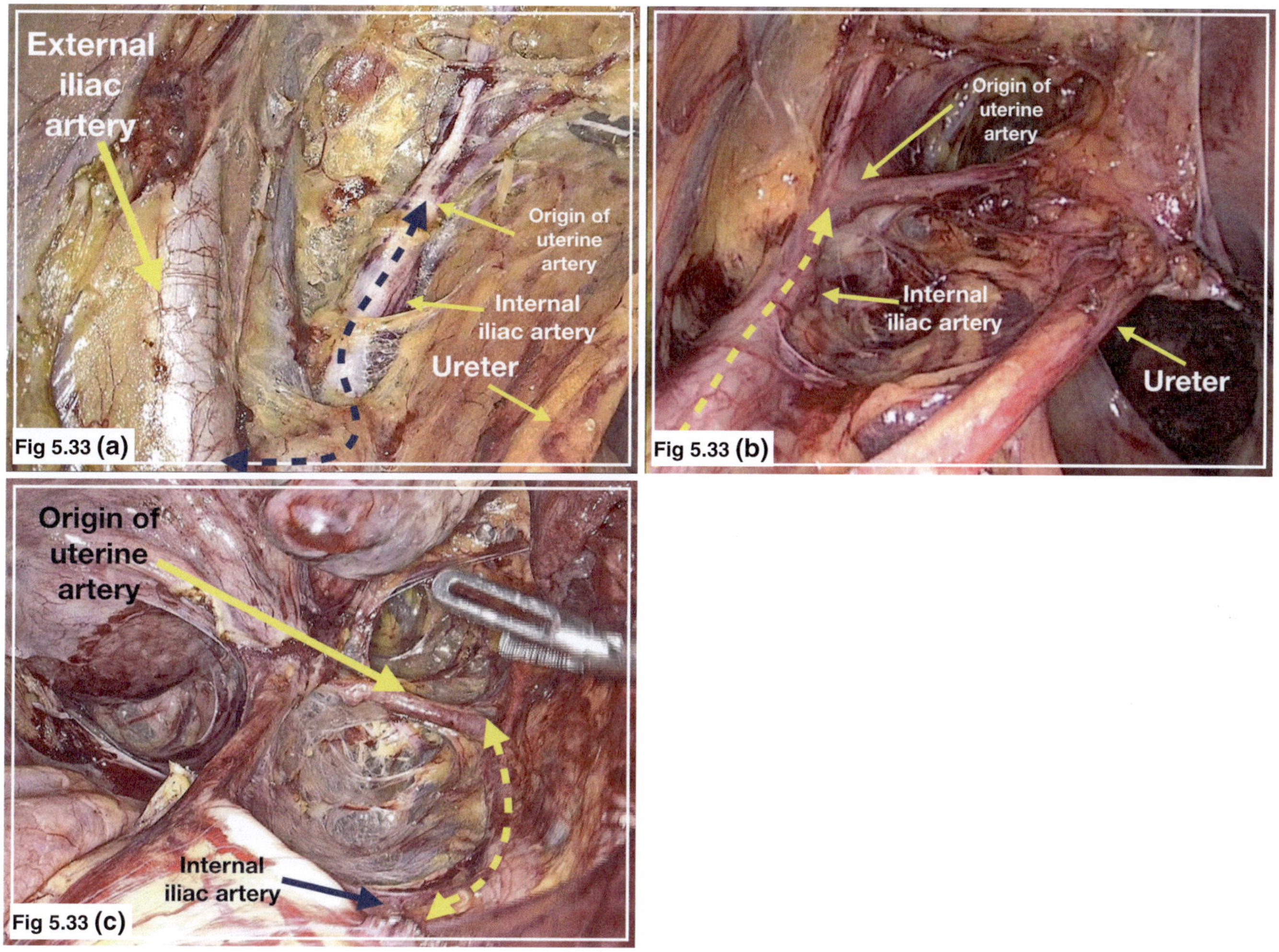

Fig. 5.33 (**a**) The uterine artery is seen arising from the anterior division of the internal iliac artery. The blue dotted line denotes the distance from the origin of internal iliac artery. If measured, the distance between the origin of the uterine artery and the origin of anterior division of iliac artery is 5–6 cm. (**b**) Similarly in another image the yellow dotted arrow represents the distance between the origin of uterine artery and the origin of the anterior division of the internal iliac artery, approximately 5–6 cm. (**c**) The image is from a case of dissection of donor for uterine transplant. The length of the internal iliac artery available for dissection can be seen in yellow dotted lines. The distance is roughly 5–6 cm. It does vary not only from person to person but also from side to side in the same person as well

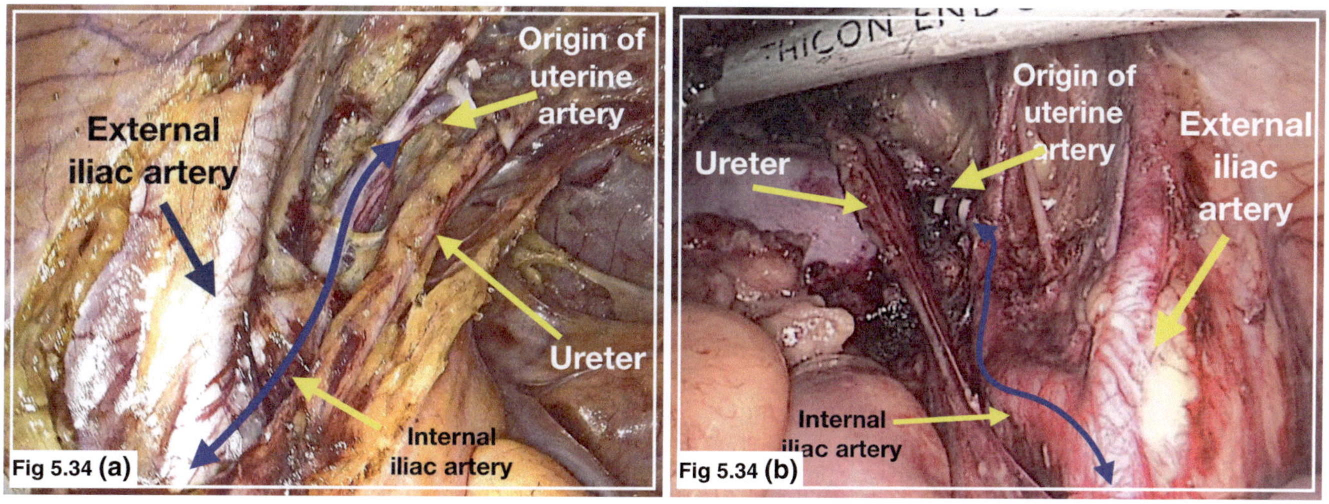

Fig. 5.34 (**a**) The blue line denotes the length of anterior division of internal iliac artery available for ligation before the first branch. (**b**) Similarly as seen on the right side, the length of the vessel available for ligation is variable in measurement, but in the range of 5–6 cm as shown in blue arrows. The uterine artery has already been clipped

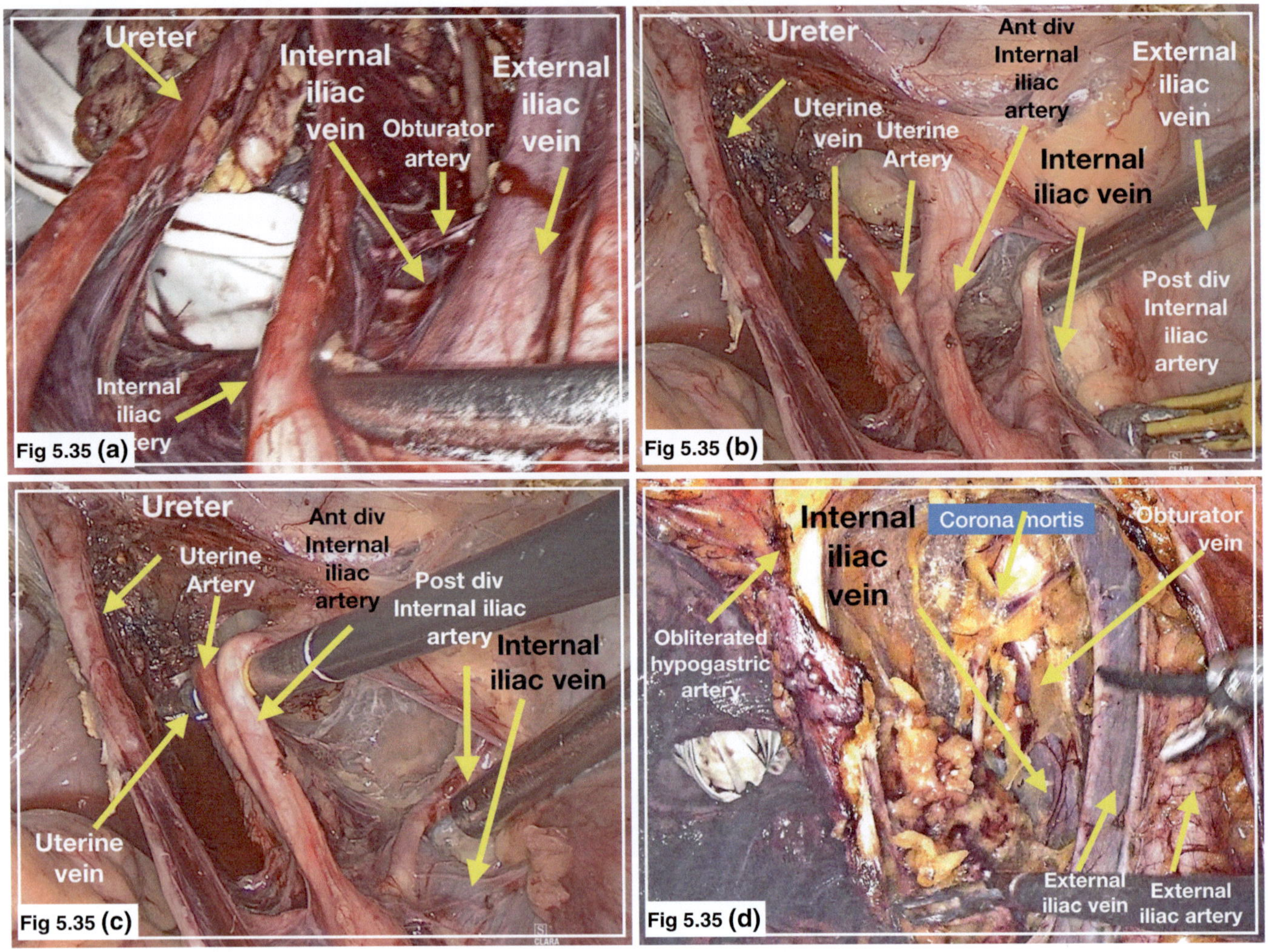

Fig. 5.35 (**a**) The internal iliac vein can be seen closely following a congruent path as that of the internal iliac artery. The internal iliac vein can be seen near the origin of the internal iliac artery under the branch of the obturator artery. (**b**) Here the internal iliac vein can be seen by dissection of the posterior division of the internal iliac artery. The uterine vein can be seen travelling along and under the uterine artery and communicating with the internal iliac vein. (**c**) The internal iliac vein can be seen more clearly under the internal iliac artery, under the posterior division near the root. (**d**) In certain cases the internal iliac vein is more closely located to the lateral pelvic wall. The internal iliac vein can be identified by its tributaries, i.e. the corona mortis draining into the obturator vein and the obturator vein draining into the internal iliac vein. The internal iliac artery can be identified by the obliterated hypogastric artery

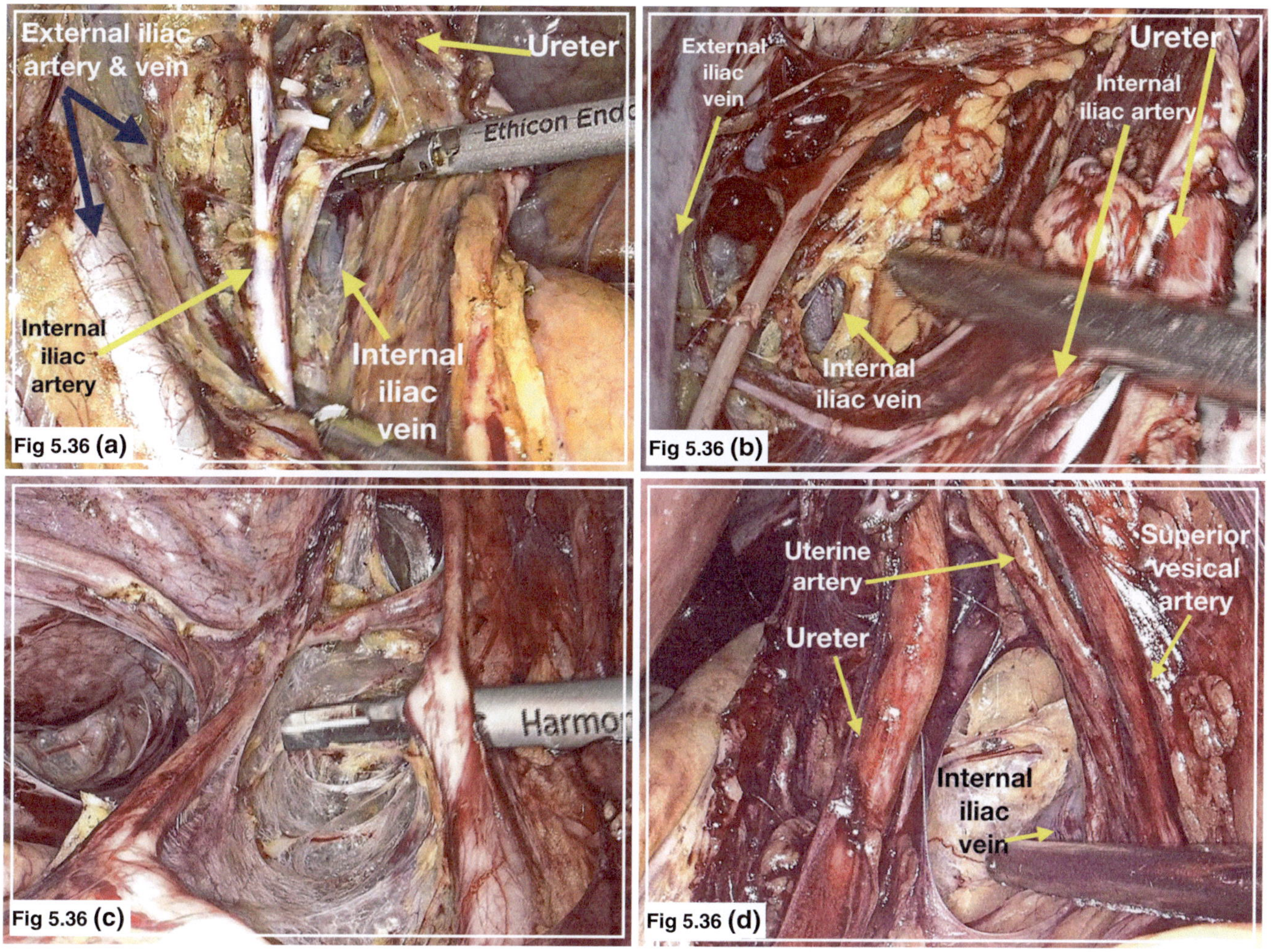

Fig. 5.36 (**a**) The more sure location for dissection of the internal iliac vein is just a few centimetres prior to the first branch of the anterior division (uterine artery) of the internal iliac artery as shown in the image. Window is seen created here underneath the uterine artery. (**b**) The internal iliac vein can be identified lateral to the internal iliac artery underneath the fibrofatty tissue. (**c**) This image shows the Harmonic scalpel blade passing under the space where there is a deficit of tissue to separate the internal iliac artery from the internal iliac vein as explained in the text. (**d**) This image shows the Harmonic scalpel blade passing under the space where there is a deficit of tissue to separate the internal iliac artery from the internal iliac vein as explained in the text

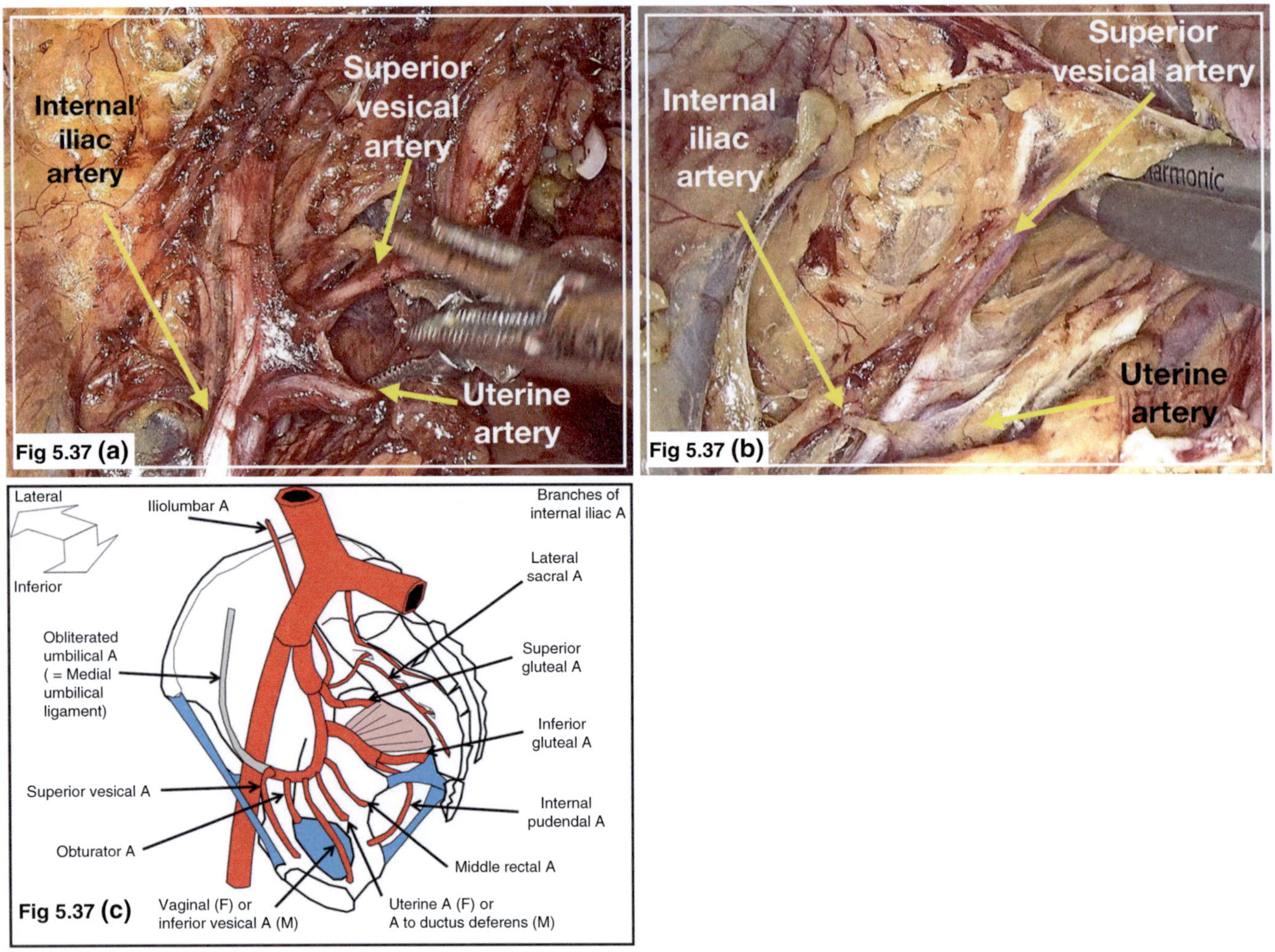

Fig. 5.37 (**a**, **b**) This pair of images show the origin and the course of the superior vesical and the uterine artery arising from the anterior division of internal iliac artery. (**c**) This is a comparative image of the difference in the vascular architecture of the internal iliac artery in the male and female pelvis. As explained in the text the superior vesical artery is the first branch from the internal iliac artery in males while it is the second branch in females with the first branch being the uterine artery

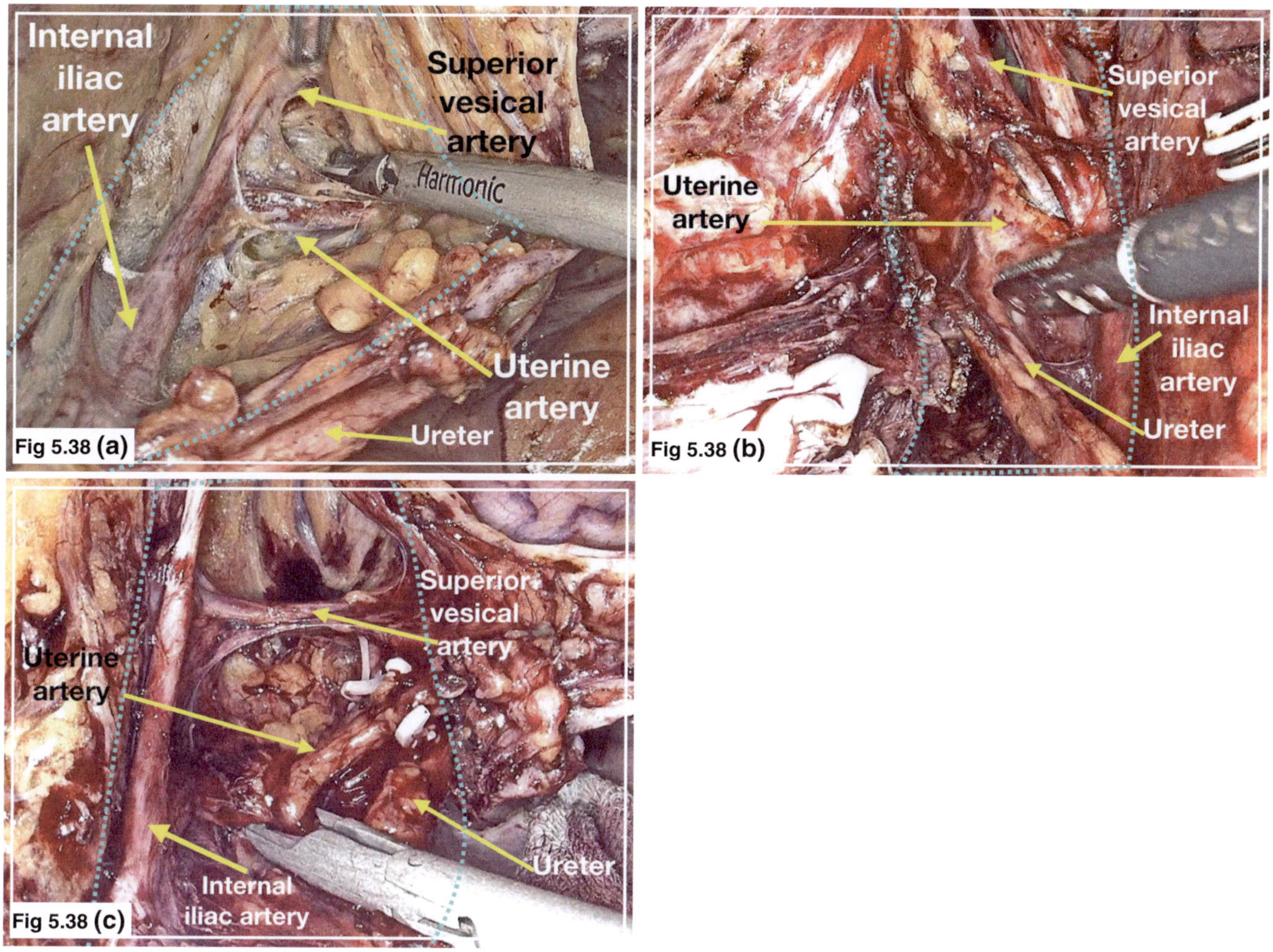

Fig. 5.38 (**a**–**c**) This series of images demonstrate the course of the internal iliac artery and their branches, the uterine and the superior vesical artery, across the pararectal space

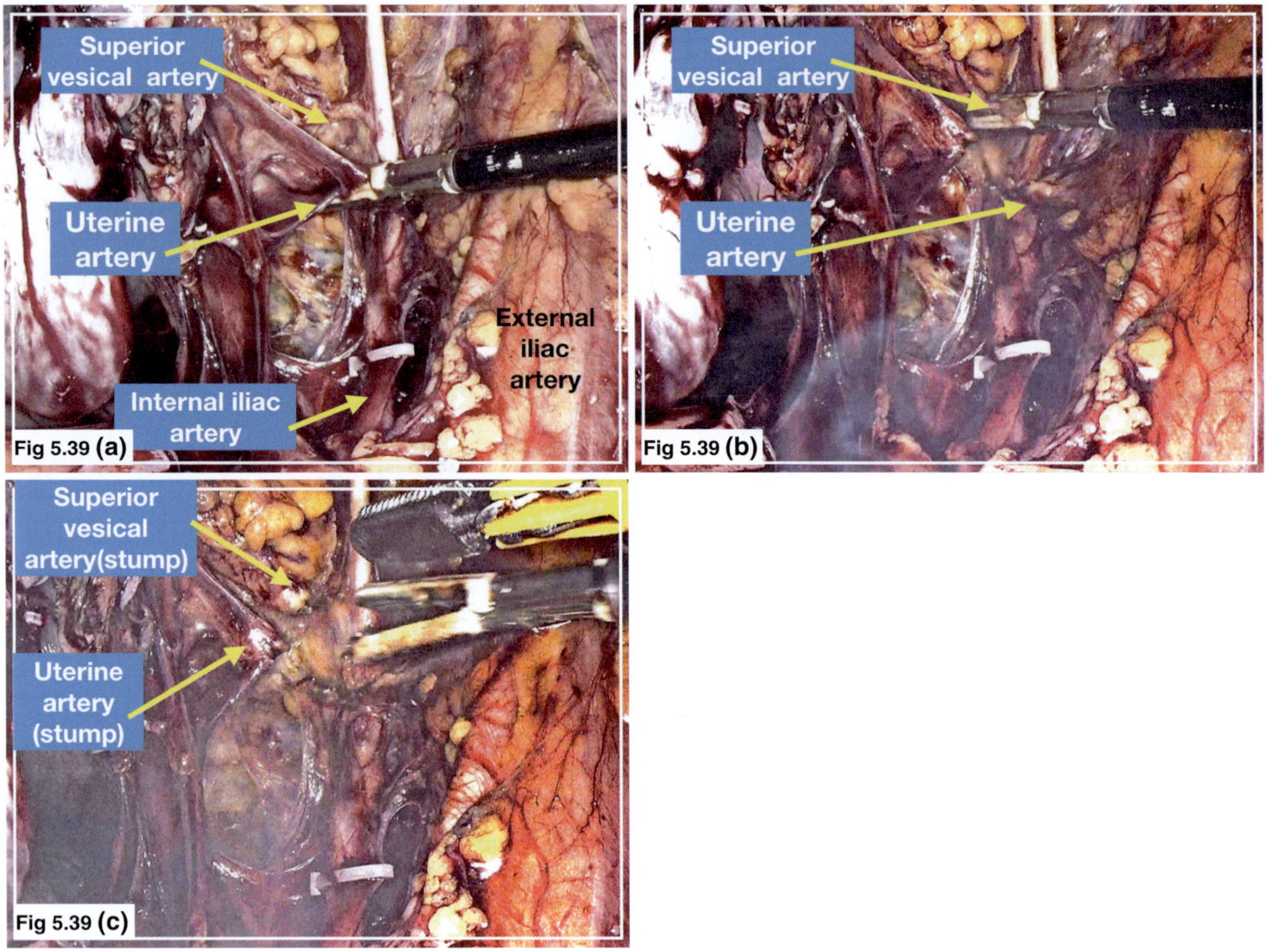

Fig. 5.39 (**a**–**c**) The series of images from a case of laparoscopic anterior exenteration show the laterality of coagulation of vessels. (**a**) Shows the uterine artery clipped and superior vesical artery above it. (**b**) The superior vesical artery is clipped and the stump of the uterine artery can be seen underneath. (**c**) The stumps of the uterine and the superior vesical artery can be seen

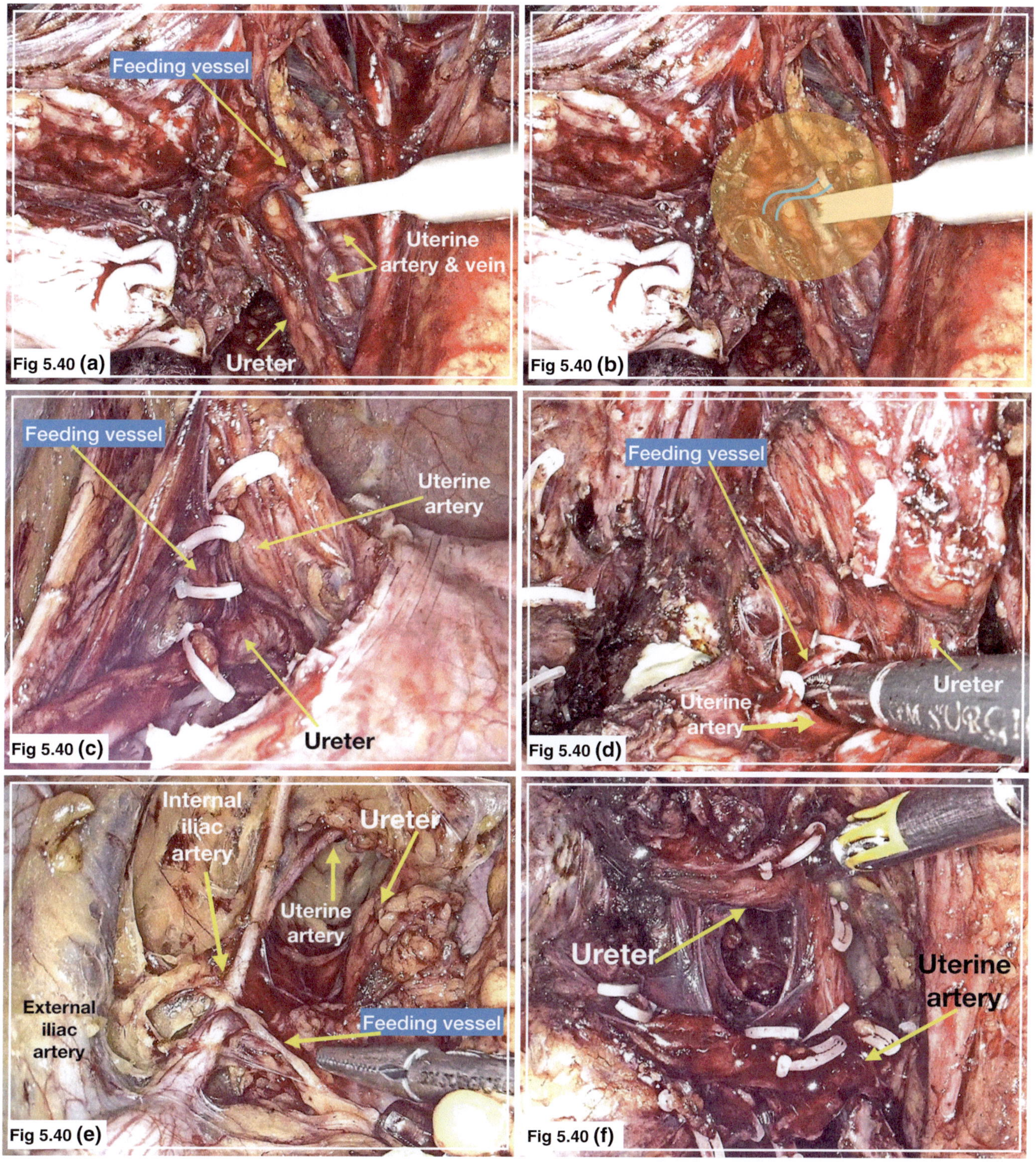

Fig. 5.40 (**a**–**e**) The series of images show the feeding vessels which contribute to the mesentery of the ureter and maintain its blood supply throughout he course. These vessels arise randomly from the uterine artery and the superior vesical artery and the internal iliac artery as well. The significance of these feeding vessels was identified during transplant surgery where these feeding vessels become leaky area leading to haemorrhage on re-anastomosis. Otherwise they are clinically insignificant. (**f**) The multiple number of such vessels can be seen on the uterine artery supplying the ureter

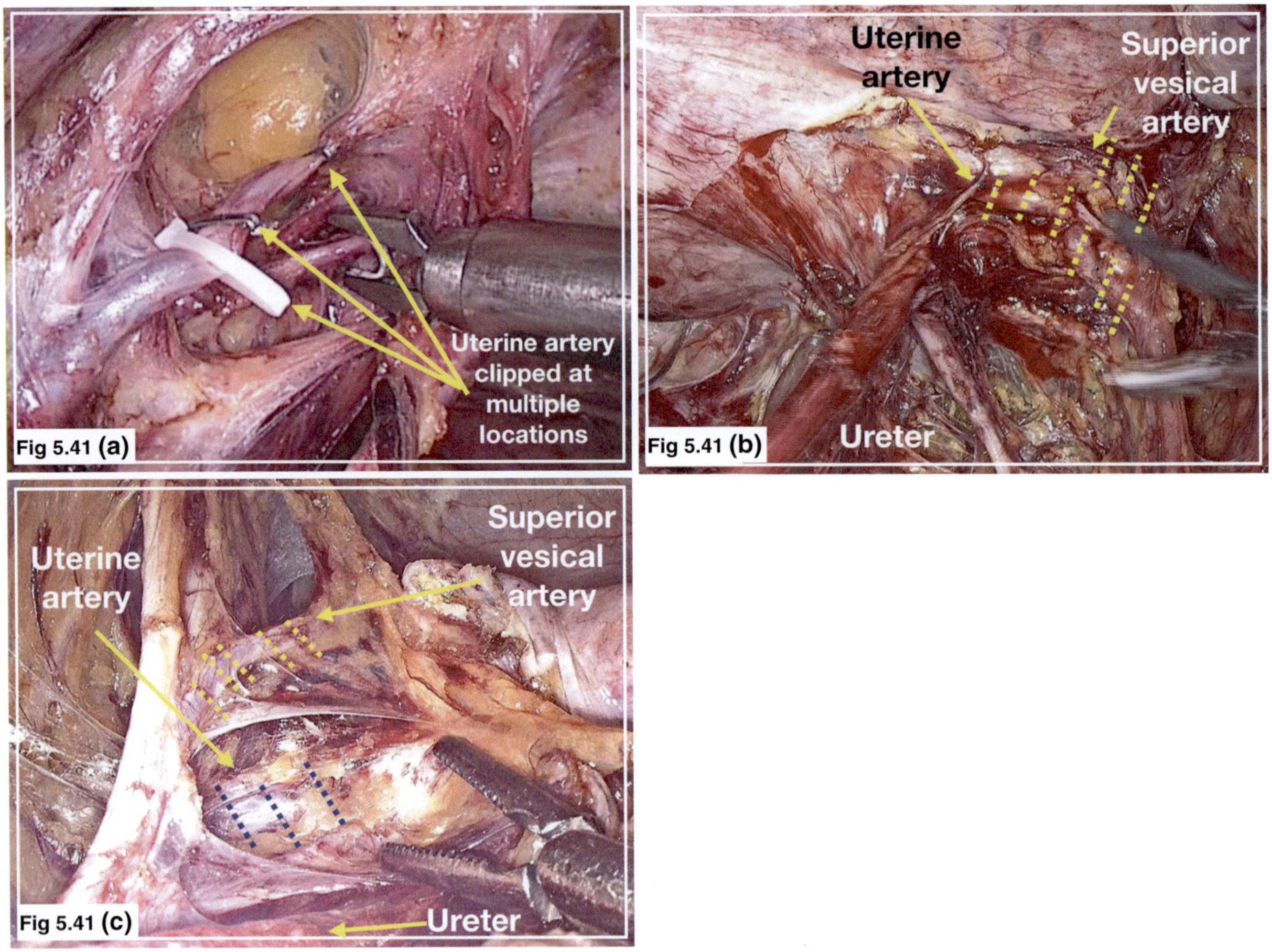

Fig. 5.41 (**a**) The image has been taken from a case of laparoscopic radical hysterectomy. The uterine artery can be seen ligated at multiple sites. This indicates that the uterine artery is available for ligation along its entire length. (**b**, **c**) Similar images of laparoscopic radical hysterectomy shows potential areas where the uterine and the superior vesical artery can be ligated as laterally as possible till its origin on the internal iliac artery

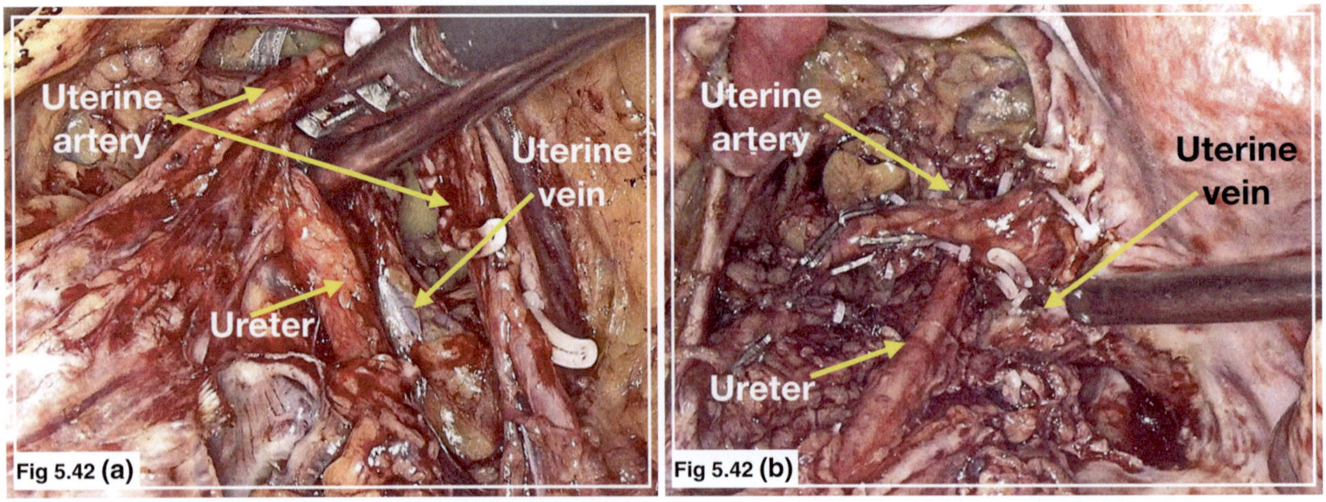

Fig. 5.42 (**a**, **b**) Images of the ureter lying in the fork between the uterine artery (above) and the uterine (below). This precise anatomy helps in understanding the source of bleeding as explained in the text

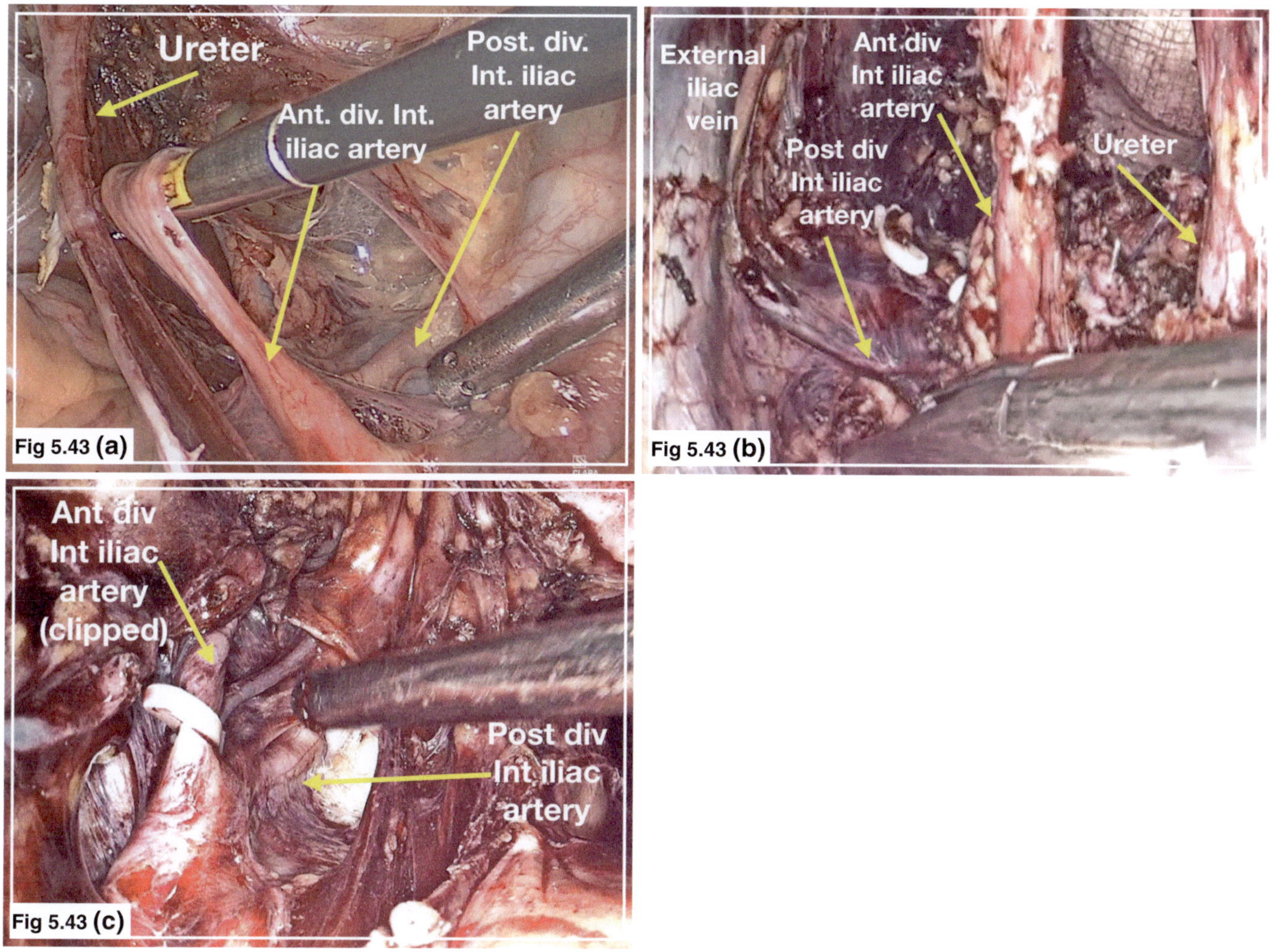

Fig. 5.43 (**a**) In this image of internal iliac artery dissection the posterior division can be seen clearly arising a few centimetres from the bifurcation of the common iliac artery and turning backwards to supply the gluteal region. (**b**) The close location of the site of ligation of the anterior division of internal iliac artery from the origin of the posterior division of the internal iliac artery can be seen clearly. The posterior division is in between the lips of the empty clip applicator to show its location more precisely. (**c**) The clips applied at the anterior division of internal iliac artery for a case of anterior exenteration where both uterine and superior vesical artery have to be sacrificed; hence the clip can be safely applied on the entire anterior division but few centimetres away to be safely away from the posterior division of the internal iliac artery

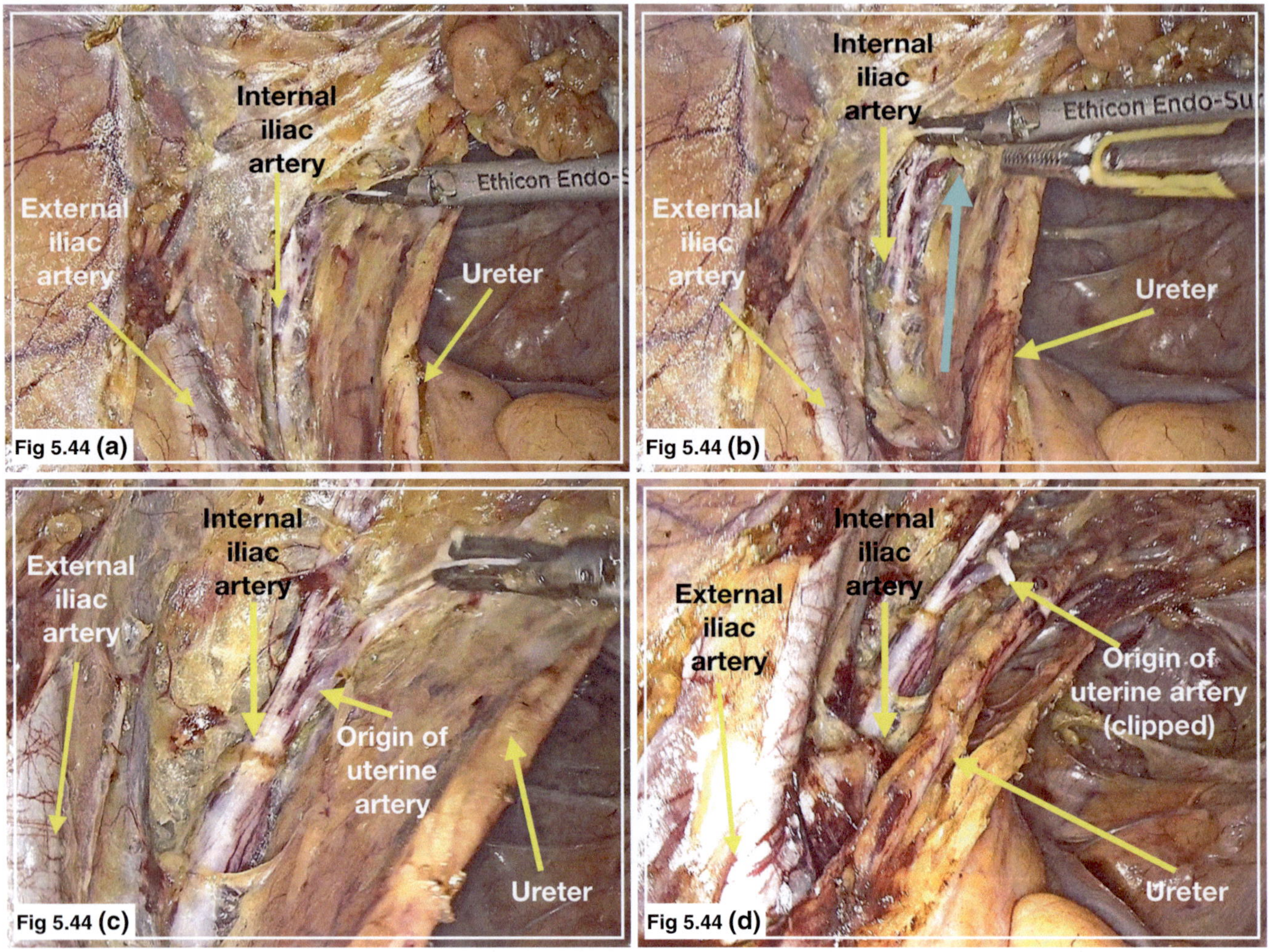

Fig. 5.44 The series of images show lateral vascular control. (**a**) Incision lateral to the sacral promontory opening the pararectal space. The external iliac, internal iliac vessels and ureter and its co-relations identified. (**b**) The direction of dissection has been shown in the light of blue arrow remaining parallel and at the same level as that of the ureter has been explained. (**c**) The origin of the uterine artery has been identified at the anterior division of internal iliac artery. (**d**) The uterine artery has been clipped at its lateral-most part, at its origin at the external iliac artery

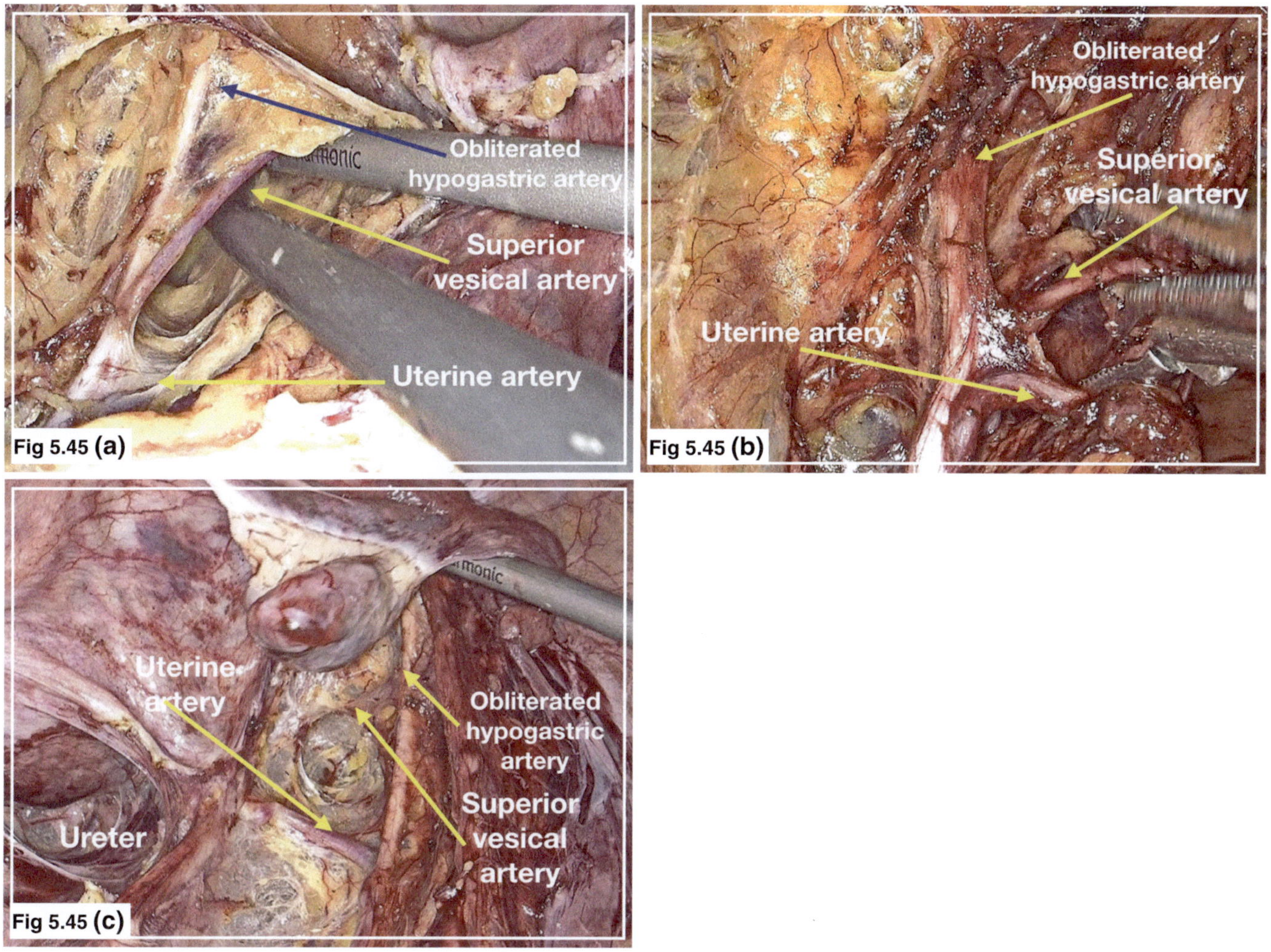

Fig. 5.45 (**a**–**c**) Series of images show that the next vessel arising from the medial side of the anterior division of the internal iliac artery is superior vesical artery in females

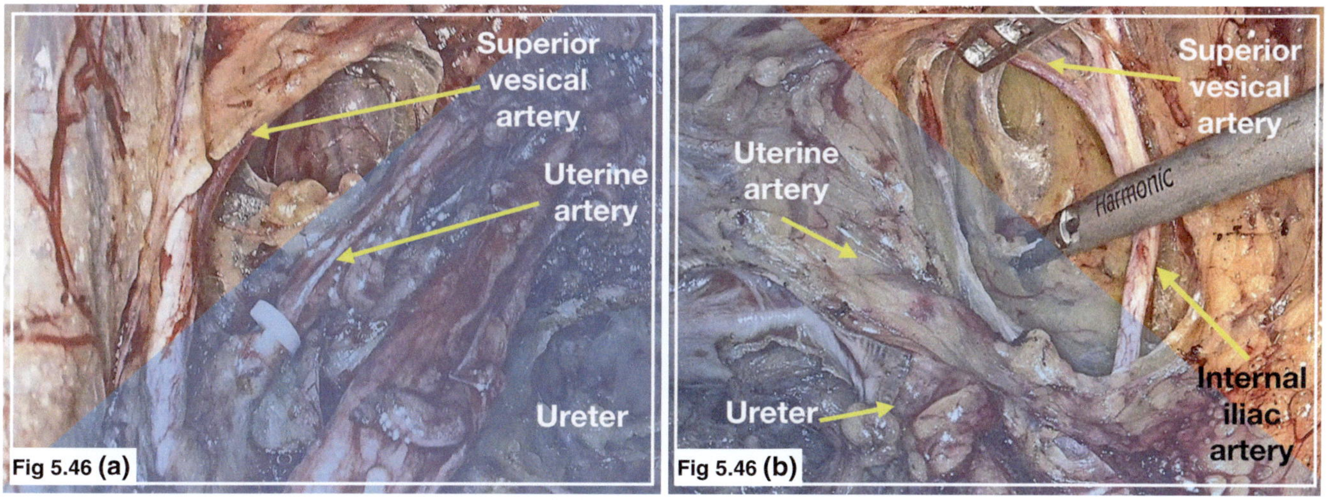

Fig. 5.46 (**a**–**d**) Series of images showing the superior vesical artery lying at a higher plane or more anterior than the uterine artery. The superior vesical artery has no clinical correlation with the ureter like the uterine eatery. Thus it is always safe in radical surgeries as most focus is towards separating the ureter from the uterine artery above it, only focussed during anterior exenterations. The operative area concerned is shaded in blue, thus keeping the superior vesical artery safe from any intervention

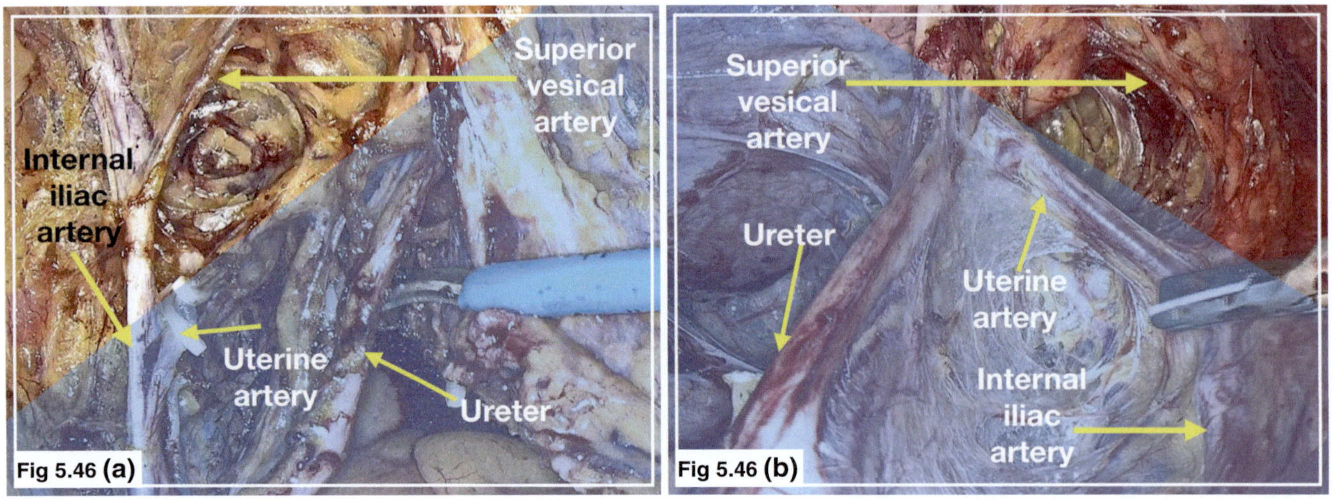

Fig. 5.46 (continued)

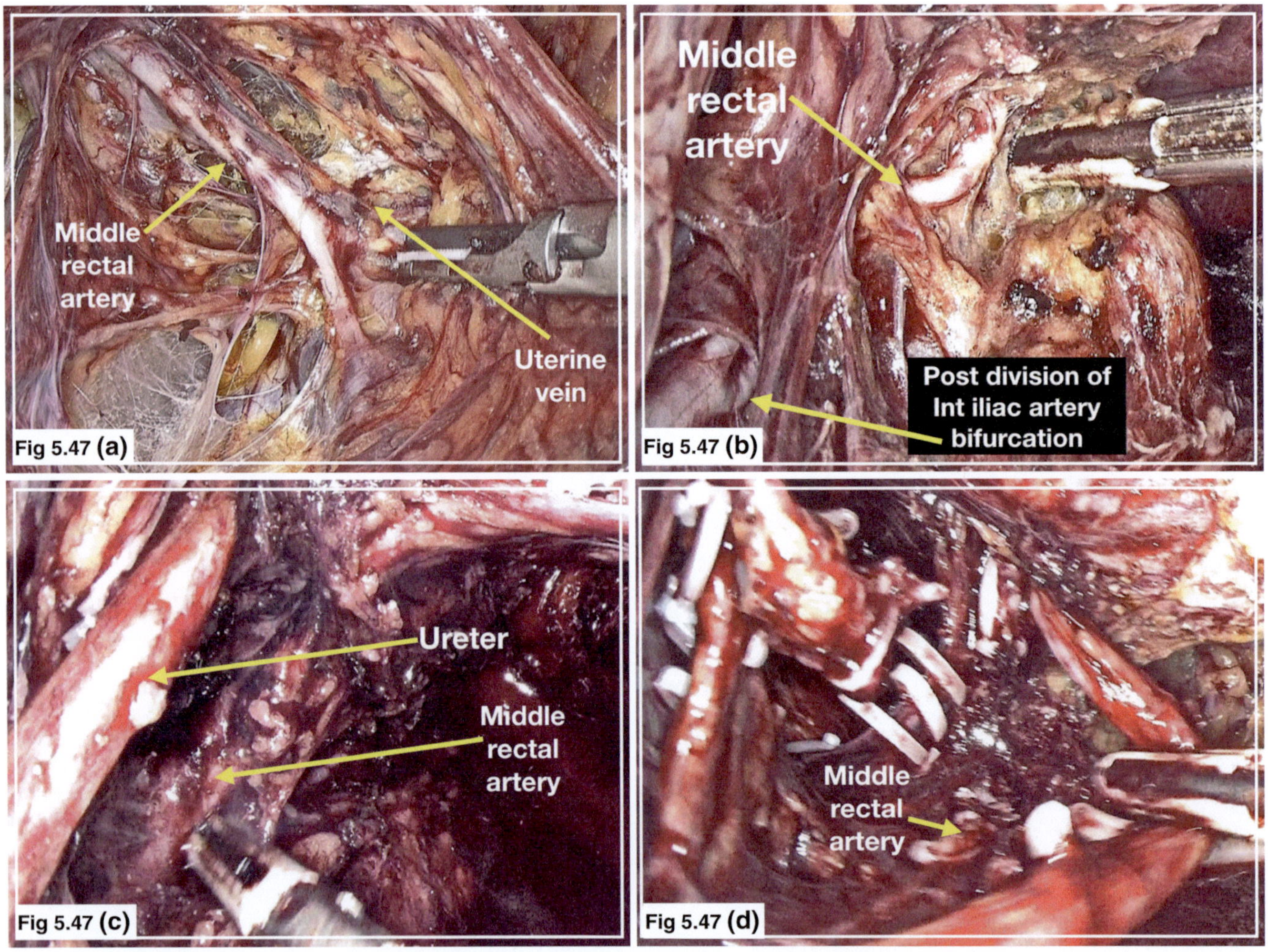

Fig. 5.47 (**a**–**d**) The middle rectal artery can be seen arising from the posterior division of internal iliac artery

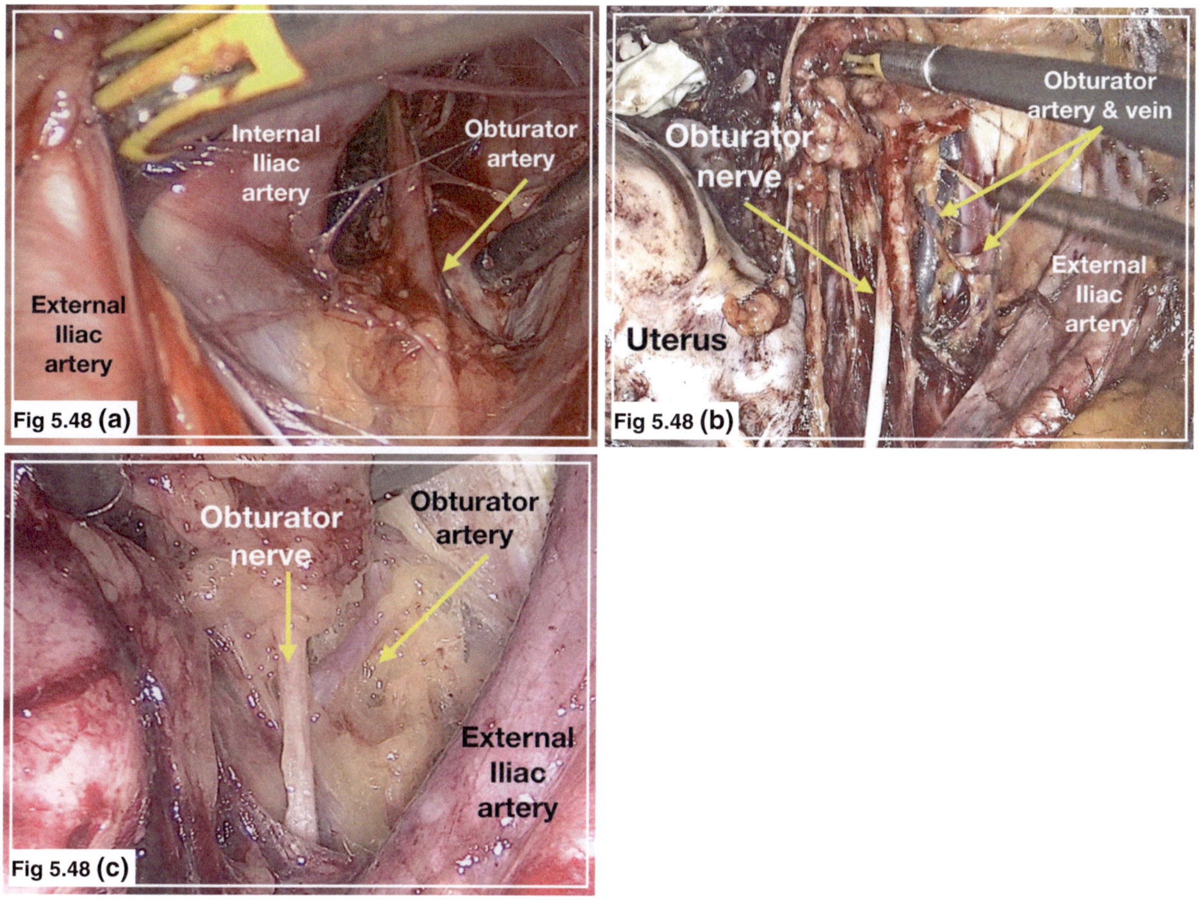

Fig. 5.48 (**a**–**c**) The series of images show the obturator artery from its origin lateral to the internal iliac artery

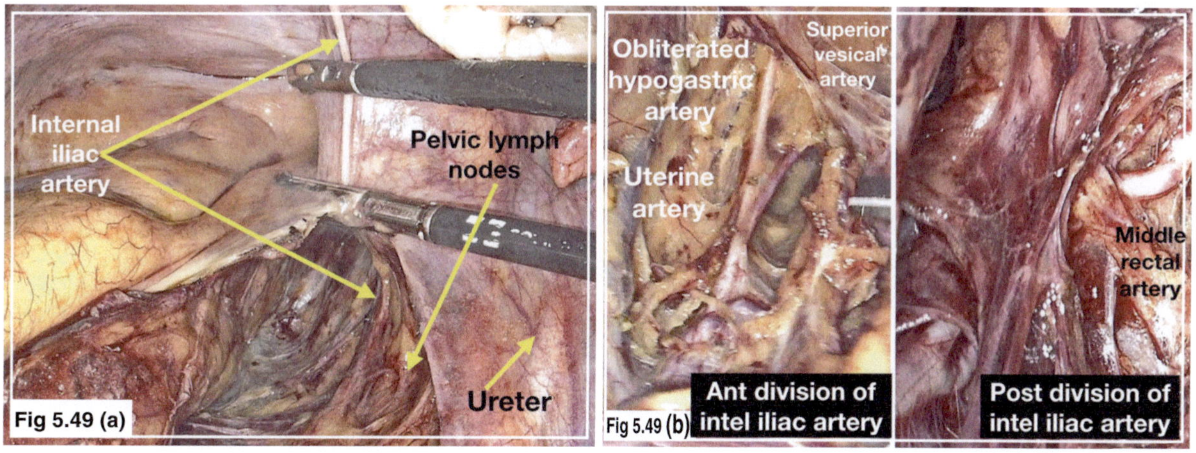

Fig. 5.49 (**a**) The image is from a case of laparoscopic low anterior resection. The ureter can be identified and the internal iliac vessel can also be identified but the obturator vessels are not visible even though the ilio-obturator nodes are visible. (**b**) Final view of the anterior and posterior divisions of internal iliac artery with its branches after dissection

5.2.3 Rules

- If one stays medial to the artery, the risk of damaging the obturator nerve or external vessels is minimal (Fig. 5.50).

During the obturator nodal dissection the artery can be salvaged by the remaining anterior to the nerve (Fig. 5.51).

There is a direct branch of internal iliac artery which supplies the ureter (Fig. 5.52).

Salient points of surgical anatomy of internal iliac artery

1. There is 6 cm length of internal iliac artery available for ligation before it gives its first branch (Fig. 5.53).
2. The uterine artery and the superior vesical traverse along a distance before they enter the organs (Fig. 5.54).
3. Obliterated hypogastric artery divides the vascular and avascular spaces (Fig. 5.55).
4. The internal iliac artery forms the lateral boundary of paravesical and pararectal spaces. The only structures which cross these spaces transversally are the arteries on their entrance to the organs (Fig. 5.56).
5. The internal iliac vein is closely hugging the artery posteriorly (Fig. 5.57).
6. The middle rectal artery is inconsistent (Fig. 5.58).

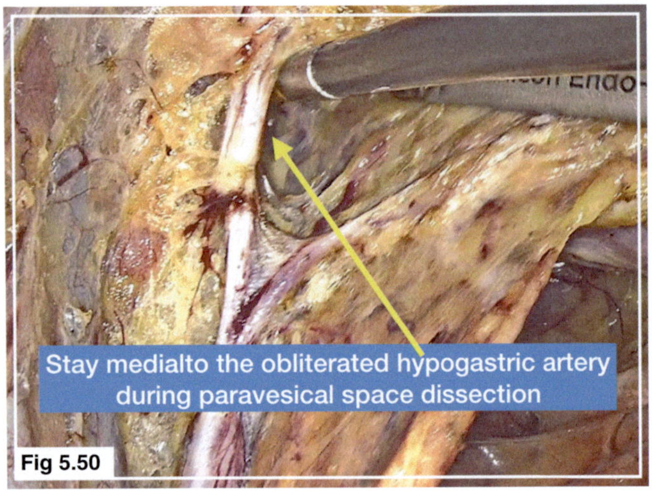

Fig. 5.50 Staying medial to the obliterated hypogastric artery during paravesical space dissection maintains a clean dissection without any haemorrhage

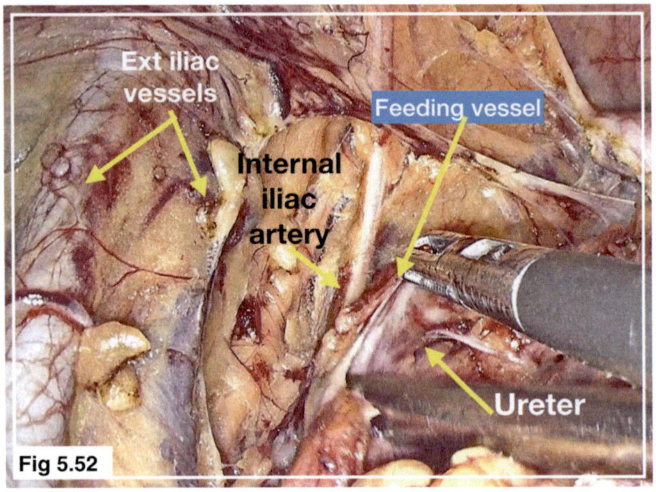

Fig. 5.52 The feeding vessel can be seen from the internal iliac artery to the ureter. The ureter receives such feeding vessels all along its entire course from nearby vessels from the ovarian artery, internal iliac artery, uterine artery and even superior vesical artery in a complex uniform mesenteric manner instead of segmental supply

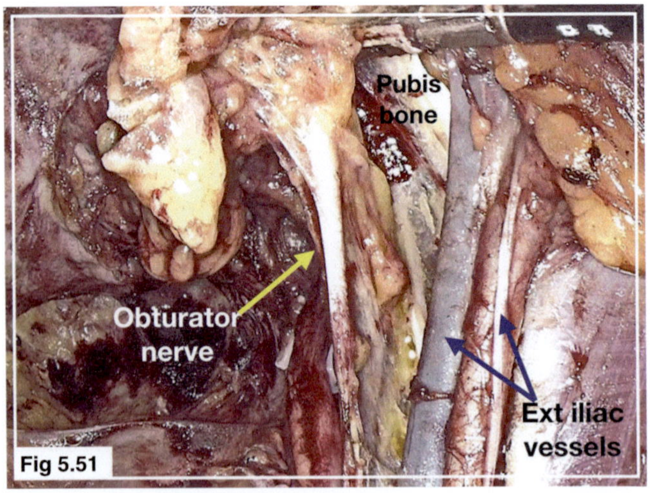

Fig. 5.51 Staying anterior to the obturator nerve prevents untoward injury to the underlying obturator artery and vein which causes significant haemorrhage

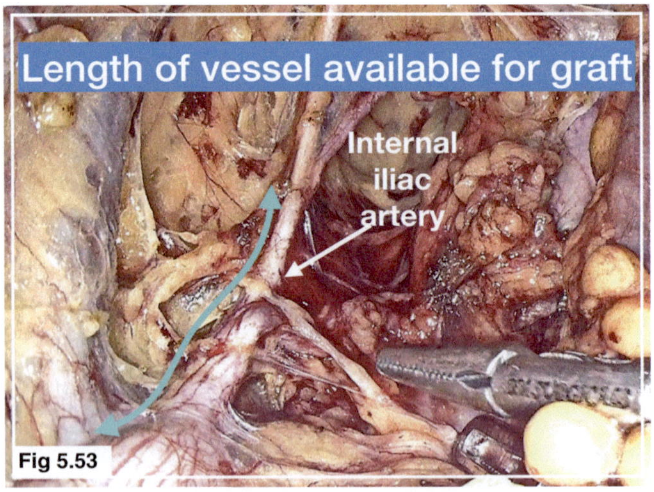

Fig. 5.53 The length of the internal iliac artery can be assessed for the purpose of harvesting vessels for uterine transplant

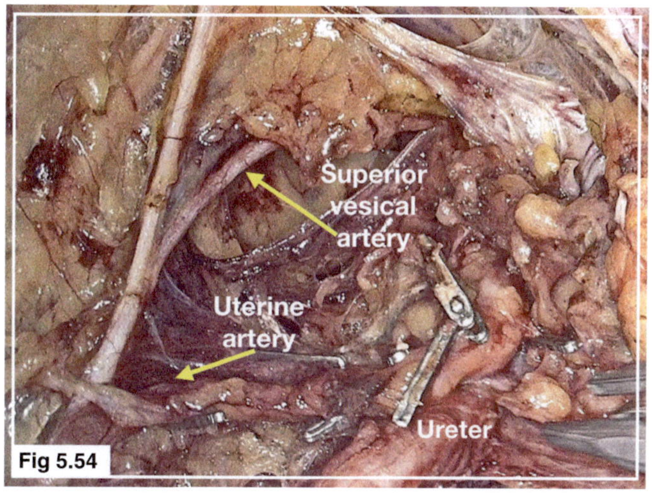

Fig. 5.54 The uterine and the superior vesical artery travel across the entire pararectal space to supply their respective organs. This provides adequate lateral coagulation in the condition of haemorrhage

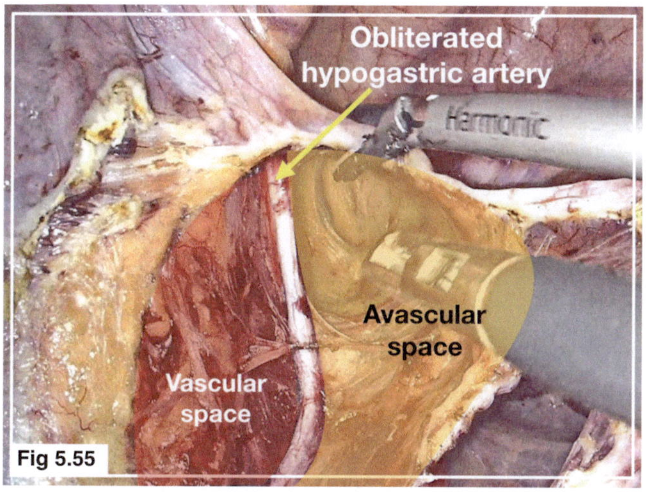

Fig. 5.55 The obliterated hypogastric artery divides the paravesical space into medial avascular and lateral vascular space. The lateral space contains lymph nodes for ilio-obturator node dissection and hence it is considered vascular

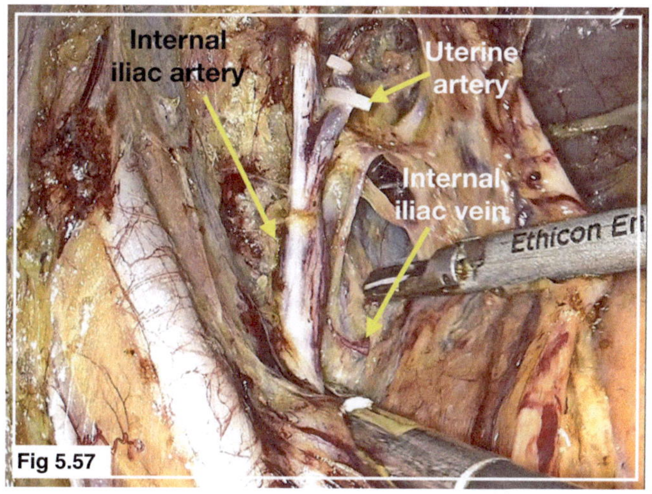

Fig. 5.57 The internal iliac vein lies very close to the internal iliac artery. It can be easily dissected from close to the origin of the uterine artery

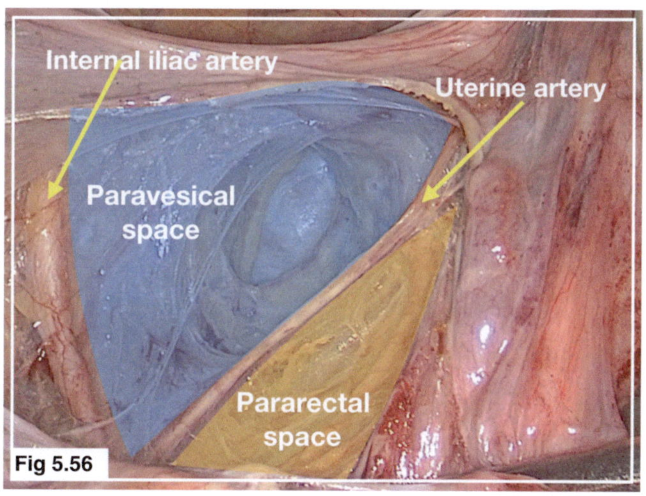

Fig. 5.56 The internal iliac artery forms the boundary for both the pararectal and the paravesical space

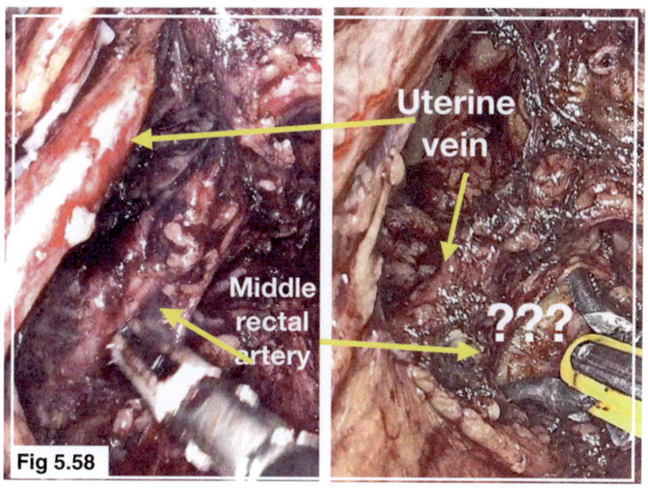

Fig. 5.58 Inconsistency of the course of the medial rectal artery can be compared in two images showing the uterine vein above in both images but only one image shows the middle rectal artery

5.3 Uterine Artery

The artery originates as the first branch of anterior division of internal iliac artery. It is tortuous and traverses a long distance transversely in the lateral pararectal space to reach the uterus. This course allows it to be accommodated during the enlargement of uterus (Fig. 5.59a–e).

The diameter of uterine artery is approximately 7 mm; thus it can be coagulated by either the Harmonic or the LigaSure (Fig. 5.60a–d).

The artery crosses the ureter anteriorly on its way to uterus. It gives a branch to the ureter. This branch needs to be separated to free the ureter (Fig. 5.61a–d).

During surgery the artery needs to be cut with scissors as any energy source will cause thermal damage to the ureter (Fig. 5.62a–c).

There are multiple small branches of the uterine artery. This is seen during its dissection from its origin till it supplies the uterus. These branches supply the ureter, mesorectum and Mackenrodt's ligament (Fig. 5.63a–c).

The artery enters the uterus at the level of internal os (Fig. 5.64a, b).

A small vein invariably accompanies the artery but it is not the uterine vein. It then divides into ascending and descending branches. The descending branch is called as cervical branch and supplies the cervix and upper vagina.

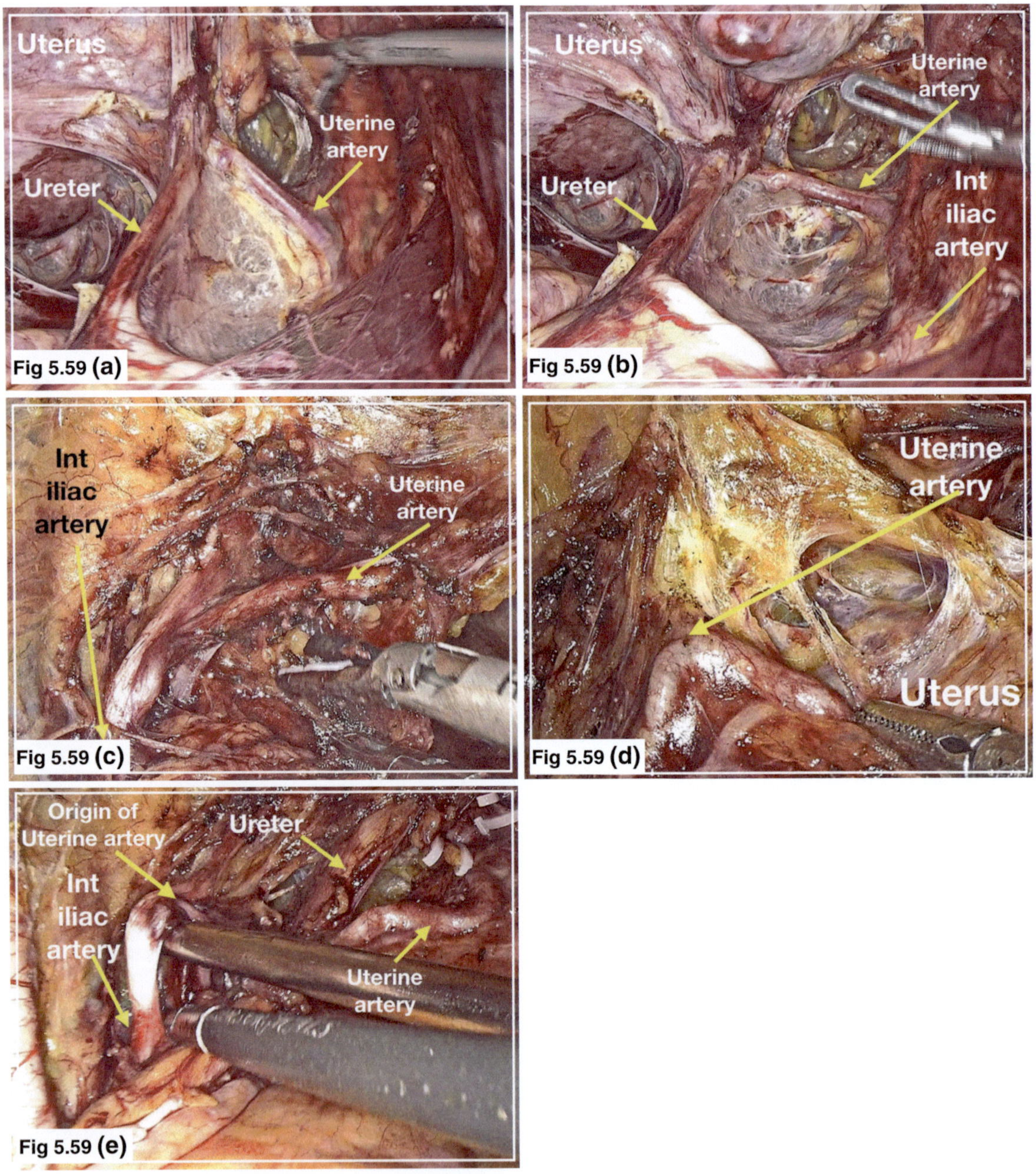

Fig. 5.59 (a–e) This series of images show the tortuous course of the uterine artery from its origin at the anterior division of the internal iliac artery to its supplying the uterus

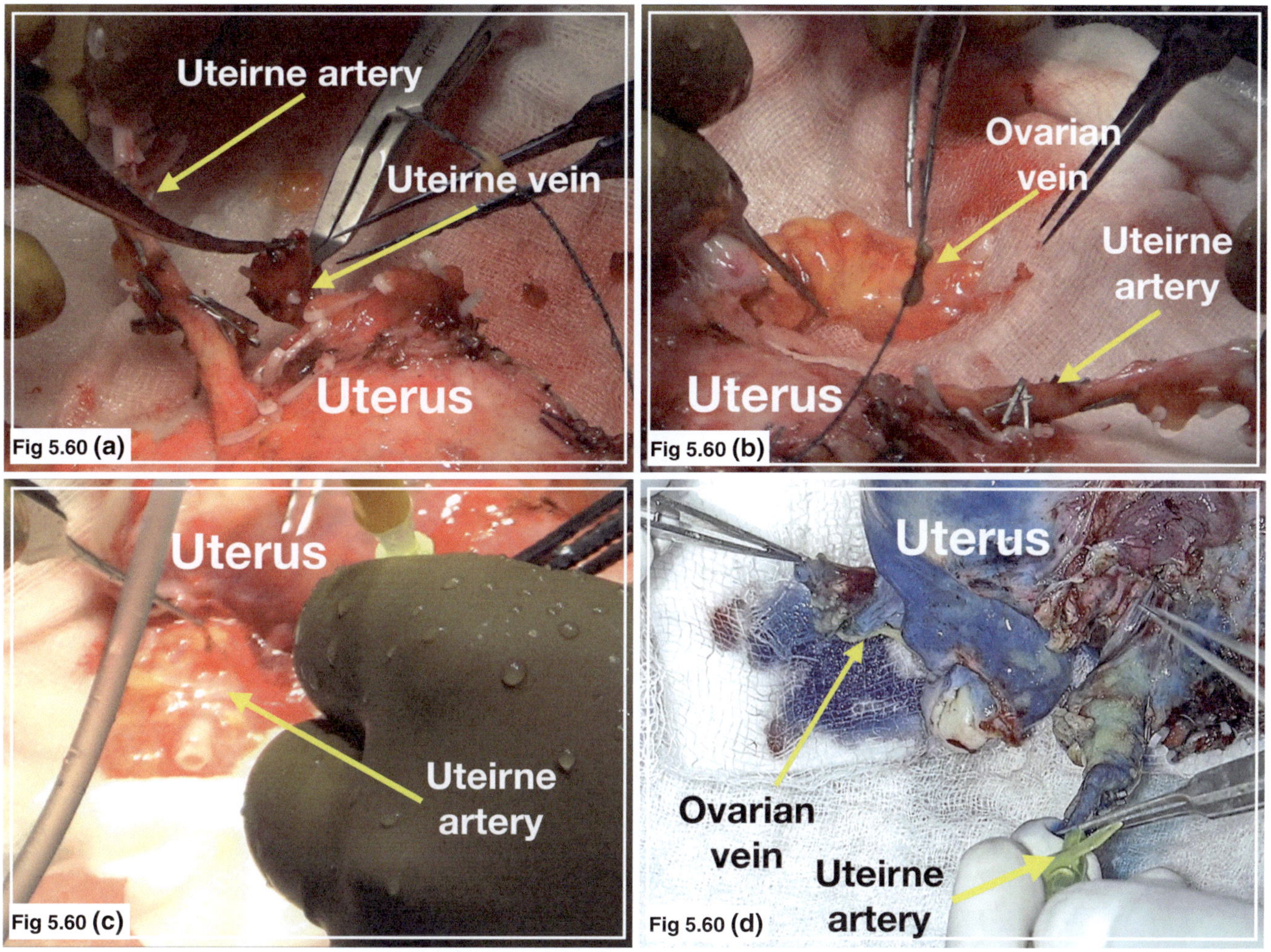

Fig. 5.60 (**a**–**c**) This series of images have been taken from the bench surgery of the donor uterus for uterine transplant. The uterine artery has been dissected in its entire length and the venous outflow is maintained by ovarian veins as shown in the image. (**d**) This image demonstrates the patency of the utero-ovarian anastomosis. Methylene blue dye has been injected into the uterine artery and its outflow can be seen in the ovarian vein

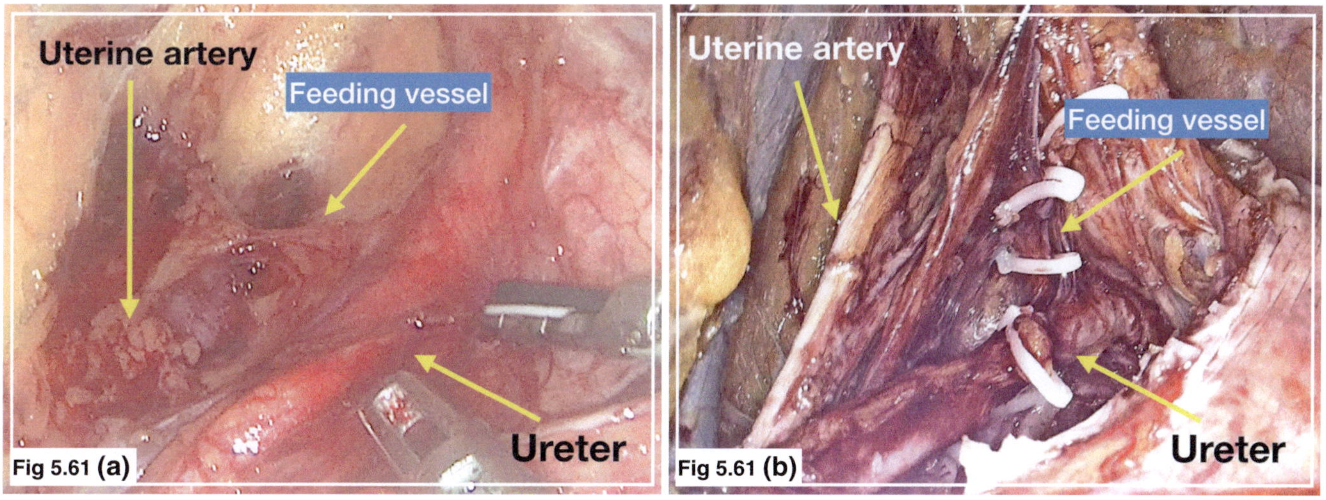

Fig. 5.61 (**a**–**d**) The series of images show the various feeding vessels from the uterine artery to the ureter. These feeding vessels are seen maximum during transplant surgery as they hold clinical significance in controlling haemorrhage during re-anastomosis

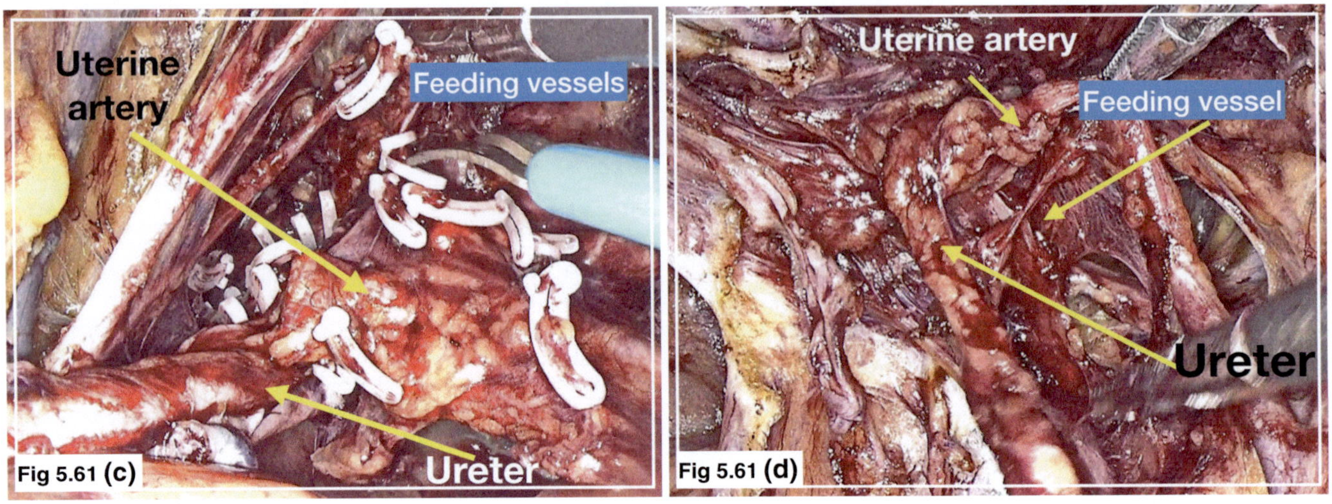

Fig. 5.61 (continued)

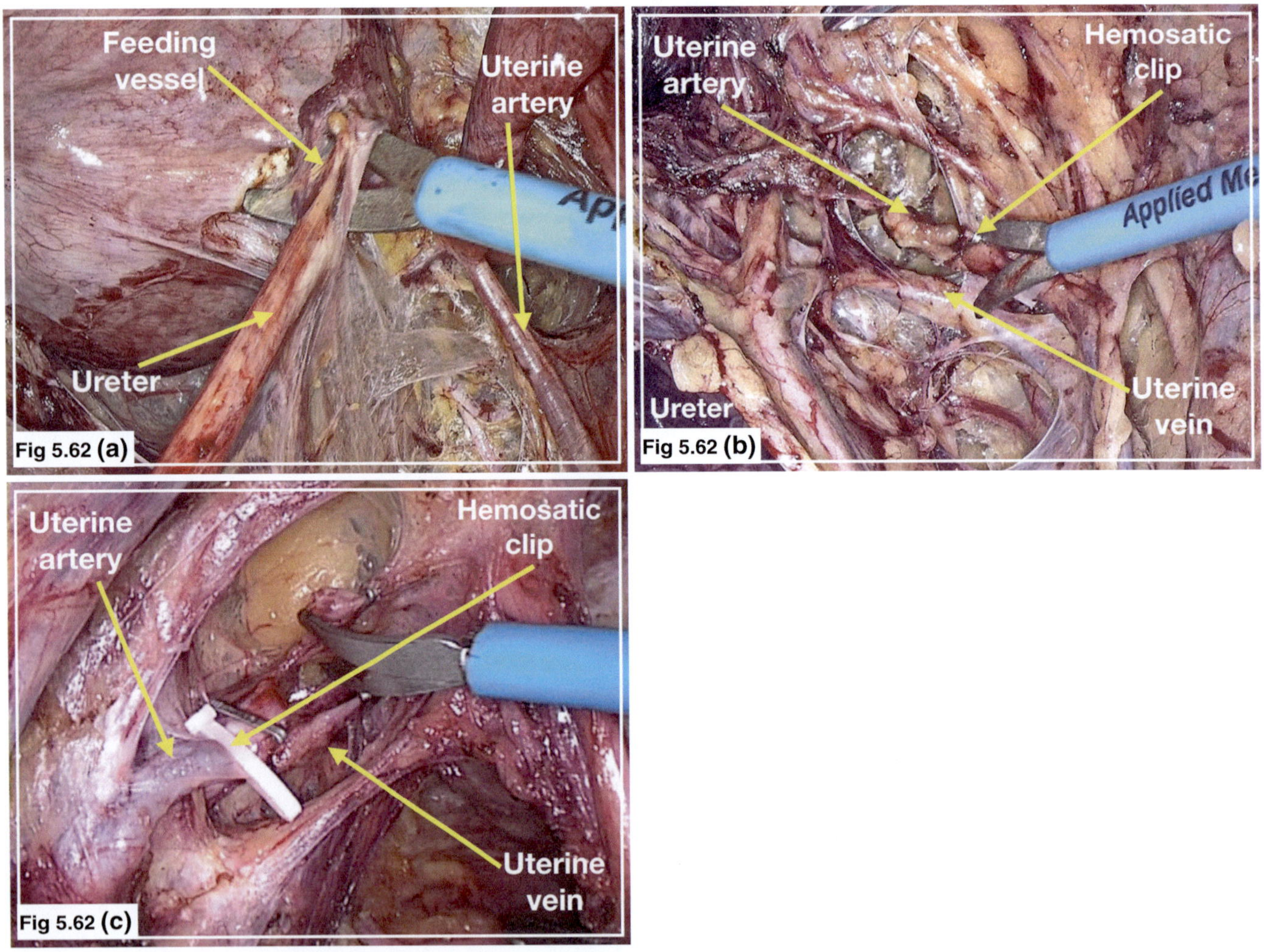

Fig. 5.62 (**a**) The image shows the feeding vessel being held between the blades of cold scissor. Uterine artery lies in close proximity to the ureter; thus it is always discouraged to use energy sources for coagulation and cutting due to the higher incidence of thermal injury due to lateral spread. (**b**) Cold scissors are almost always used in conjunction with homeostatic clips to prevent bleeding as shown in this image. (**c**) The clips can be applied at multiple locations and without the use of any motorised instruments making it very compliant with the surgeon and cold scissors

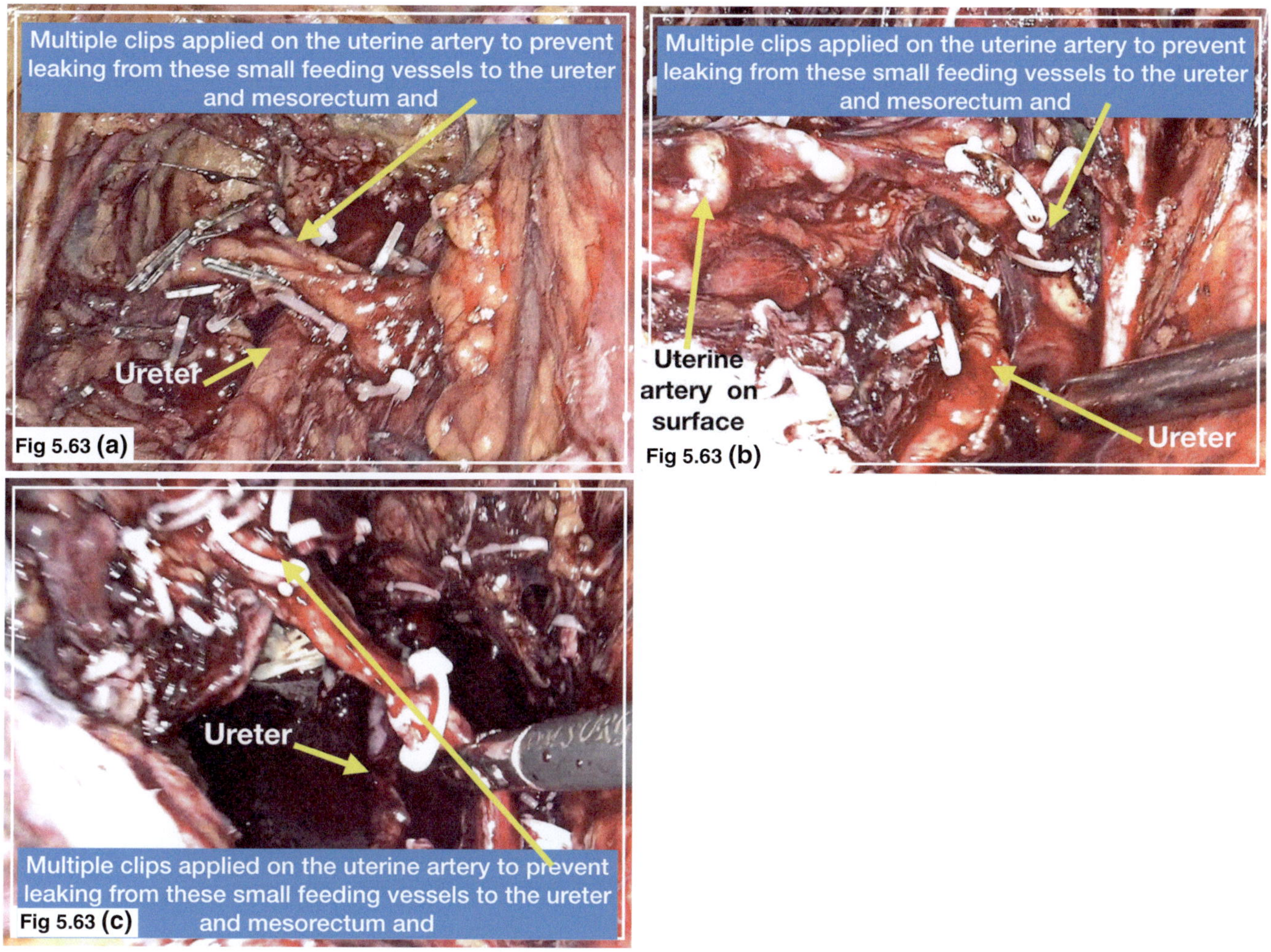

Fig. 5.63 (**a**–**c**) The series of images taken in cases of dissection of donor uterus for uterine transplant which show the multiple small feeding vessels arising from the uterine artery supplying the mesorectum, Mackenrodt's ligament and ureter which have been clipped and cut to prevent leakage during re-anastomosis

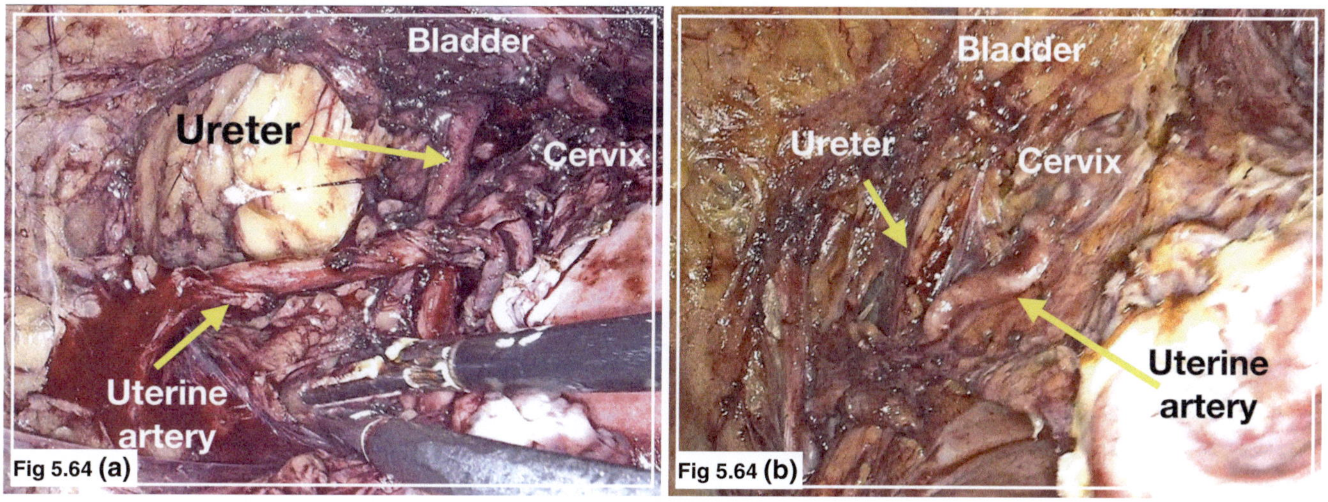

Fig. 5.64 (**a**, **b**) These two images show the uterine artery entering the uterus above the level of the cervix. This corresponds to the level of the internal os. The ureter can be seen below the uterine artery travelling straight and inserting into the bladder

The ascending branch runs paracervically upwards for some distance before entering the uterus (Fig. 5.65a–e).

This allows the surgeon to clamp only the ascending branch to uterine proximally, way above the internal os. The main advantage of taking the artery higher up is avoiding the descending branch and having a long stump of the artery. The descending cervical can be avoided by staying medial to the uterine artery after cutting (Fig. 5.66a, b).

The main supply to the uterus comes from the ascending branch and hence all the fibroids grow in the upward direction. The arterial supply thus comes from below. This allows the entire separation of the myoma till the base. Had there been supply coming from all around the myoma separation would not have been possible. Also due to the blood supply coming from the base, the depth of the cavity needs to be closed carefully to avoid secondary haemorrhage (Fig. 5.67a–d).

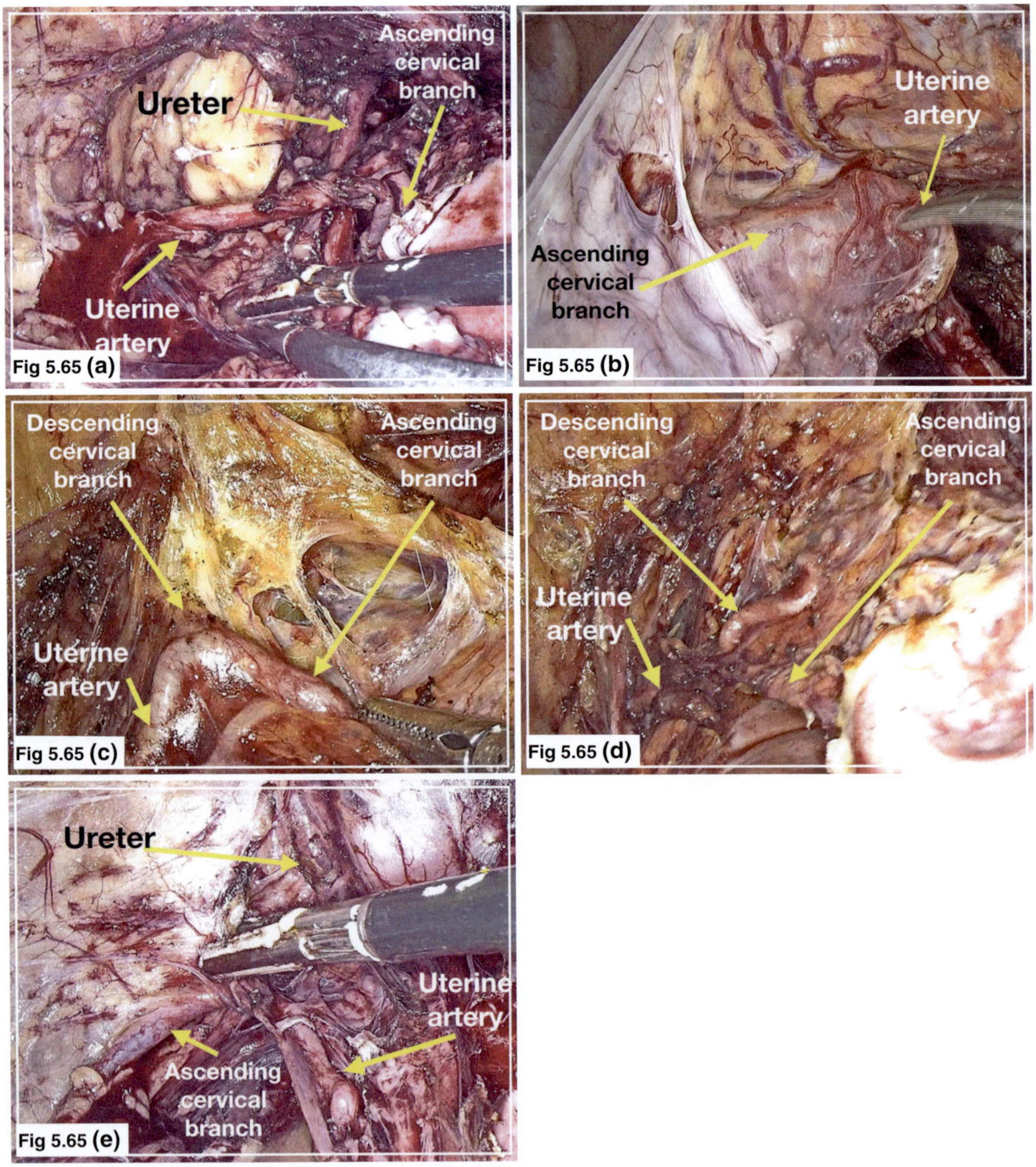

Fig. 5.65 (a–e) This series of images show the uterine artery dividing into ascending and descending branches. The descending branch is called as the descending cervical branch while the ascending branch is the uterine artery proper

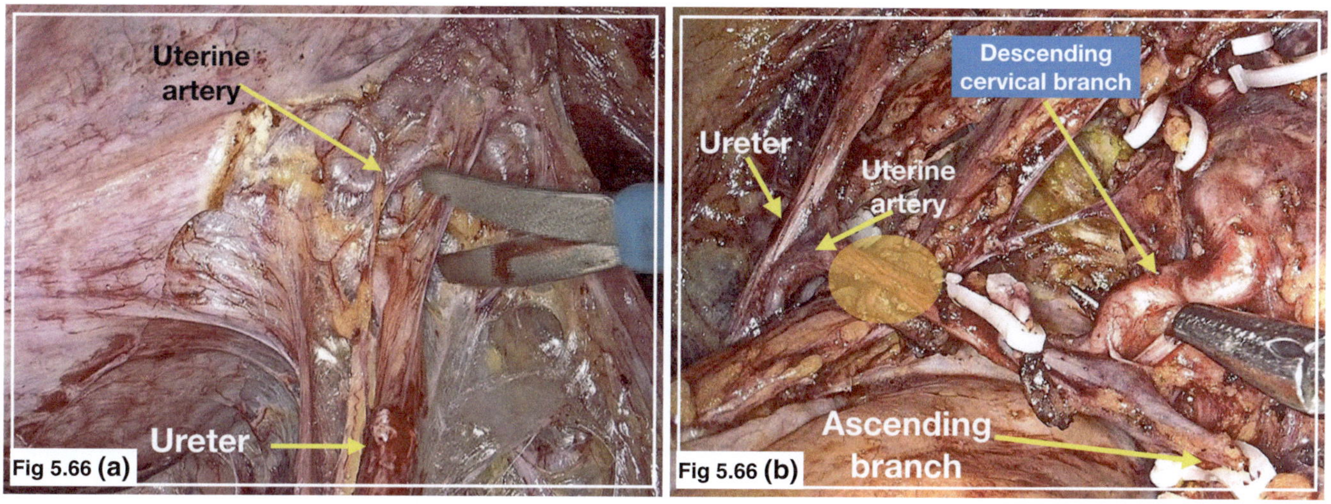

Fig. 5.66 (**a**) The uterine artery can be seen travelling over the ureter and into a further tortuous course as the ascending branch. The best place to ligate the uterine artery is before it gives off the descending cervical branch and after it crosses over the ureter. (**b**) Both the branches of the uterine artery can be seen here as ascending and descending cervical branches. The ureter can be seen inserting into the bladder and the uterine artery can be seen changing its course towards the uterus. The area shaded in yellow is the best area to clamp and cut the uterine artery. It is away from the ureter and before the descending cervical branch

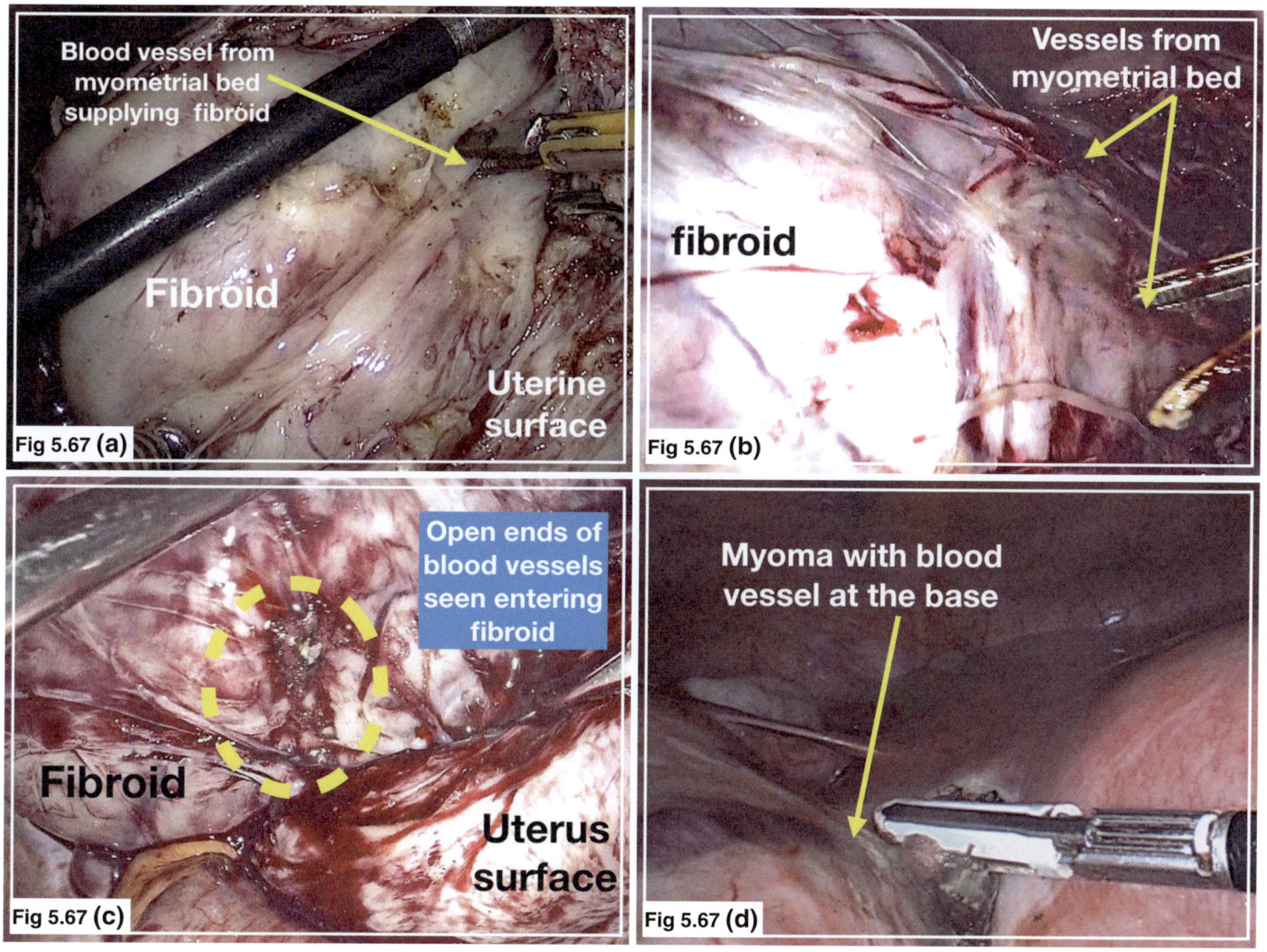

Fig. 5.67 (**a**–**d**) Series of images showing the fibroid with their blood vessels arising from the myometrial bed underneath. The vessels always lie below the fibroid or the fibroid always grows over the vessel

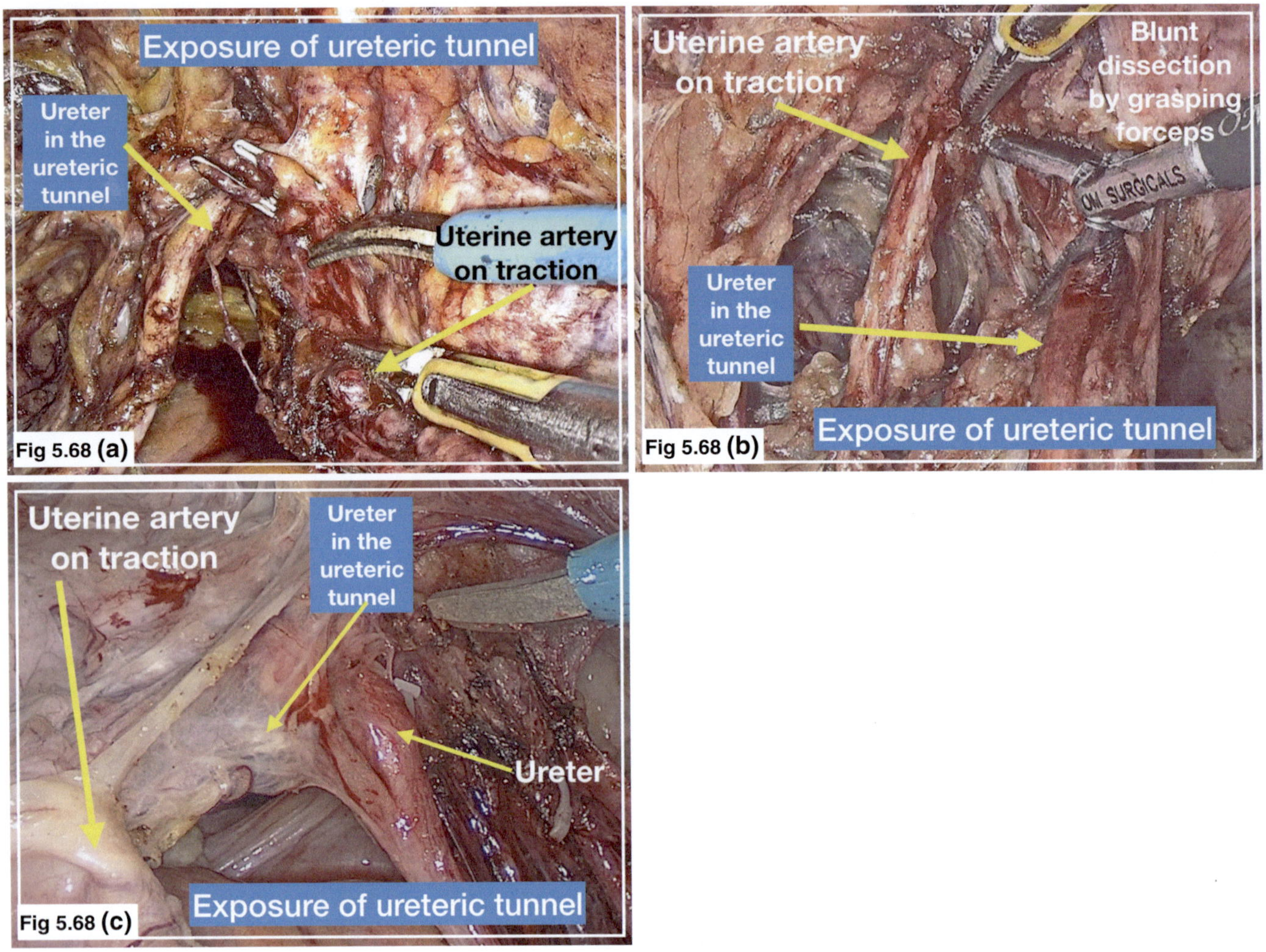

Fig. 5.68 (**a**–**c**) The series of images are from different cases of laparoscopic radical hysterectomy where dissection at the ureteric tunnel is shown by providing traction to the uterine artery stump and exposing the ureteric tunnel or the Wertheim's tunnel

In a radical hysterectomy the stump of the uterine has to be carefully reflected medially to lateralise the ureter (Fig. 5.68a–c).

5.3.1 Rules

1. Since the uterine artery traverses a long distance before reaching the organ, the artery can be clamped at multiple levels (Fig. 5.69a, b).
2. The pararectal space is the best place to ligate or clip the uterine artery (Fig. 5.70a, b).
3. All the subserosal fibroids of the uterus grow cranially; it is said that the growth of the fibroid over the uterine is like that of a tree over a stem. Thus by clamping uterine artery laterally during myomectomy, the blood supply of the fibroid can be decreased (Fig. 5.71).

5.4 Superior Vesical Artery

The superior vesical artery is the first branch of anterior division of internal iliac artery in males. It crosses the ureter anteriorly to reach the bladder (Fig. 5.72).

In females it is the second branch and arises at an anterior plane than the uterine artery (due to the fact that the bladder is anterior to the uterus). It therefore doesn't cross the ureter. Thus it can be avoided when opening the pararectal space (Fig. 5.73a–e).

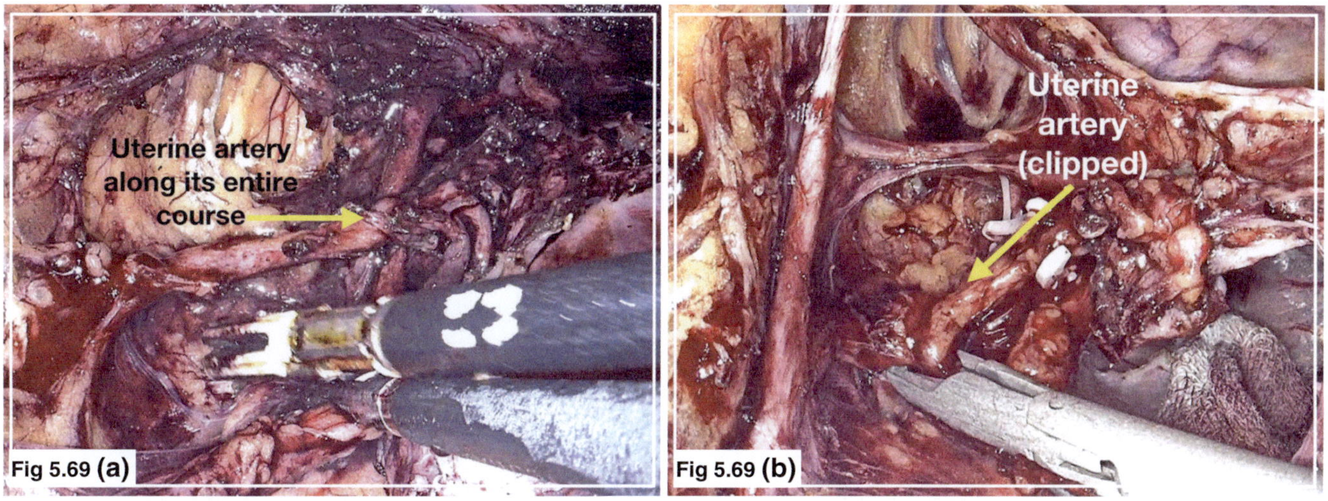

Fig. 5.69 (**a**, **b**) The images show the uterine artery along its entire course and thus all the various possible locations where the vessel can be clamped depending upon the surgeon's preference and comfort

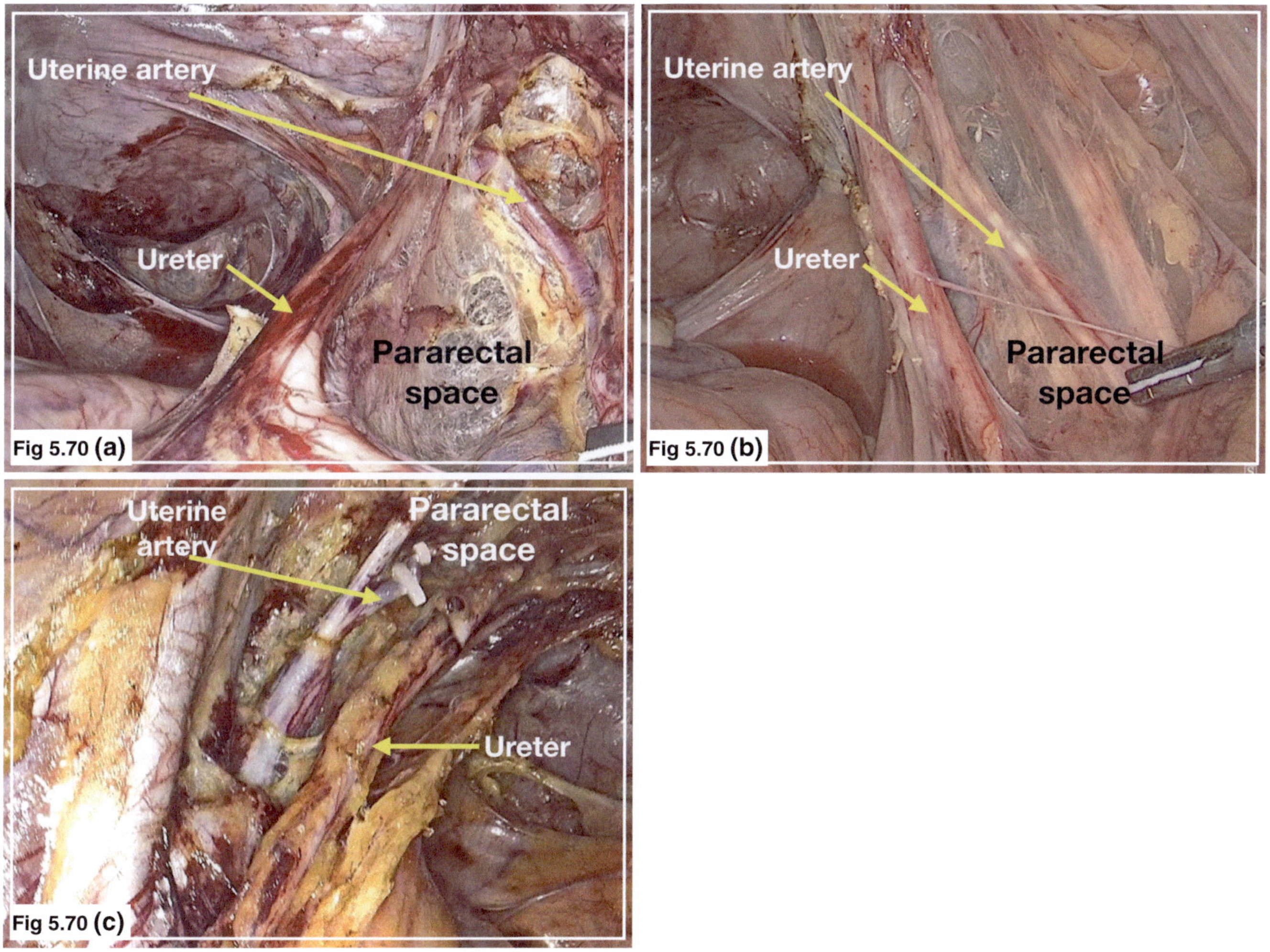

Fig. 5.70 (**a**–**c**) The uterine artery can be seen traversing across the entire pararectal space. Thus pararectal space is the best area for clamping the uterine artery at desired locations

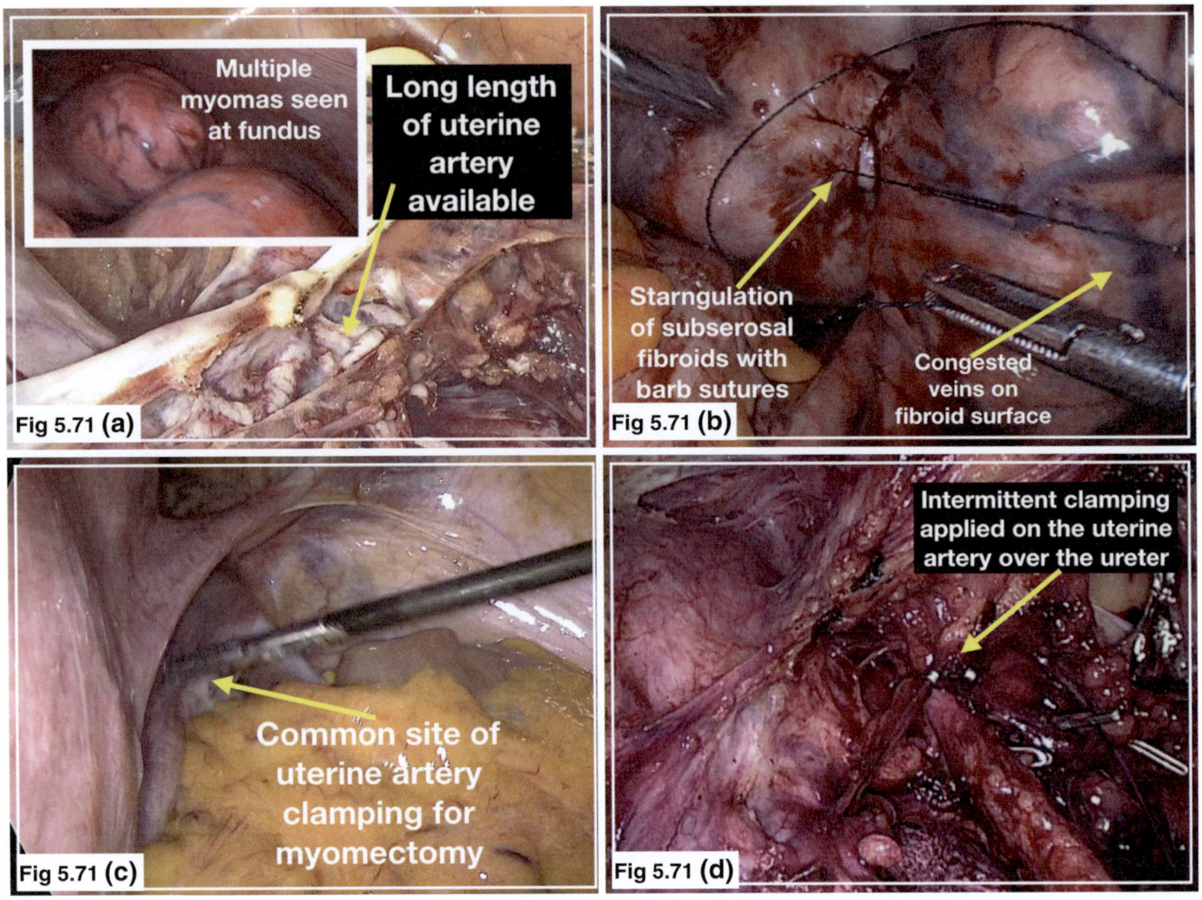

Fig. 5.71 (**a**) The long length of the uterine artery can be appreciated which is commonly clamped intermittently with temporary clips during myomectomy to reduce blood loss. Inset images show that most fibroids grow higher up in the uterus and mostly subserosal. (**b**) In case of small pedunculated subserosal fibroids with small stalk, the fibroid can be strangulated from the base with the help of barb sutures. The veins can be seen congested in their initial stages. This is followed by blanching of the fibroid and at this the myomectomy can be done. (**c**) Common site for intermittent clamping of the uterine artery for myomectomy. (**d**) The uterine artery has been clamped above the ureter for myomectomy. The steel clips are temporary and can be removed easily with laparoscopic forceps

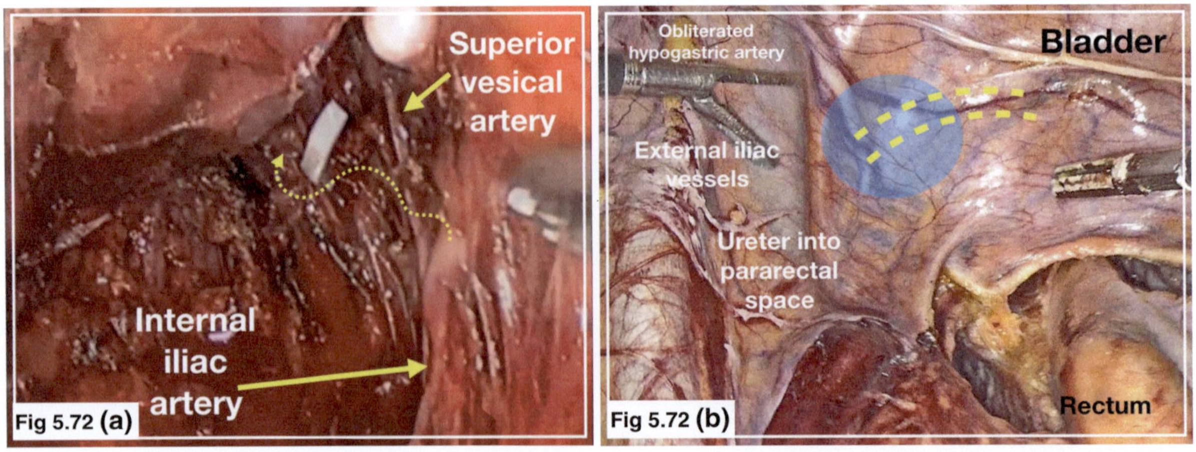

Fig. 5.72 (**a**) Image from a case of laparoscopic radical prostatectomy showing the superior vesical artery being the first branch of the internal iliac artery in males. (**b**) The image has been taken from a case of laparoscopic low anterior resection in a male patient. The ureter can be seen on the side dipping acutely into the pararectal space. The obliterated hypogastric artery can be seen travelling upwards. The area shaded in blue is the potential space for the organ of the superior vesical artery. The bladder in males is closely applied to the pubis bone and attached to the rectum in a shallow rectovaginal space or pouch of Douglas. Thus the ureter seldom encounters the superior vesical artery

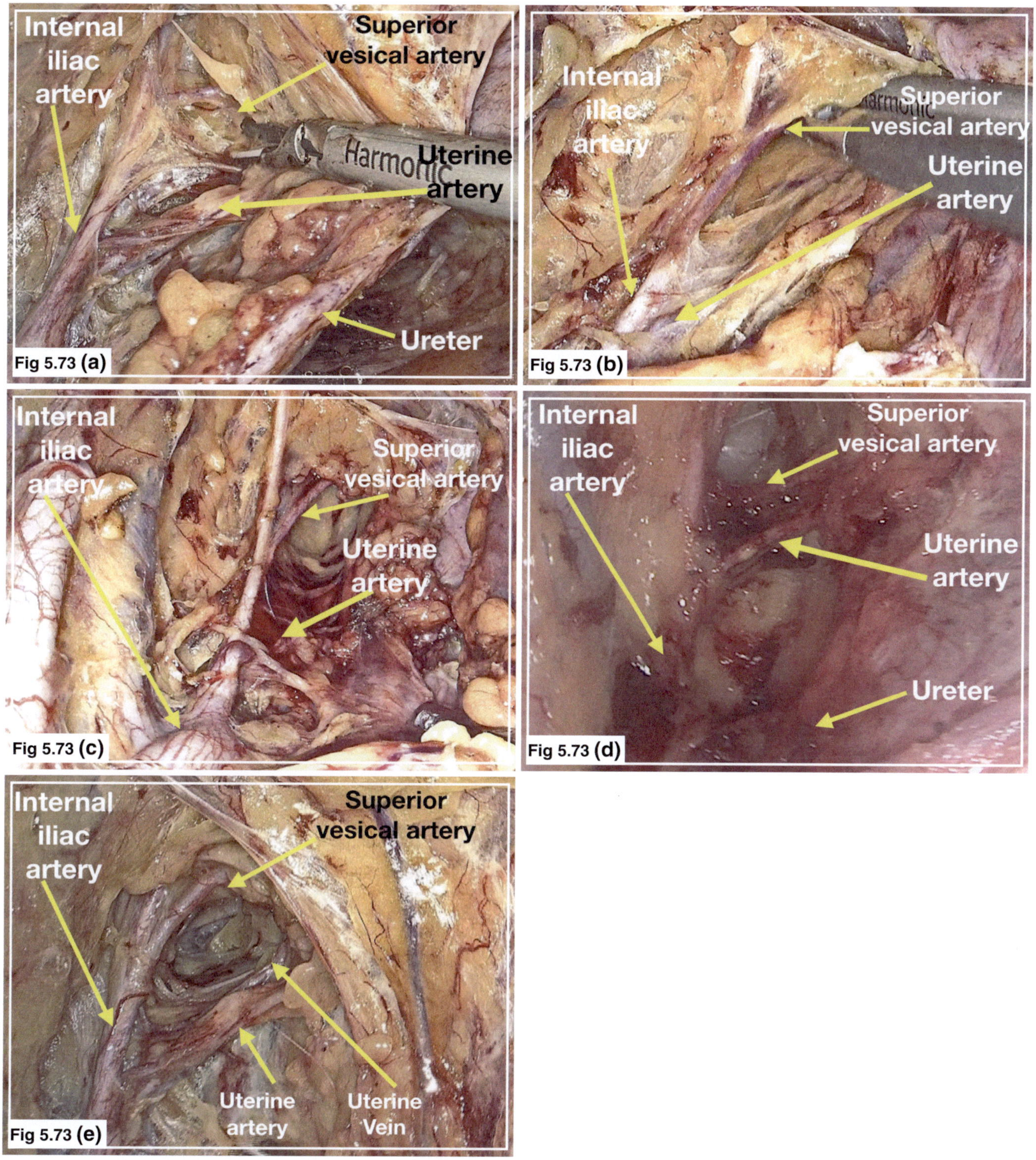

Fig. 5.73 (**a**) The supervesical artery is the second branch arising from the anterior division of internal iliac artery. It lies in the same plane but anterior to the uterine artery. (**b**) The superior vesical artery and the uterine artery form the boundaries of the paravesical space. The ureter has no relations with the paravesical space. Hence it is seldom encountered during ureteric dissection. (**c**) Though the superior vesical artery lies away from the ureter, it lies in the same plane as that of the uterine artery. It lies above the ureter and supplies the bladder anteriorly as seen in the image. (**d**) The superior vesical artery at times may be confused with the uterine vein. But the uterine vein lies underneath the uterine artery and is below the ureter. (**e**) In this image the uterine artery and the uterine vein and the superior vesical artery can also be seen in the same frame. Thus the correlation is explained here

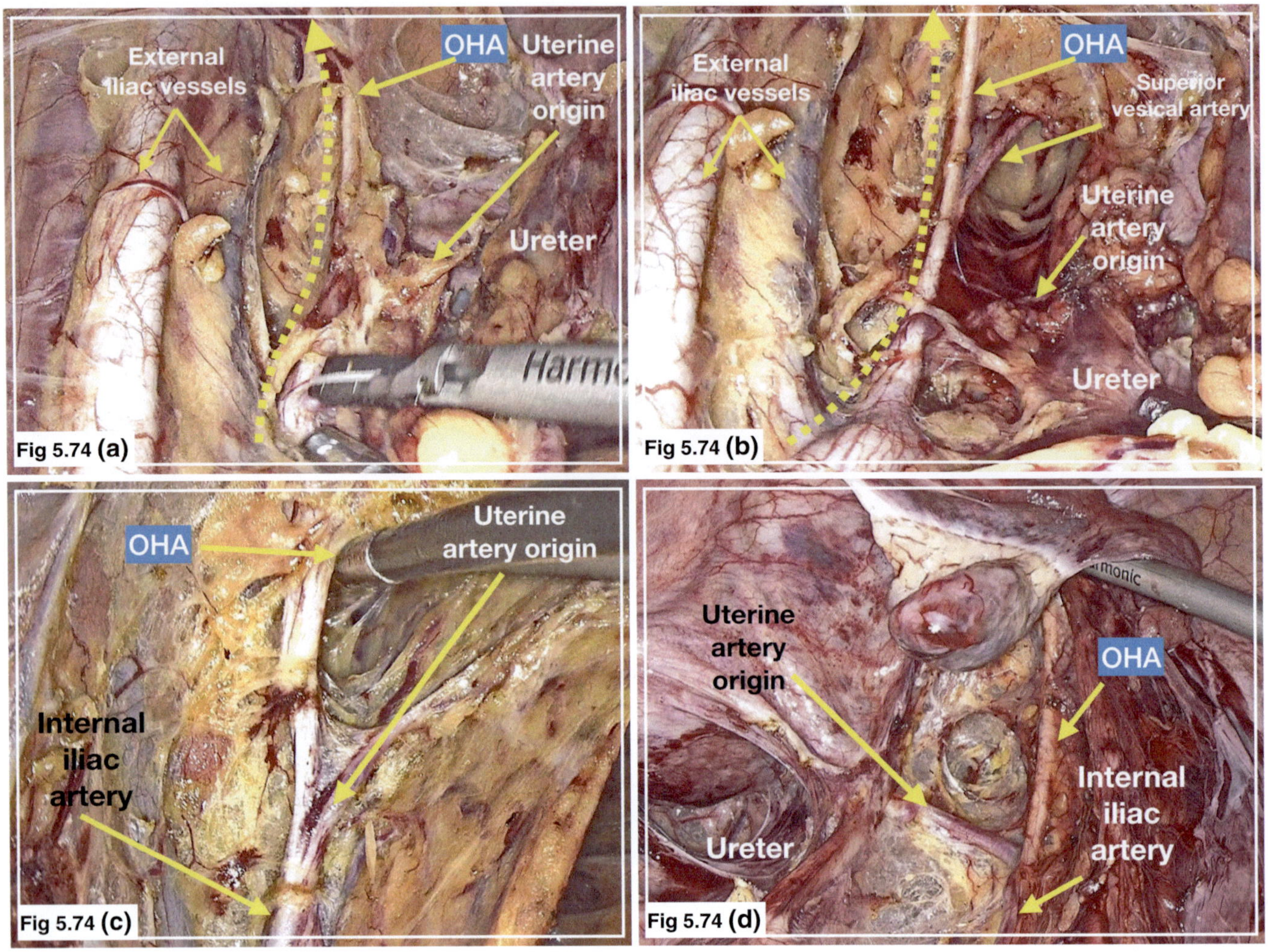

Fig. 5.74 (**a–d**) The series of images show the anterior division of internal iliac artery along its entire course and branches in the pararectal space and terminating as the obliterated hypogastric artery (OHA in blue) as it exits the pelvis at the level of the pubis bone

5.5 Obliterated Hypogastric Artery

The anterior division of the internal iliac artery ends as the obliterated hypogastric artery (Fig. 5.74a–d).

This forms the medial umbilical ligament on either side of the bladder. It ends by entering the bladder at the level of urethra (Fig. 5.75).

The paravesical space lies medial to it. The paravesical space is divided by the artery into lateral and medial paravesical space (Fig. 5.76).

The obturator fossa lies lateral to it. To avoid damage to the obturator vessels and nerves the dissection should remain medial to the artery (Fig. 5.77a).

5.5.1 Rules

1. The lateral limits for dissection in benign gynaecological surgery are obliterated hypogastric artery on either side.
2. The obturator nerves and veins are lateral to the artery; thus remaining medial avoids damage to these structures (Fig. 5.78).

The bladder lies between the two obliterated hypogastric arteries. To enter the prevesical space, one has to remain superomedial to the obliterated hypogastric artery (Fig. 5.79).

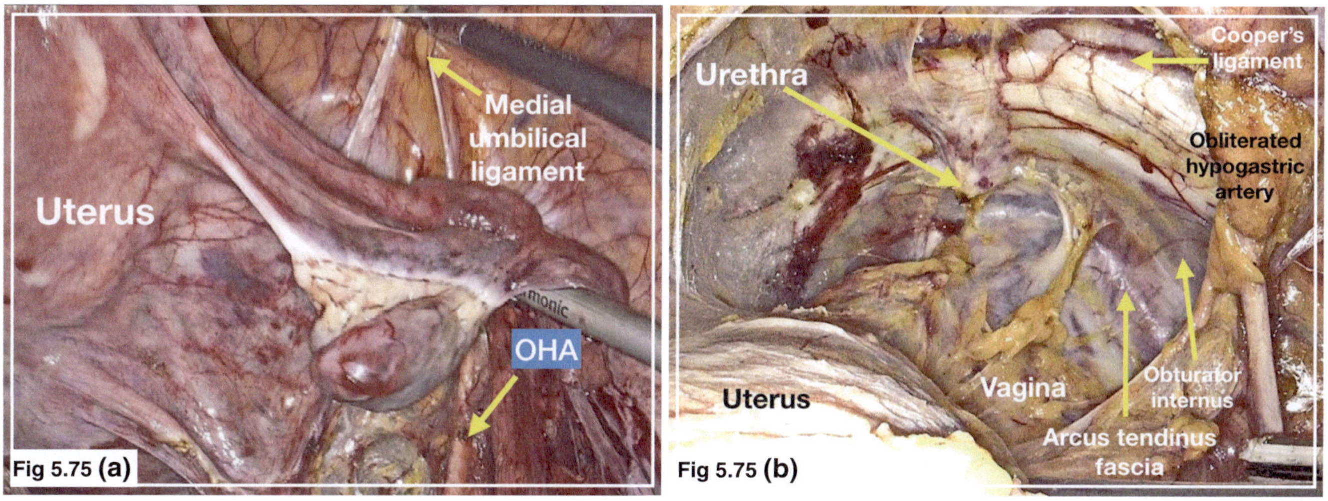

Fig. 5.75 (**a**) The obliterated hypogastric artery is seen as a continuation into the medial umbilical ligament on the posterior surface of the anterior abdominal wall. (**b**) In a case of anterior exenteration the prevesical space is opened. The pubic bone can be seen. Superior border comprises the Cooper's ligament where colposuspension surgery sutures are attached and the inferior border shows a mild swelling in the form of a minor branch of the obliterated hypogastric artery ending at the level of the urethra. The arch tendon fascia is a fascia where the pelvic floor muscles insert into a common aponeurosis. The obturator internus muscle lies between the obliterated hypogastric artery and the arch tendons

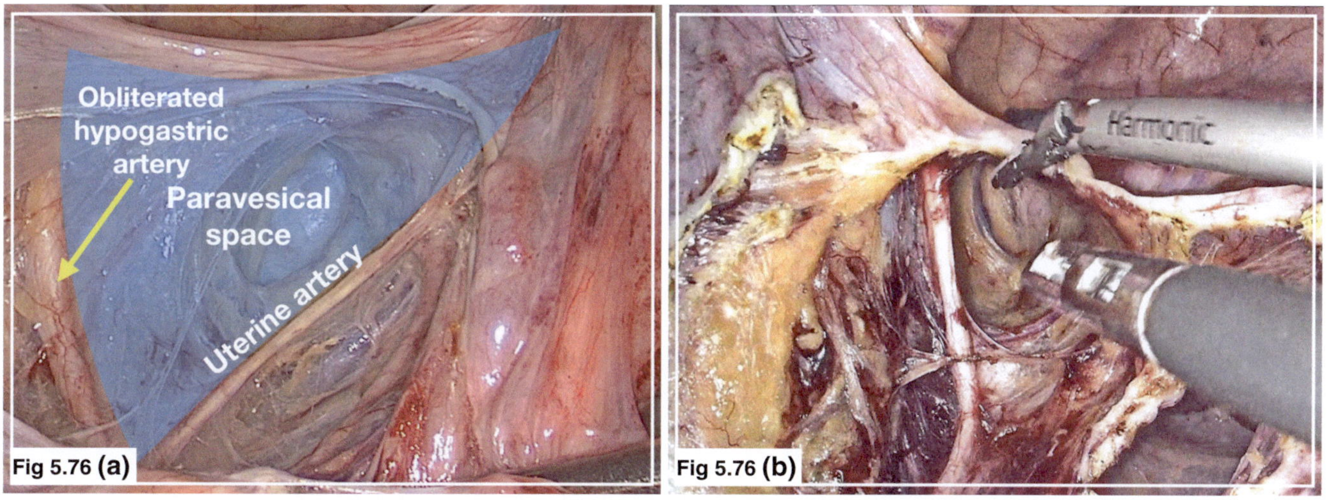

Fig. 5.76 (**a**) The paravesical space, a retroperitoneal space, lies medial to the obliterated hypogastric artery. It is surrounded by the obliterated hypogastric artery and the uterine artery. (**b**) The obliterated hypogastric artery divides the paravesical space into medial and lateral paravesical space. The medial paravesical space is avascular and is essential in the resection of the paracolpos during laparoscopic radical hysterectomy while the lateral paravesical space is essential in lymph node dissection. This area is also called as the obturator fossa

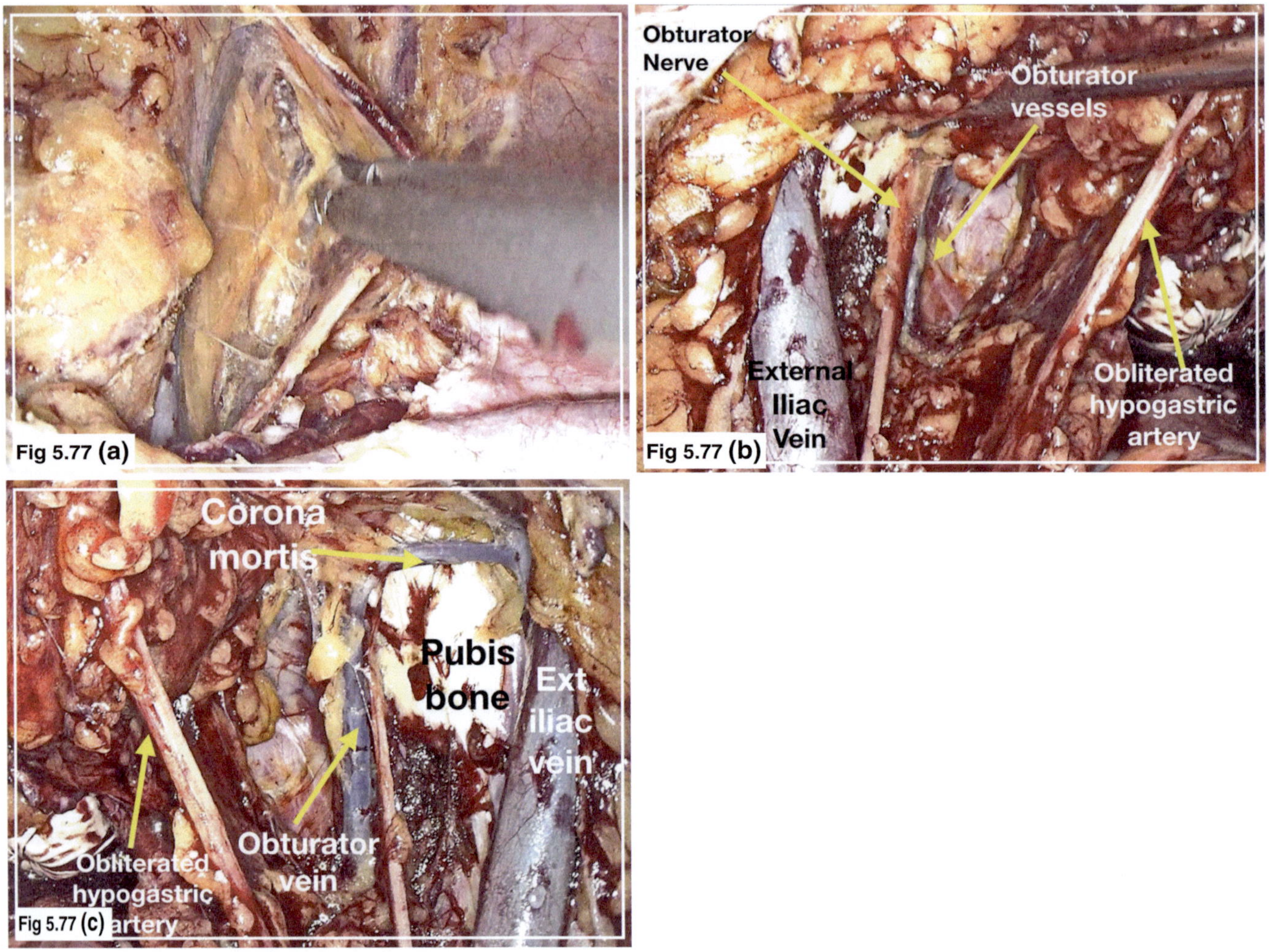

Fig. 5.77 (**a**) The lateral paravesical space or the obturator fossa contains the ilio-obturator group of lymph nodes essential for radical hysterectomy. (**b**, **c**) The images demonstrate the obturator fossa on the lateral side of the obliterated hypogastric artery. Dissection in this area is prone to injury to obturator vessel which leads to significant bleeding

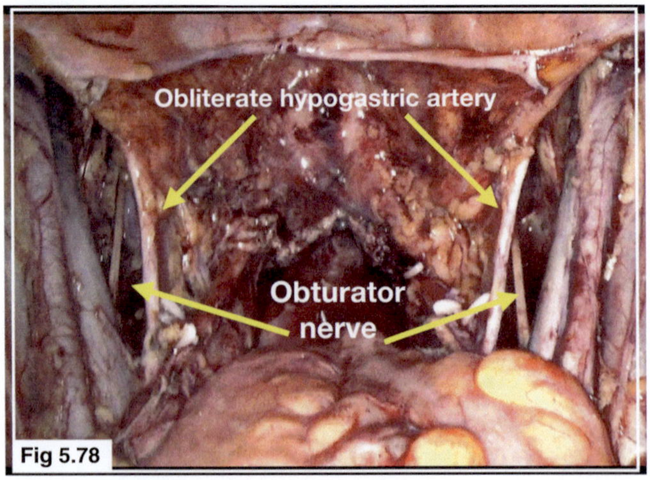

Fig. 5.78 The image is the final end view of a case of laparoscopic radical hysterectomy. The vault is in centre with the exposed retroperitoneal spaces. The lateral limit of dissection is the obliterated hypogastric artery. The obturator nerve can be seen emerging lateral to the obliterated hypogastric artery

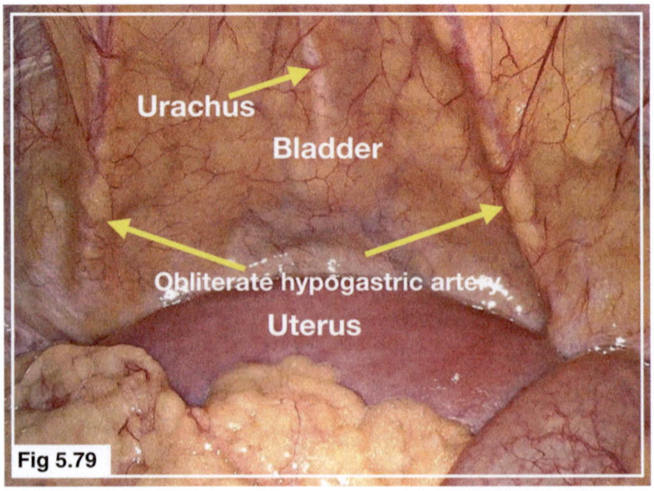

Fig. 5.79 The bladder is seen confined between the two obliterated hypogastric arteries for the medial umbilical ligament on the posterior surface of the anterior abdominal wall

5.5.2 Obturator Artery

The obturator is the only lateral branch of the internal iliac artery. It runs parallel and posterior to the obturator nerve in the obturator fossa (Fig. 5.80).

Thus it can be damaged during lymph node dissection. The plane of dissection should always be superficial and parallel to the nerve and artery (Fig. 5.81).

5.5.3 Ovarian Artery

The artery arises as a direct branch on either side of aorta. There is always a single artery. The artery travels along a distance before it reaches the ovary and fallopian tubes (Fig. 5.82a–f).

The ovarian artery gives one or two branches to supply the ureter very close to their origin from the aorta and always above the pelvic brim. The presence of this supply along with the mesentery ensures a good blood supply to the ureter even after its complete dissection from the pelvic brim to the ureterovesical junction (Fig. 5.83a–e).

The ovarian artery on either side is enough to supply the uterus and also maintain the pregnancy in the absence of supply from the uterine artery. Thus the uterine artery can be sacrificed as in trachelectomy and clipped in large fibroids without the fear of necrosis of the uterus (Fig. 5.84a, b).

The ovarian artery supplies fallopian tube and the ovary through separate branches. Thus the fallopian tubes or the ovaries can be removed independently without affecting the supply to the remaining part. Salpingectomy can be done without the fear of compromising the blood supply to the ovary and vice versa (Fig. 5.85a–i).

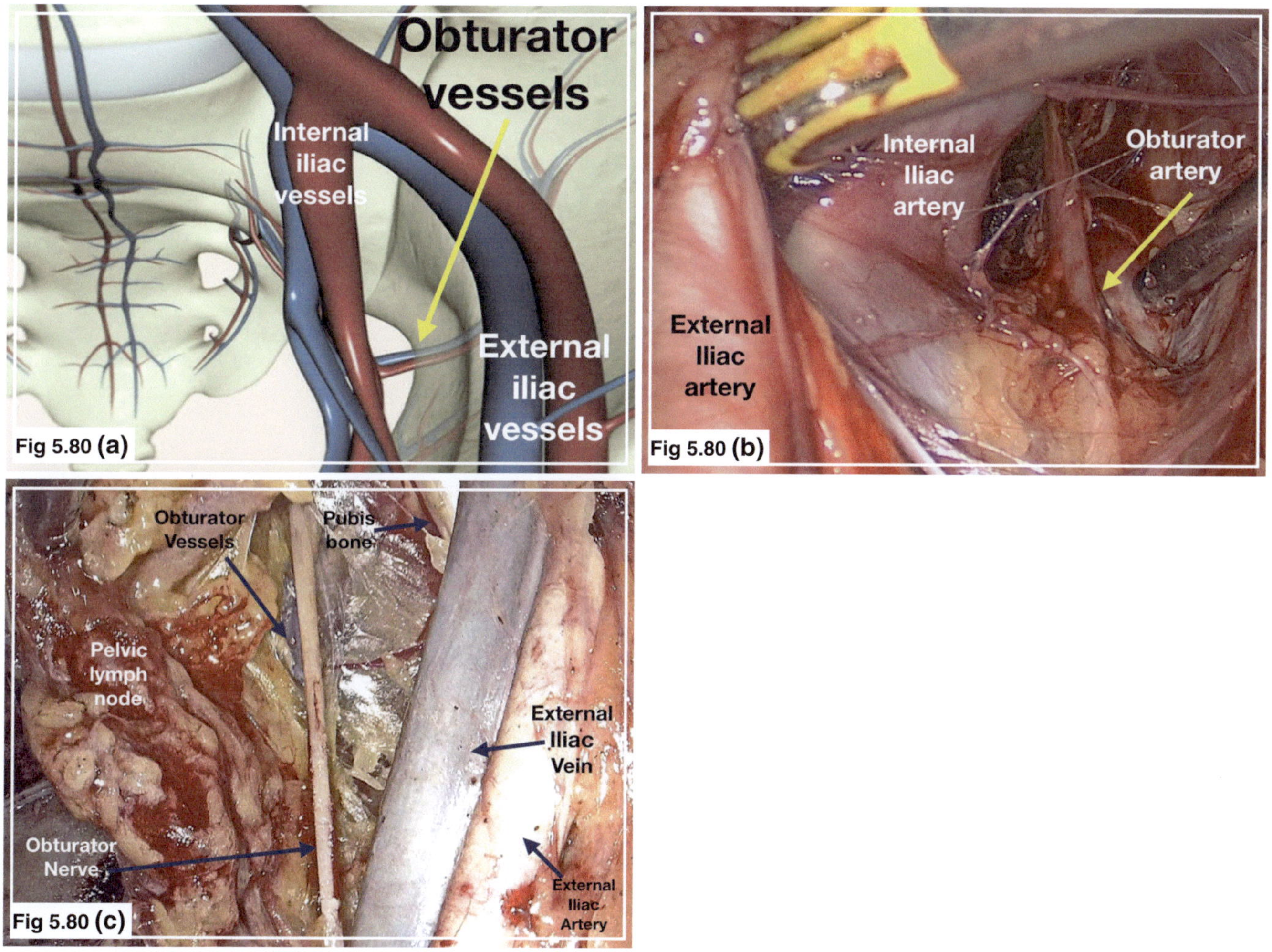

Fig. 5.80 Obturator artery. (**a**) Diagrammatic representation of the obturator vessels arising from the internal iliac artery. (**b**) Image from Fig. 5.48a has been used to explain the origin of the obturator vessels. It is the only branch of the internal iliac artery which travels laterally towards the pelvic wall unlike other branches. (**c**) The obturator vessel can be seen closely associated with the obturator nerve. Thus it is important to do lymph node dissection with utmost caution

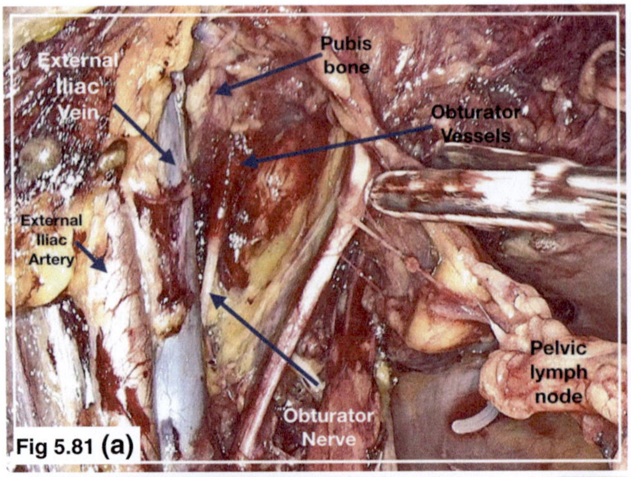

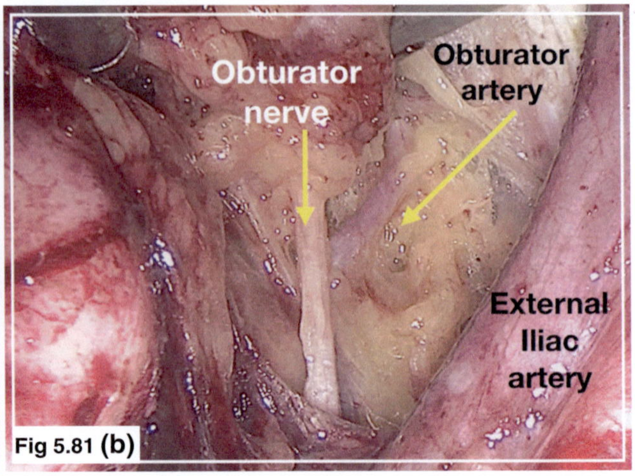

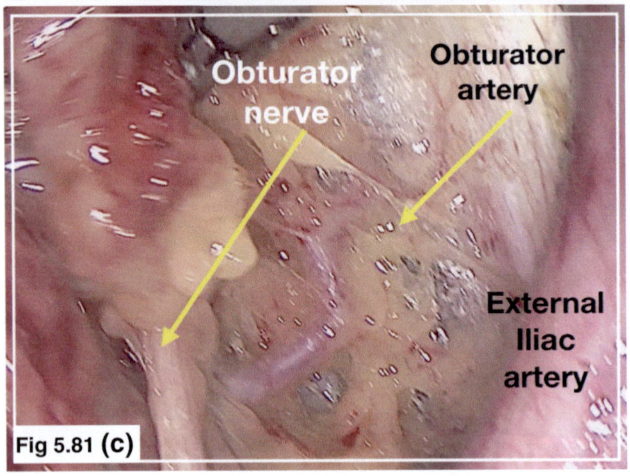

Fig. 5.81 (**a**) Image shows bleeding from the obturator artery due to iatrogenic injury due to excessive force used during lymph node dissection. (**b**, **c**) These images show the course of obturator artery under the obturator nerve. Often the vessel traverses in a congruent path with respect to the nerve. Here the vessels have been seen in a tortuous course

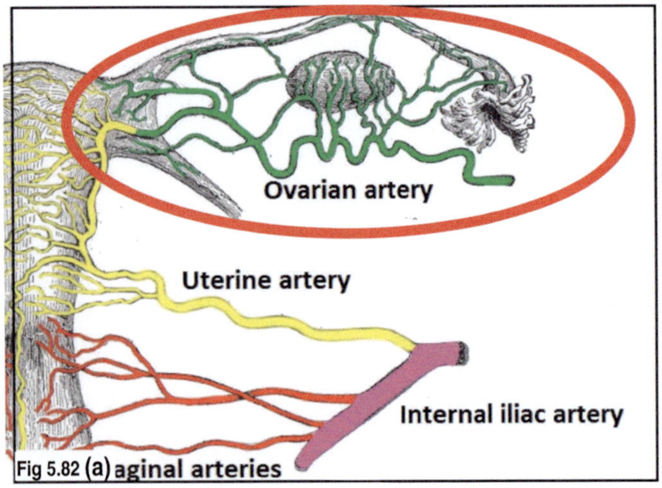

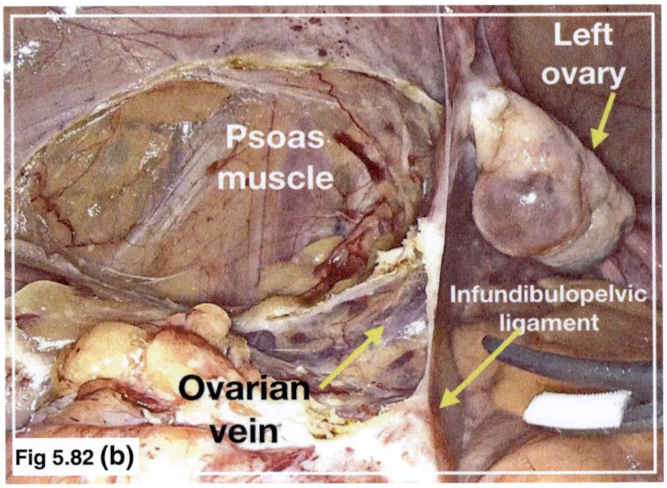

Fig. 5.82 (**a**) The ovarian artery has been labelled/encircled in this image as amongst the most important vessel in the pelvic cavity supplying the female genital tract. (**b**) The image shows the left ovarian vessel at the level of the left infundibulopelvic ligament. The ovarian vein is seen here. The pararectal space has been opened by the lateral approach. (**c**) The left ovarian artery is seen on further dissection (medial traction of the infundibulopelvic ligament) and exposure of the left pararectal space. (**d**) The ovarian artery and vein dissected at a singular unit at the level of the infundibulopelvic ligament. (**e**) The ovarian vessels have a long meandering course before they supply the ovaries and the fallopian tubes. The ovarian vessels however do not end there. They anastomose with the ascending branches of the uterine artery at the level of the isthmus of the fallopian tube. (**f**) The entire ovarian vessel has been dissected off its peritoneal covering at the infundibulopelvic ligament. The ovarian vessels travel along their own fascia

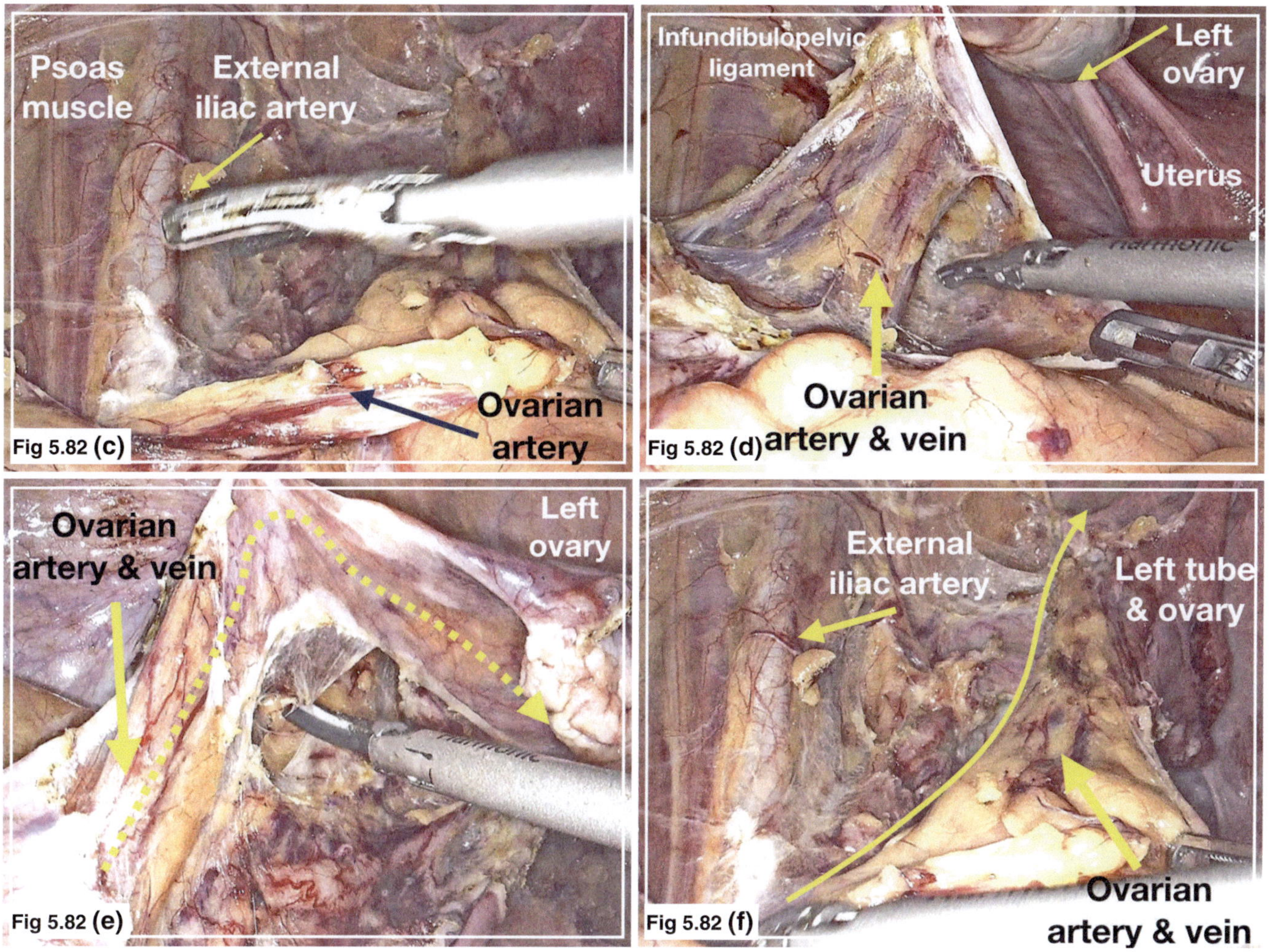

Fig. 5.82 (continued)

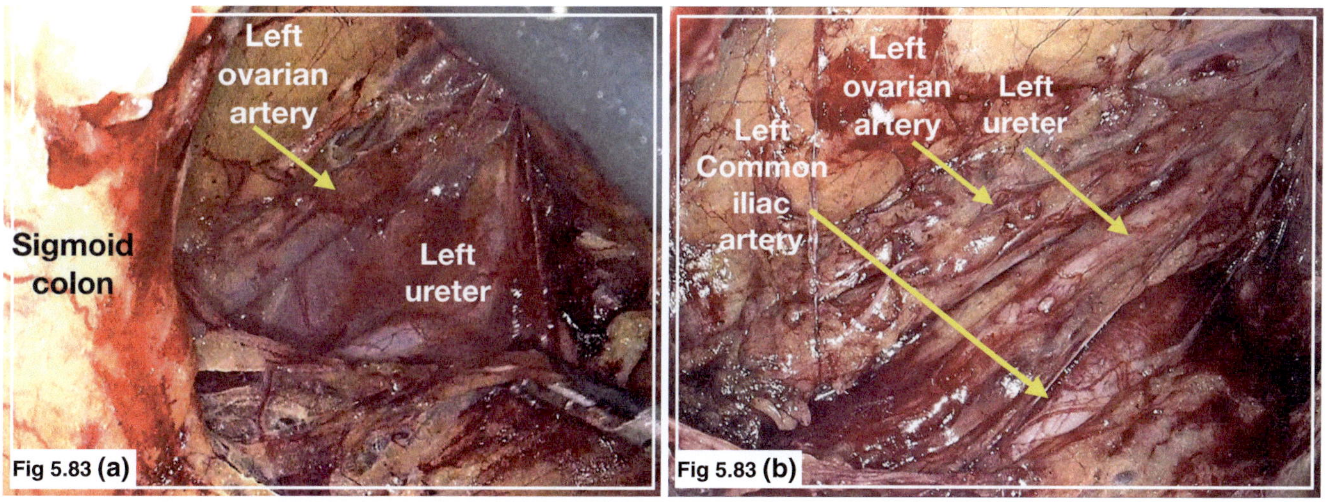

Fig. 5.83 (**a**) In a case of laparoscopic low anterior resection the sigmoid colon is mobilised up to the splenic flexure. The ureter here can be seen travelling along the ovarian vessel in a parallel manner upto the pelvic brim. (**b**) The abdominal ureter, the ovarian vessels and the common iliac artery can be seen in this image as parallel vascular structures. (**c**) In a case of laparoscopic low anterior resection, the contralateral ureter is visualised at the level of the origin of the inferior mesenteric artery. It lies lateral and parallel to the ureter. (**d**) The ureter is seen dipping deep into the pelvis at the pelvic brim while the ovarian vessels continue further into the uterus at the cornea. Thus the ureter is not anatomically related to the ovarian vessels after entering the pelvis. (**e**) The pelvic ureter can be seen clearly free of all attachments in the pelvis from the pelvic brim to the insertion into the bladder

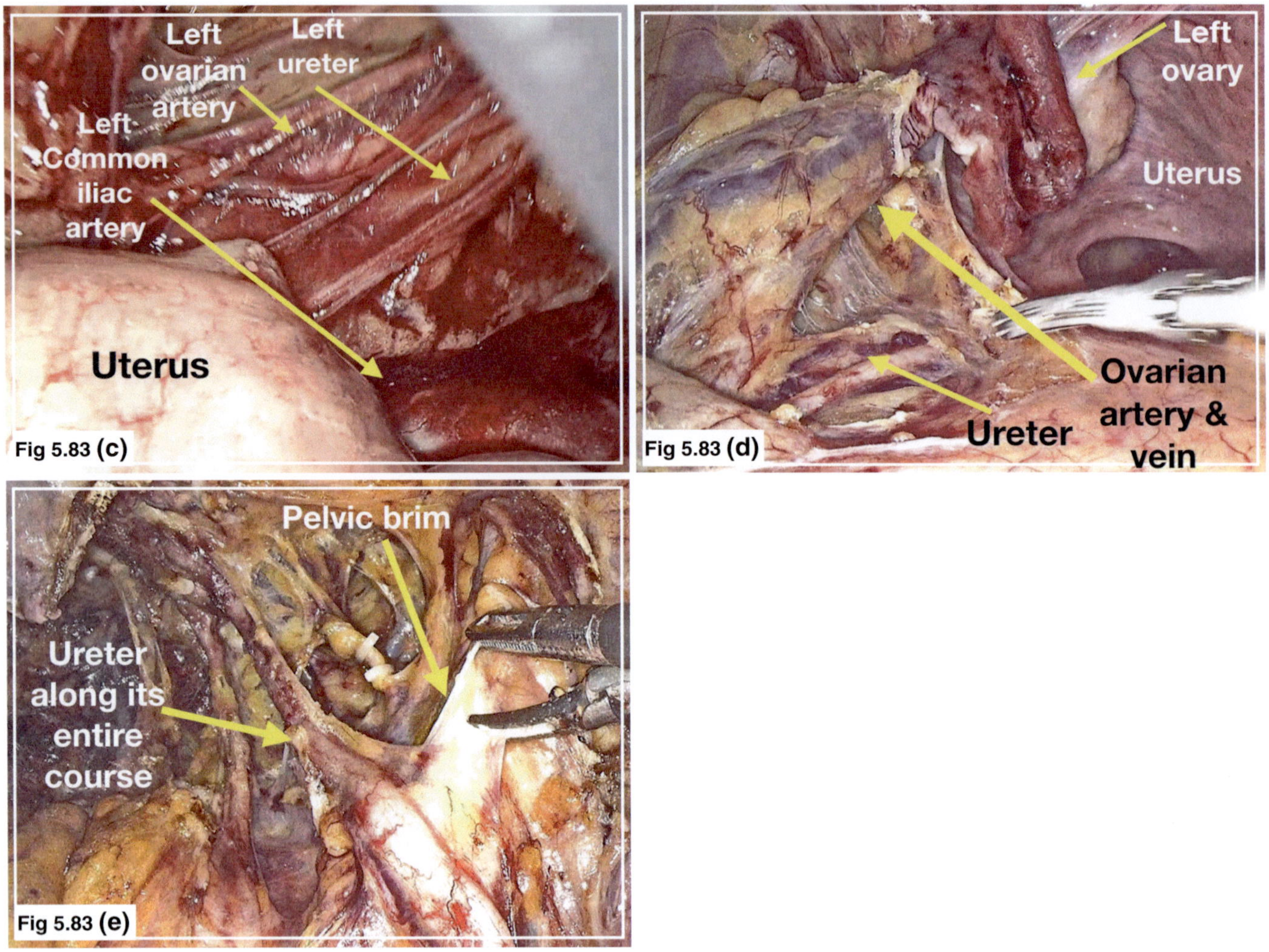

Fig. 5.83 (continued)

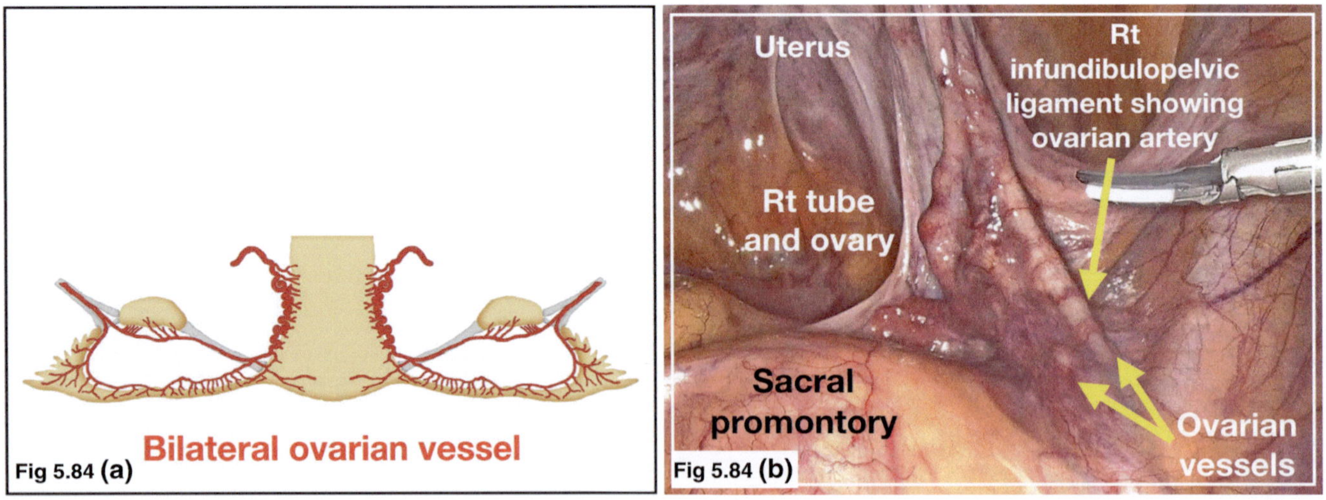

Fig. 5.84 (**a**) Image of the bilateral ovarian vessels anastomosing with the bilateral uterine arteries on either side. (**b**) The ovarian artery can be seen through the translucent peritoneal covering at the infundibulopelvic ligament. The calibre of the vessel is compatible to sustain the uterus without the uterine artery. (**c**) Schematic representation of trachelectomy. (**d**) Compensation of blood supply by the ovarian vessels has been explained with this schematic image

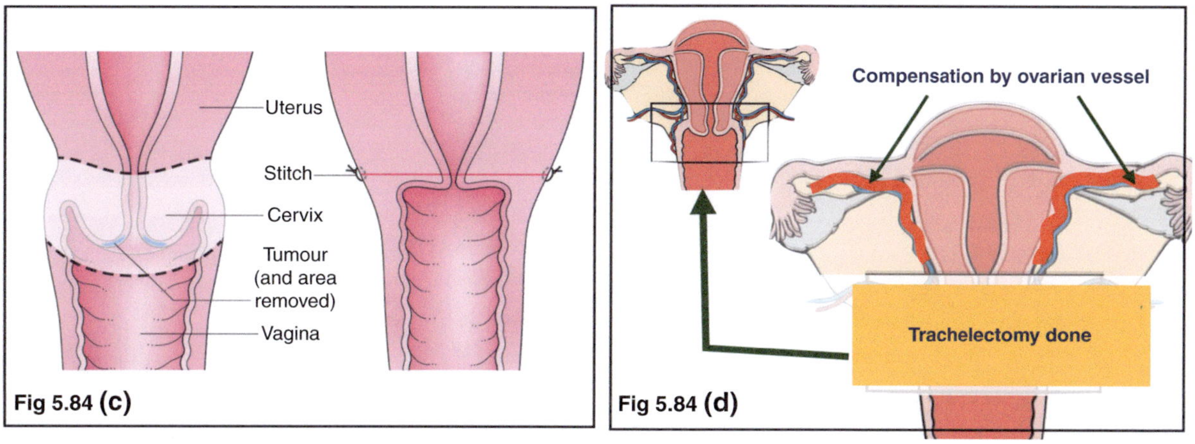

Fig. 5.84 (continued)

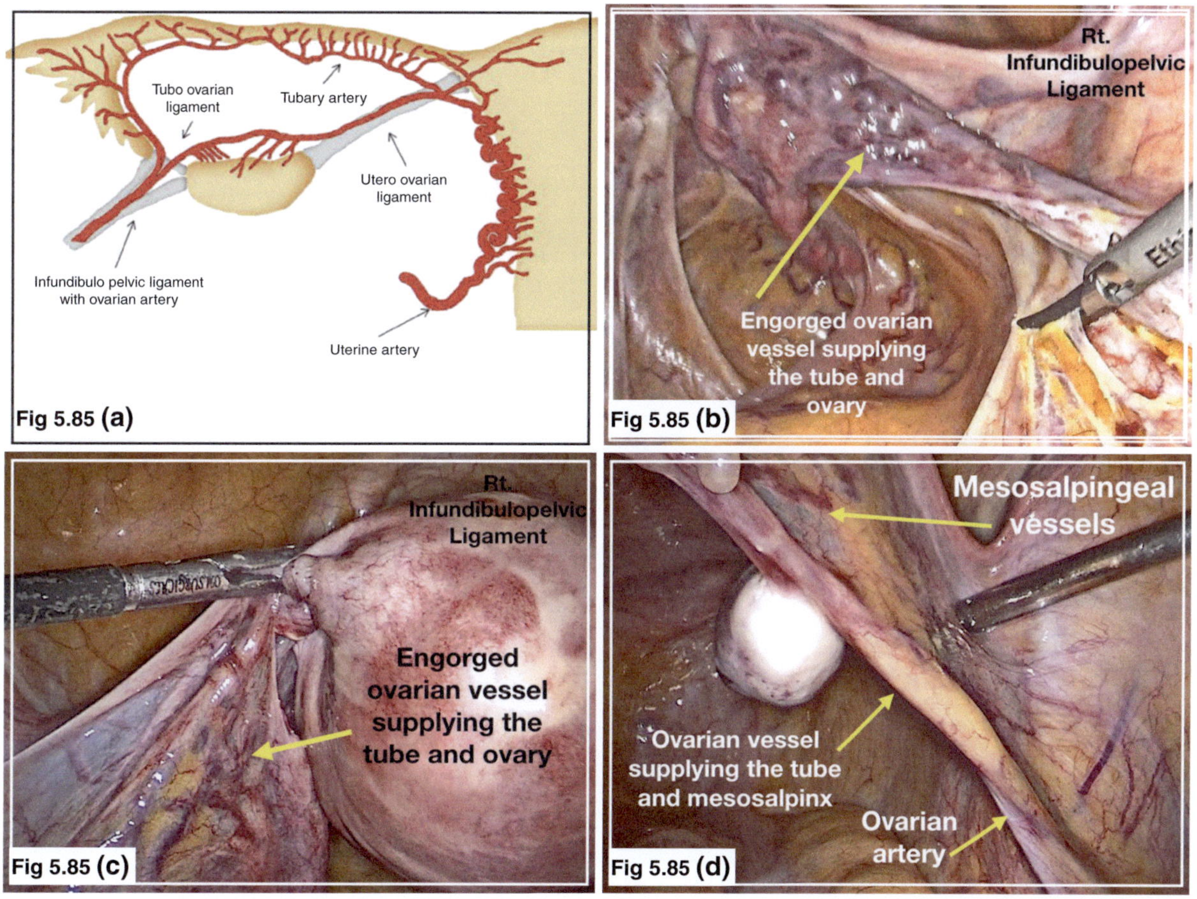

Fig. 5.85 (**a**) The image shows the division of the ovarian artery at the infundibulopelvic ligament into vessels supplying the ovary and fallopian tubes separately. (**b**) The engorged veins seen on the surface of the mesosalpinx of the right tube can be traced to its origin at the ovarian vessels. (**c**) The similar picture can be seen on the left fallopian tube and its mesosalpinx. (**d**) At the outer border the mesosalpinx the ovarian artery gives a branch which traverses the mesosalpinx and supplies the fallopian tube and the mesosalpinx. The ovarian artery continues to supply the ovary and later meets the uterine artery branch near the cornea at the utero-ovarian anastomosis. (**e**) Similar image as the previous one. (**f**) Salpingectomy can be done without compromising the blood supply to the ovary as shown in image. (**g**) The vessel mentioned in the previous images is the first to be clamped and coagulated and dissected in the plane between ovary and fallopian tube along the mesosalpinx. The dissection is carried out till the insertion of the fallopian tube at the cornea. (**h**) Bilateral salpingectomy is often done in case of large bulky fallopian tubes which obstructs the view of posterior surface dissection of the uterus. This does not affect the functioning of ovaries in any manner. (**i**) Similar to the salpingectomy the ovaries can be removed individually without involving the fallopian tube. This image has been taken from the case of dissection of donor uterus for uterine transplant to remove ovaries from the procedure. However in common practice the ovaries are always removed along with the tube. The tube however can be removed individually. But with respect to ovaries the tubes are removed along with ovaries

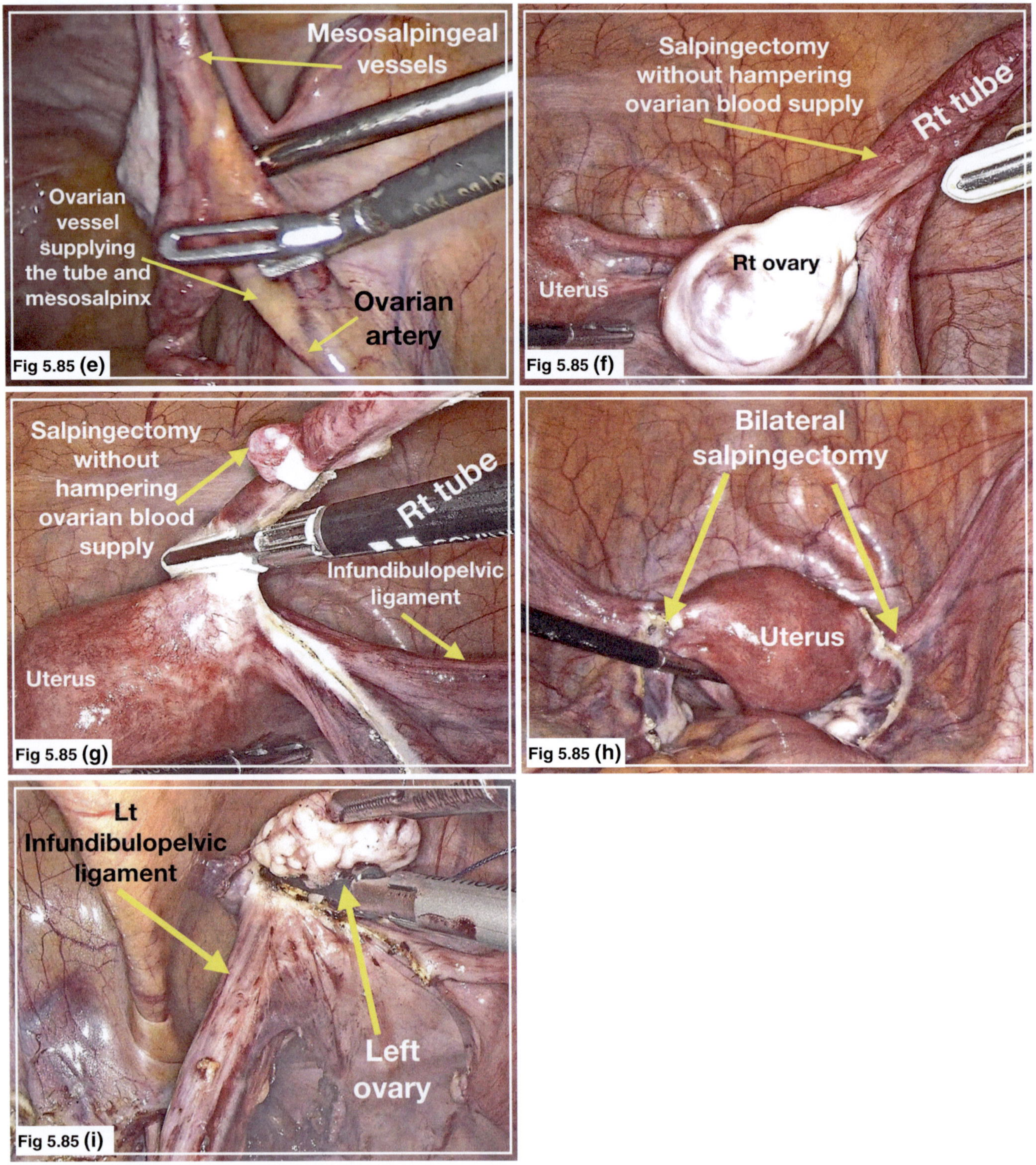

Fig. 5.85 (continued)

5.5.4 Ovarian Vein

The ovarian vein drains in the inferior vena cava on either side. There may be more than one ovarian vein and invariably there are two on either side (Fig. 5.86a–d).

The calibre of the uterine veins is about 3 mm (Fig. 5.87).

The ovarian veins drain the fallopian tubes, ovary and also uterus. This anatomical knowledge of uterine venous drainage allows for sacrifice of the uterine veins in trachelectomy without the fear of uterine congestion (Fig. 5.88).

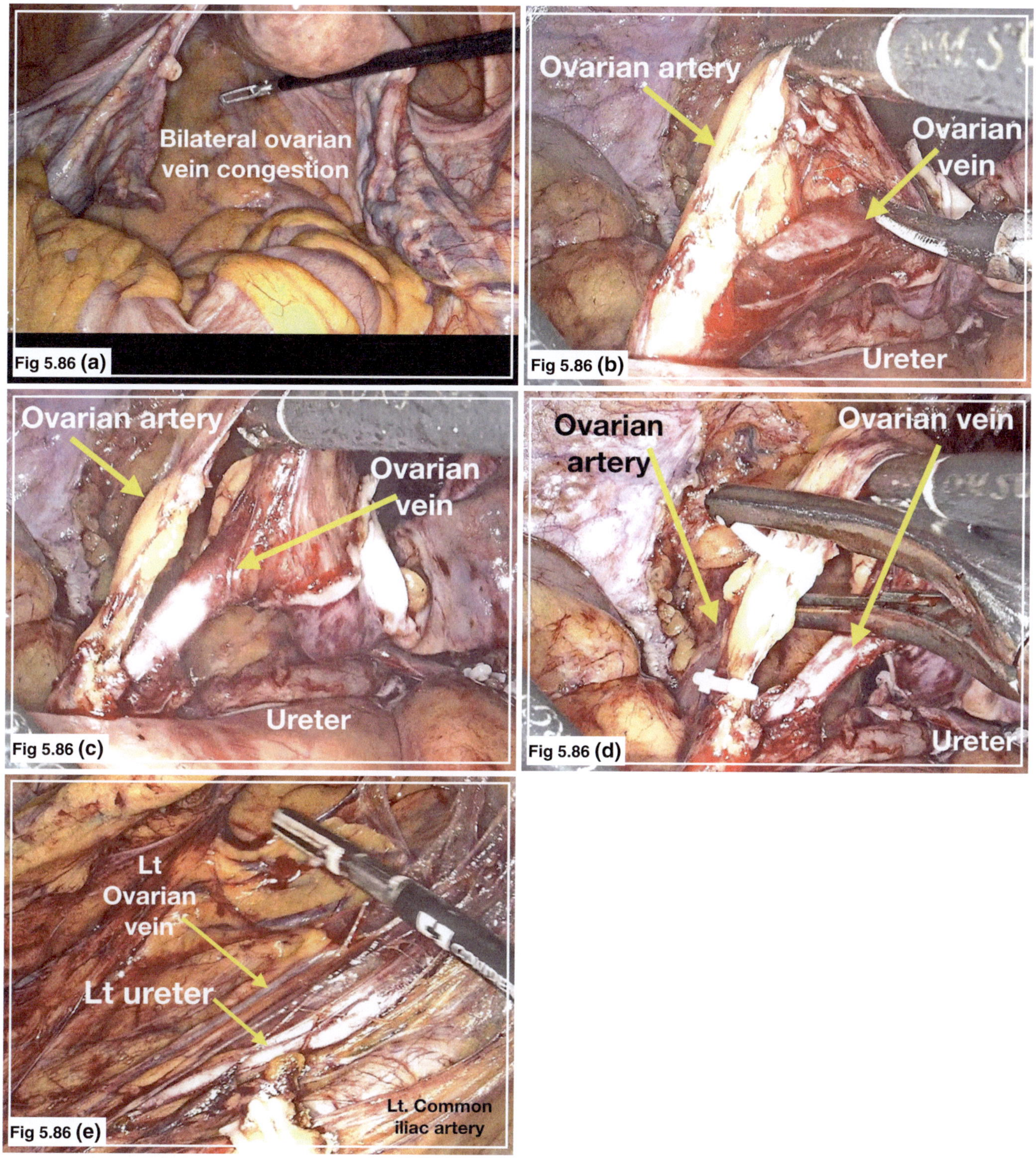

Fig. 5.86 (**a**) Bilateral ovarian vein congestion noticed which helps distinguish artery from veins in the infundibulopelvic ligament. (**b–d**) These images show harvesting of the ovarian vein from the pedicle at the infundibulopelvic ligament. The ovarian vein is separated from the artery without clamping and only the ovarian artery is clamped. (**e**) This image shows the relation of the ureter with the ovarian vein in the retroperitoneal region behind the abdomen. The vein lies lateral to the ureter till the pelvic brim after which the ureter crosses over to the lateral side keeping the ovarian vessels medial to the ureter

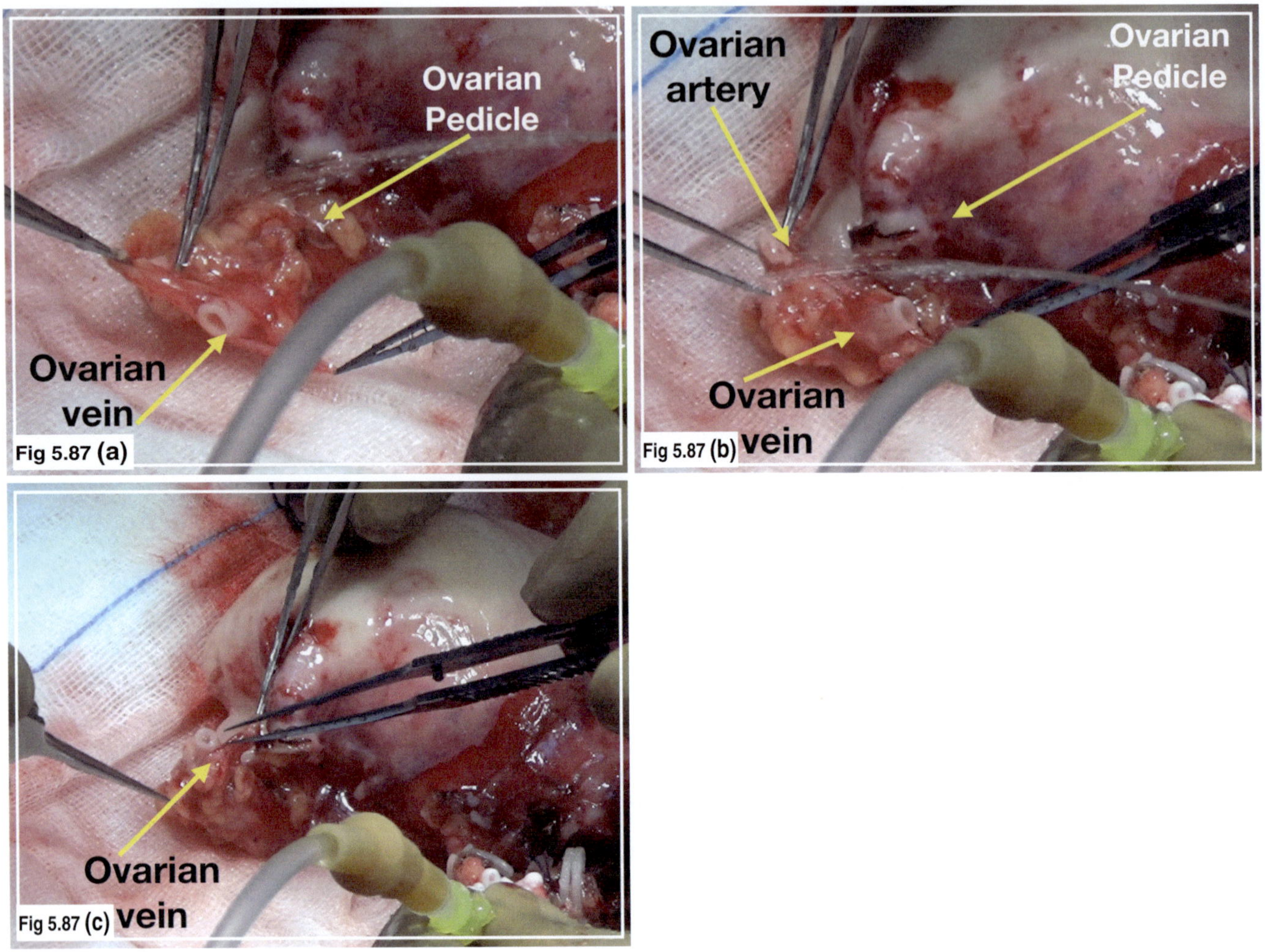

Fig. 5.87 (**a–c**) The series of images are from the bench surgery on the donor uterus for uterine transplant. The ovarian pedal is first isolated and cleaned and the ovarian artery is separated from the vein. The ovarian vein is cleaned and identified. The flow of fluid from the uterine artery is assessed at the end of the ovarian vessels to establish the utero-ovarian anastomosis and to rule out leakage of fluid

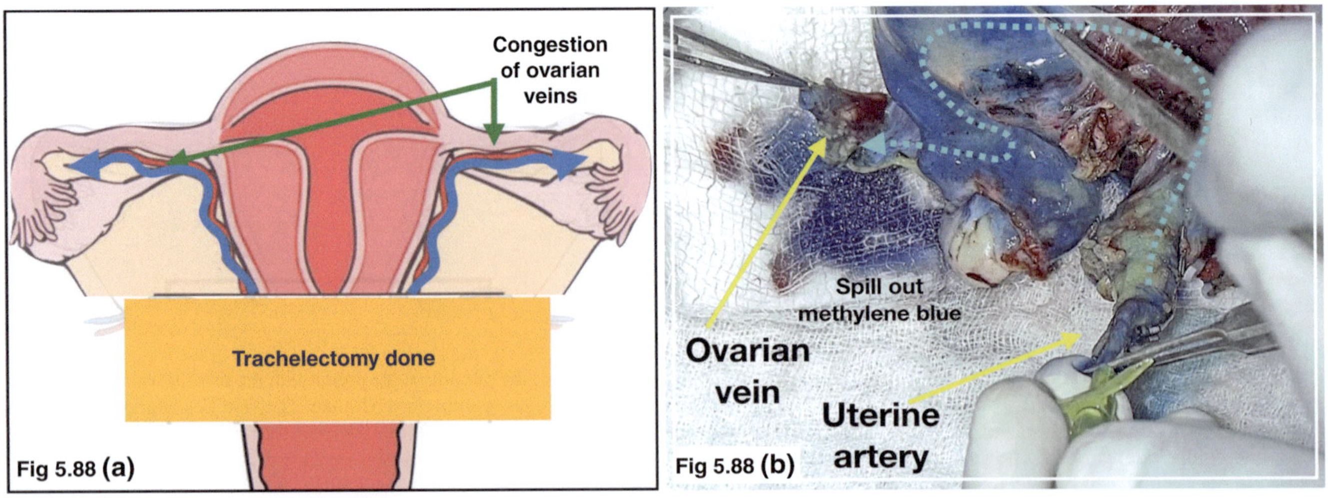

Fig. 5.88 (**a**) The compensated blood supply to the uterus by ovarian artery has its effects on the engorged or enlarged ovarian veins often seen post-trachelectomy. (**b**) This image is from a trial of bench surgery during the preparation of uterine transplant. Vessels of routine radical hysterectomy specimens were dissected at long lengths and then on bench surgery the uterine artery was infused with diluted methylene blue dye to see if they flowed out of the ovarian veins as the uterine vein was pre-emptively clamped. But dye is seen flowing out of the ovarian veins, thus establishing utero-ovarian anastomosis and thus confirming our fact that the ovarian vessels can sustain circulation in the uterus in the absence of the uterine artery

The ovarian vein drains the ureter above the pelvic brim (Fig. 5.89a, b).

The long length of the ovarian vessels ensures tension-free blood supply to the uterus not only during pregnancy but also in large uterine pathologies (Fig. 5.90) (figure from transplant when we dissect the ovarian pedicle and also ovarian masses).

The ovarian vessels lie in a fascial covering. This fascial covering ensures separation of these vessels easily during colonic and sigmoid resections (Fig. 5.91a, b).

Except a few arteries and veins that supply the ureter at the level of kidney the ureter is an independent plane always being medial to the infundibulopelvic ligaments. This allows

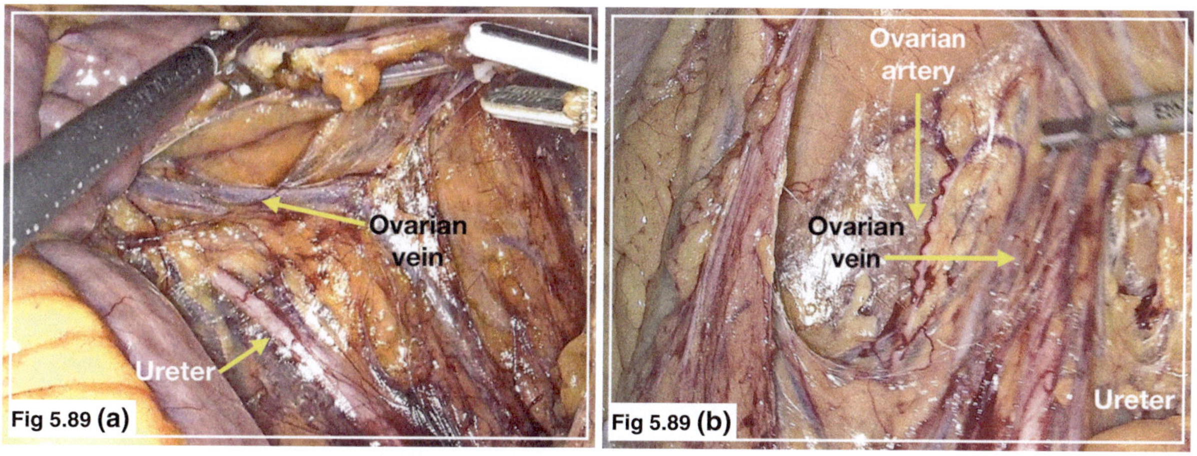

Fig. 5.89 (**a**, **b**) These images taken from a case of laparoscopic low anterior resection show the relation of the ureter with the ovarian vein above the pelvic brim

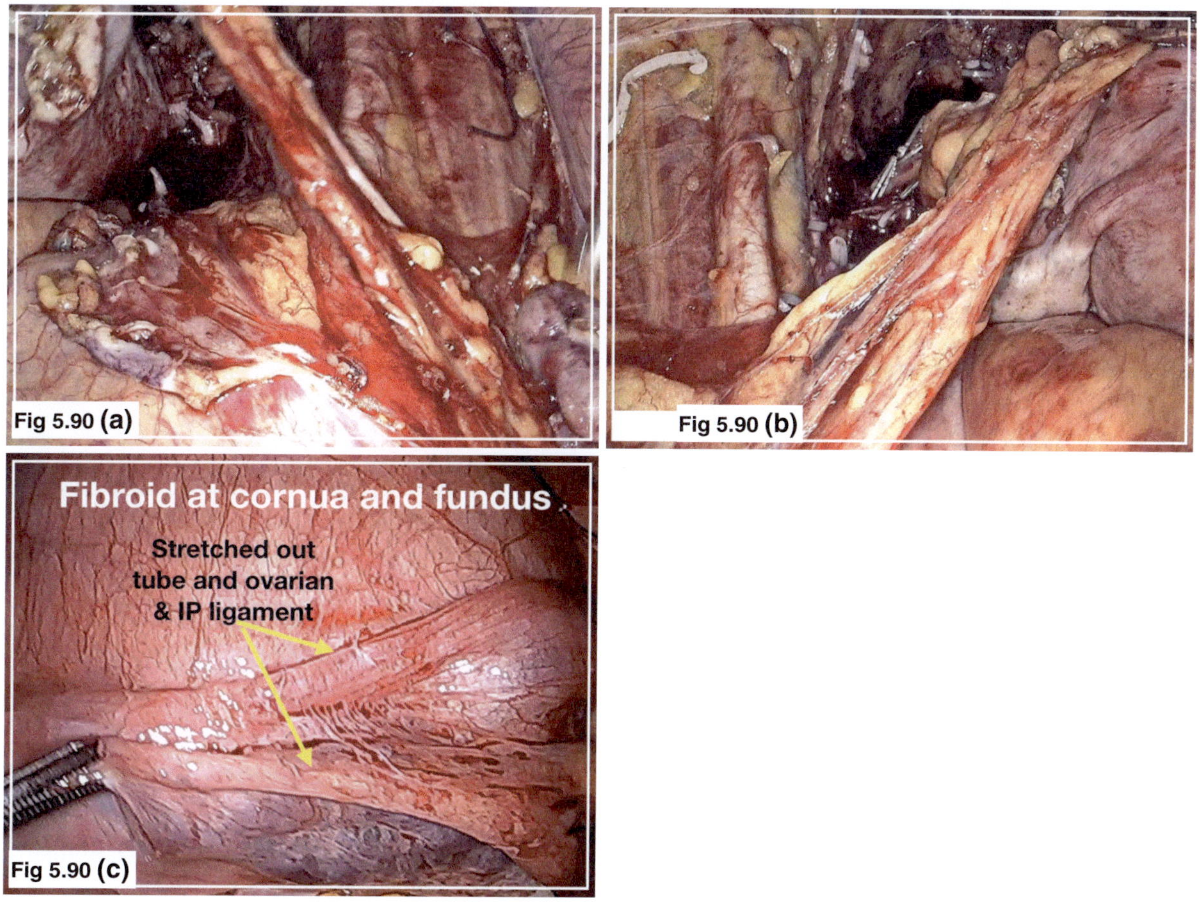

Fig. 5.90 (**a**, **b**) These images have been taken from a case of dissection of donor uterus for uterine transplant. (**c**) The image for a case of fundal fibroid at the cranial region showing the adaptive measures taken by the road ligament and ovarian vessel in terms of lengthening themselves for support and vascularity to the uterus, respectively

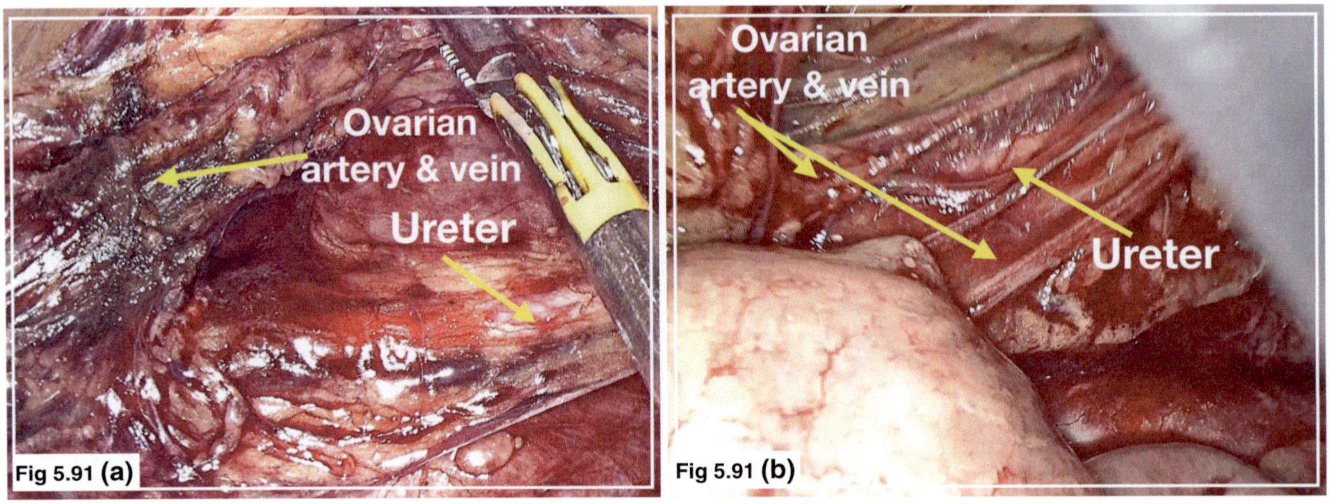

Fig. 5.91 (**a**, **b**) View of the ovarian vessel and the ureter during sigmoid resection

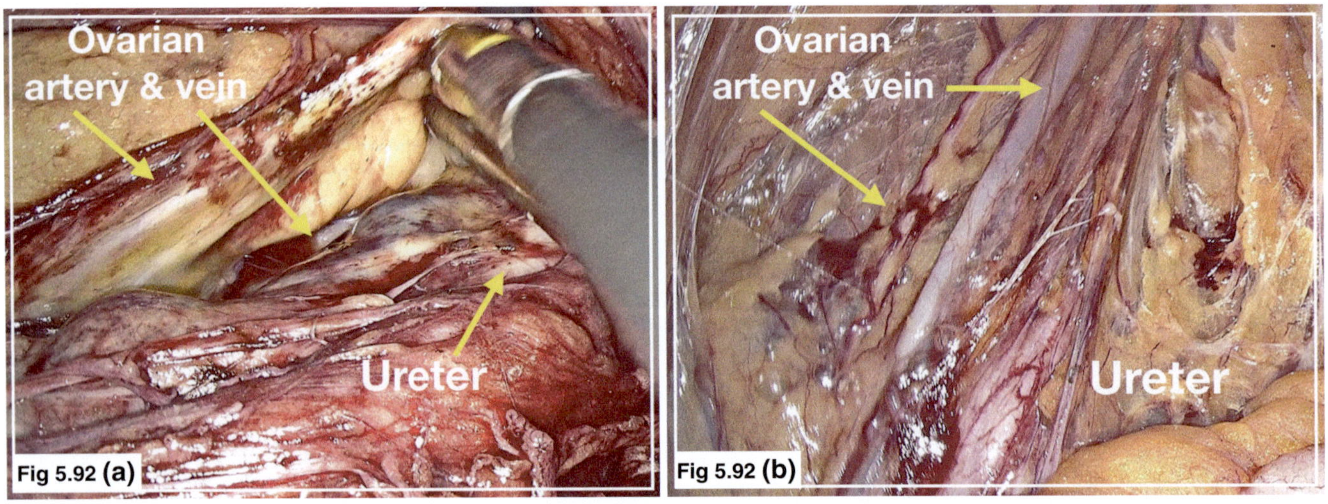

Fig. 5.92 (**a**) The relation of the ovarian artery and vein with the ureter has been demonstrated in this image from a case of para-aortic lymph node dissection for a case of Ca endometrium. (**b**) The image from a case of low anterior resection done laparoscopically demonstrates the relation between the ureter and the ovarian artery and vein in the abdominal retroperitoneal region

complete separation of these two structures independently below the pelvic brim (Fig. 5.92a, b).

Since there is no supply from ovarian vessels to any organ below the pelvic brim the dissection of these vessels should be done remaining parallel to the external iliac vessels (Fig. 5.93a–c).

5.6 Veins

5.6.1 Common Iliac Vein

The common iliac vein divides into the internal and external vein at caudal to the division of common iliac artery (Fig. 5.94).

The veins essentially lie medial or posterior to the main arteries as surrounded by some free space. This is due to the reason that the veins have to adjust the diameter as per the venous blood while the arteries can accommodate the increased volume without increasing the diameter (Fig. 5.95).

There are no tributaries of common iliac vein. It is closely approximated to the presacral fascia and thus rarely damaged during surgery (Fig. 5.96).

5.6.2 Internal Iliac Vein

This is closely applied to the anterior branch of internal iliac artery and is posterior to it. It drains the veins of pelvic organs. The main tributaries: 2–3 medial, 2 lateral, 2 posterior (Fig. 5.97).

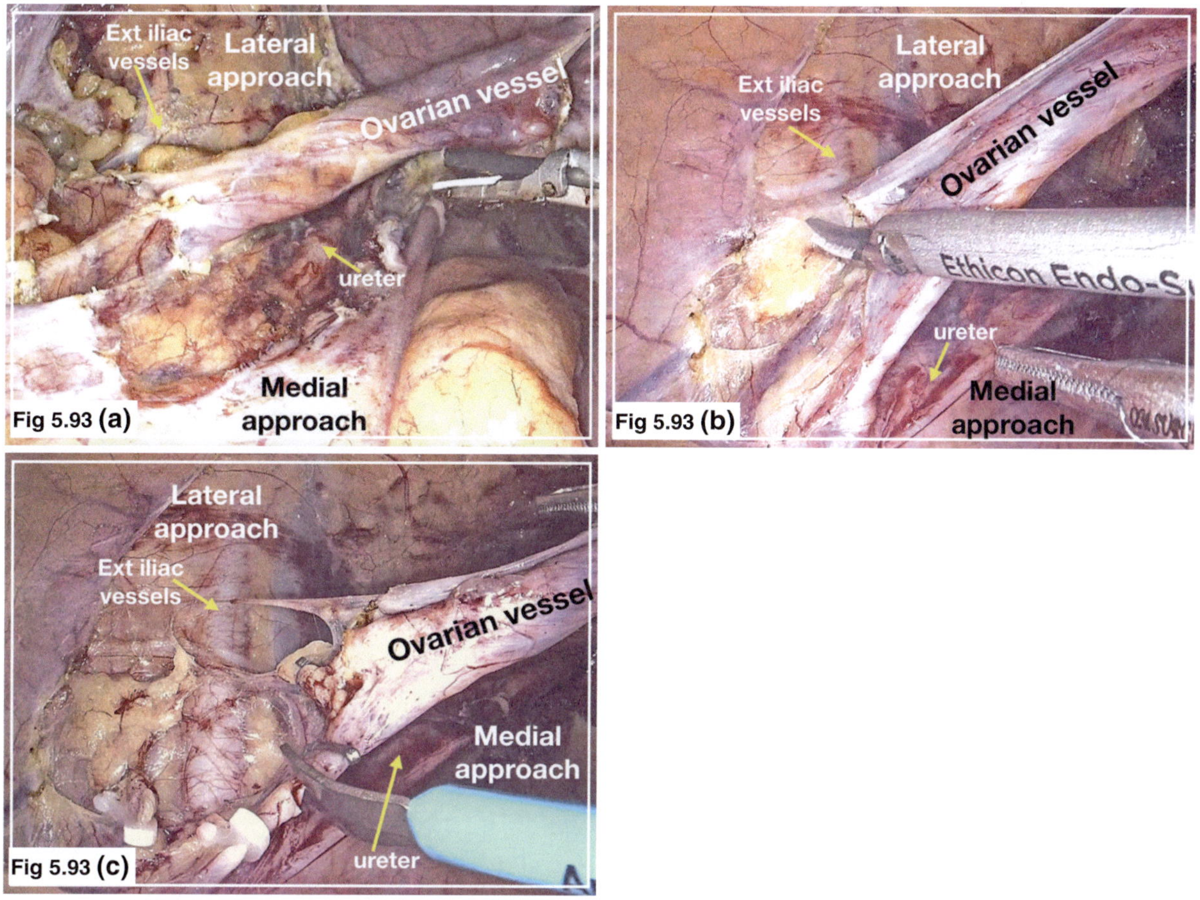

Fig. 5.93 (**a**–**c**) These images are from different cases of laparoscopic radical hysterectomy where the pararectal space has been approached medially and laterally with respect to the infundibulopelvic ligament. In both approaches the direction is done parallel to the ovarian vessels. The external iliac vessels are clearly visible as per the lateral approach and the ureter is visible as per the medial approach

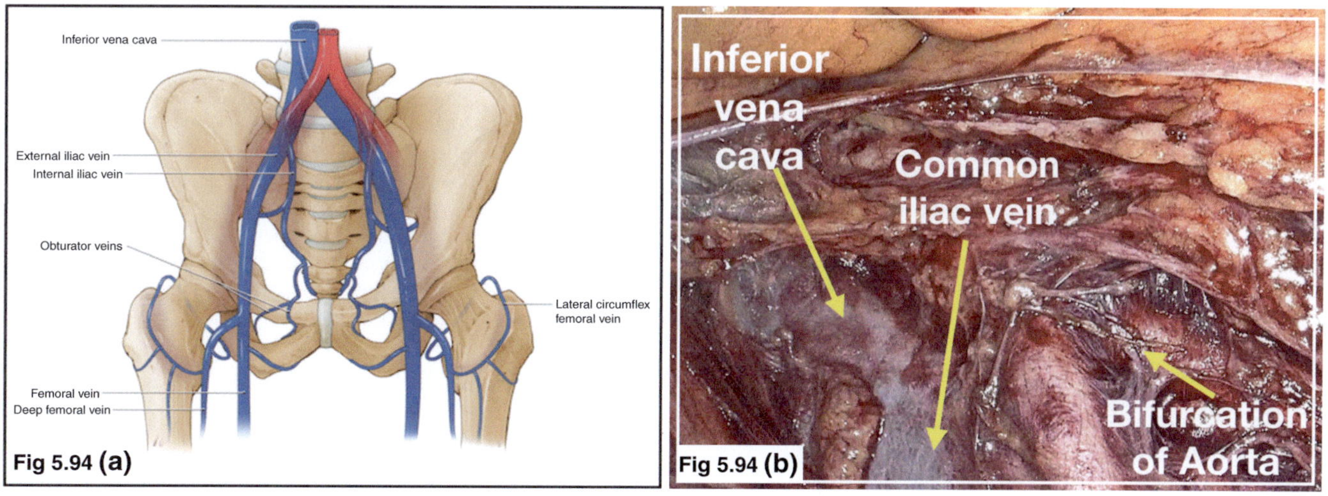

Fig. 5.94 (**a**) Diagrammatic representation of the common iliac vein. The inferior vena cava is formed by the union of the two common iliac veins at the level of L4 vertebra. (**b**) The image from a case of para-aortic lymph node dissection shows the common iliac veins draining into the inferior vena cava. They lie under the arterial counterparts. The bifurcation of the aorta leading to the common iliac arteries can be seen as well. (**c**) The image is from a case of ilio-obturator lymph node dissection where the internal iliac is dissected to its origin and the external, internal and common iliac veins can be seen. The veins lie high in the pelvis and the external and internal iliac veins communicate to form the common iliac vein at the lateral pelvic wall

Fig. 5.94 (continued)

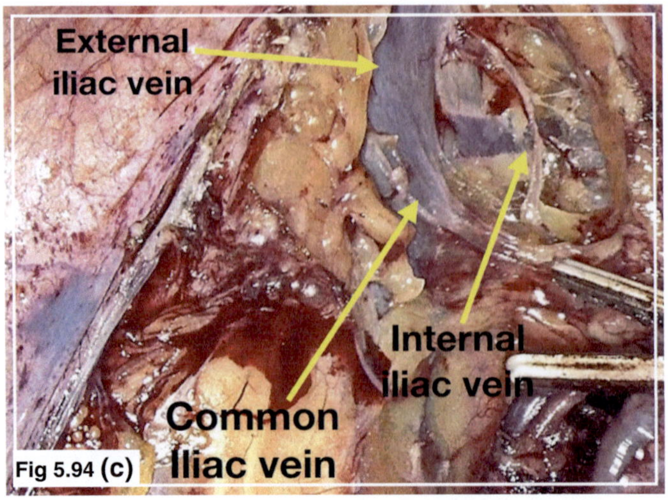

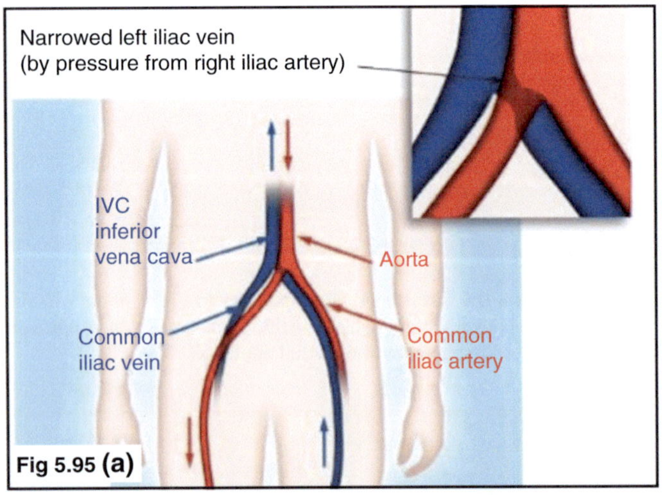

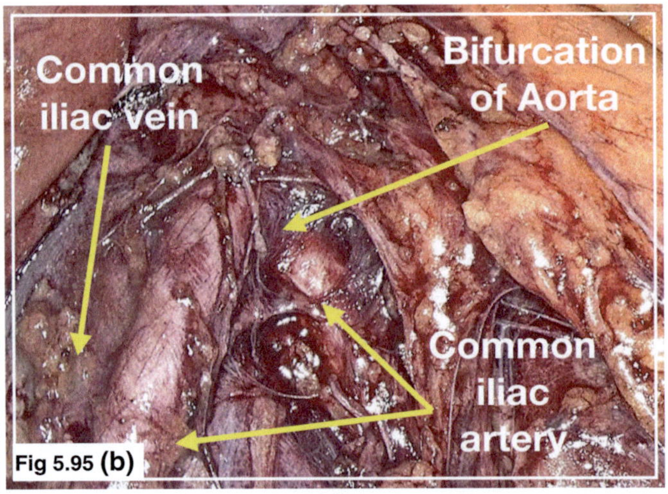

Fig. 5.95 (**a**) Diagrammatic representation of the orientation of common iliac veins with arteries. Often compression of the left iliac vein by the right iliac artery leads to intermittent claudication called as May-Thurner syndrome. (**b**) The bifurcation of the inferior vena cava occurs posterior and towards the right side of the aorta and thus the veins lie accordingly posterior and lateral towards the right side. (**c**) The common iliac vein can also be accessed from behind the bifurcation of the common iliac artery. As the veins follow the common path of the arteries but below and to the right the common iliac vein can be reached from a few centimetres just below the origin of the external iliac artery. (**d**) The common iliac vein is exposed in conditions of lymphadenectomy of the inter iliac group of lymph nodes. (**e**) The common iliac vein can also be seen below the external iliac artery at the region where the external iliac vein meets the internal iliac vein as shown in the figure

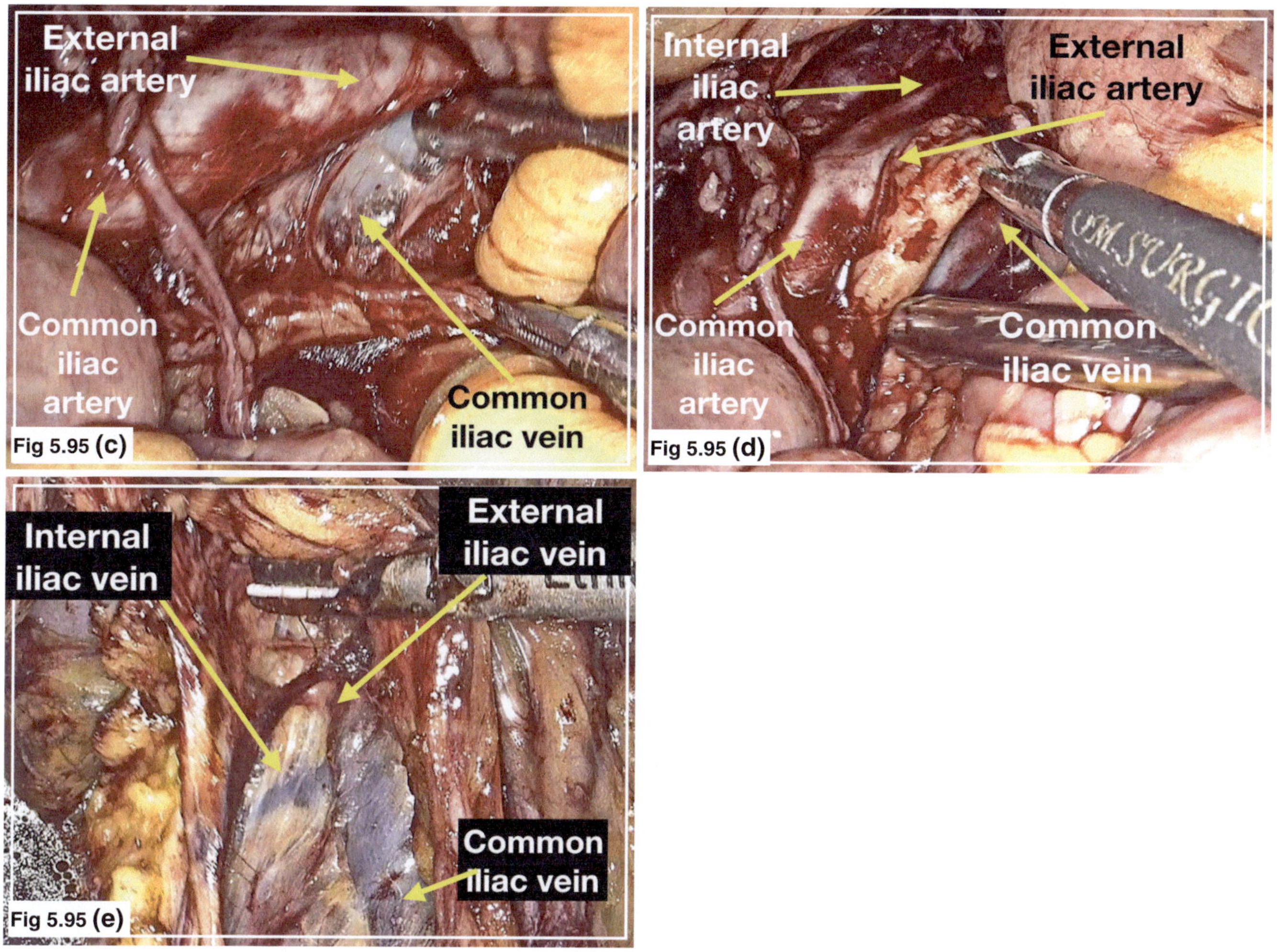

Fig. 5.95 (continued)

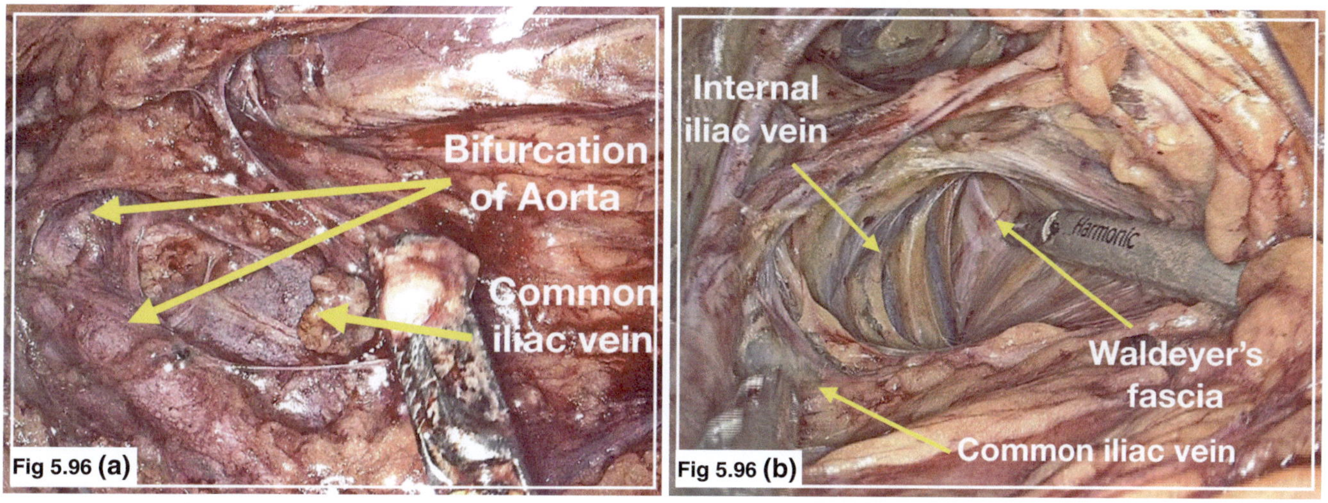

Fig. 5.96 (**a**, **b**) The common iliac vein has no tributaries. It is drained only by the internal and external iliac veins, following which it remains close to the Waldeyer's fascia and communicates with the contralateral common iliac vein for the inferior vena cava

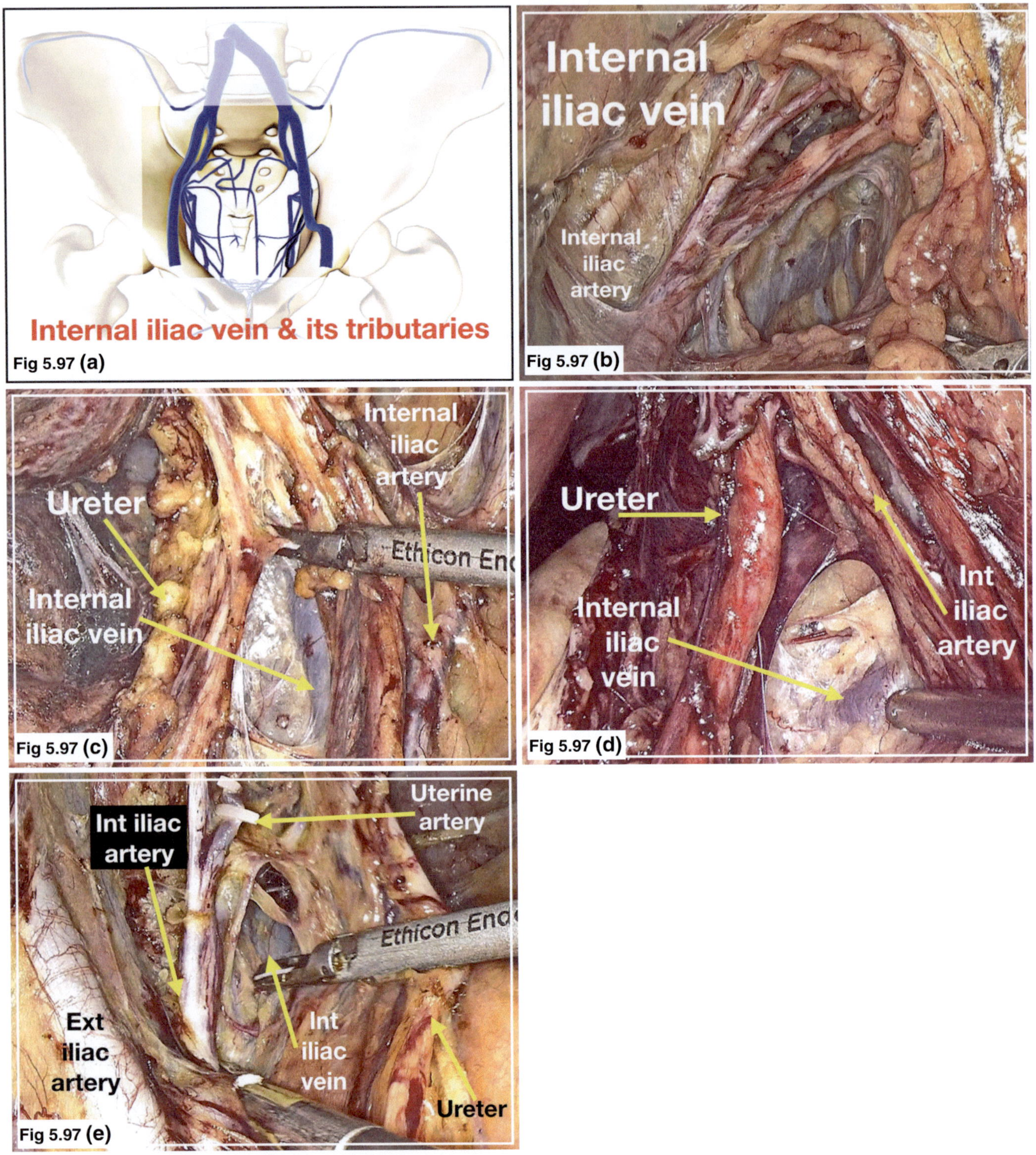

Fig. 5.97 (**a**) The schematic representation of the internal iliac vein and the communication with the external iliac vein (corona mortis) (**b**) The internal iliac vein can be seen under the internal iliac artery in a case of laparoscopic radical hysterectomy. The internal iliac vein receives many tributaries from the pelvic organs. It is the chief vein into which pelvic organs drain their venous blood. (**c–e**) The internal iliac vein seen deep in the pararectal space. The vein remains lateral to the ureter in the lateral pelvic wall. The uterine vein which travels parallel and under the uterine artery drains into the internal iliac vein directly

Medial

- Deep uterine vein: 2–3 in number
- Superior vesicle vein: In females it invariably drains into the deep uterine vein
- In males the superior vesicle veins drain directly into the internal iliac vein (Fig. 5.98).

Lateral

- Obturator
- Ilio-inguinal vein

These drain the veins of the inferior extremities (Fig. 5.99).

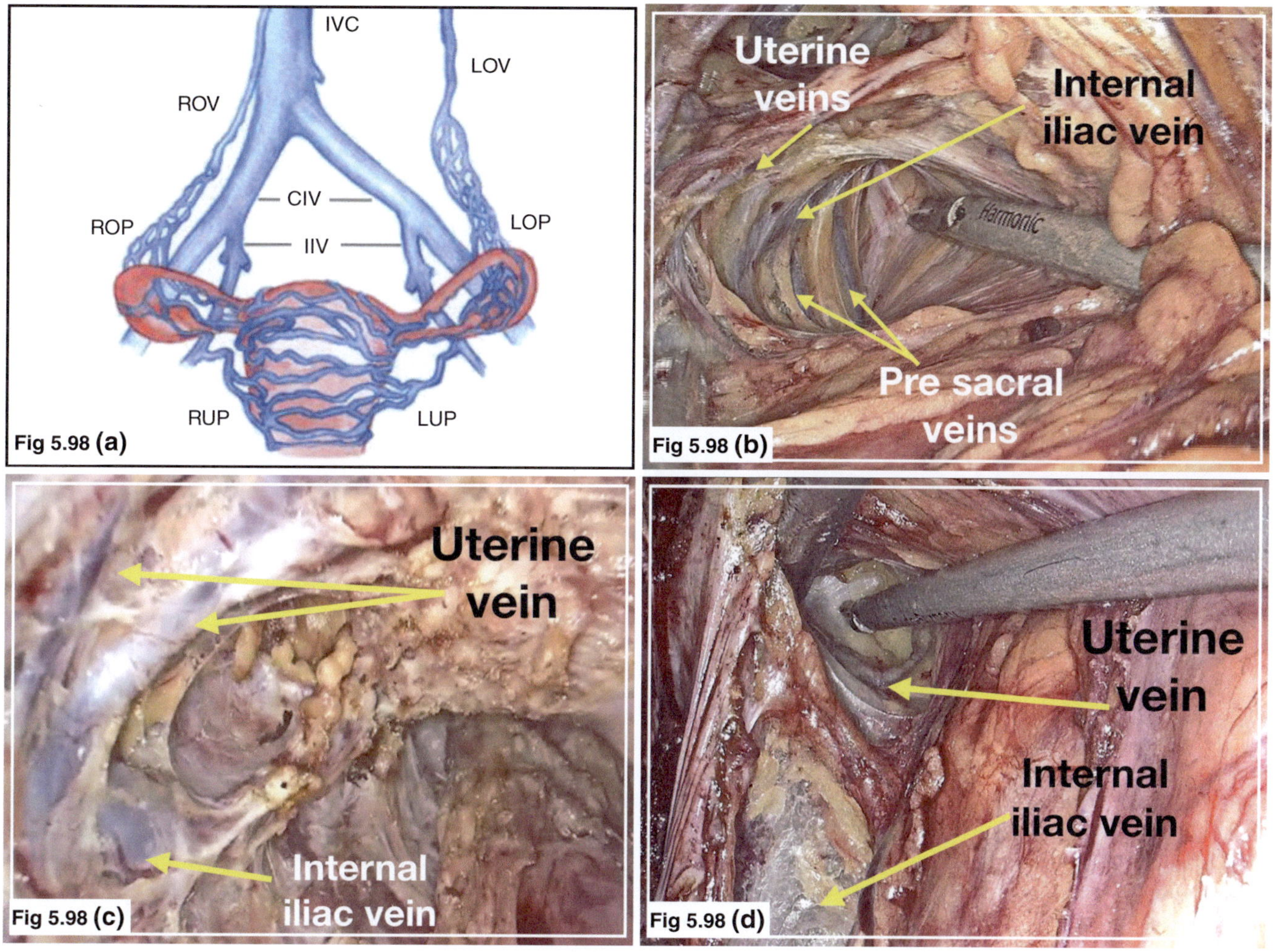

Fig. 5.98 (**a**) Schematic representation of the internal iliac veins and its tributaries from the uterus, namely, the ovarian vein and the uterine vein have been displayed. (**b**) In a case of laparoscopic radical hysterectomy the dissection of the sacral region of the pararectal space exposes the Waldeyer's fascia and the presacral veins. The presacral veins drain into the internal iliac veins as seen in this image. (**c**) The uterine vein is of two kinds, the short superficial veins and the deep uterine veins. The short superficial veins drain into the deep veins which then drain into the internal iliac veins. The discrepancy lies in the number of veins. There is no fixed number of deep uterine veins. They range from one to three. In this image two uterine veins can be seen draining into the internal iliac veins. (**d**) In this image as compared to the previous image there is only a single uterine vein which drains into the internal iliac veins. (**e**) Similarly in this image the right uterine vein drains into the right internal iliac vein. (**f**) The uterine vein seen travelling parallel to the uterine artery but underneath it eventually drains into the internal iliac vein as seen in the next image. (**g**) The uterine vein can be traced cranially to drain into the internal iliac vein as seen in this image. The posterior division of the internal iliac artery can be seen crossing over the internal iliac vein while the anterior division travels steadily anteriorly to the anterior abdominal wall. The uterine artery can be seen branching out from the internal iliac artery

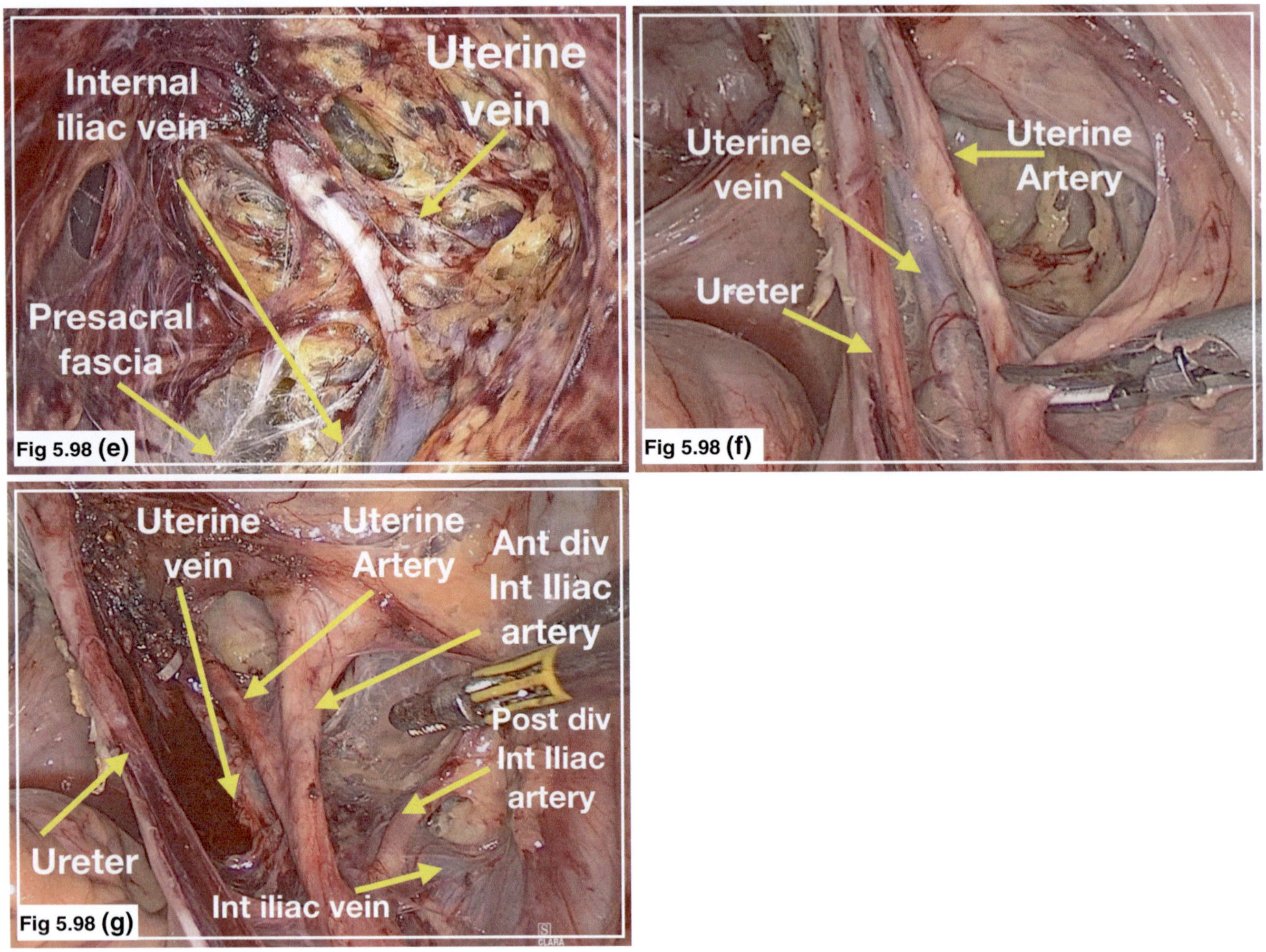

Fig. 5.98 (continued)

Posterior

- Two presacral veins which enter the internal iliac vein posteriorly.

  The presacral veins also drain into this. Hence damage to the presacral veins is difficult to control as the tributaries retract. The parasympathetic fibres arise medial to the vein on their way to the pelvic organs (Fig. 5.100).

The junction of the obturator vein with the circumflex iliac vein is seen on the pelvic bone. This is the only connection between the external and internal iliac vein. This junction is called as corona mortis, as damage to any of these veins can lead to direct bleeding from external and internal iliac veins.

This can be damaged during the surgery if care is not taken (Fig. 5.101).

5.6.2.1 Rules

Understanding the anatomy of the internal iliac veins and its tributaries is of great importance for harvesting the vein during uterine transplant (Fig. 5.102).

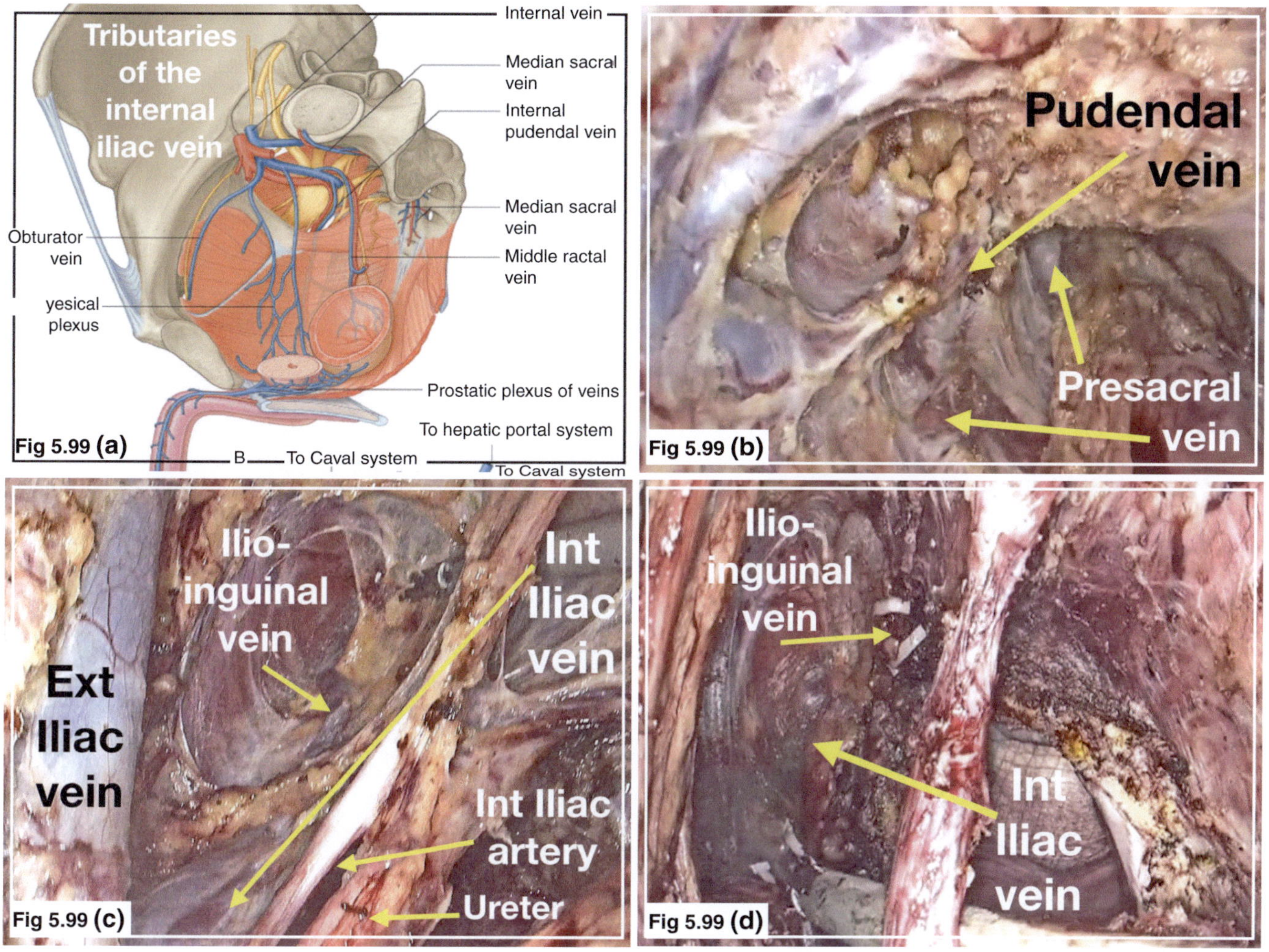

Fig. 5.99 (**a**) The tributaries drawing into the internal iliac vein can be seen in this image. (**b**) The vesico-vaginal-venous complex or the Santorini venous complex drains venous blood into the pudendal vein. The pudendal vein then drains inferiorly into the internal iliac vein as seen in the image. This image has been taken from a case of dissection donor for uterine transplant. The internal iliac vein was harvested through the pudendal vein. (**c**) The ilio-inguinal vein drains into the internal iliac vein from the lateral side travelling under the levator ani. (**d**) The ilio-inguinal vein has been clipped as shown in the image. It drains into the internal iliac vein

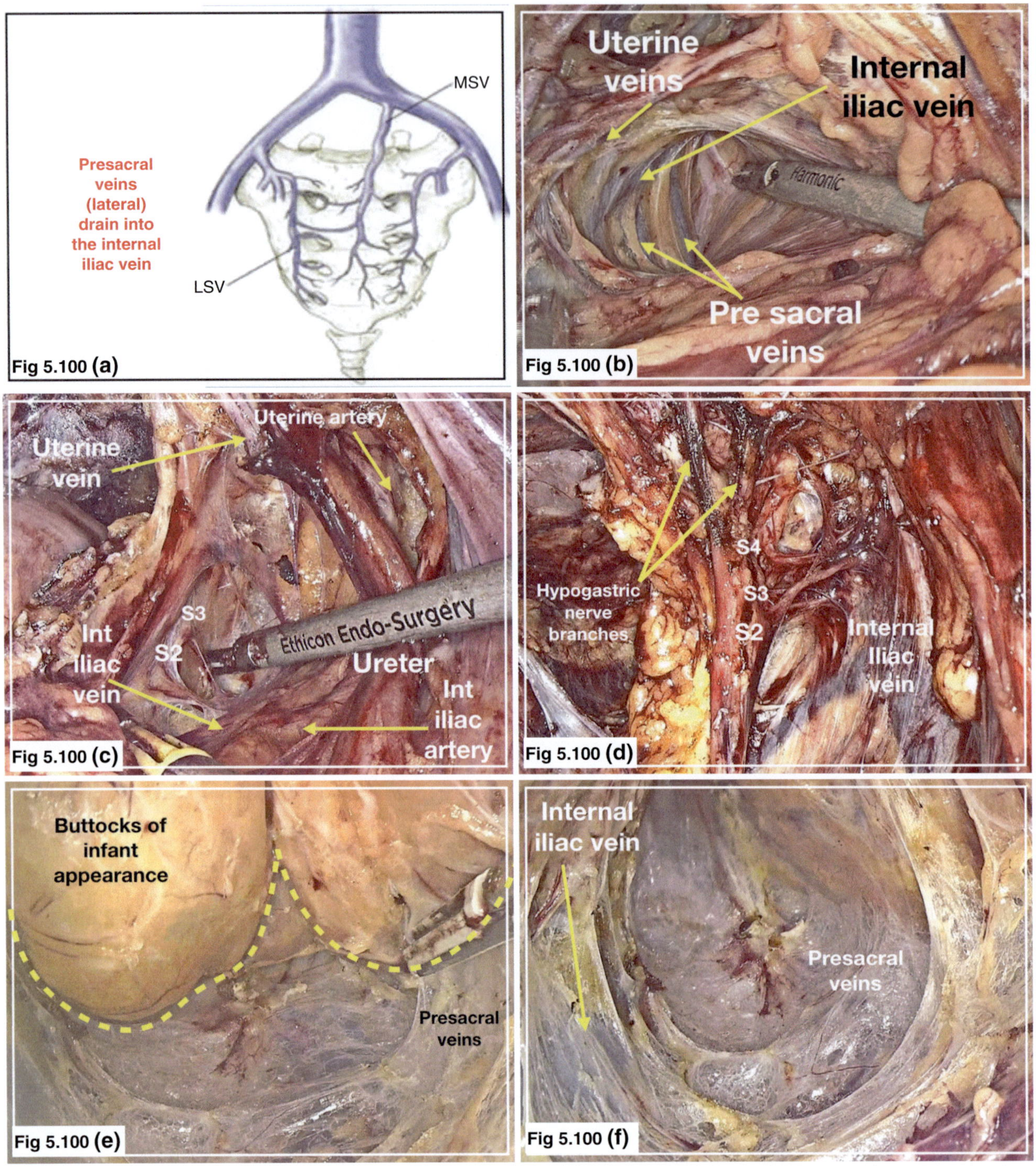

Fig. 5.100 (**a**) The presacral veins comprise the medial and the lateral presacral veins. While the medial sacral vein drains directly into the inferior vena cava or the left common iliac vein, the lateral sacral vein drains into their ipsilateral internal iliac veins. (**b**) Here the presacral veins can be seen draining into the internal iliac veins as seen in the case of laparoscopic radical hysterectomy previously shown. (**c**) The parasympathetic fibres S2, S3 and S4 lie above prior to the Waldeyer's fascia. Underneath these lie the presacral veins. They are exposed by dissecting the pararectal space more sacrally. (**d**) The internal iliac vein is seen and a single branch of the presacral vein is visible. The S2, S3 and S4 nerves can be seen lying above the venous structures. (**e**) The presacral veins are commonly encountered in rectal surgeries. In this image from a case of laparoscopic low anterior resection the rectum is mobilised from the Waldeyer's fascia. This is done also in the condition of posterior exenteration and in case of deep infiltrating endometriosis. The appearance similar to the buttocks of an infant is seen. The presacral veins can be seen underneath the fascia. (**f**) The internal iliac vein is also visible at the sides of the dissection of the bowel as shown in the image. The more superficial vessels are minor veins which drain into the presacral veins. Their bleeding can be controlled with energy sources. (**g**) In this image the diagrammatic representation has been shown where the presacral veins drain intercommunicated with the intervertebral veins which flow independently. Thus in case of presacral vein injury bleeding is torrential and not controlled easily

Fig. 5.100 (continued)

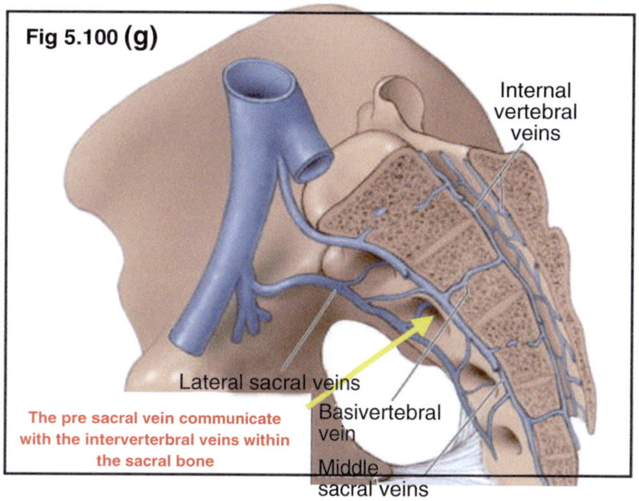

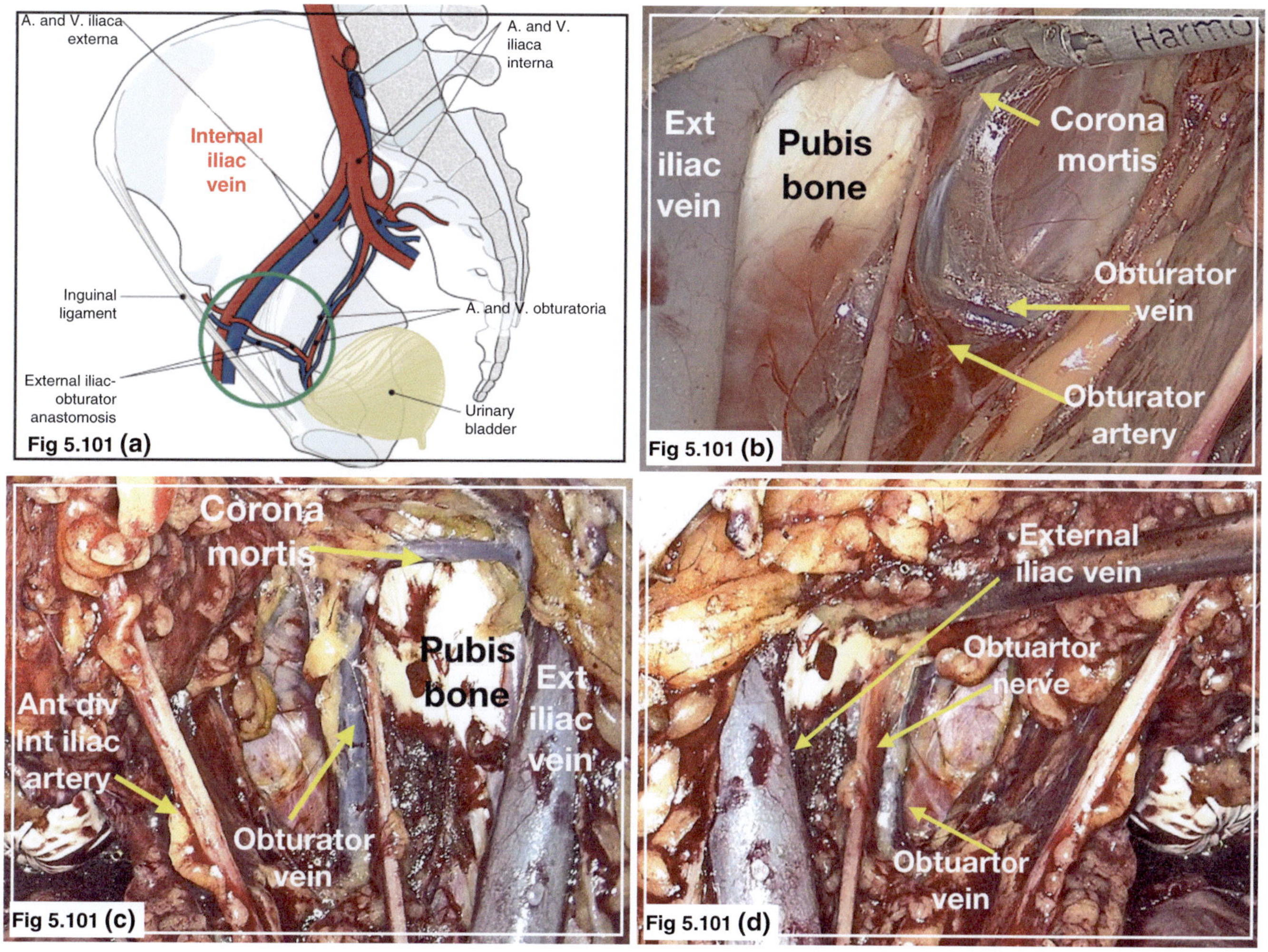

Fig. 5.101 (**a**) The image of corona mortis has been demonstrated here. The only intercommunication between the internal and the external iliac vein. (**b**) Corona mortis is an aberrant communication between the internal and external iliac vein via the obturator vein (internal iliac vein) and the deep circumflex iliac vein (external iliac vein). This is commonly encountered during pelvic lymph node dissection. (**c**) The corona mortis seen on right pelvic lymph node dissection. It lies on top of the pubic bone. (**d**) The obturator vein is seen travelling upwards towards the external iliac vein. It communicates with the deep circumflex iliac vein. (**e**) The obturator vein lies under the obturator nerve. Hence the lower limit of dissection during lymphadenectomy is the obturator nerve. Forceful dissection on the nerve leads to injury to the veins which leads to significant haemorrhage

Fig. 5.101 (continued)

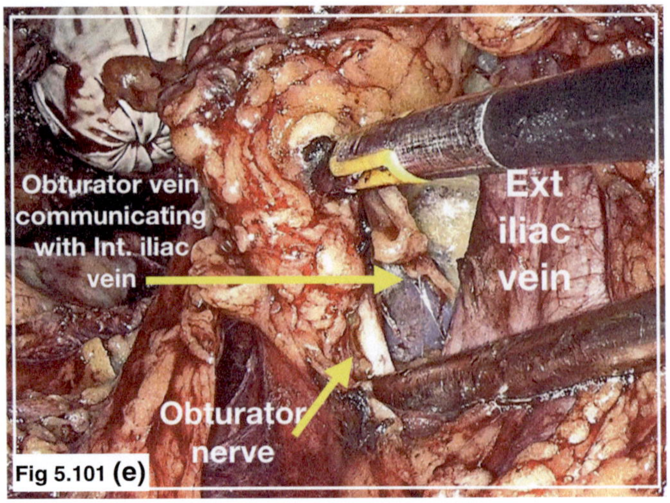

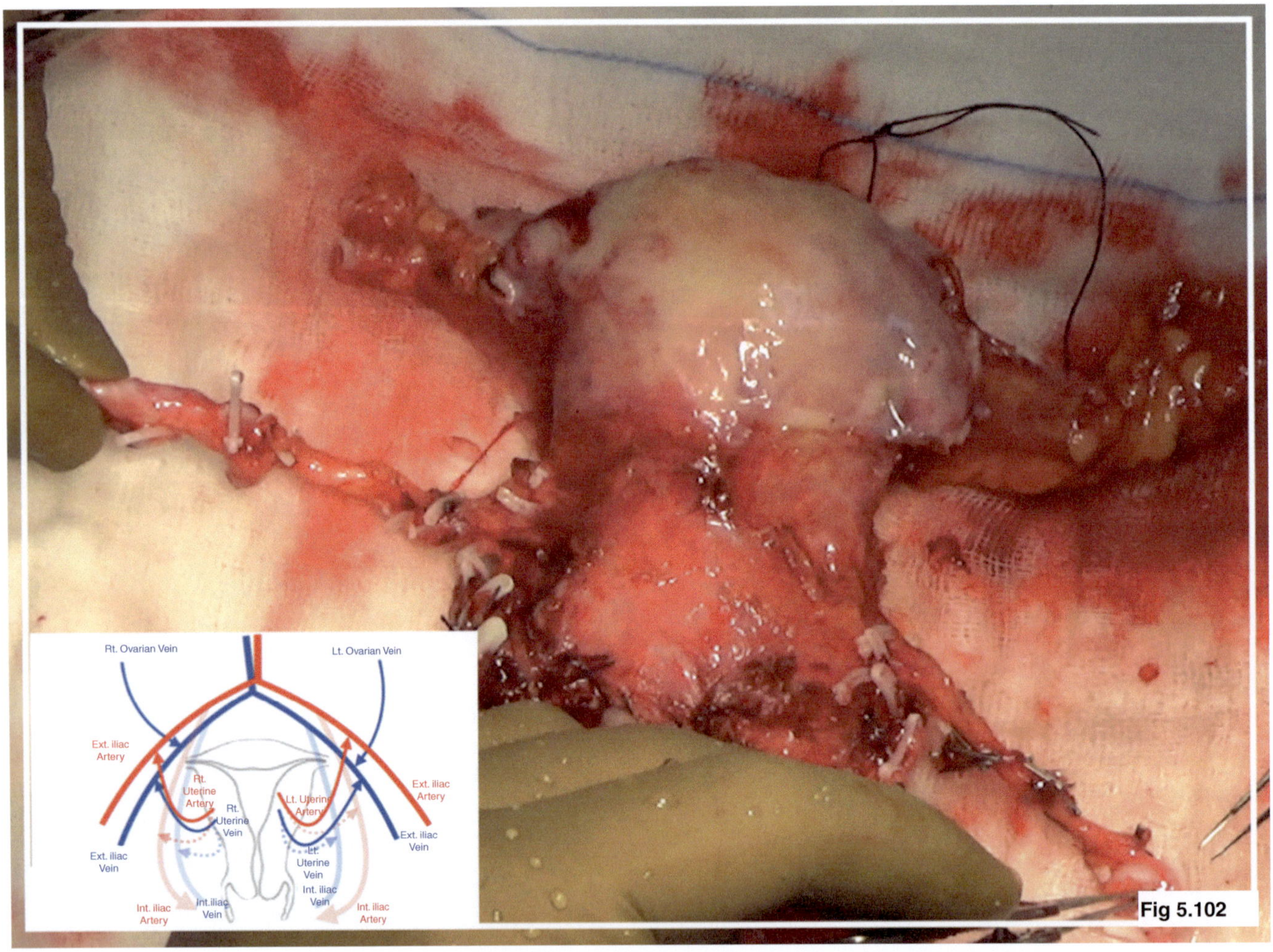

Fig. 5.102 The uterus dissected laparoscopically for uterine transplant has been brought for bench surgery where the anatomises with vessels is done prior to transplant in the recipient. The schematic diagram of the uterine transplant and their vascular anastomosis is shown in the inset

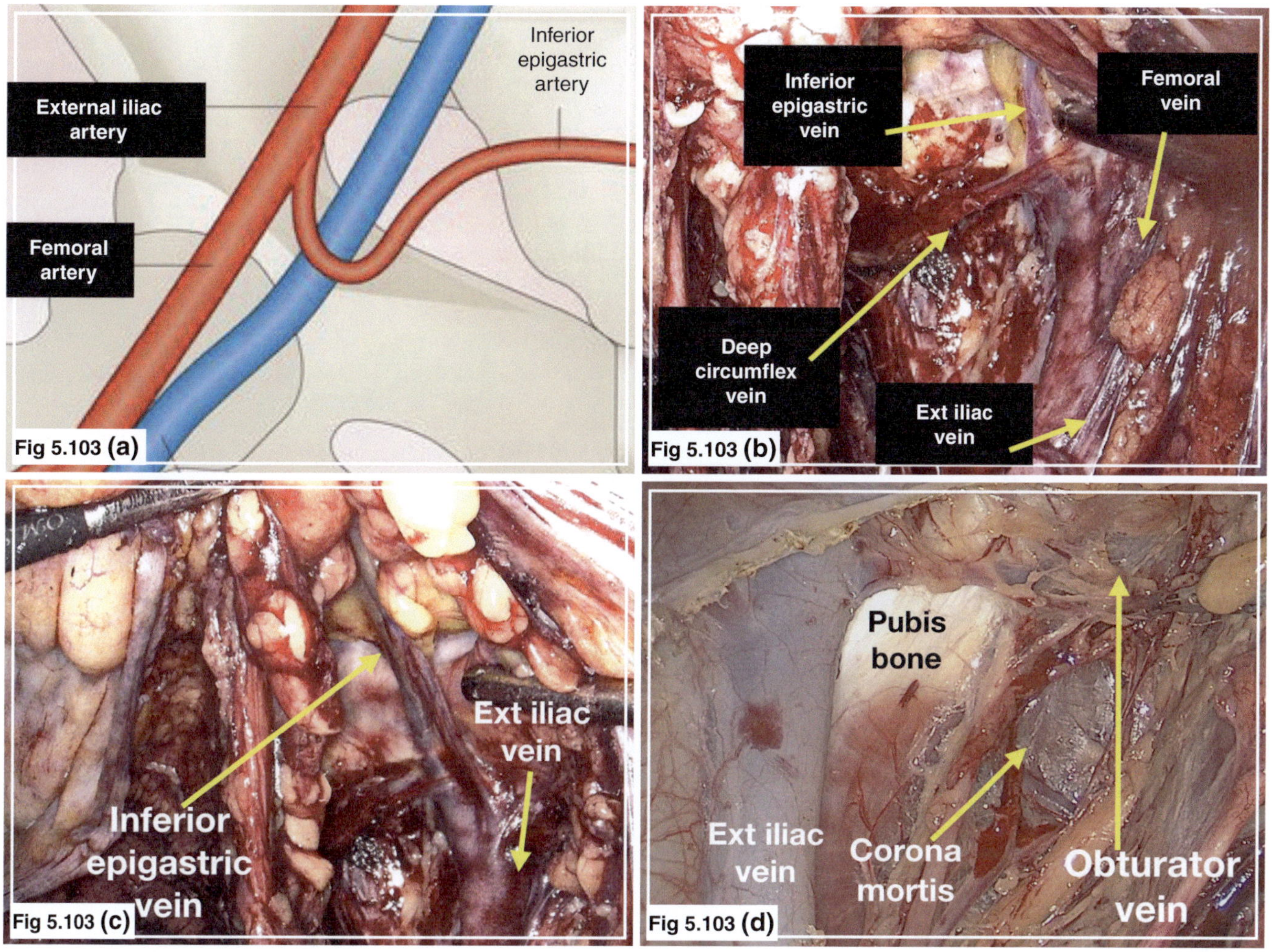

Fig. 5.103 (**a**) Diagrammatic representations of the external iliac vein and its course beyond the pelvis. (**b**) The external iliac vessels are seen giving off branches at the level of inguinal ligament, the inferior epigastric vessels. The deep circumflex iliac vein is seen communicating with the obturator vein downward. After passing through the inguinal ligament the external iliac vessels are labelled as femoral vessels. (**c**) Similar image seen on the interior abdominal wall. (**d**) Corona mortis is shown which has been explained previously

5.6.3 External Iliac Vein

The external iliac vein runs medial to the artery and continues as femoral vein. The only tributaries are inferior epigastric and circumflex iliac vein which joins the obturator vein (already discussed earlier) (Fig. 5.103).

5.6.3.1 Rules

Since there are no branches to the artery and vein, remaining parallel to these is of utmost importance during nodal dissection (Fig. 5.104).

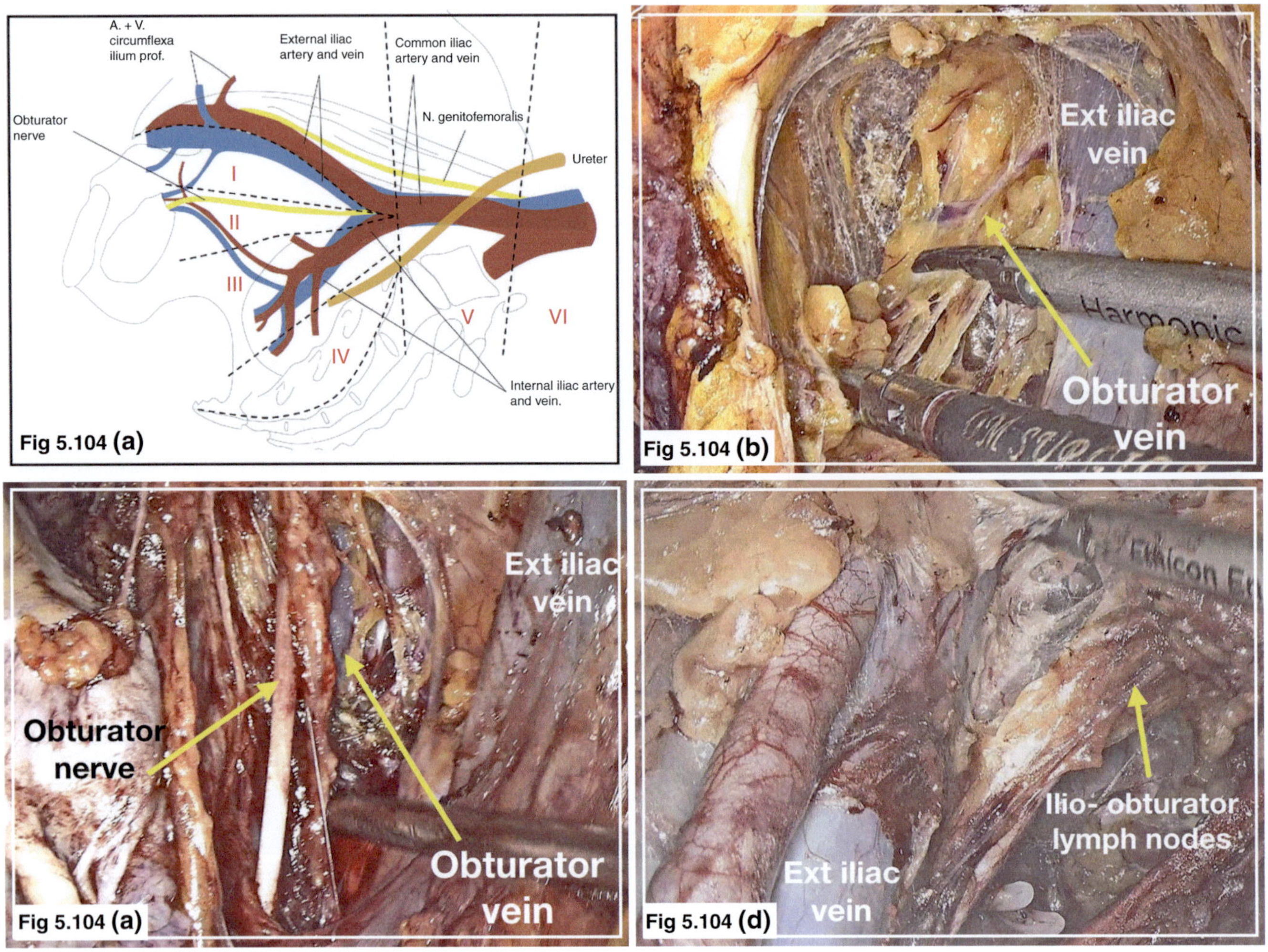

Fig. 5.104 (**a**) Diagrammatic representation of the clinical significance of the external iliac vessel in lymph node dissection. (**b**–**d**) Real-time images of the external iliac vein which shows the lack of any branches on its anterolateral surface along its entire length until the anterior abdominal wall near the inguinal ligament where it gives branches (inferior epigastric and deep circumflex iliac vessels)

6 The Spaces

6.1 Pouch of Douglas or the Rectovaginal Space

The pouch of Douglas is bounded by cardinal and uterosacral ligaments on either side, the uterus anteriorly and rectum posteriorly. It is a deep space. The peritoneum reflects in the pouch of Douglas on the anterior part of the rectum (Figs. 6.1, 6.2, 6.3, and 6.4b).

The rectum below the pouch of Douglas and the vagina are devoid of the peritoneum. Opening of the peritoneal reflection exposes the Denonvilliers' fascia (Fig. 6.4c–f).

There are two layers of Denonvilliers' fascia. One layer covers the rectum completely while the other lies on the posterior vaginal wall. The rectal fibres are protected by this fascia. The veins of the vagina lie between the fascia and the posterior vaginal wall (Fig. 6.4g, h).

There is an avascular plane between the two Denonvilliers' fascia. Any dissection between the fascia and the posterior vaginal wall leads to haemorrhage, while that between the Denonvilliers' fascia and the anterior wall

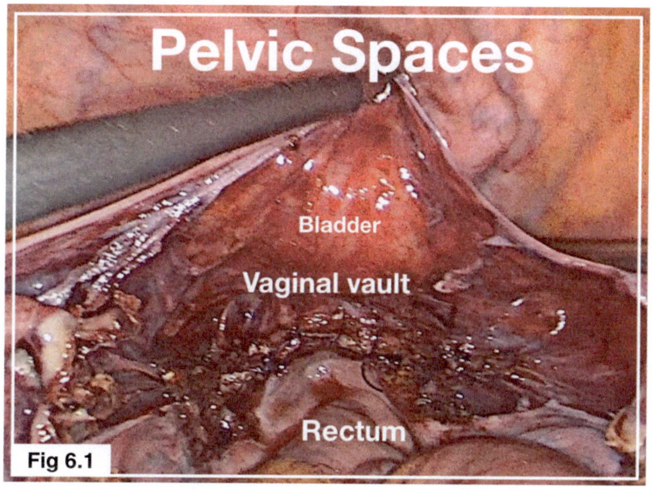

Fig. 6.1 The image has been taken from a case of intrafascial hysterectomy for a benign condition. The only spaces seen are the area mildly exposed by resecting the broad ligament and the bladder peritoneum. The purpose of this chapter is to understand deeper retroperitoneal spaces. These retroperitoneal spaces discussed ahead will aid the surgeon/gynaecologist in conducting difficult hysterectomies due to endometriosis or even operating for oncological cases

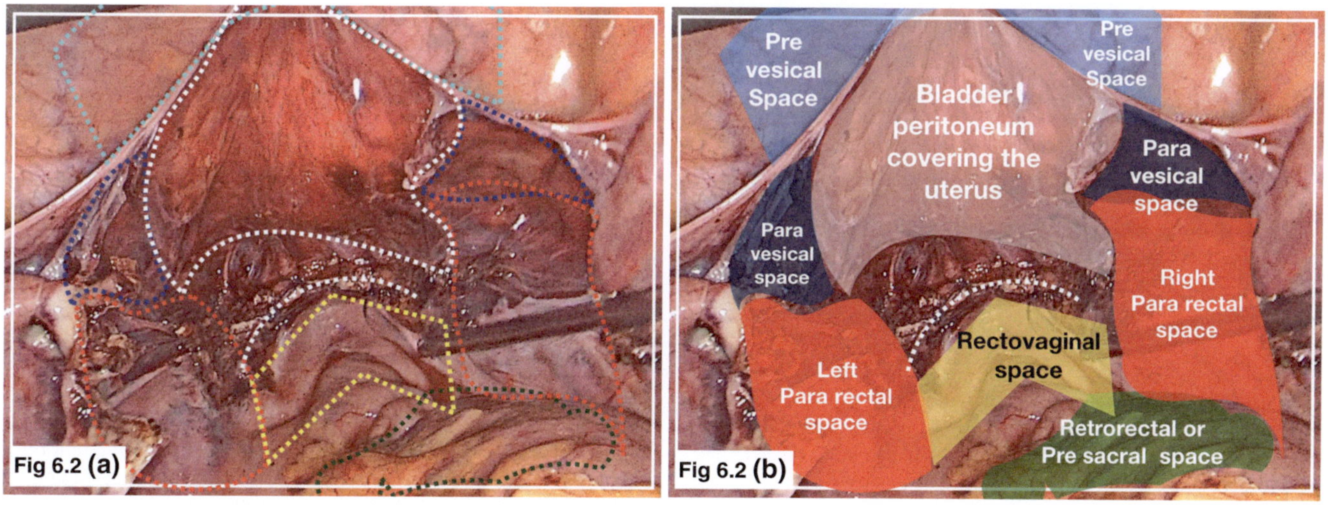

Fig. 6.2 (**a**, **b**) The dotted line denotes the potential retroperitoneal spaces to be dissected. The areas are shaded in the next image. When compared to the first image it gives a fair idea of the amount of difference between the intrafascial hysterectomy and radical hysterectomy

S. Puntambekar et al., *Laparoscopic Pelvic Anatomy in Females*, https://doi.org/10.1007/978-981-13-8653-4_6

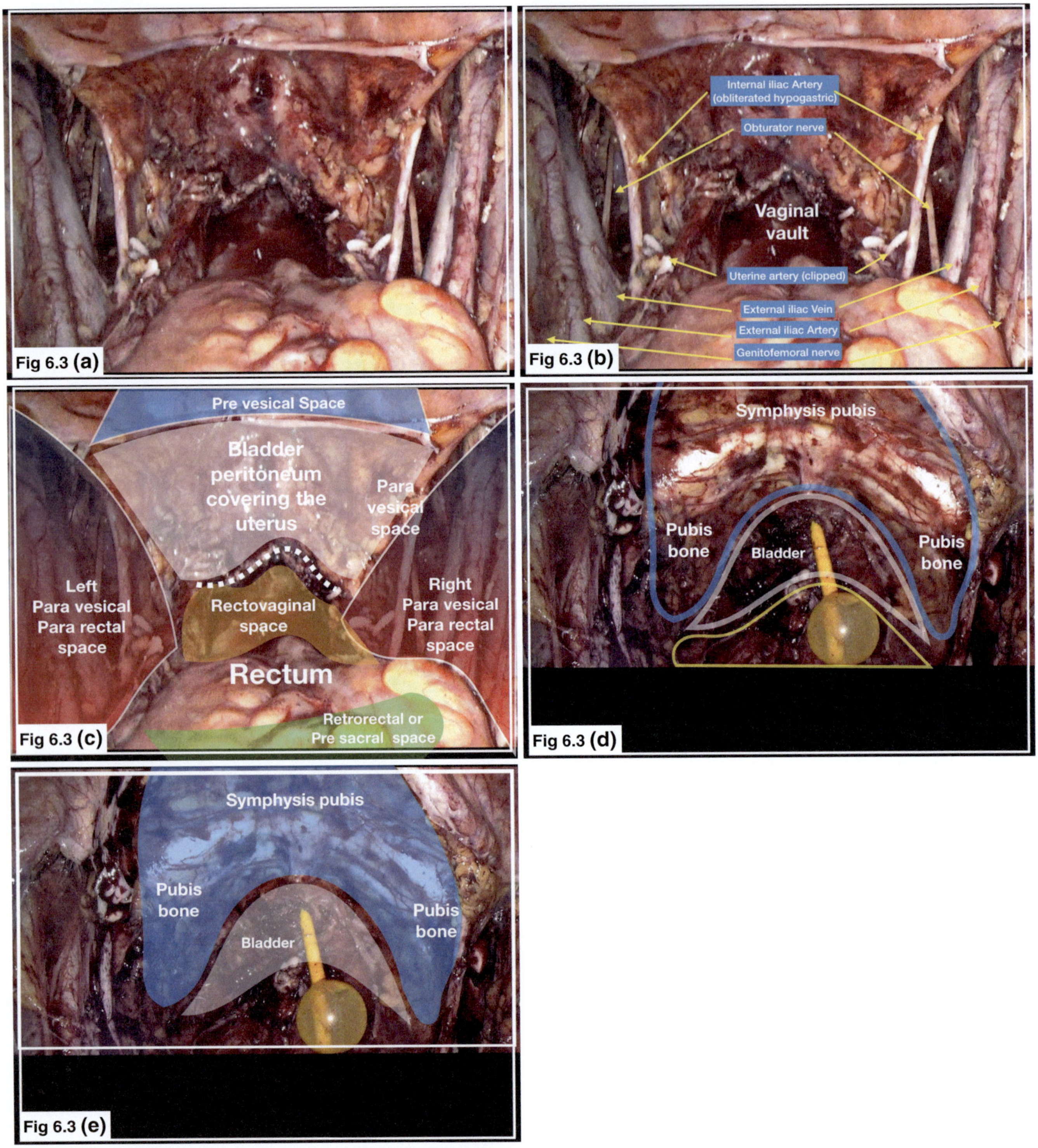

Fig. 6.3 (**a**) This is an image from the final view after a case of laparoscopic radical hysterectomy for a case of Ca cervix. The image points out at the extensive amount of retroperitoneal dissection done posteriorly to the vault as well as on the lateral sides where the Mackenrodt's ligament has been dissected to expose various structures. (**b**) All visible structures have been labelled in this image. The amount of retroperitoneal dissection can be comprehended while comparing with previous images where the literal pelvic wall is completely concealed with the Mackenrodt's ligament. (**c**) Just like Fig. 6.2b, c explain the retroperitoneal spaces in the form of territorial marking, this image also demarcates the pelvic spaces which will be discussed in the subsequent images. However the paravesical space is still marked falsely only disclosing the location without actually revealing how it appears. (**d**) In this image of anterior exenteration done for a case of Ca cervix, the Foley's catheter can be used to trace the remnant stump of urethra. Dissection done here is at a much deeper level considering that only the endopelvic fascia is visible on all sides. (**e**) The area shaded in blue represents the paravesical space. It is often exposed in case of Burch's colposuspension and in anterior exenteration. Further details to be explained later in the chapter

of the rectum leads to rectal damage. The Denonvilliers' is a tough fascia which prevents the cervical pathologies from invading into the rectum. The dissection in the pouch of Douglas is done with the dictum "fat belonging to the rectum" (Fig. 6.4i–k).

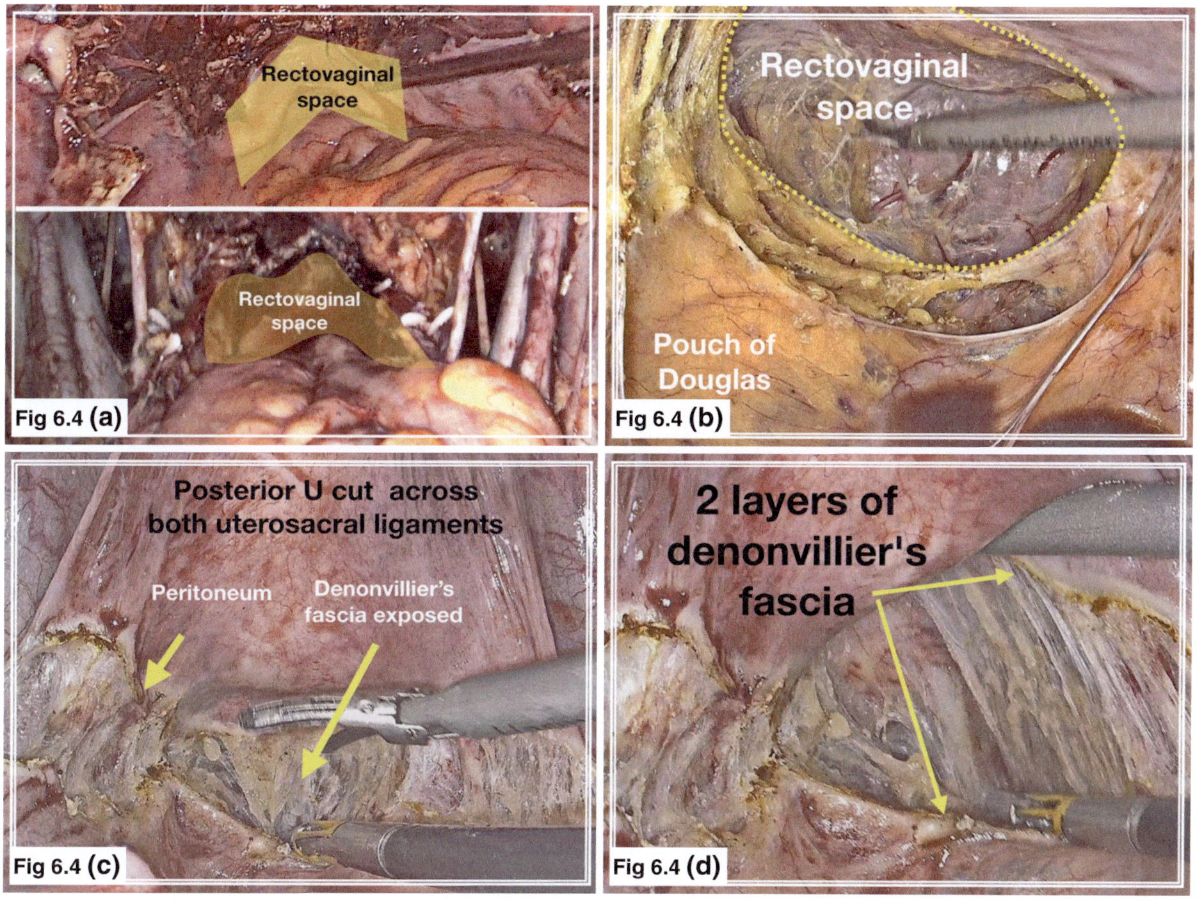

Fig. 6.4 (**a**) Rectovaginal space: The image shows rectovaginal space dissection previously explained in two chief images. Here on the details of the images will be explained. (**b**) Rectovaginal space is the retroperitoneal space under the fold of peritoneum of the pouch of Douglas. It is a midline space and is bounded by the uterosacral ligaments on either side. The peritoneum covers the area like a sheath and the Denonvilliers' fascia forms its two walls. Above the sheath the space is called the pouch of Douglas, and underneath the peritoneum (retroperitoneum) it is called the rectovaginal space (**c**) The first step of dissection of rectovaginal space is cutting open the peritoneum between the two uterosacral ligaments as shown in the image. The ultimate goal of rectovaginal space dissection is to separate the rectum from the vagina completely till the level of the endopelvic fascia. Beyond the endopelvic fascia the fibres of pubovaginalis and puborectalis completely separate the organs. (**d**) The Denonvilliers' fascia is in two layers always. Either side of the layers is covered by veins. The vaginal veins lie between the vagina and the Denonvilliers' fascia while the presacral or rectal veins lie between the rectum and the Denonvilliers' fascia. The goal here is to remain between the layers so that neither of the vessels are injured. (**e**) The presacral veins can be seen intermittently visible during the dissection of the rectovaginal space. The presacral veins drain into the internal iliac vein. Hence it is of utmost importance not to injure the veins. (**f**) The endopelvic fascia is the lower of dissection of the rectovaginal space. At this point the uterus/vagina can be seen completely separated from the rectum. (**g**) This image has been taken for the viewers to assess the depth to which the dissection has taken place, and also to make the viewers realise the close proximity of the vagina with the rectum. Once the dissection is done the uterosacral ligaments are cut and the entire paracolpium can be easily separated from the pelvis as now the resection will be done at the level of as low as the endopelvic fascia instead of the peritoneum like done in intrafascial hysterectomy. (**h**) Similar images of laparoscopic radical hysterectomy from another case have been taken to show the amount of dissection required for separating the rectum from the vagina in rectovaginal space dissection. The uterosacral ligament is respected till the level of the endopelvic fascia for aiding the resection of the paracolpium. (**i**) The direction of the dissection is of importance here. Dissection is carried in a bidirectional fashion as shown in the image. It is important to remain between the two layers of Denonvilliers's fascia and separate at right angles to the plane in both directions making the instruments move in opposite directions. (**j**) The two layers of Denonvilliers' fascia are surrounded by vaginal and rectal and presacral veins on either side. But the space between the layers remains avascular. This is the plane of dissection. Presacral veins often encountered during the space dissection need to be cauterised immediately to prevent blood loss and obscuration of the vascular plane. (**k**) The end point of dissection is the appearance of shiny surface underneath. This is the endopelvic fascia. It is best to reach the endopelvic fascia on either side of the rectum and then cautiously approach dissecting the rectum from the vagina finally. The confines of the rectum have been defined by white dotted lines

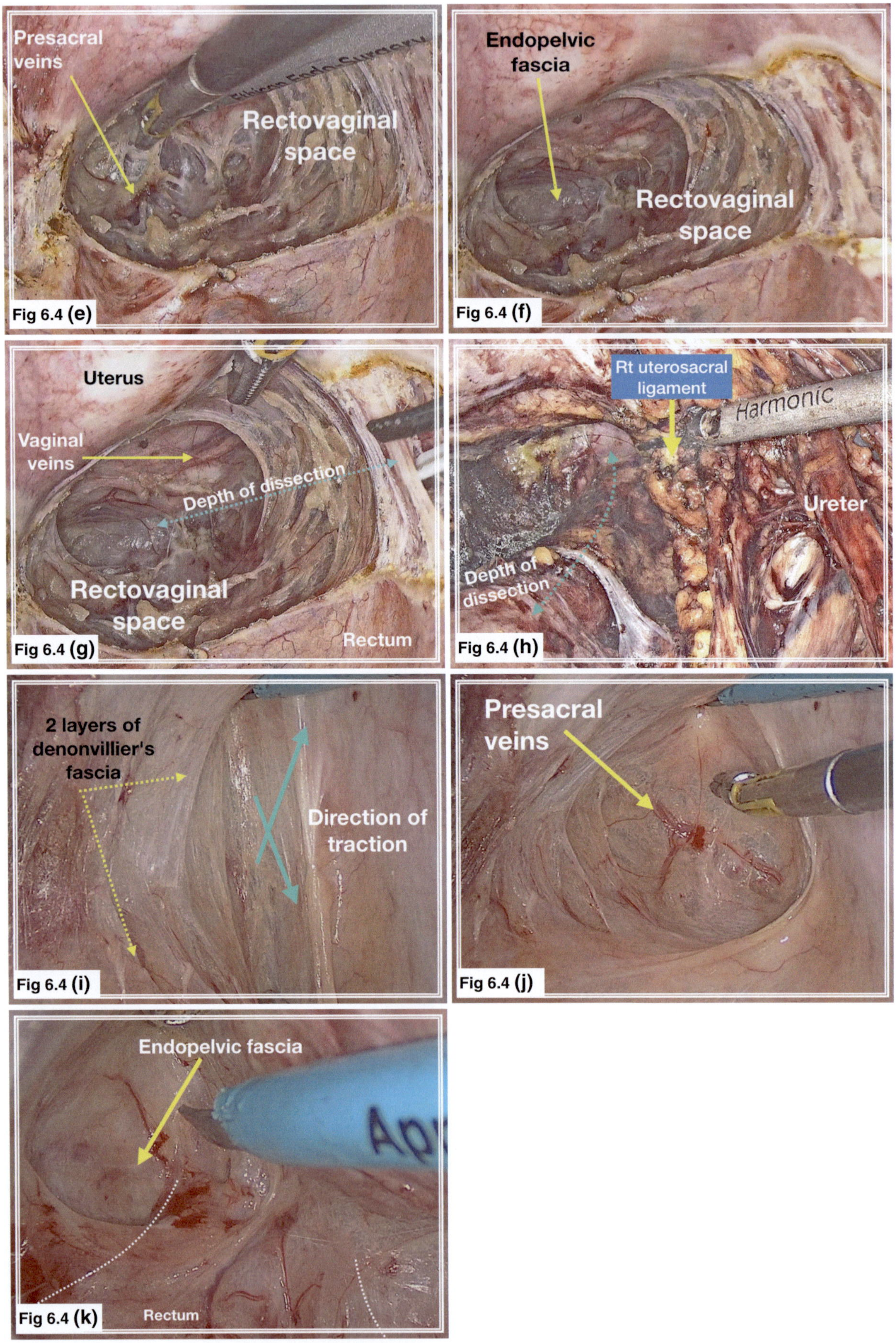

Fig. 6.4 (continued)

6.2 Pararectal Space

The pararectal space is a potential space lateral to the ureter. It needs to be exposed surgically and this can be achieved by opening the peritoneum at the level of sacral promontory. The pararectal space is divided into medial and lateral spaces by the ureter (Fig. 6.5a–d).

The boundaries of lateral pararectal space or Latzko space are ureter medially, and internal iliac artery. It is a pyramidal space, the apex of which is at the level at which the ureter crosses the common iliac and the base is formed by the levator ani muscle, with its covering endopelvic fascia. The only structure that crosses this space transversely is the uterine vessels and superior vesical vessels in females and males, respectively. The parasympathetic nerves from S to 3 and 4 also traverse this space on their way to the pelvic organs. The supports of uterus and bladder also traverse this space (Fig. 6.5e–g).

The boundaries of medial pararectal space or Okabayashi space are uterosacral medially and ureter laterally. The structures in the medial pararectal space are the hypogastric nerve which traverses longitudinally and the uterine vein which traverses transversely (Fig. 6.5h–p).

Rules: The lateral pararectal space can be exposed by beginning the dissection at the level of sacral promontory and remaining parallel and lateral to the ureter. The only structure which prevents further caudal dissection would be the uterine artery or the superior vesical artery in males. These vessels can be easily clipped or ligated in this space (Fig. 6.5q–z).

Fig. 6.5 Pararectal space dissection: (**a**) Perhaps the most important of all retroperitoneal space is the pararectal space. It is the deciding factor for operability in cases of radical hysterectomy, anterior exenteration, posterior exenteration and total pelvic exenteration. The pararectal and paravesical spaces are interconnected from under the peritoneum. They are only divided by the uterine artery under the peritoneum. Thus exposure often opens both spaces simultaneously. (**b**) This is a real-time image of the pararectal space depicting ureter dissection. The pararectal space is also important from benign surgery point of view in cases of ureter mobilisation in endometriosis, cervical fibroids and broad ligament fibroids alike. The pararectal space is the first window to the lateral pelvic wall. (**c**) Here the ureter can be seen retracted medially to the bipolar energy source. And the Harmonic scalpel is used to direct and single out the uterine artery. Here the dissection has been carried out at a level deeper between the external iliac artery and the ureter. (**d**) The medial and the lateral pararectal space has been shown in this image. The pararectal space is divided into medial and lateral by the ureter, and is also common to both oncological and benign cases. The pararectal space is the gateway to exposing the nerves in nerve-sparing surgeries, be it nerve-sparing radical hysterectomy or selective uterosacral nerve ablation for endometriosis(**e**) The uterine artery is dissected out from loose areolar connective tissue and traced up to the ureter. One of the identifying points is to see it cross the ureter. (**f**) The superior vesical artery can be seen getting exposed above the uterine artery. The blade of Harmonic scalpel is exactly in the paravesical space. The uterine artery is a common boundary shared between the pararectal and the paravesical space. (**g**) The bifurcation of the common iliac artery can be traced by dissecting both the external and the internal iliac artery further cranially. Thus pararectal space is the key deciding factor of operability, as it opens the paravesical space caudally and exposes the bifurcation of the iliac artery and gives a detailed assessment of the lateral pelvic wall. (**h**) The following series of images are taken in a sequential manner so as to explain viewers the step-by-step dissection of pararectal spaces. It is taken from a case of a postmenopausal bleeding in a 75-year-old patient with biopsy suggestive of complex endometrial hyperplasia with atypia and focal areas of carcinoma of endometrium. Owing to the extreme old age the uterine artery in further images appears to be shrunken and the planes appear avascular which forms the best condition to explain the spaces and the fascias in the next chapter. (**i**) There are two approaches to the pararectal space. In this image the medial approach is explained. The incision is made medial to the infundibulopelvic ligament. The posterior surface of the broad ligament is incised. (**j**) The incision is extended caudally towards the apex of the uterosacral ligament. The foamy appearance of the retroperitoneum is often regarded as "the champagne effect". Due to raised intra-abdominal pressure the air enters the spaces and spreads out across the loose areolar tissue forming foamy or champagne bubble-like effect. Medial traction is given to the leaf of peritoneum to open the pararectal space as we dissect further. (**k**) The incision is extended caudally towards the apex of the uterosacral ligament. The foamy appearance of the retroperitoneum is often regarded as "the champagne effect". Due to raised intra-abdominal pressure the air enters the spaces and spreads out across the loose areolar tissue forming foamy or champagne bubble-like effect. Medial traction is given to the leaf of peritoneum to open the pararectal space as we dissect further. (**l**) Just like the principles of open surgery, an opening is made across on the anterior leaf of the broad ligament; this ensures that no other structure passes in between. The anterior leaf window should be made above the level of the ureter. (**m**) The external iliac artery can be seen lateral to the infundibulopelvic ligament by retracing the ligament laterally and visualising the vessel laterally. Dissect the space between the vessel and the ureter gently and remain at the same plane as the ureter exposes the internal iliac artery as shown in the image. (**n**) Further dissection is carried out in a plane between the internal iliac artery and the ureter by maintaining the same plane of ureter. The first structure to obstruct the dissection of the ureter is the uterine artery crossing over the ureter to supply the uterus. This is one of the chief identifying points. (**o**) It is of utmost importance to remain in the same plane as that of the ureter. Deeper dissection below the level of the ureter is highly discouraged. This is because of the presence of uterine vein which travels parallel and below the uterine artery. In other conditions the internal iliac vein can also be present at the level below the ureter. Both veins are prone to injury depending upon where the depth has crossed the safe plane of dissection. (**p**) In this image injury to the uterine vein can be clearly seen leading to significant haemorrhage. The primary aim of pararectal space dissection is to expose the uterine artery. The lateral pararectal space is the best area to coagulate and cut the uterine artery from its origin till it crosses the ureter. (**q**) The lateral approach has been explained in this sequence of images here on. The incision is made lateral to the infundibulopelvic ligament. The ligament is given a medial traction to expose its lateral area. (**r**) The incision begins from the lateral side of the infundibulopelvic ligament (without involving the ovarian vessels) and is extended up to the round ligament involving the round ligament as well. The direction of dissection has also been explained in this image with the yellow arrows. (**s**) The first structure to be exposed here in the lateral approach is the external iliac artery and vein. They along with the psoas muscle form the lateral border of the pararectal space. Often the peritoneum can be dissected in the direction (yellow arrow) to open the peritoneum further and expose the pararectal space further. Similar image can be seen previously in (**g**). (**t**) Similar to the previous steps, gentle blunt dissection between the external iliac artery and the ureter exposes the internal iliac artery and the thus the uterine artery in a similar manner. The internal iliac artery terminates as the obliterated hypogastric artery. (**u**) Dissection between the uterine artery and ureter is carried out in the same plane so as to separate the uterine artery from the surrounding areolar tissue. Yellow arrow denotes the direction of dissection. (**v**) As discussed previously the ureter divides the pararectal space into medial and lateral pararectal space. The lateral space is called the Latzko space while the medial is called the Okabayashi space. The lateral space is for dissecting the uterine artery while the medial space is for identification and dissection of hypogastric nerves. (**w**) In this image the ureter can be seen dividing the pararectal space into medial and lateral spaces. The nerve fibres are seen around the ureter. These are the pelvic splanchnic nerves which travel in close proximity to the uterine vein which is also seen under the ureter here. More images of these nerves can be seen in theatre chapter on nerves. (**x**) The hypogastric nerves seen on the medial pararectal space lie along the peritoneum and the ureter. They are formed of fusion of nerve fibres of the superior hypogastric plexus. They later communicate with pelvic splanchnic nerves to form the inferior hypogastric plexus. Thus dissection of medial parental space is essential for nerve-sparing surgeries. (**y**) The hypogastric nerve can be seen being formed by fusion of the nerve fibres of superior hypogastric plexus, which is seen as converging fibres above the nerve itself. The leaf of the peritoneum is dissected completely. This completes the medial and pararectal space dissection. (**z**) This image explains the relation of the pararectal space with the paravesical space. The paravesical space is explained later in the following series of images

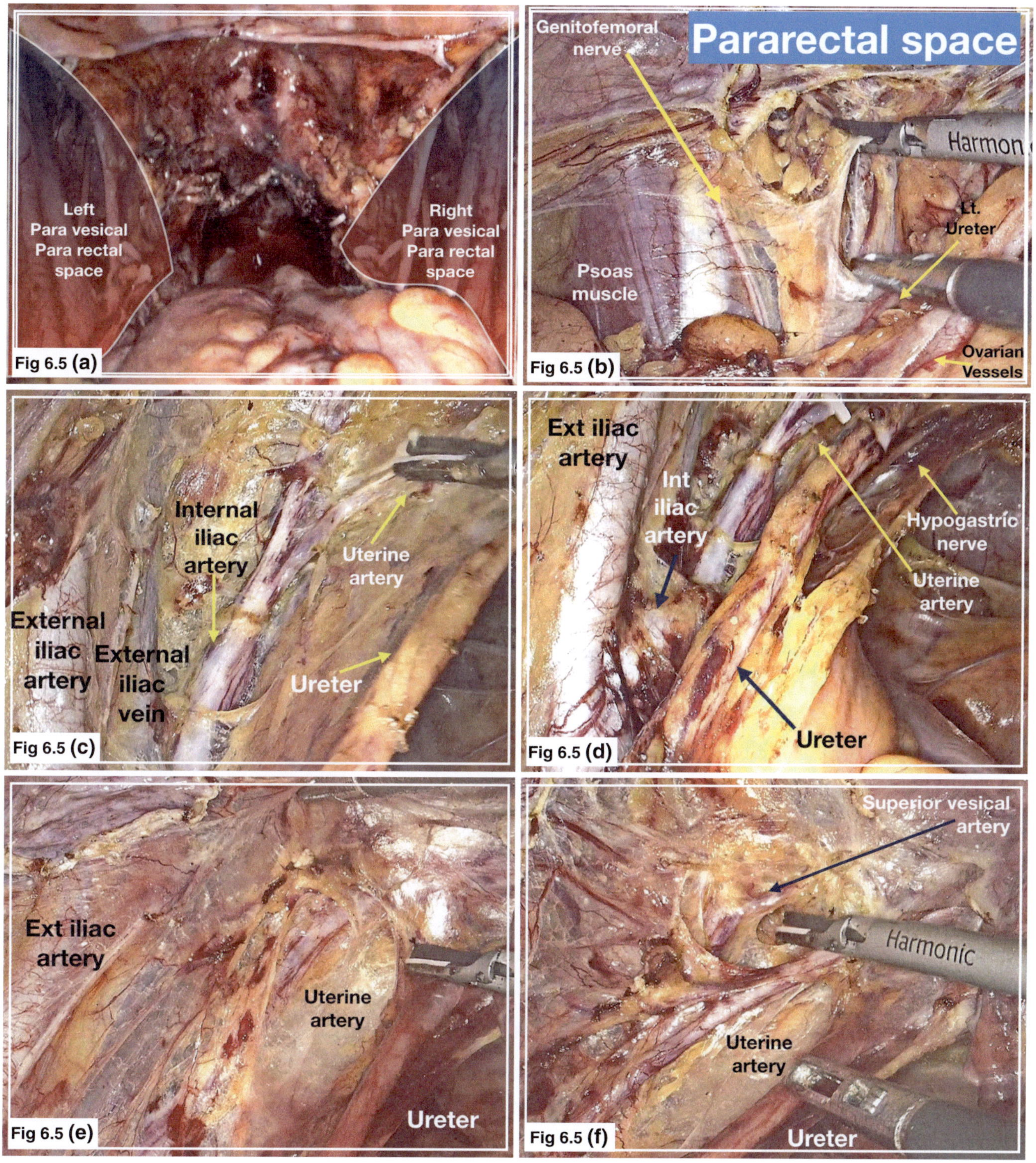
Left
Para vesical
Para rectal
space
Right
Para vesical
Para rectal
space
Fig 6.5 (a)
Genitofemoral
nerve
Pararectal space
Harmon
Lt.
Ureter
Psoas
muscle
Ovarian
Vessels
Fig 6.5 (b)
Internal
iliac
artery
Uterine
artery
External
iliac
artery
External
iliac
vein
Ureter
Fig 6.5 (c)
Ext iliac
artery
Int
iliac
artery
Hypogastric
nerve
Uterine
artery
Ureter
Fig 6.5 (d)
Ext iliac
artery
Uterine
artery
Ureter
Fig 6.5 (e)
Superior vesical
artery
Harmonic
Uterine
artery
Ureter
Fig 6.5 (f)

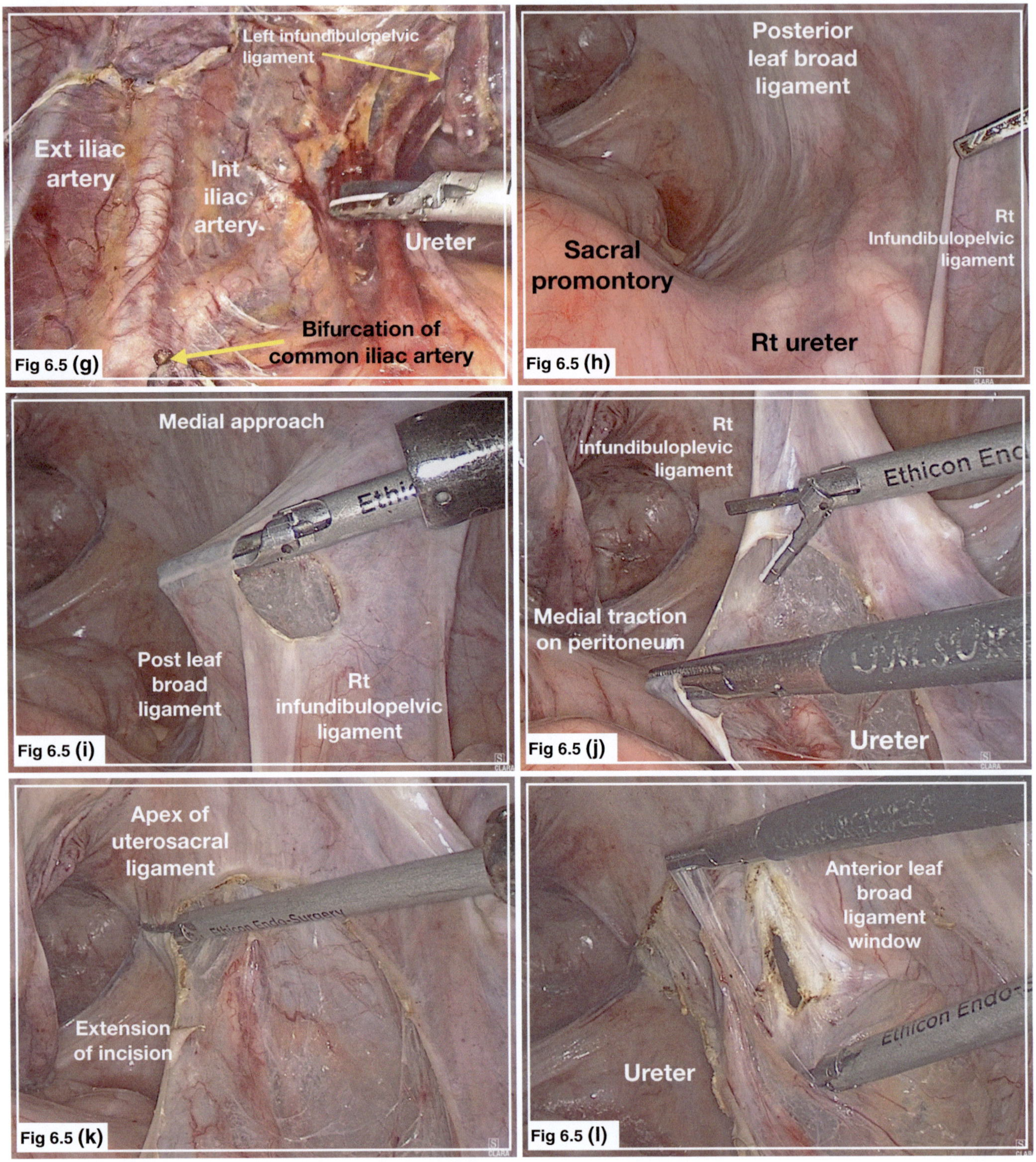

Fig. 6.5 (continued)

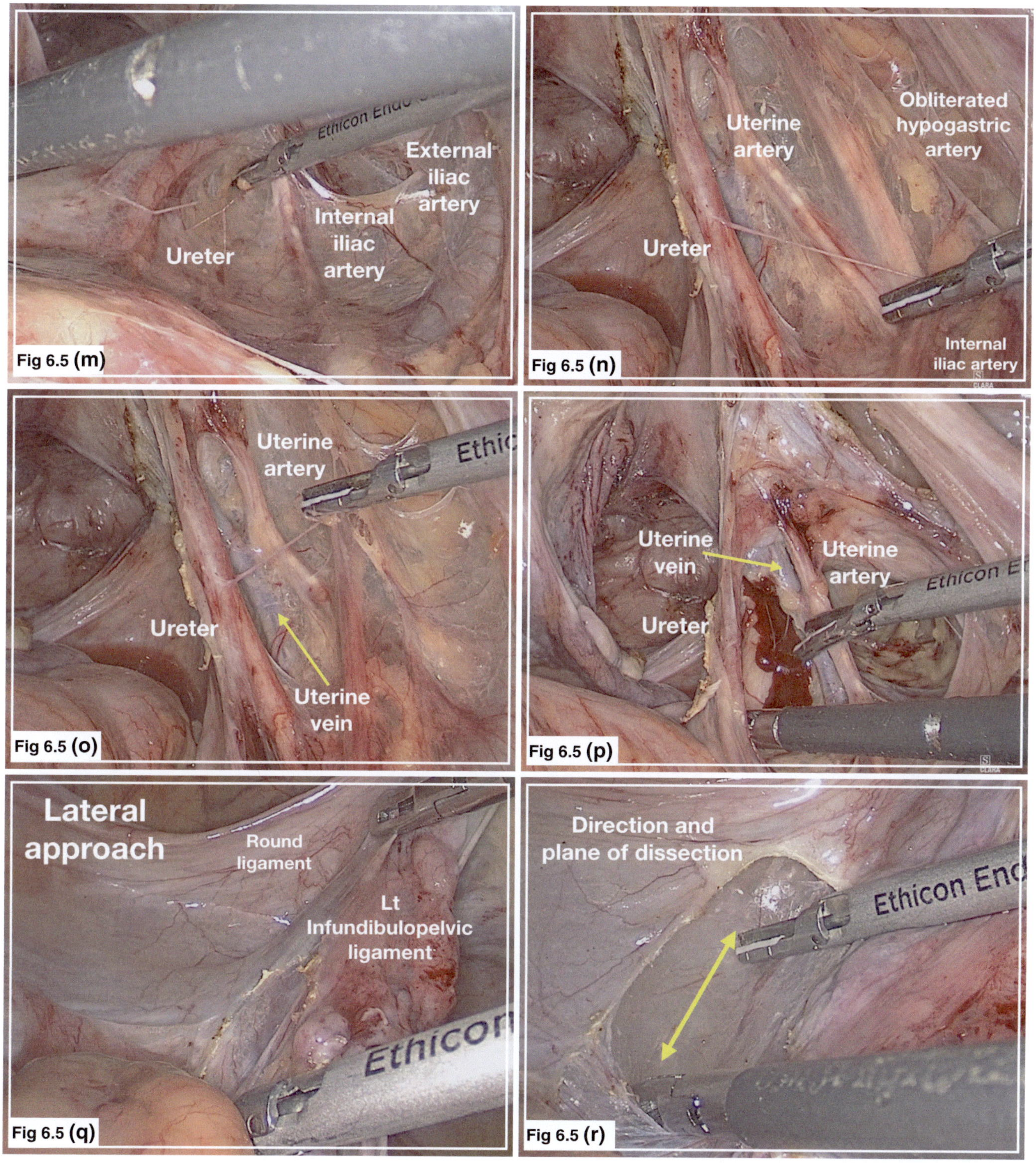

Fig. 6.5 (continued)

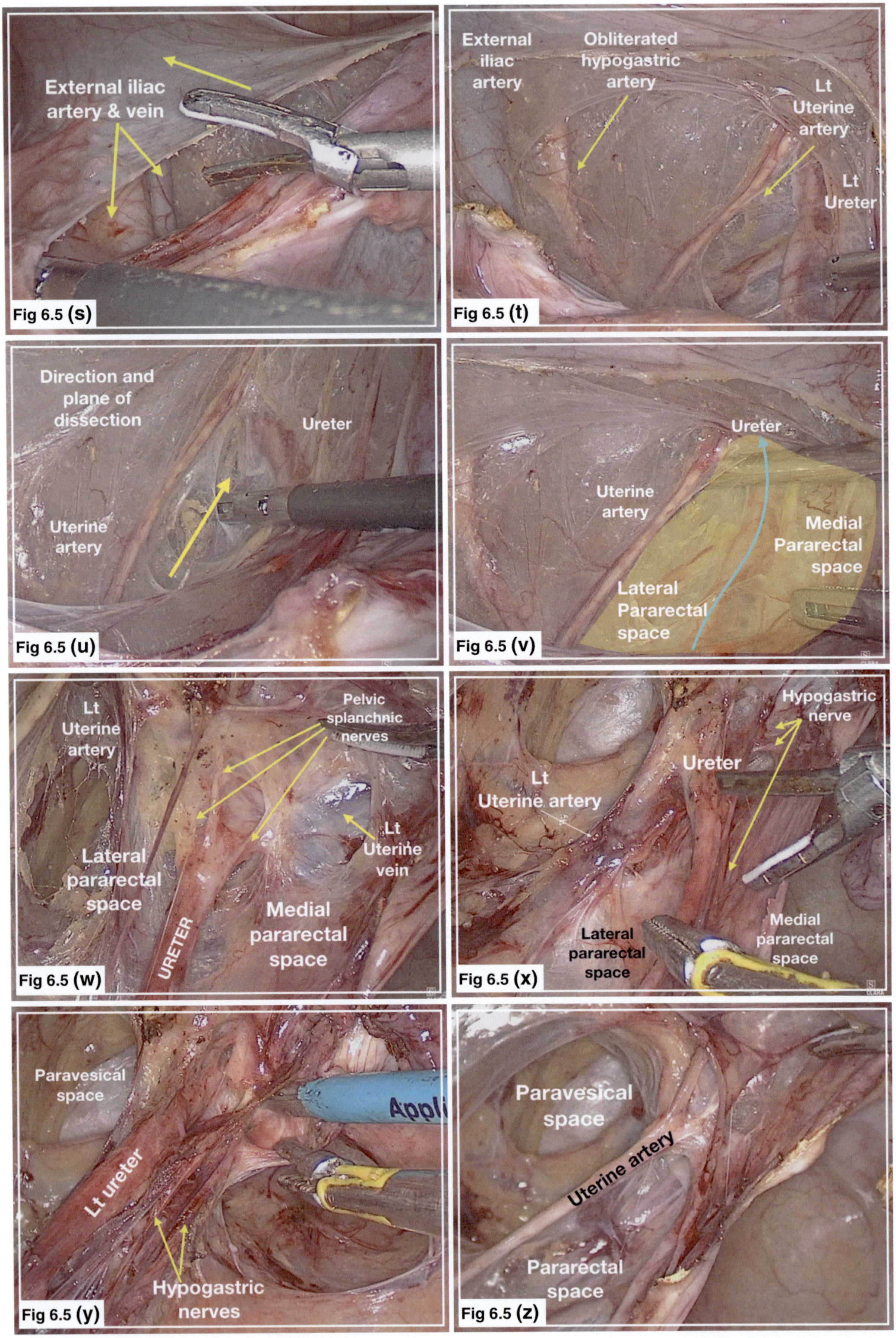

Fig. 6.5 (continued)

6.3 Paravesical Space

The paravesical space lies lateral to the urinary bladder and the boundaries are laterally the obliterated hypogastric artery, medially the urinary bladder, inferiorly the pubic bone and superiorly the pararectal space. Both these spaces are connected to each other and hence the entire vascular structures can be separated from the solid organs (Fig. 6.6a–d).

During the radical surgeries this space needs to be opened to reach the lateral side wall and achieve an optimum oncological clearance. The obliterated hypogastric artery is also called as the lateral umbilical ligament (hernia surgery—transperitoneal) (Fig. 6.6e–o).

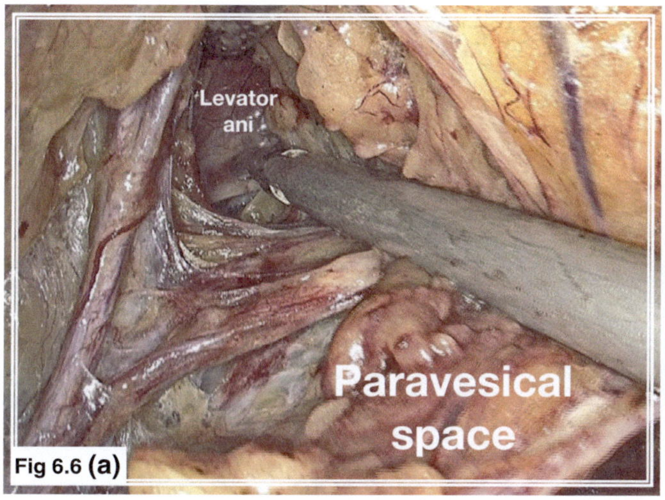

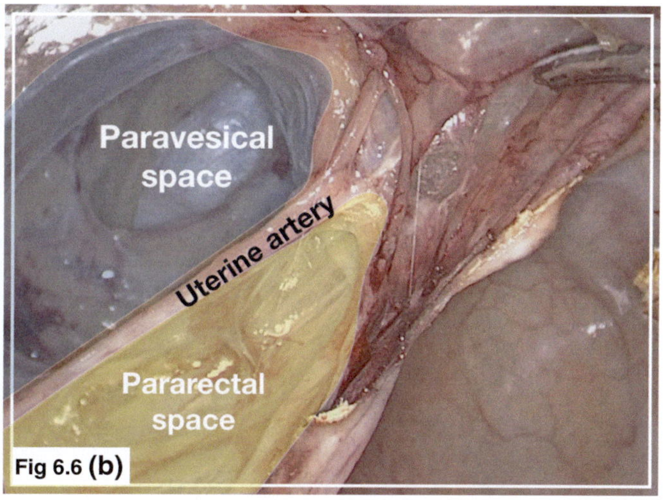

Fig. 6.6 Paravesical space: (**a**) The paravesical space has been shown in this image with its lower limit as the levator ani also visible. (**b**) The relation of the pararectal space with the paravesical space has been demonstrated with this image. The paravesical space is shaded in blue while the pararectal space is shaded in yellow. (**c**) The image shows the right paravesical space which is bounded by a distinct uterine artery separating it from the pararectal space. The uterine artery is seen crossing over the ureter. (**d**) This is the final image of the complete paravesical space dissection. Step-by-step image of dissection has been explained further in the next series of images. The purpose of paravesical space dissection is to ensure complete resection of the uterosacral and Mackenrodt's ligament during radical hysterectomy. Hence it is important to reach till the levator ani during paravesical space dissection. (**e**) From the case mentioned in pararectal space dissection the same case is carried further to explain paravesical space dissection. Here the boundaries of the paravesical space can be identified: the uterine artery below, the obliterated hypogastric artery on the lateral side and the peritoneum extending over the bladder anteriorly. (**f**) Paravesical space dissections are easiest after identification of the uterine artery. Here onwards, the dissection is carried out parallel to the uterine artery and deeper till the end point is reached as explained with the yellow arrow. (**g**) Though the direction of the dissection is bidirectional, for a case of oncological significance it is always advisable to dissect in the direction towards the uterus. This makes all the fat in the paracolpium shift towards the uterus, thus increasing lymph node yield and improving oncological clearance. (**h**) The end point of paravesical space dissection is the exposure of shiny pearly white surface of the endopelvic fascia. Often the levator ani can be seen in thin endopelvic fascia like in (**a**). (**i**) As explained above this is the end point of dissection of the paravesical space. The endopelvic fascia is exposed. The uterine artery is dissected and the fat is separated and towards the uterus. (**j**) Similar steps are done on the right side in this image. Always remain parallel and above the uterine artery during dissection. (**k**) The direction of dissection has been shown in this image. The fat is operated and towards the uterus. (**l**) The uterine artery, vein, ureter and obliterated hypogastric artery can be seen. The end point of dissection, the endopelvic fascia, can be seen. (**m**) This image has been taken from a case of anterior exenteration. Medial and anterior to the paravesical space lies the prevesical space. The paravesical space becomes an access to enter the prevesical space in case of anterior exenterations and total pelvic exenterations. (**n**) This image shows how the prevesical space can be approached from the lateral side from the paravesical space. Always remain medial to the obliterated hypogastric artery. The obliterated hypogastric artery which is the terminal structure of the internal iliac artery continues on the anterior abdominal wall as the median umbilical ligament. Thus it is important for bladder dissection to remain medial to the median umbilical ligament. (**o**) The image shows the final view after complete dissection of the paravesical and the prevesical space. Both the spaces share a common endopelvic fascia. The prevesical space is only in its pelvic phase

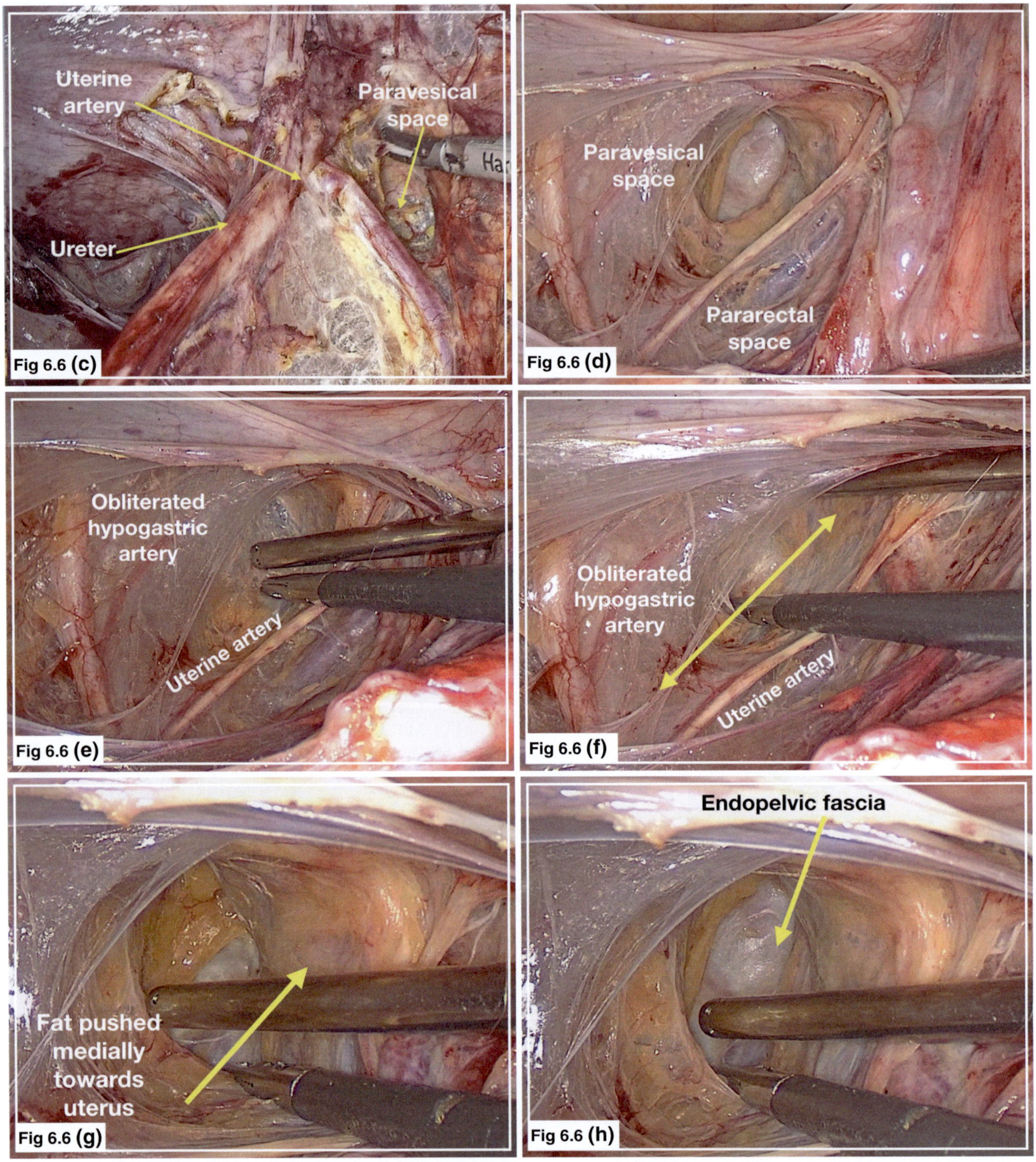

Fig. 6.6 (continued)

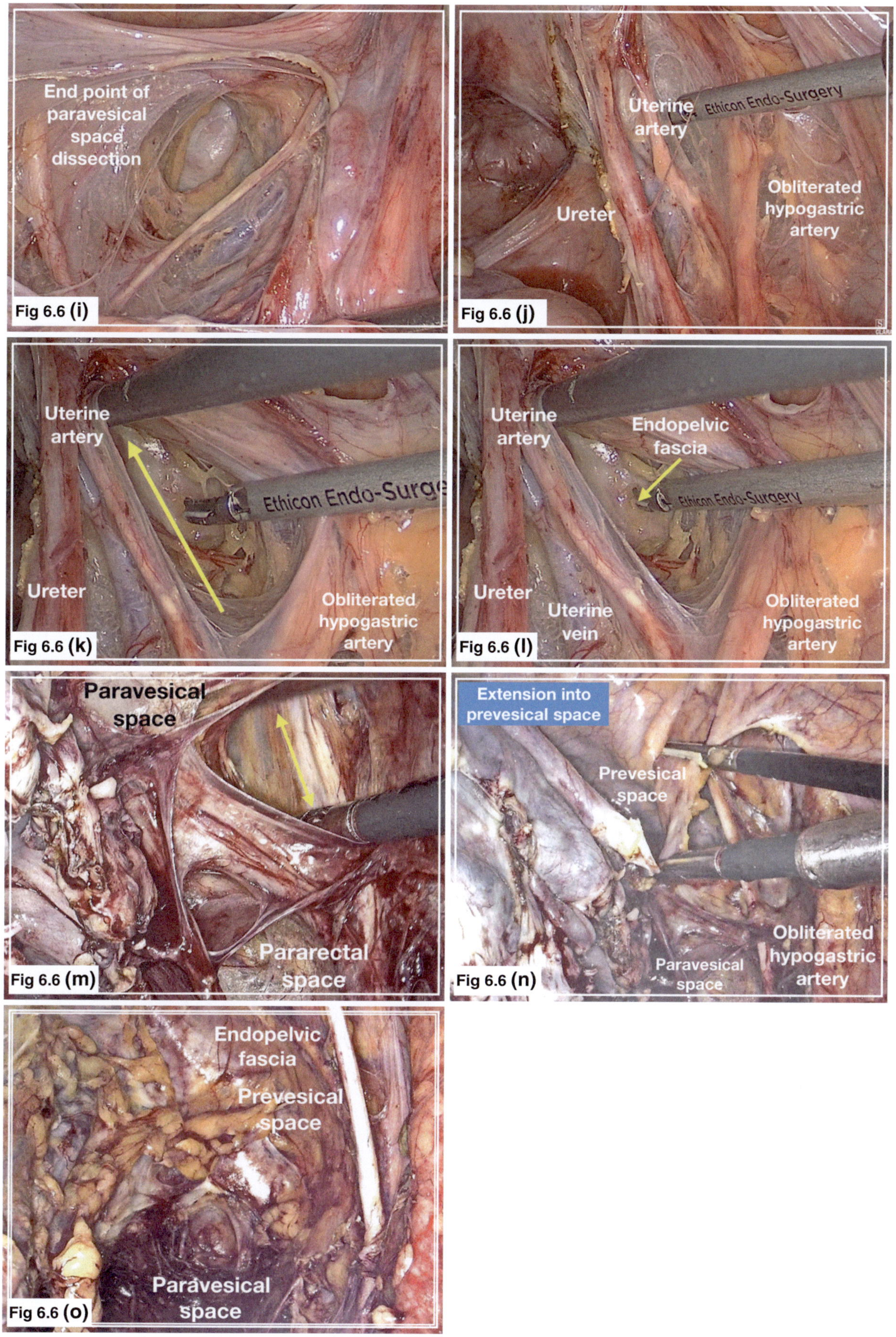

Fig. 6.6 (continued)

6.4 Prevesical Space

The prevesical space lies anterior to the urinary bladder and is bounded by pubic symphysis anteriorly and bladder neck and urethra posteriorly. It is a continuous space which communicates with the paravesical spaces on either side. The base is formed by the levator ani muscles (Fig. 6.7a–g).

This space is important during the extraperitoneal as well as transperitoneal hernia surgery. The opening of this space ensures the safety of bladder and the mesh is placed in this space (Fig. 6.7h–n).

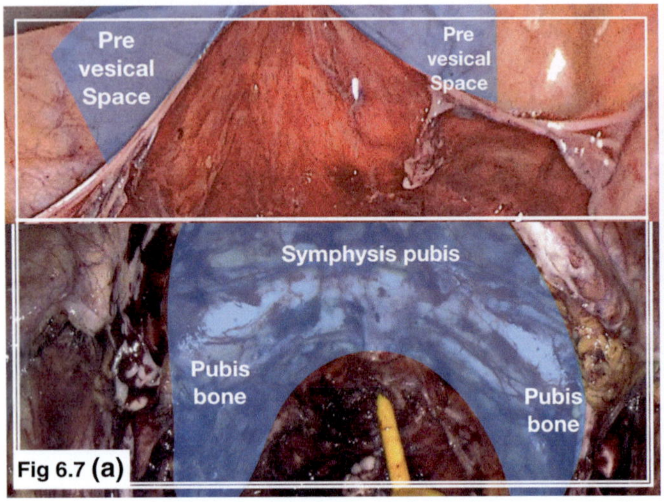

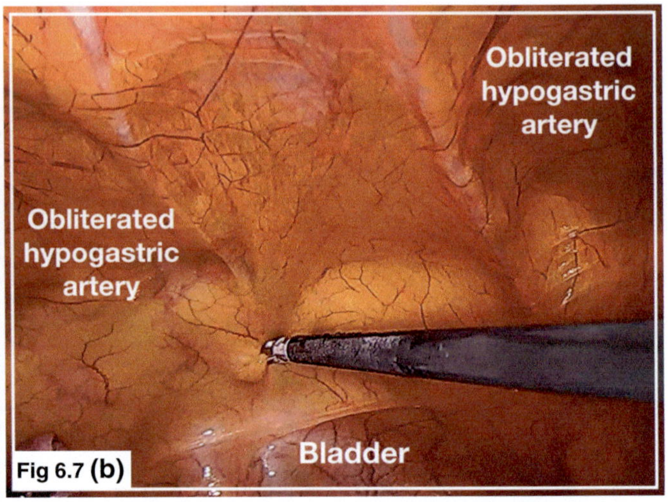

Fig. 6.7 Prevesical space. (**a**) The following series of images will pertain to prevesical space and its dissection. The image shows the previously explained areas of prevesical space. It is seldom opened in oncological cases, except during exenteration, and even more rarely in benign condition of SUI for Burch's colposuspension. (**b**) The prevesical space is under the anterior abdominal wall and tears down along the midline behind the pubic symphysis and up to the bladder neck region. It is bounded on both sides by the respective obliterated hypogastric artery or the median umbilical ligament. (**c**) Traction on the bladder from midline downwards pulls the median umbilical ligament towards each other. It should be kept in mind that at all times the dissection should not cross the median umbilical ligaments as it increases the risk of injury to the inferior epigastric artery lying lateral to the median umbilical ligament. (**d**) The urachus may or may not be definitively seen as an impression over the anterior abdominal wall. However it is important to identify the urachus. The champagne effect of pneumoperitoneum can be seen in mild variety on either side of the folder bladder under traction. This is a telltale sign that dissection is being carried out in the correct plane. (**e**) The correct plane lies between two different types of fat: the fat of the anterior abdominal wall and the fat covering the bladder. The plane lies between these two planes of fat. This is a vascular plane. Thus lack of vascularity during dissection also helps in surveillance of the plane of dissection. (**f**) The champagne effect of pneumoperitoneum can be clearly seen as two separate layers of fat separating from each other. The bladder is completely almost freed from the anterior abdominal wall. (**g**) Similar to the dissection done in rectovaginal space. The direction of traction and dissection is bidirectional and at right angles to the plane. Thus this helps operate the bladder from the anterior abdominal wall. Yellow arrow indicates direction of traction and dissection. This can be done with blunt instruments. (**h**) The prevesical space is also called as the space of Retzius. The space of Retzius is different from the cave of Retzius. The space of Retzius lies just posterior to the pubic symphysis. The cave lies superior to the space of Retzius. (**i**) Boundaries of the space of Retzius: The urethra and the bladder rest on anterior vaginal wall (floor). The vagina attaches itself to the arch tendon fascia pelvis laterally (inferiorly). The iliopectineal line or the Cooper's ligament is seen under the pubic tubercle on the inner aspect. The sutures for Burch's colposuspension are taken here. The inguinal ligament lies on the top at the pubic tubercle. The obturator neurovascular bundle is present along with the vesico-vaginal-venous complex (Santorini) plexus at the floor near the vagina and a small segment the external iliac vessel where they give branches, i.e. inferior epigastric vessels, and continue towards the inguinal ligament. (**j**) The Foley's catheter impression can be seen through the bladder. This is the urethrovesical junction and the part of bladder which remains extraperitoneal. The vagina is exposed and sutured to the iliopectineal line for paravaginal defects and urinary incontinence surgeries. (**k**) The bleeding seen in this image belongs to the Santorini plexus of veins which is seen at the floor of the prevesical space. The vascular structures are present laterally and seldom encountered in Burch's colposuspension. (**l**) The diagrammatic representation of the Burch's colposuspension where sutures have been taken on the Cooper's ligament and the fascia. The obturator neuromuscular bundle can also be seen. But it passes above the obturator internus muscle. The Santorini plexus lies below the obturator internus muscle. (**m**) The image is from a case of Burch's colposuspension. The bladder is completely mobilised anteriorly and the fascia planes are tightened by taking serial sutures with the periosteum of the pubis in a manner of strengthening the fascia. (**n**) As explained previously the paravesical space lies on either side of the prevesical space. Thus the prevesical space can be accessed through the paravesical space as well in cases of anterior exenteration. (**o**) In this image, a case of anterior mobilisation of bladder for exenteration of the urachus can be identified as a chord-like structure in the midline. It is important to stay above the urachus. This ensures that the dissection is in the correct plane. (**p**) Going below the urachus would lead to entering the urinary bladder superiorly and hence staying above urachus helps maintain the correct plane of dissection. (**q**) The bladder separated from medial sides of the obliterated hypogastric artery. Pubic bones can be seen all around the anterior boundary. (**r**) The final view of the pelvis after anterior exenteration with the prevesical space opened and continuing as the endopelvic fascia. The Foley's catheter is the remnant urethra stump left in situ. (**s**) Anterior mobilisation of bladder is also done in case of UVF repair for ureteroneocystostomy as shown in the image. This helps in reducing tension between the ureter and the bladder and gives the ureter more area to implant the ureter

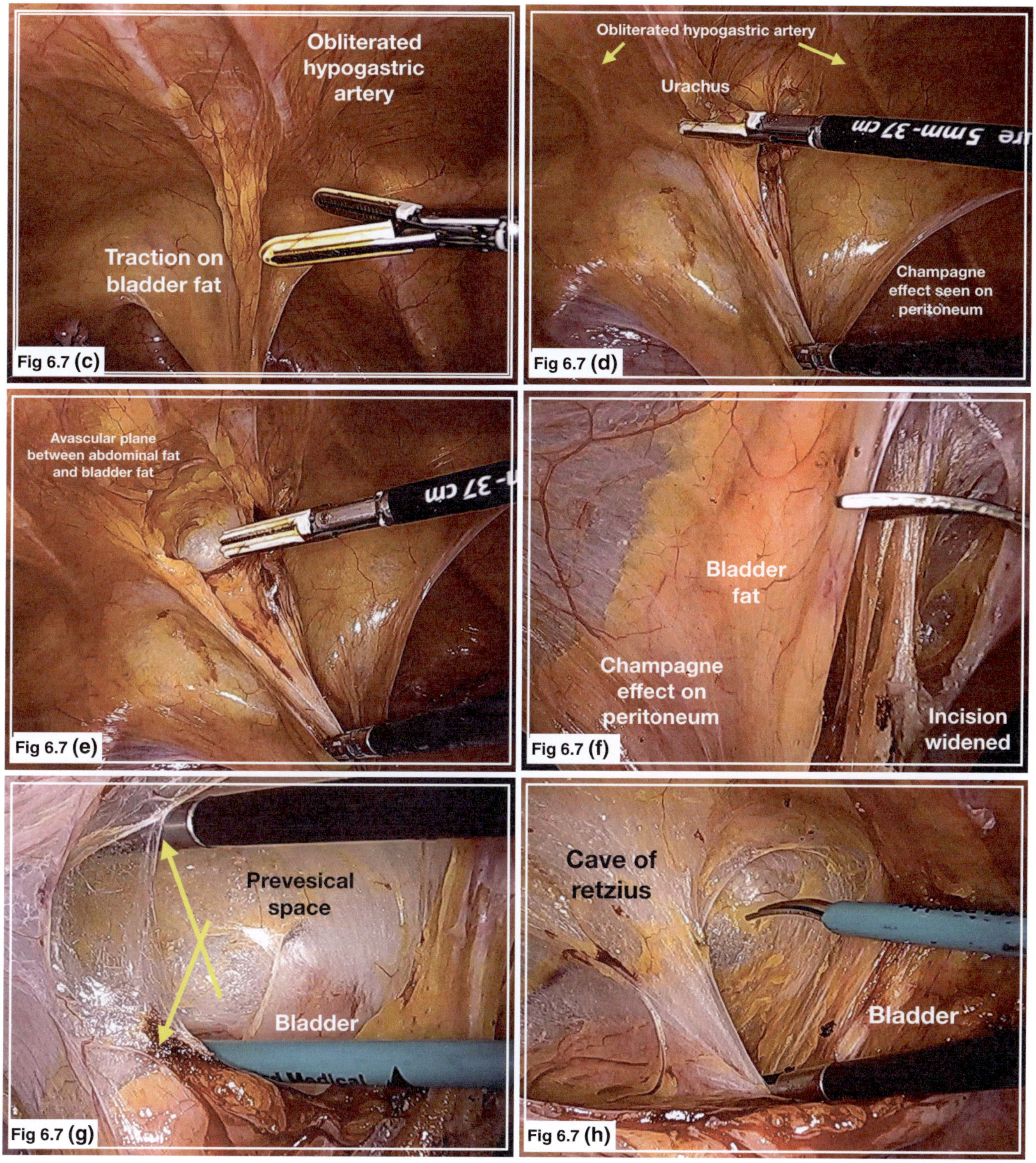

Fig. 6.7 (continued)

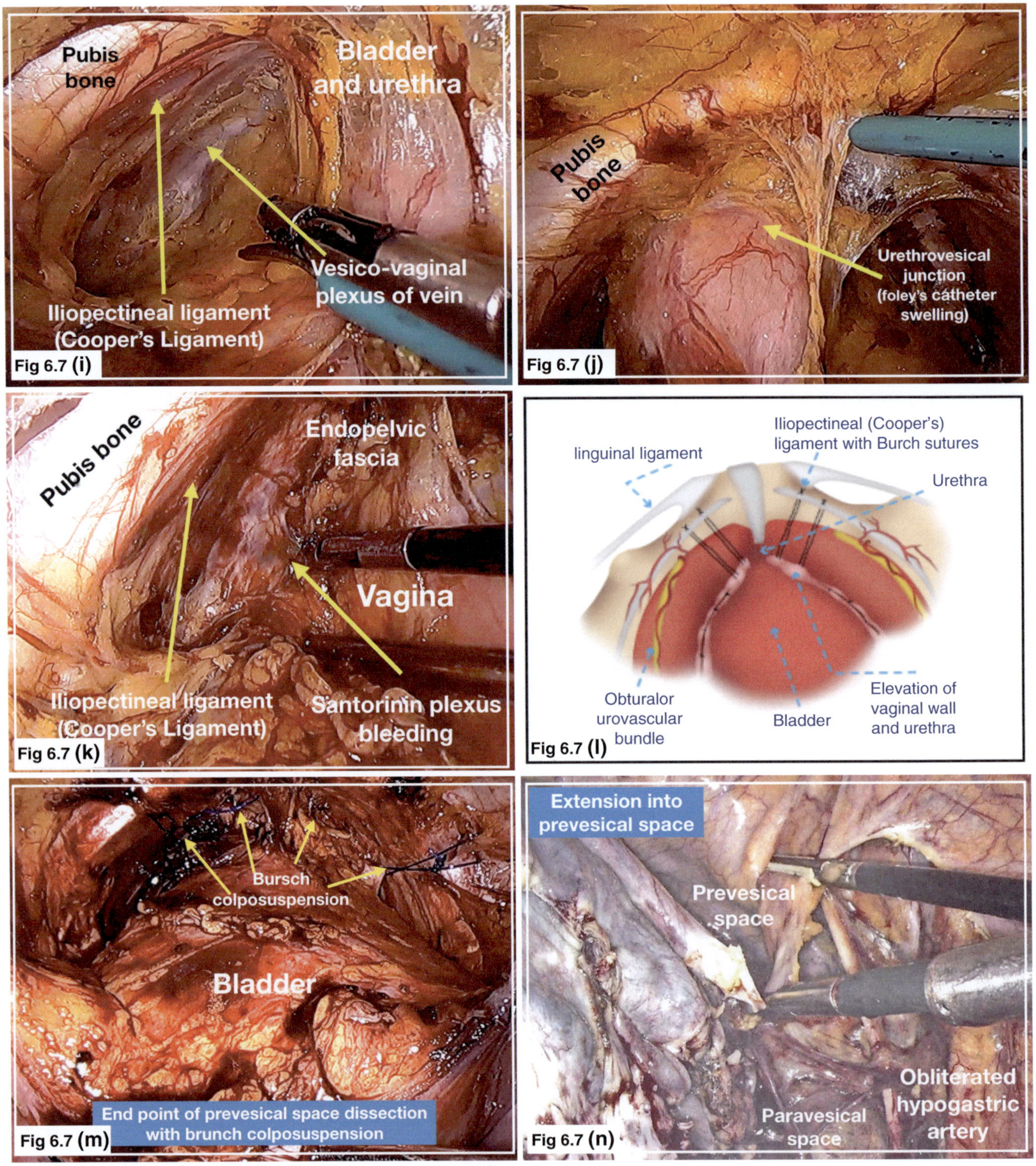

Fig. 6.7 (continued)

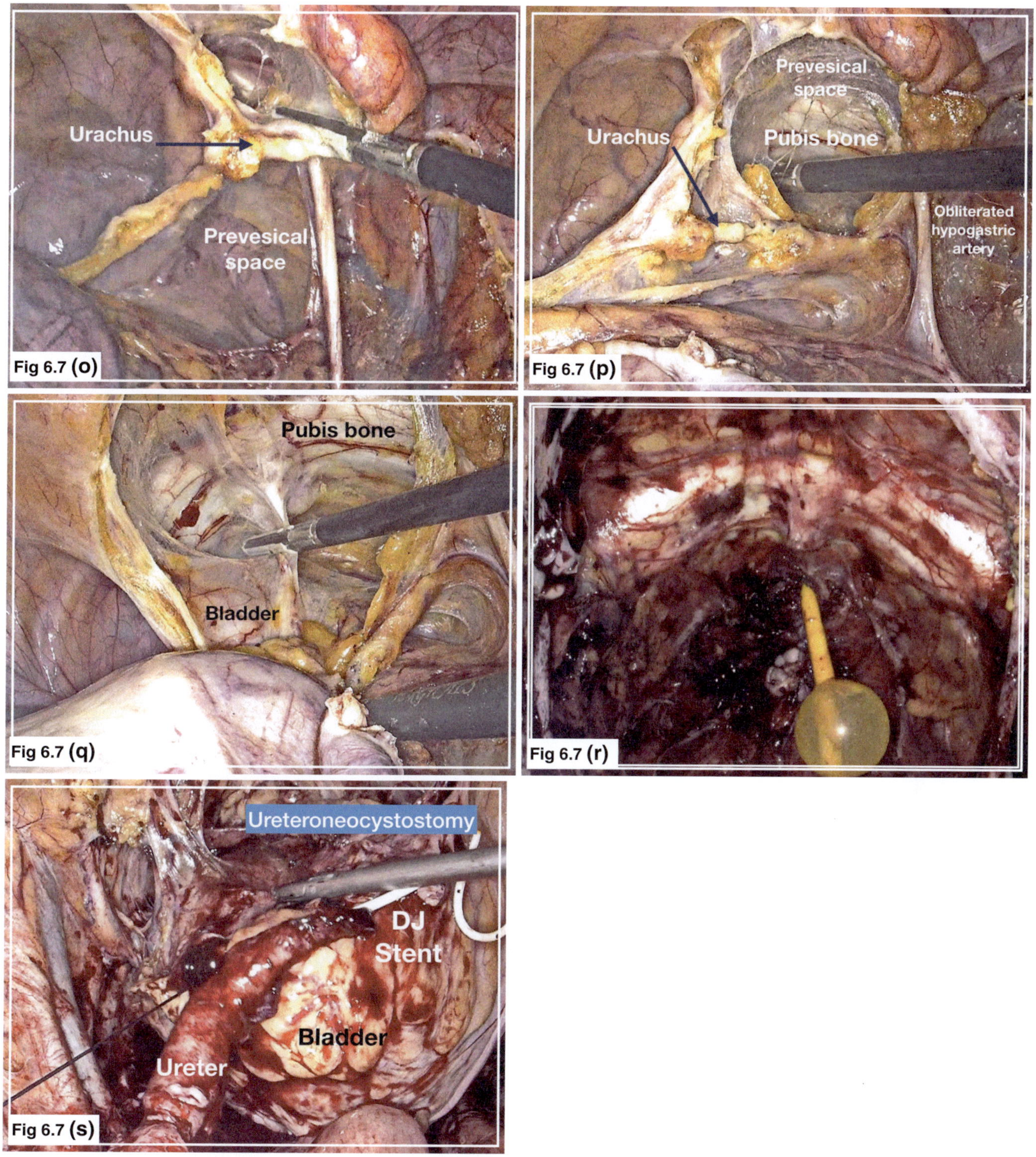

Fig. 6.7 (continued)

This space is also opened selectively in Burch's repair and radical prostatectomy. The space can be opened by taking a peritoneal cut on the urachus and then dissecting the space bluntly as this space is completely avascular (Fig. 6.7o–s).

Presacral space: It is behind the rectum and is bounded anteriorly by the mesorectum and posteriorly by the Waldeyer's fascia. The Waldeyer's fascia covers the presacral veins. Any breach in this fascia leads to torrential bleeding. This space is opened during sacrocolpopexy and presacral neurectomy. This space is also opened for posterior and total pelvic exenteration (Fig. 6.8a–j).

Rules: The organs of the pelvis are bounded by two avascular spaces anteriorly and two avascular spaces posteriorly. Understanding the anatomy of these spaces is the key to good surgery (Fig. 6.9a–c).

Yabuki space: This space is medial to the ureter proximal to the cervicovesical ligaments. This is an avascular space and contains the pelvic splanchnic nerves on its way to the bladder innervation. These fibres have to be carefully dissected off the uterine cervix to achieve a nerve-sparing surgery (Fig. 6.10a–k).

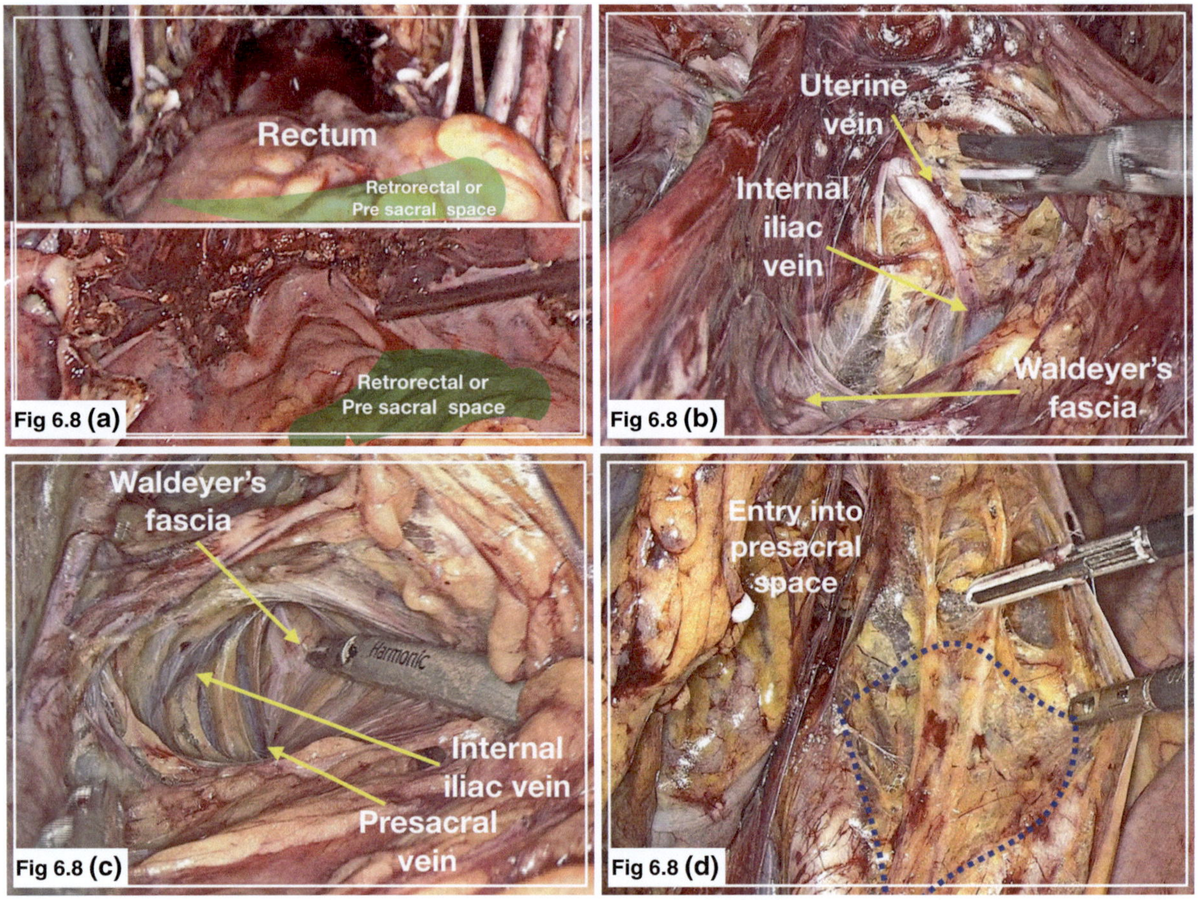

Fig. 6.8 Presacral or retrorectal area: (**a**) The previously explained images never clearly demarcated the presacral space as it lied behind the rectum. Hence it is also called as retrorectal space or presacral space as it lies ahead of the sacral region. (**b**) The presacral area is covered by Waldeyer's fascia. It can be seen in small amounts during the cranial end of the pararectal space near the bifurcation of the common iliac artery. The Waldeyer's fascia covers the presacral veins and part of internal iliac vein. Thus the area is exposed during dissection of the internal iliac vein. (**c**) As seen in the image the presacral veins are the chief components of the presacral space. The presacral veins drain into the internal iliac veins. This communication is covered by the Waldeyer's fascia which is present in the presacral space. (**d**) The presacral space is most commonly and clearly visible during the mobilisation of the rectum and sigmoid colon during posterior exenteration. As shown in the image the area lies just ahead of the sacrum and can be accessed just ahead of sacral promontory. Bifurcation of the aorta can be seen. The superior hypogastric plexus fibres can be seen on the peritoneal reflections. The area lies between these boundaries. The area is marked with blue dotted lines. (**e**) The area demarcated in the previous image is dissected further deeper in the same region as shown in the image. The principle followed is "fat belongs to rectum". Thus avascular plane is maintained. (**f**) The white arrow in the image represents the depth of dissection at the level of sacral promontory. The acute depth of dissection is achieved. Dissection is carried out nearly at right angles to the plane of dissection. (**g**) The presacral veins and the internal iliac veins are the most vital structures to be kept in mind during dissection at all times. Injury to these structures can lead to torrential and uncontrollable haemorrhage. (**h**) Clusters of minor branches of presacral veins can be seen in the presacral space. Haemostasis of these minor vessels can be managed with energy sources but injury to major vessels requires more aggressive measures. (**i**) The characteristic image of the presacral space dissection is "buttocks of infant" appearance. This is seen in the condition of correct avascular plane of dissection. (**j**) The buttocks of infant are demarcated with yellow dotted lines

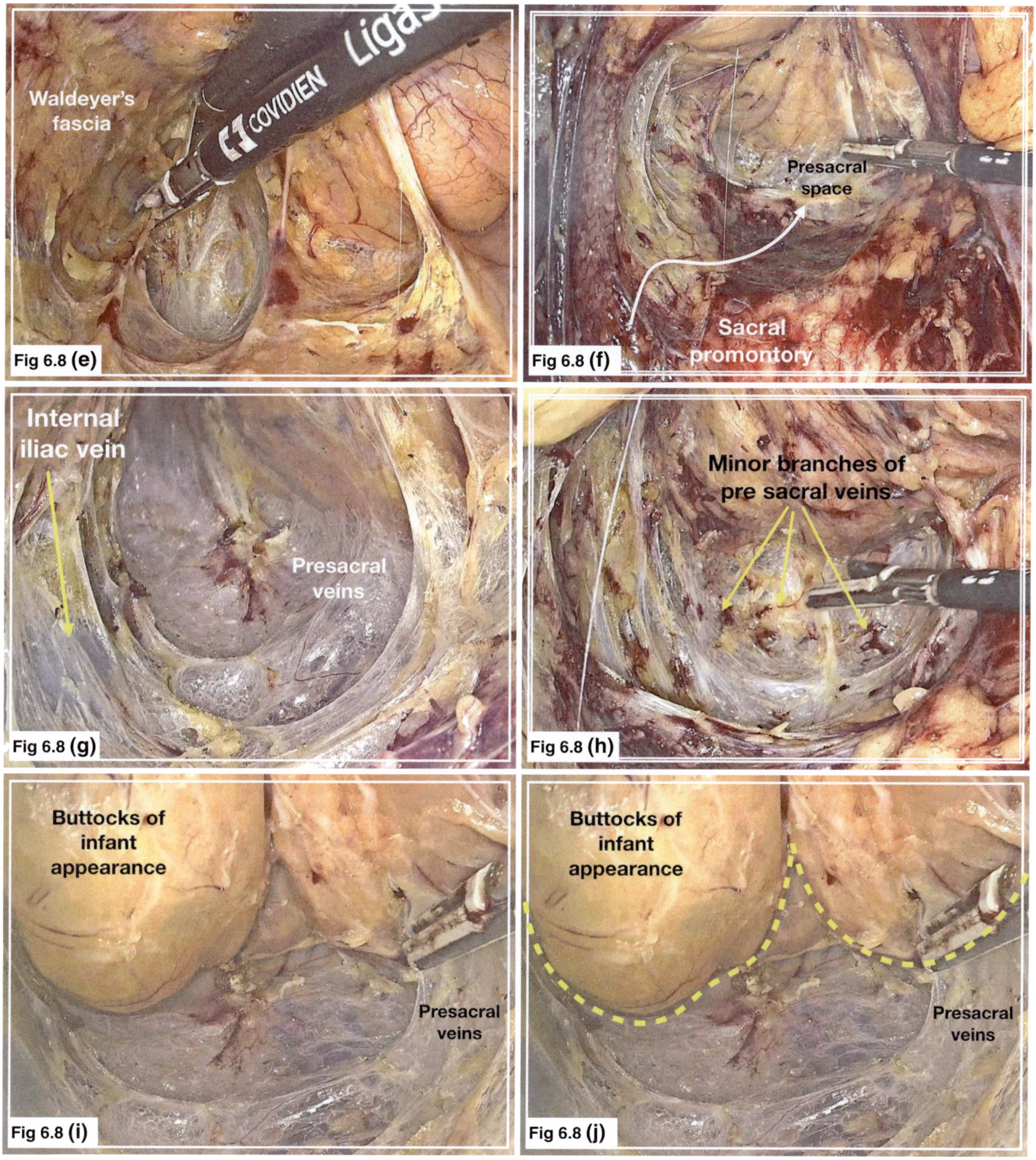

Fig. 6.8 (continued)

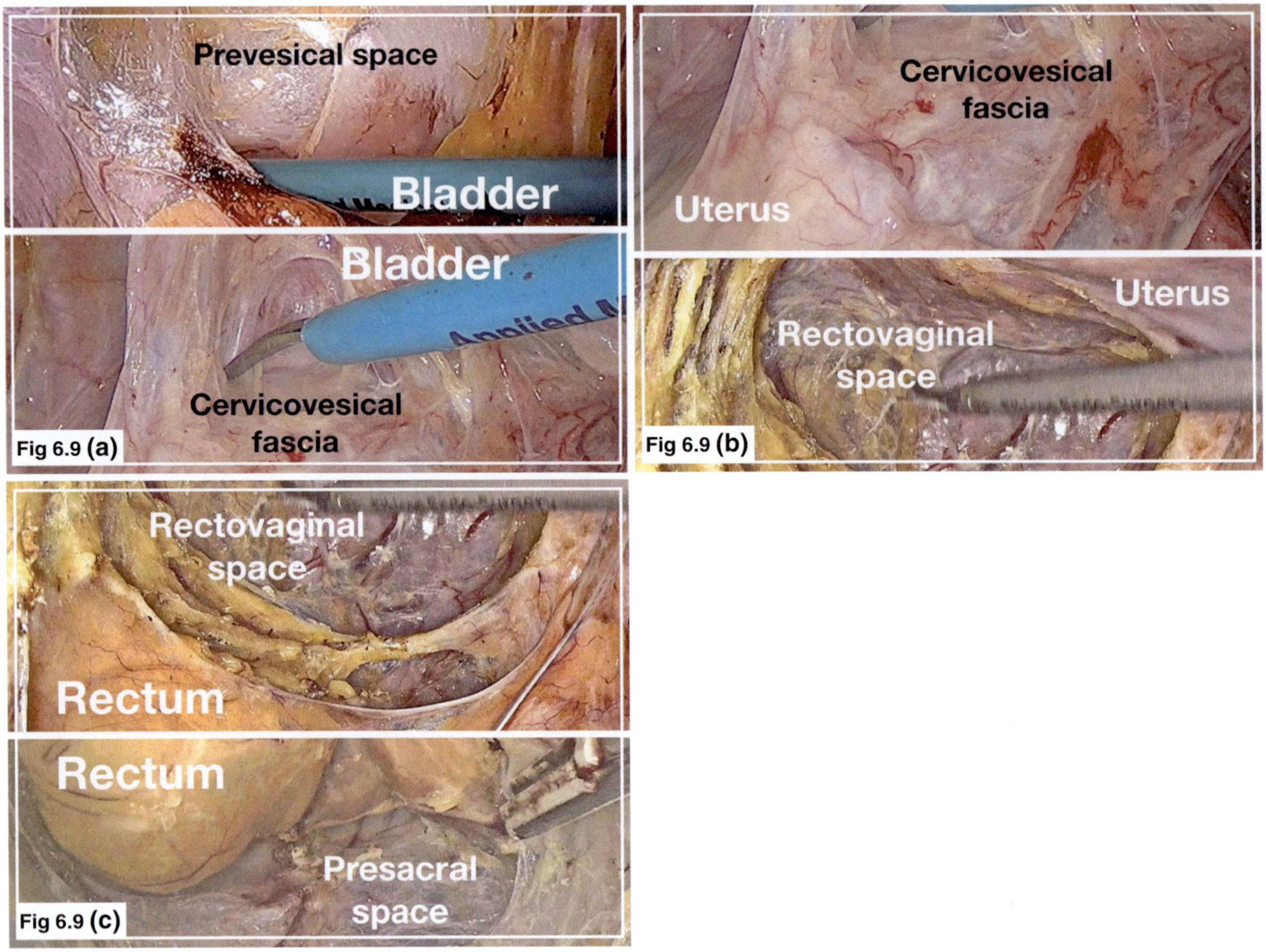

Fig. 6.9 (**a**–**c**) These images are of the rule where the pelvic organs are surrounded by avascular planes for dissection. And finding the right place is the key to good clean and bloodless surgery

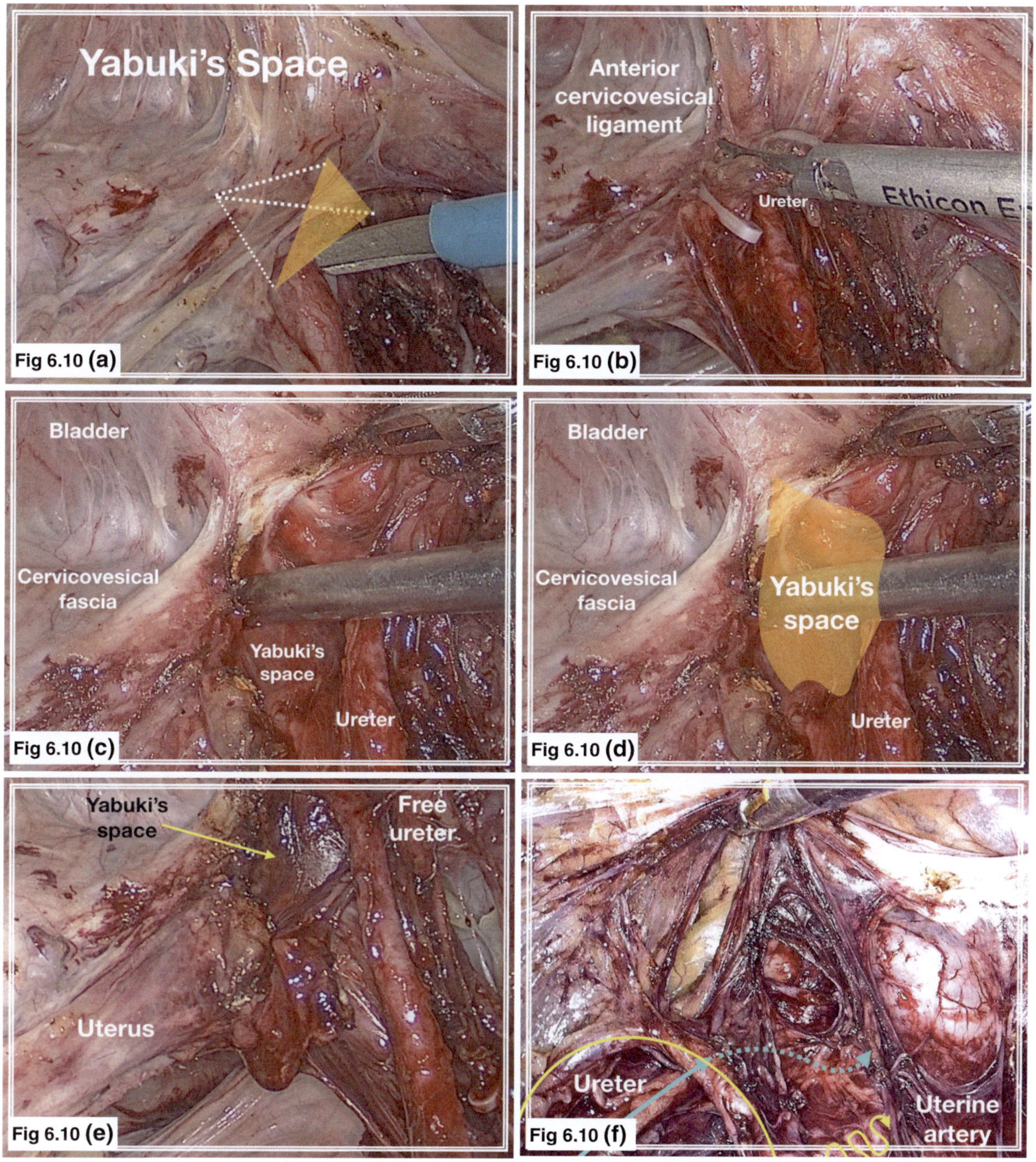

Fig. 6.10 Yabuki space. (**a**) The right-angled triangular space between the uterus surface, bladder surface and anterior cervicovesical ligament is called as the Yabuki space. The hypotenuse is composed of the anterior cervicovesical ligament. It contains the ureter and the pelvic splanchnic nerves which supply the bladder. The pyramidal space with its tip pointing inwards to the medial midline side. (**b**) The anterior cervicovesical ligament contains two veins which need to be clipped prior to dissecting the ligament. This maintains vascularity in the operating field and enhances clearer dissections. (**c**) The ureter is completely dissected off at this space. It is free from all sides. The ureter can be seen up to its insertion into the bladder. (**d**) Dissection of this space is important in nerve-sparing surgeries. While routine radical hysterectomies dissect the uterine veins lateral to the ureter, there is no need of Yabuki space dissection as the nerve fibres have been dissected off laterally. But in cases of nerve-sparing surgeries, attempts can be made to preserve these nerves as the counterpart nerves have been preserved. The space is shaded in yellow. (**e**) The ureter has been completely mobilised and retracted upwards comfortably without any strain on the ureter. The avascular space identified here is the Yabuki space. (**f**) The ureter and the uterine artery have been labelled in this image. The Yabuki space is labelled in the next image. The anterior cervicovesical ligament is tethered and covers the ureter. This is the point of identification. (**g**) It is to be noted that the Yabuki space lies on the surface of the uterus but it lies below the level of uterine artery always as shown in the image. (**h**) The anterior cervicovesical ligament is marked in bracket-like structures and the arrows indicate the empty avascular space underneath. Dissection of the ligament frees the ureter completely. (**i**) The anterior cervicovesical ligament viewed from another angle. (**j**) Similar image can be seen on the right side. (**k**) The yellow dotted area is the Yabuki space on the right side. The pelvic splanchnic nerves can be seen in the Yabuki space

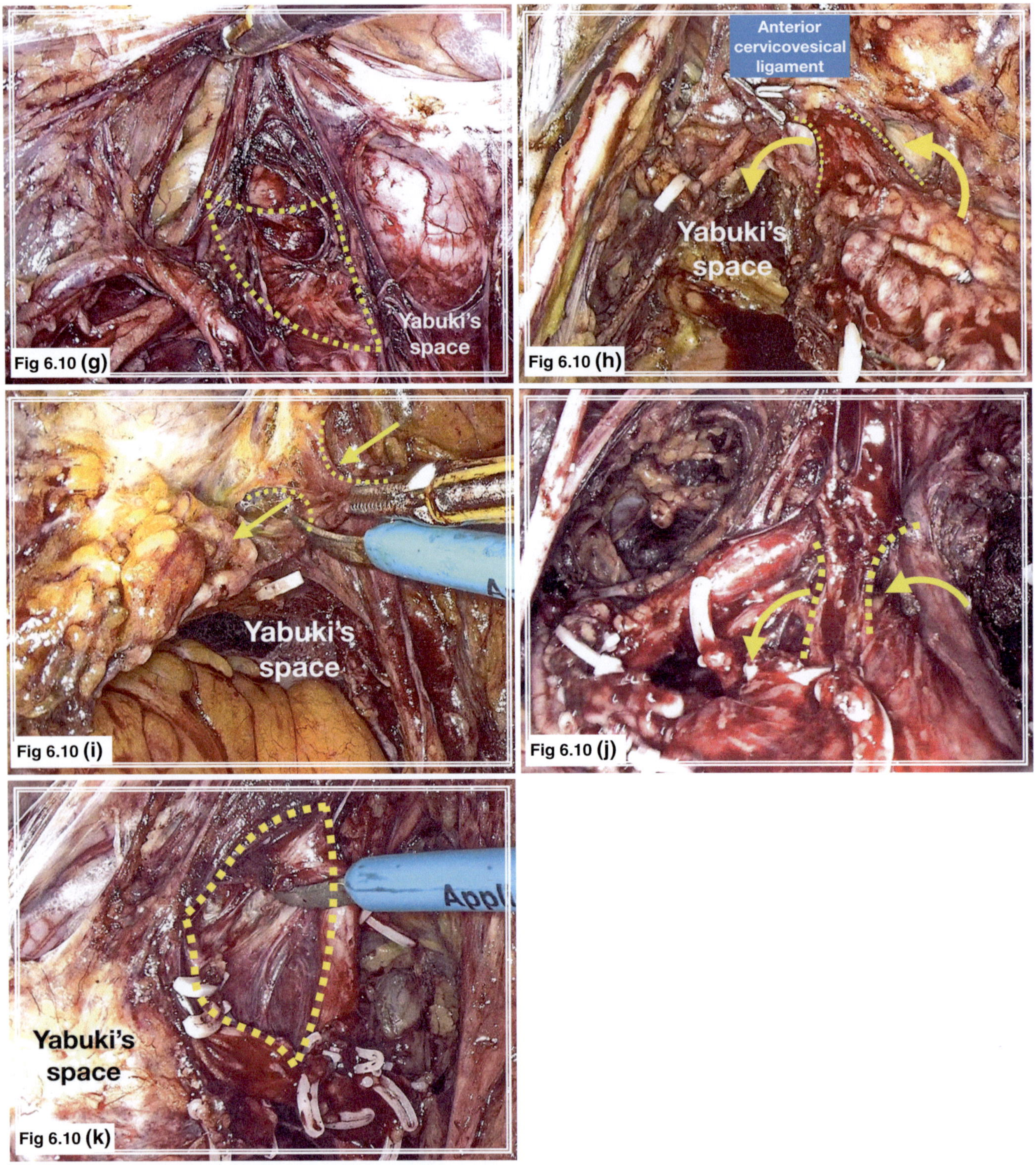

Fig. 6.10 (continued)

7 Fascial Anatomy

The fascias covering the pelvis (Fig. 7.1):

- Cervicovesical fascia
- Denonvilliers' fascia
- Endopelvic fascia
- Waldeyer's fascia

7.1 Cervicovesical Fascia

Covers the anterior vaginal wall and continues on the lateral side. The veins of the vagina lie between the fascia and the vagina. The bladder is dissection from the anterior vaginal wall by remains above the cervicovesical fascia. Any breach of the fascia leads to bleeding (Fig. 7.2a–j).

Intrafascial hysterectomy is done by cutting the vagina below the fascia at the level of the apex of the uterosacrals (Fig. 7.2k, l).

The cervicovesical fascia splits into anterior and posterior cervicovesical ligament. This is to allow the ureter to go through the ureterovesical junction. Anterior cervicovesical ligament is commonly called as the ureteric tunnel. It drains two veins from the cervix into the bladder and is hence tried vascularly (Fig. 7.2m–o).

The posterior cervicovesical ligament continues laterally and merges with the endopelvic fascia. There are two veins in this ligament which are the inferior vesicle and vaginal veins. Thus there is a potential gap on the lateral side of the vagina due to splitting of these fascia. This probably leads to the spread of cervical and vaginal pathologies into pararectal and paravesical spaces (Fig. 7.2p–u).

Since the endopelvic fascia continues on the obturator internus this is probably the anatomical space through which the transobturator tape traverses to remain at the mid-urethral level. The ureter is held by few strands of endopelvic fascia on the medial side just proximal to its entry into the bladder. These strands have to be transacted to lateralise the ureter in radical hysterectomy. The plane between the cervicovesical fascia and the bladder is understood to be covered by fat. Thus the bladder is directed by the dictum "fat belongs to the bladder". The laxity of the cervicovesical fascia leads to cystocele (Fig. 7.2v, w).

7.2 Denonvilliers' Fascia

Explained earlier. The laxity of this fascia leads to enterocoele (Fig. 7.3a–v).

7.3 Endopelvic Fascia

Covers the obturator interns and the levator ani. This fascia is the key to support the pelvic diaphragm and the pelvic organs. Thus this is the basis for repairs for prolapse and incontinence surgeries (Fig. 7.4a–o).

7.4 Waldeyer's Fascia

The Waldeyer's fascia covers the presacral space and the presacral veins. Any breach in this fascia leads to torrential bleeding (Fig. 7.5a–q).

Cardinal Rules (Fig. 7.6)

S. Puntambekar et al., *Laparoscopic Pelvic Anatomy in Females*, https://doi.org/10.1007/978-981-13-8653-4_7

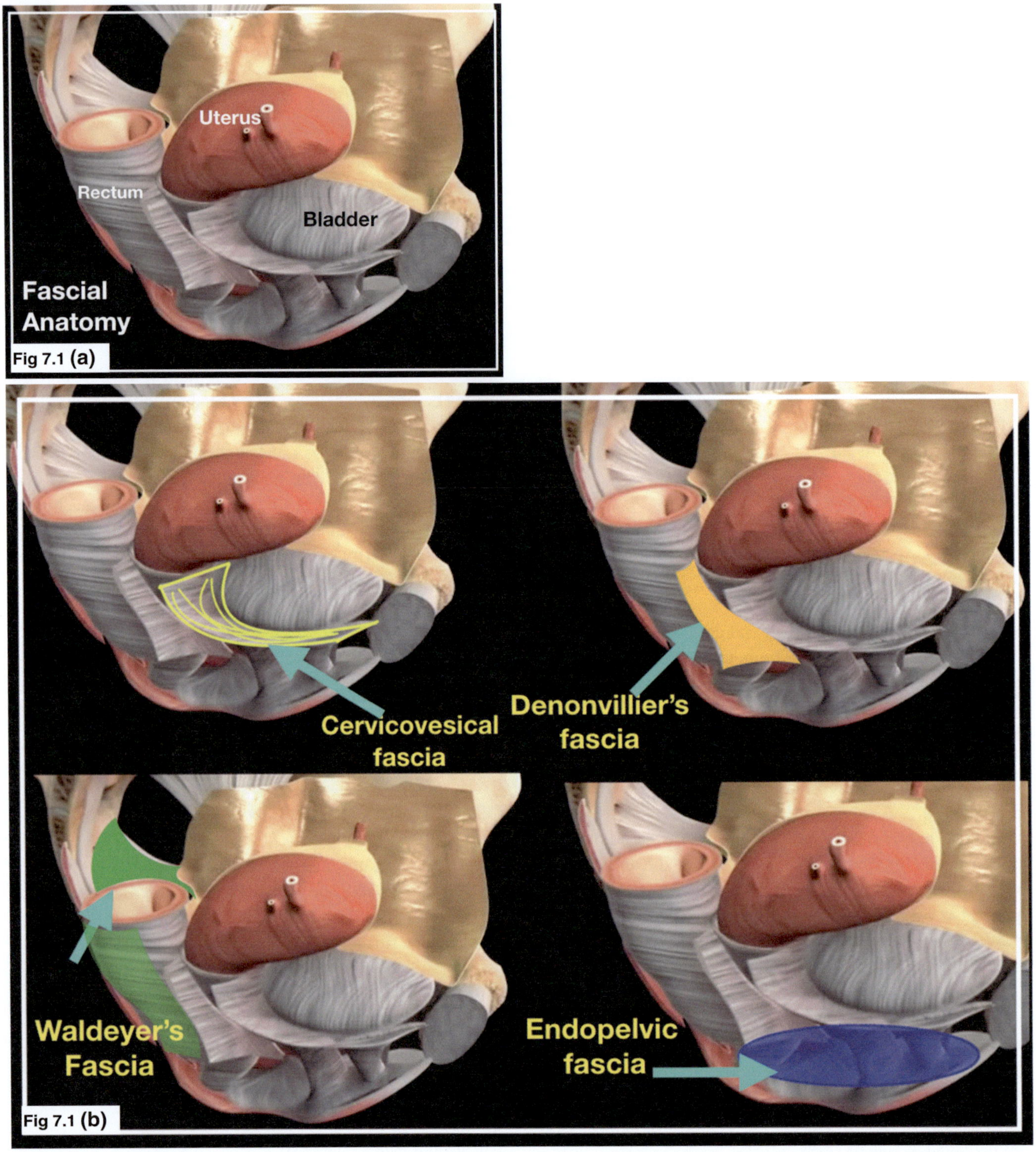

Fig. 7.1 Fascial anatomy: (**a**) As discussed in the previous chapter, it is considered that all organs of the pelvis are wrapped around avascular spaces and between fascias. Remaining in between these safety zones provide clean, surgically precise, and bloodless surgery. In this chapter fascias important of surgical importance are discussed. (**b**) This collage is a diagrammatic representation of the four fascia to be discussed individually, namely, the cervicovesical fascia, Denonvilliers' fascia, endopelvic fascia, and Waldeyer's fascia. (**c**) Real-time images of the four fascia have been shown in this collage. (**d**) The concept of fascial anatomy is important for various factors. Firstly the fascia lacks fibroblast tissue; thus chance of adhesions post-operatively is reduced significantly if dissection is done along the plane of the fascia. Secondly the veins always lie underneath the fascia. Venous haemorrhage is more difficult to manage than arterial haemorrhage. (**e**) Arteries have a thicker muscular support while veins have very little thickness of vascular smooth muscles. Thus by remaining under the fascia, the fascia itself provides mechanical support which the veins mechanically lack since the beginning. Due to lack of support the veins often collapse while arteries do not collapse. The fascial support hinders complete collapse of the veins

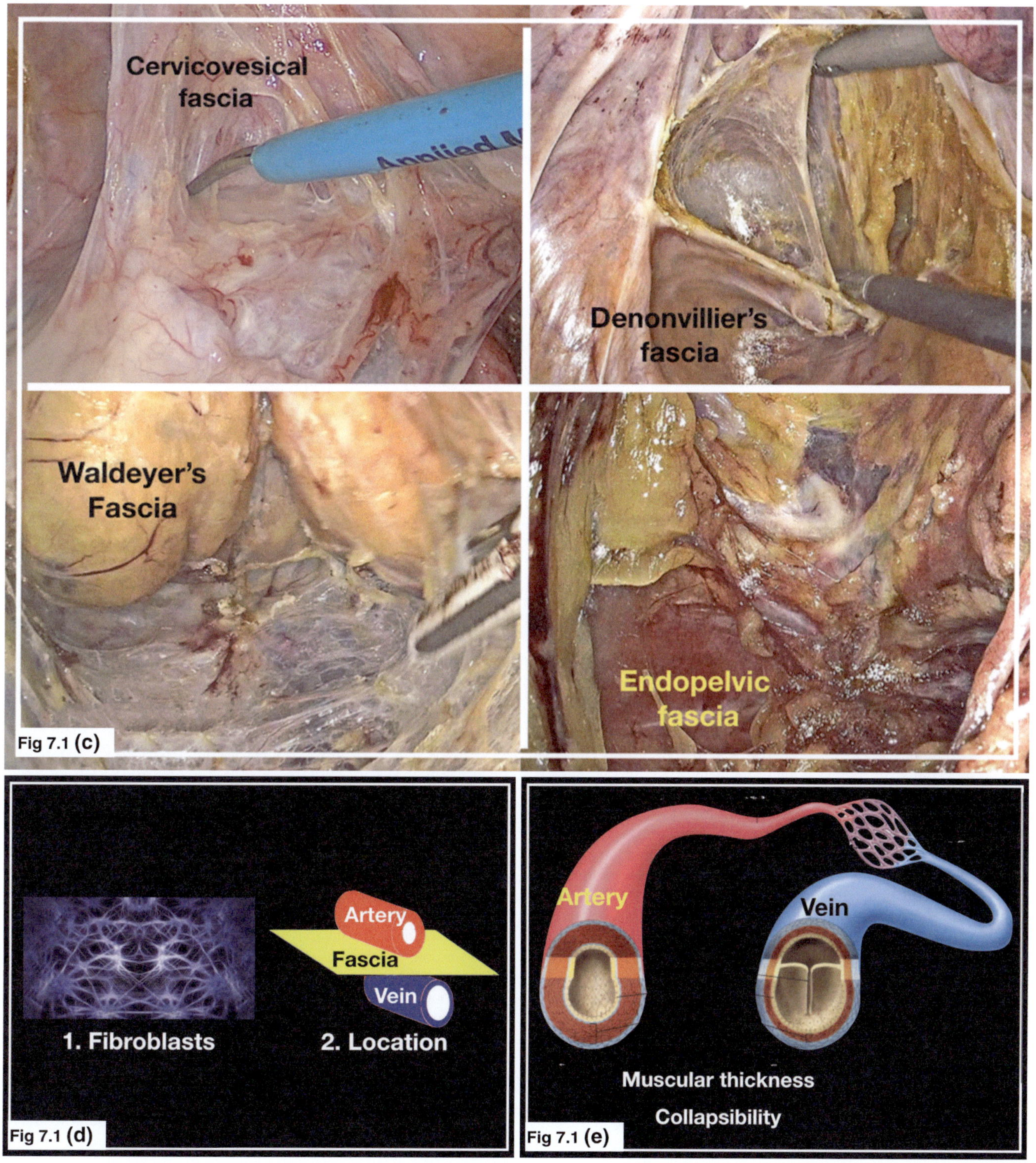

Fig. 7.1 (continued)

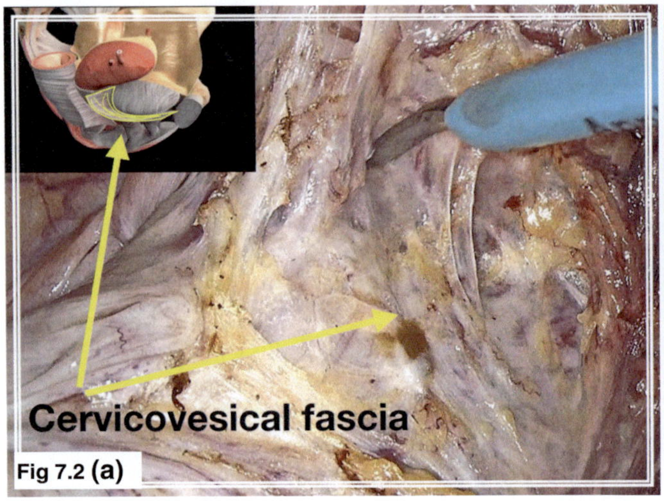

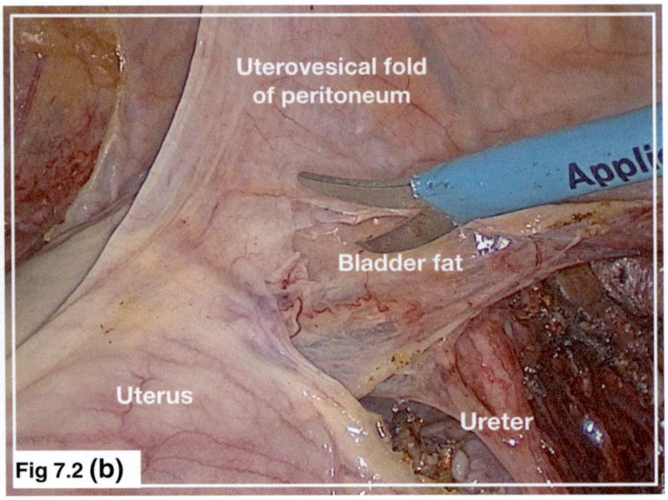

Fig. 7.2 (**a**) The image is of the cervicovesical fascia. Its name comes from its anatomical location. This fascia lies on the inferior aspect of the bladder and the anterior aspect of the uterus. (**b**) The chief role of the cervicovesical fascia appears in its relation to bladder dissection and in the ureteric tunnel dissection. It provides an avascular plane for separating the bladder from the anterior surface of the uterus during bladder dissection while it engulfs the ureter from all sides to form the ureteric tunnel which helps in dissection. (**c**) This fascia helps separate the bladder from the uterus. *Fat belongs to bladder* is the dictum to be followed here. Forceful encroachment into the fascia leads to haemorrhage. (**d**) The yellow-headed zone explains the exact location of the fascia. Condensation of the fascia at the ends to accommodate the ureter through it leads to formation of the anterior and posterior cervicovesical ligament. (**e**) This is a diagrammatic and schematic representation of the layers of tissue over the bladder and the uterus. The left-side image is a cross-sectional image while the right-side image is schematically drawn as per seen on laparoscopy. The bladder is unclothed with fat from all sides. The green arrow points at the exact plane where bladder dissection is to be carried out. The image will be explained in detail with real-time images in the following series of images. (**f**) Anterior U-cut of Pune technique is an integral step in conducting laparoscopic radical hysterectomy. In this image we see that incision has been made across lateral 1/3rd of both round ligaments dissecting only the peritoneum. The bladder dissection and importance of cervicovesical fascia will be explained in a stepwise manner. In this case the LRH is conducted on a patient with cervical cancer with a history of previous caesarean section. (**g**) The white fibrous tissue held between the blades of the scissors is the dense adhesions of the peritoneum. It must be kept in mind always that *fat belongs to bladder*. The yellow-coloured fat which appears underneath the white fibrous peritoneal adhesions must be reflected upend away from the uterus to visually consider bladder dissection in the respective area. (**h**) In this image dissection is done in a way to separate the fat from the uterus. The avascular plane underneath the fat is the cervicovesical fascia. The dissection is to be carried out in a particular plane. The image also explains the previously repeated rule *fat belongs to the bladder*. (**i**) The dissection is done at the base of the uterus and then pushed away from the uterus in an upwards direction. The dissection is always carried out anterior to the uterine artery. (**j**) The fat of bladder and cervicovesical fascia dissection are relatively easier at the centre region. Towards the sides/edge of the fascia the bladder pillars exist along the side the anterior and poster cervicovesical ligament. (**k**) Posterolateral colpotomy done for a case of benign hysterectomy at the level above the apex of uterosacral ligaments. This is the safest place for colpotomy. (**l**) Posterior colpotomy done solely for retrieval specimen vaginally without conducting a hysterectomy. This is also done at the level of apex of the uterosacral ligament. (**m**) Resecting the anterior cervicovesical ligament is the most important step in completing the bladder dissection and beginning the ureteric tunnel dissection. In several occasions it is advised to apply haemostat clips at the cervicovesical ligament to prevent retrograde bleeding. Cutting the ligament frees the bladder from the pillars and opens the Yabuki space to dissect the ureter and free the ureter from all its sides till its insertion into the bladder. (**n**) A homeostatic clip has been applied on the anterior cervicovesical ligament as explained in the previous image. The ureter here is separated anteriorly from the cervicovesical fascia. (**o**) Once freed from the anterior surface the Yabuki space is completely exposed and the ureter is attempted to free from the posterior surface. The cervicovesical fascia completely engulfs the ureter near its insertion, at the ureteric tunnel. It is from this side that malignant cells from the cervix can metastasise locally to cause obstruction of the ureter. (**p**) The posterior cervicovesical ligament can be seen after exposing the Yabuki space. The anterior and posterior cervicovesical ligaments contain small veins which drain the bladder. Thus it is important to clip the ligaments before resecting them. (**q**) The posterior cervicovesical ligament lies in close proximity to the uterine vein which originates from the lower side of the uterus on the lateral side. It has been clipped here in the image. The ureter can be seen free from all sides. (**r**) Similar series of images show the association of the ureter with the cervicovesical fascia on the left side. The anterior cervicovesical ligament can be seen clipped with haemostat clips. The blades of the scissors pass through the space between the anterior cervicovesical ligament and the ureter. (**s**) The cervicovesical ligament held between the blades of the scissor, when cut, will release the bladder pillars above it (seen as clips applied) and also free the ureter from its anterior attachment on to the uterus. The uterine vein is clipped and cut as seen under the ureter. (**t**) The posterior cervicovesical ligament can be seen under the ureter. The uterine vein has already been clipped and cut. Resecting the posterior cervicovesical ligament will release the ureter completely as seen in the next image. (**u**) The ureter is free of all attachments. The ureteric tunnel dissections have been completed. The cervicovesical fascia and its ligaments have been resected. (**v**) Diagrammatic representation of transobturator sling for urinary incontinence surgeries. The sling is applied at the obturator muscle plate. (**w**) Diagrammatic representation of cystocele. (**x**) *Fat belongs to bladder*: Principle for clean bladder dissection

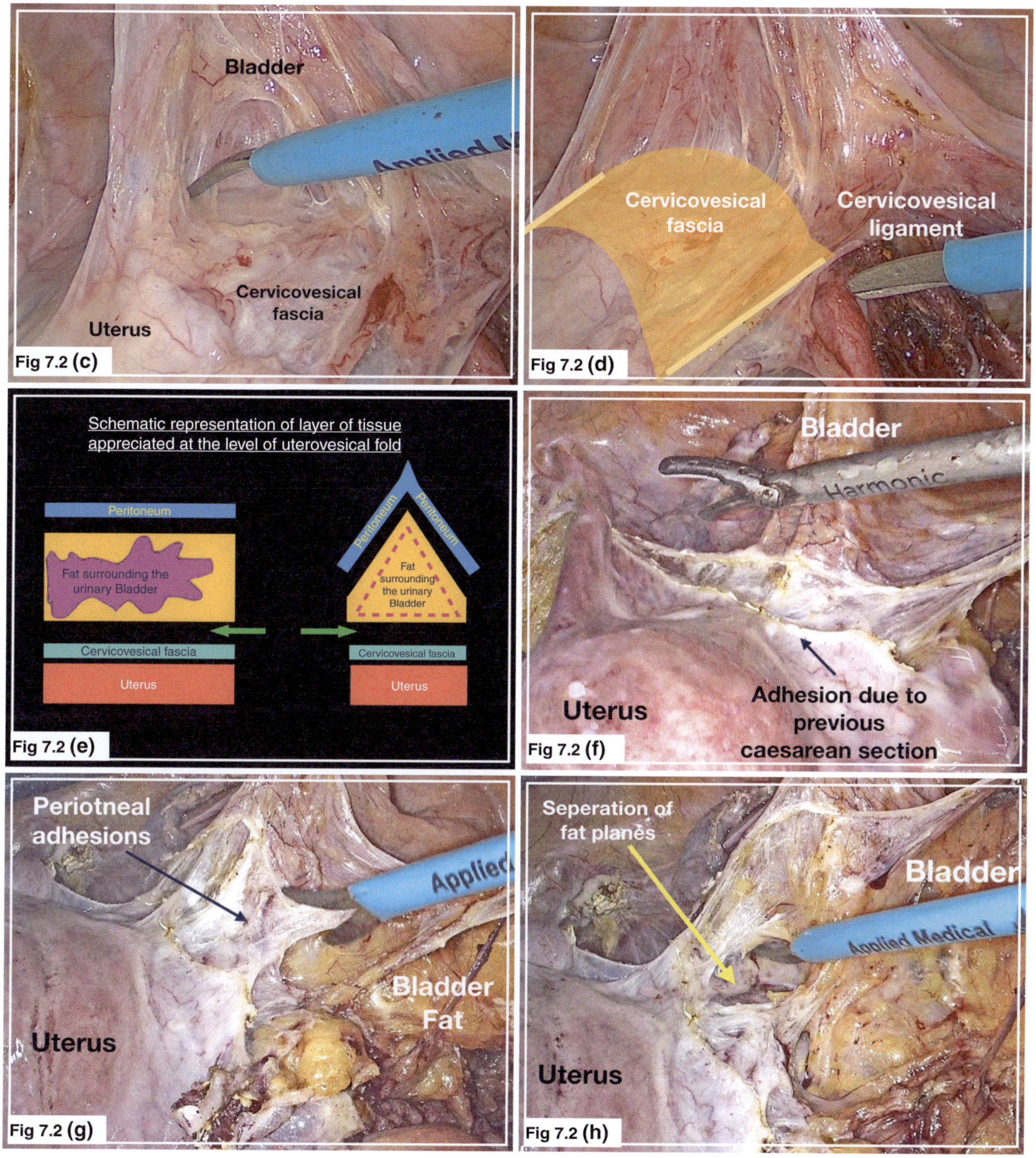

Fig. 7.2 (continued)

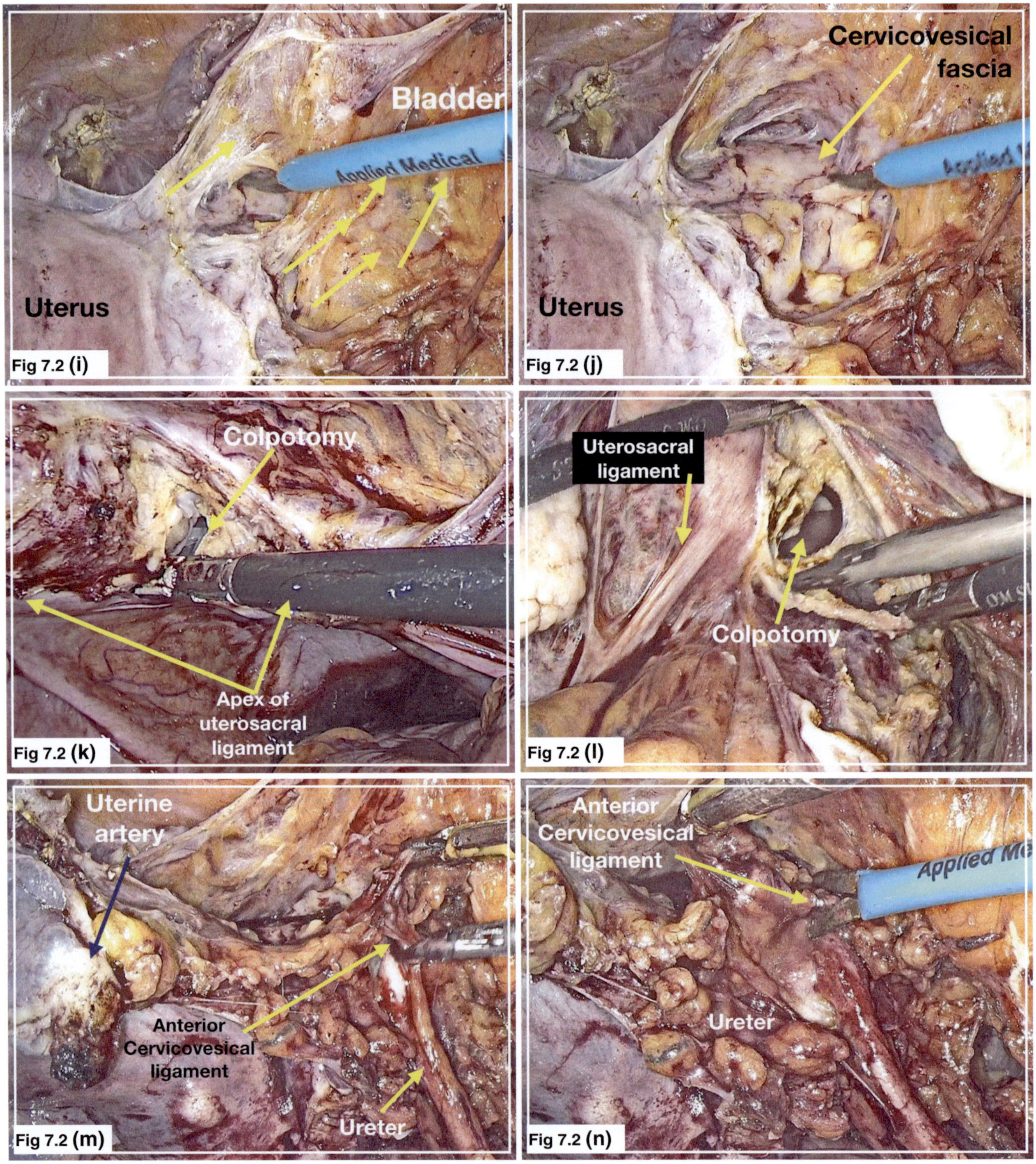

Fig. 7.2 (continued)

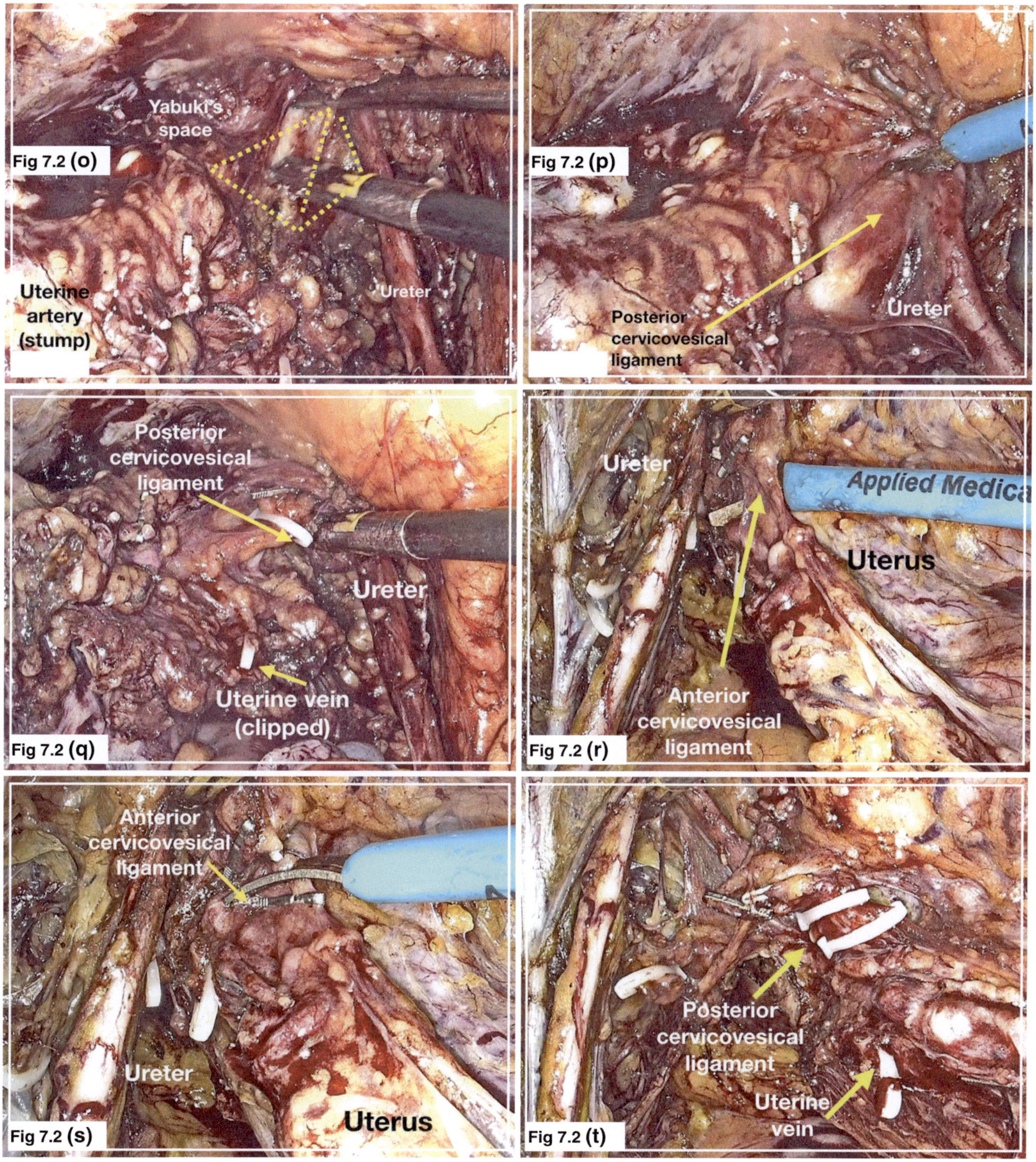

Fig. 7.2 (continued)

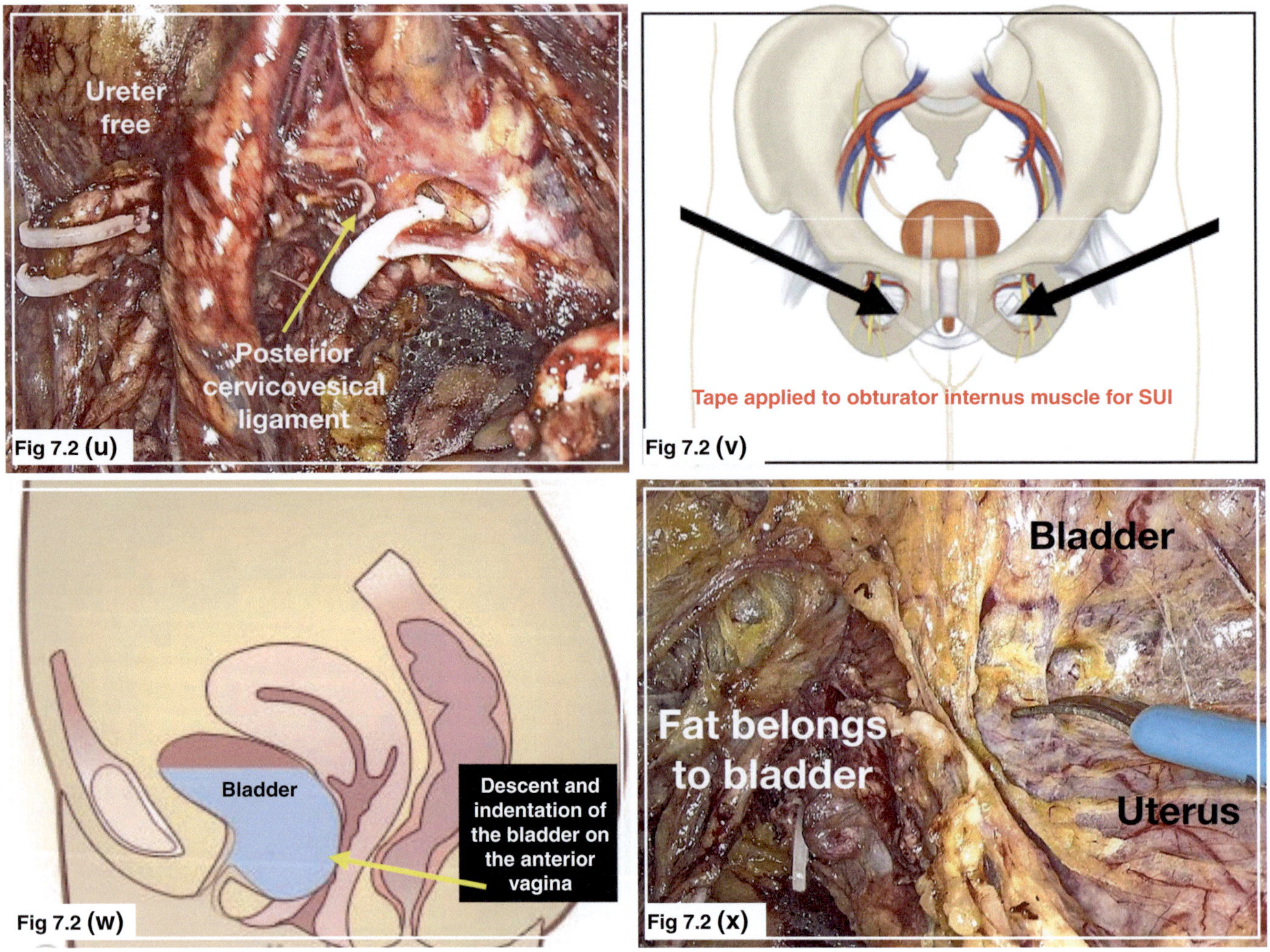

Fig. 7.2 (continued)

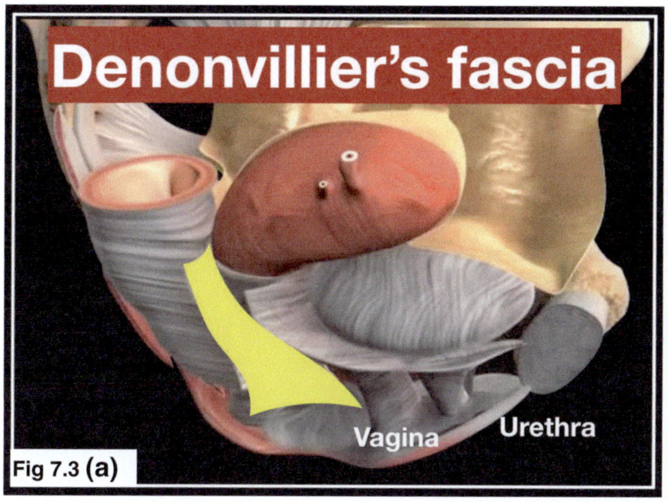

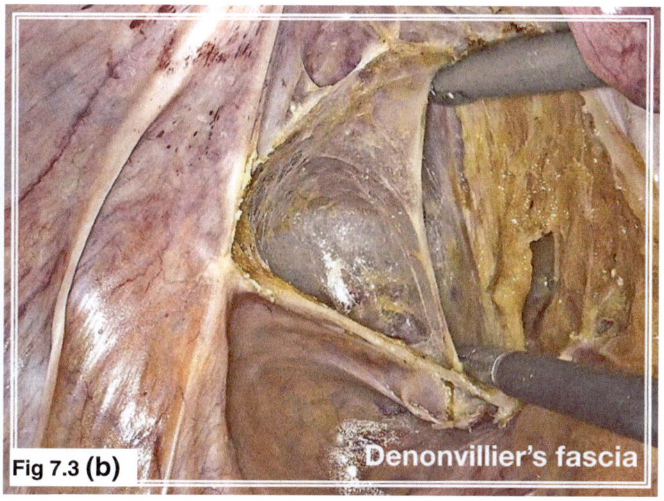

Fig. 7.3 Denonvilliers' fascia. (**a**) The image is a diagrammatic representation of the Denonvilliers' fascia. It lies between the uterus and the rectum and terminates at the level of vagina at the endopelvic fascia. (**b**) The image is the real-time image of the Denonvilliers' fascia during the rectovaginal space. The Denonvilliers' fascia is two layered and the desired plane of dissection lies between the two layers of the fascia. (**c**) The first step of the Denonvilliers' fascia dissection is the posterior U-cut (explained later). Traction at the midline backwards opens the rectovaginal space. However the area is covered with fat. It is important to find an avascular plane between the layer of fat. (**d**) *Fat belongs to rectum* is the dictum followed for safe and clean Denonvilliers' fascia dissection. Always bear in mind that the dissection should occur above and away from the layer of fat. (**e**) The Denonvilliers' fascia lies in the rectovaginal space. Hence the dissection is to be carried out between both the apexes of the uterosacral ligaments as shown in the image. The yellow dotted arrow denotes the course of dissection. (**f**) *Fat belongs to rectum*. Always dissect above the level of fat so that the fat falls down as a part of the rectum as shown in the image. This ensures a complete avascular plane of dissection. (**g**) In this image there are two "apparent" avascular planes seen but the correct and the incorrect planes are labelled. Dissection in the wrong plane increases the chances of entering the rectum (perforation). Thus in conditions of doubt always choose the plane above the fat and away from the rectum and rectal fat. (**h**) Even though initially avascular plane there is certain significant amount of fat seen above the plane in the lower region as compared to the higher plane. Thus the correct plane can be differentiated from the wrong ones. (**i**) The method or the direction of dissection of the Denonvilliers' fascia has been explained in the previous chapter in the rectovaginal space. (**j**) Similar steps of the dissection can be carried out in the whole area of the space not just the centre. Even at the edges of the fascia, dissection is carried out perpendicular to the plane. (**k**) The main motive of the Denonvilliers' fascia dissection is to expose the rectovaginal space completely and separate the uterus from the rectum completely at the level of vagina and rectum. Thus it is important to dissect in the correct plane of dissection. The rectum can be seen falling away from the uterus. (**l**) The lower end point of dissection is the shining appearance of the endopelvic fascia as shown in the image. (**m**) This image explains the difference between the rectal fat and the Denonvilliers' fascia. The Denonvilliers' fascia appears as a translucent layer and separates from the fat which belongs to the rectum. (**n**) The concept of the fascia covering the vessels has been explained here. In this image we can see the dissection done in the correct plane. Stay above and away from fat. Avascular plane has been maintained. (**o**) In this image overzealous and forceful dissection through the Denonvilliers' fascia on the uterine surface leads to bleeding from the site of entry. Veins are thin and thus fascia provides mechanical support to them. (**p**) However in such conditions instead of reaching for the vein itself dissecting deeper leads to more bleeding owing to more injury sustained on the fascia. Thus it is best to cauterise the fascia itself with energy source instead of desperate attempts to reach the vessel. (**q**) Another example of wrong plane of dissection has been demonstrated in the image. Thus it is always important to bear in mind to dissect above and away from the fat, and *fat belongs to rectum*. (**r**) The correct avascular plane has been demonstrated with the instrument entering the plane without any bleeding. All fat remains under the space. (**s**) The Denonvilliers' fascia has been completely dissected and the endopelvic fascia is visible at the lower end of the rectovaginal space. The depth can be viewed from the level of the uterosacral ligament. (**t**) The Denonvilliers' fascia and the endopelvic fascia can be seen as separate fascial structures in the image. (**u**) The image represents diagrammatic representation of the two fascias; the endopelvic fascia is shaded in yellow and the Denonvilliers' fascia is shaded in blue. (**v**) Diagrammatic representation of the Denonvilliers' fascia meets the endopelvic fascia. (**w**) Real-time image of Denonvilliers' fascia meeting the endopelvic fascia. This image has been taken from a case of laparoscopic low anterior resection of a case of Ca rectum. The rectum is completely separated from the vagina and the uterus. Similar dissection is also done for posterior exenterations

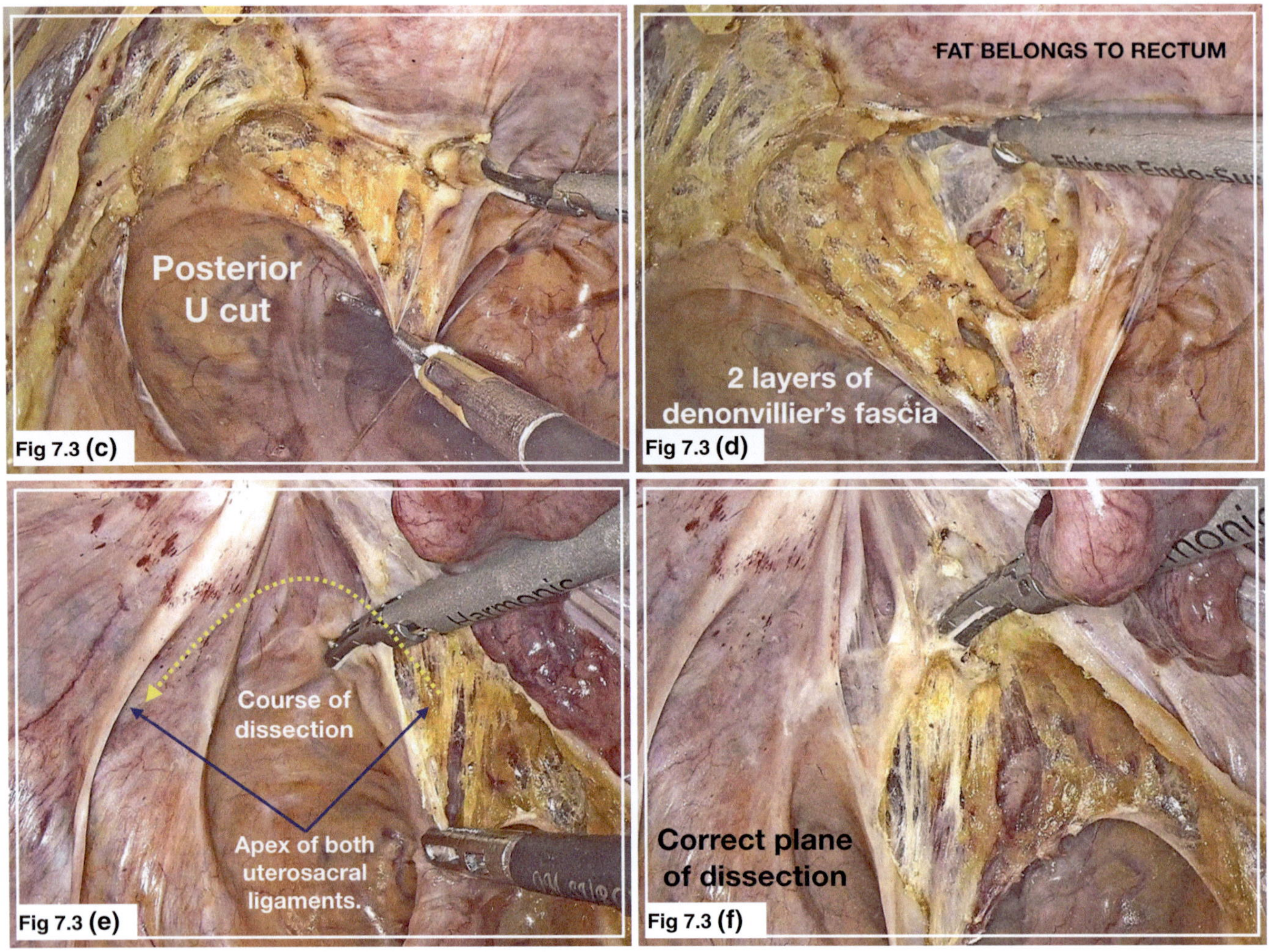

Fig. 7.3 (continued)

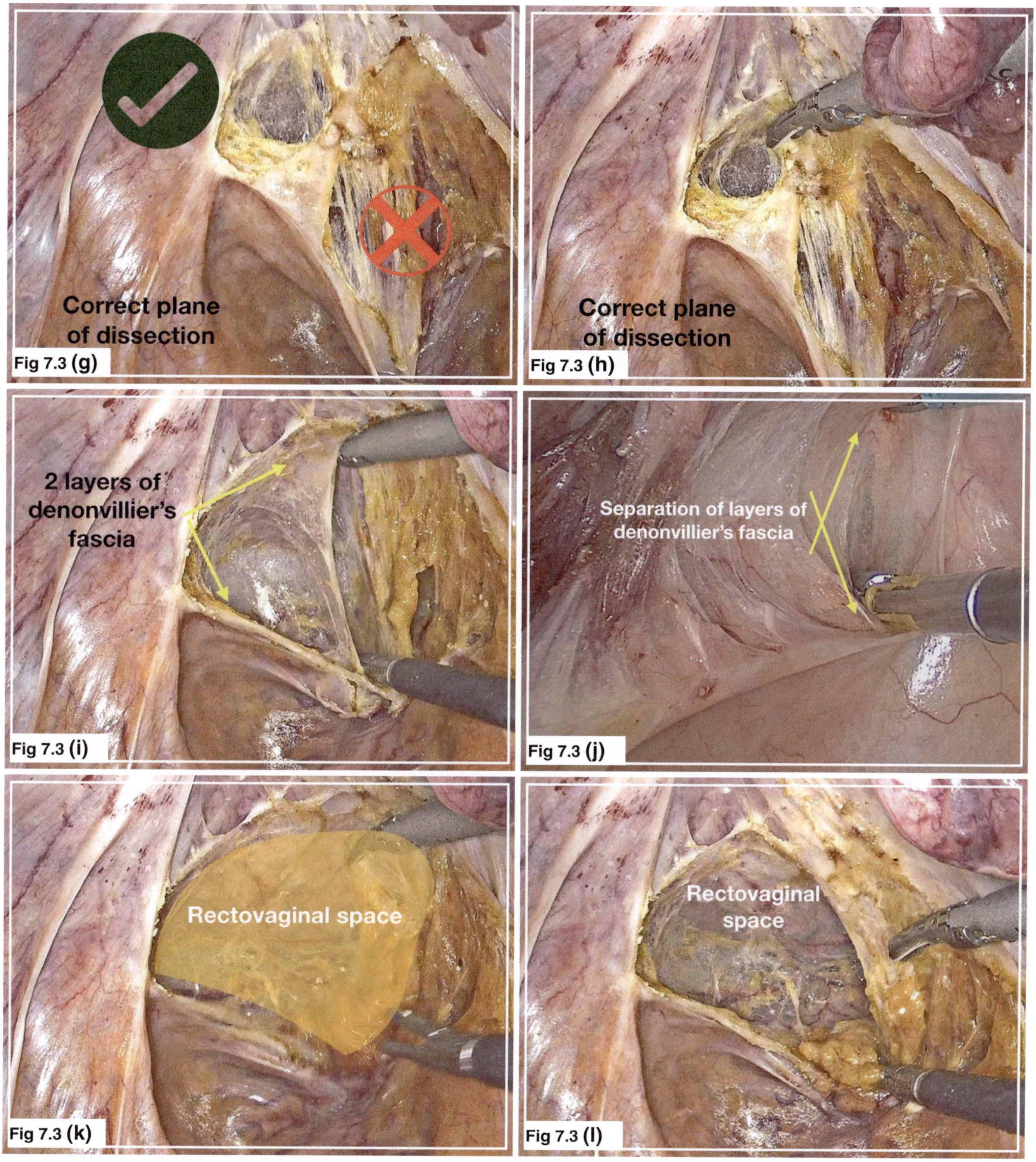

Fig. 7.3 (continued)

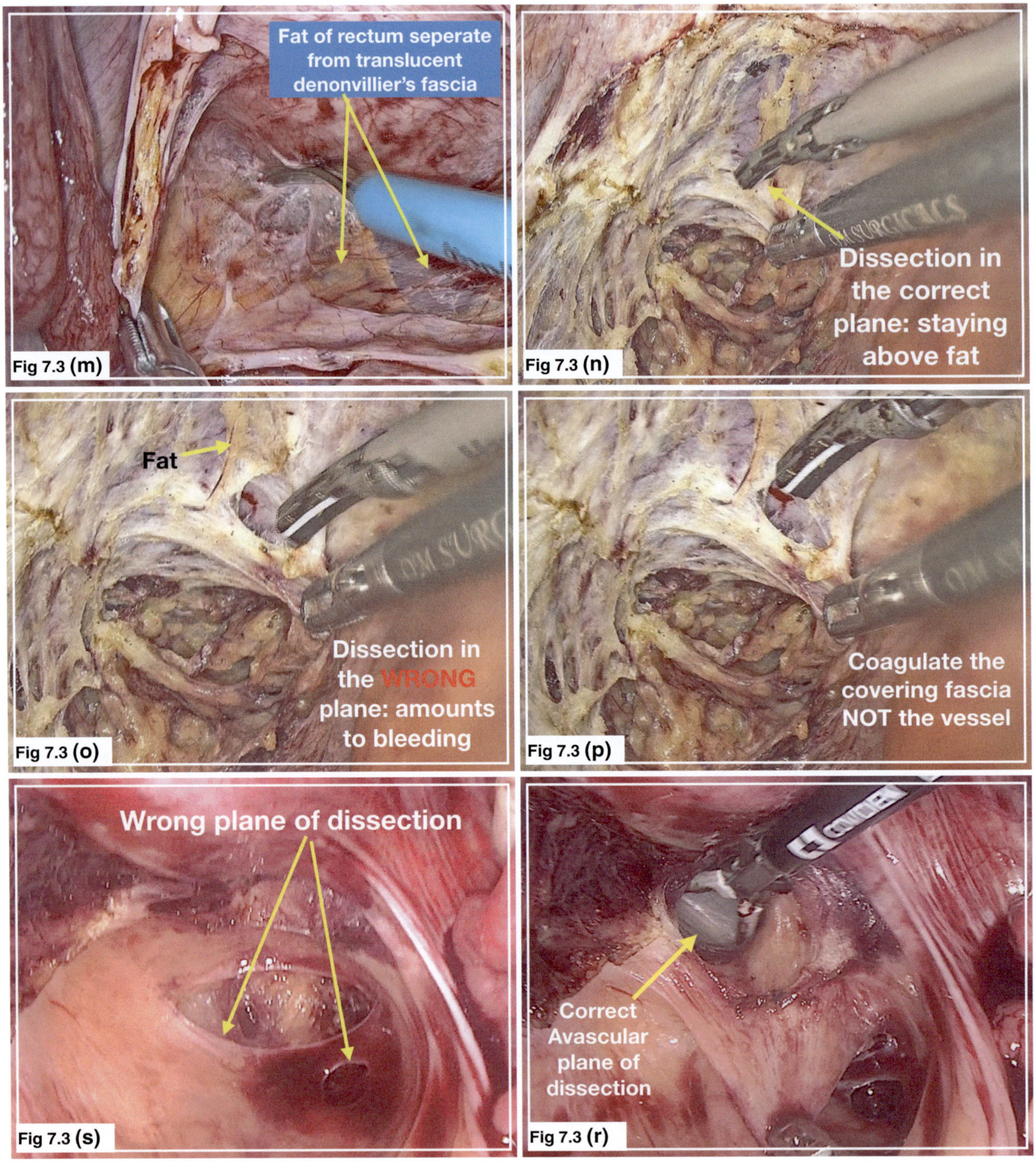

Fig. 7.3 (continued)

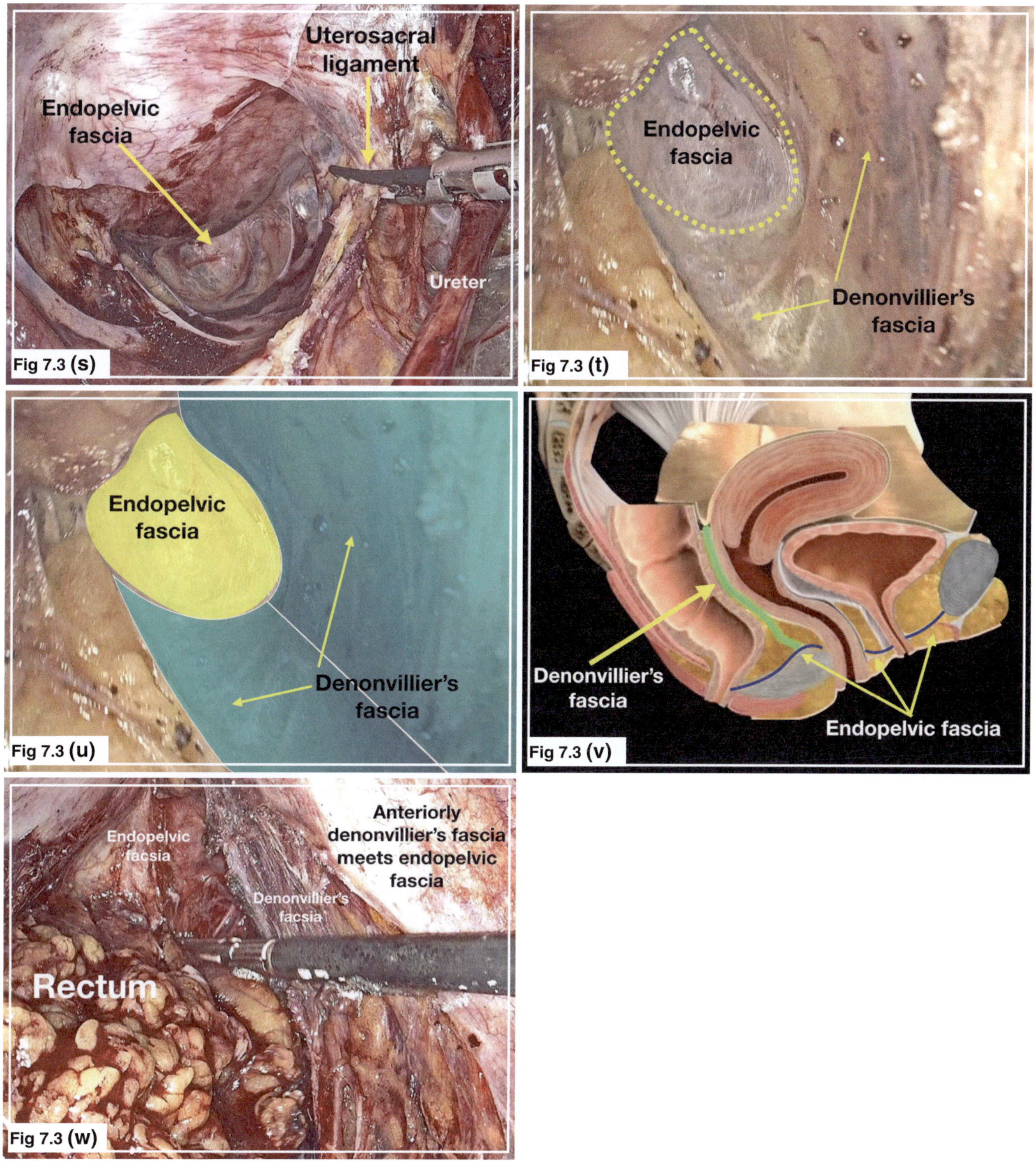

Fig. 7.3 (continued)

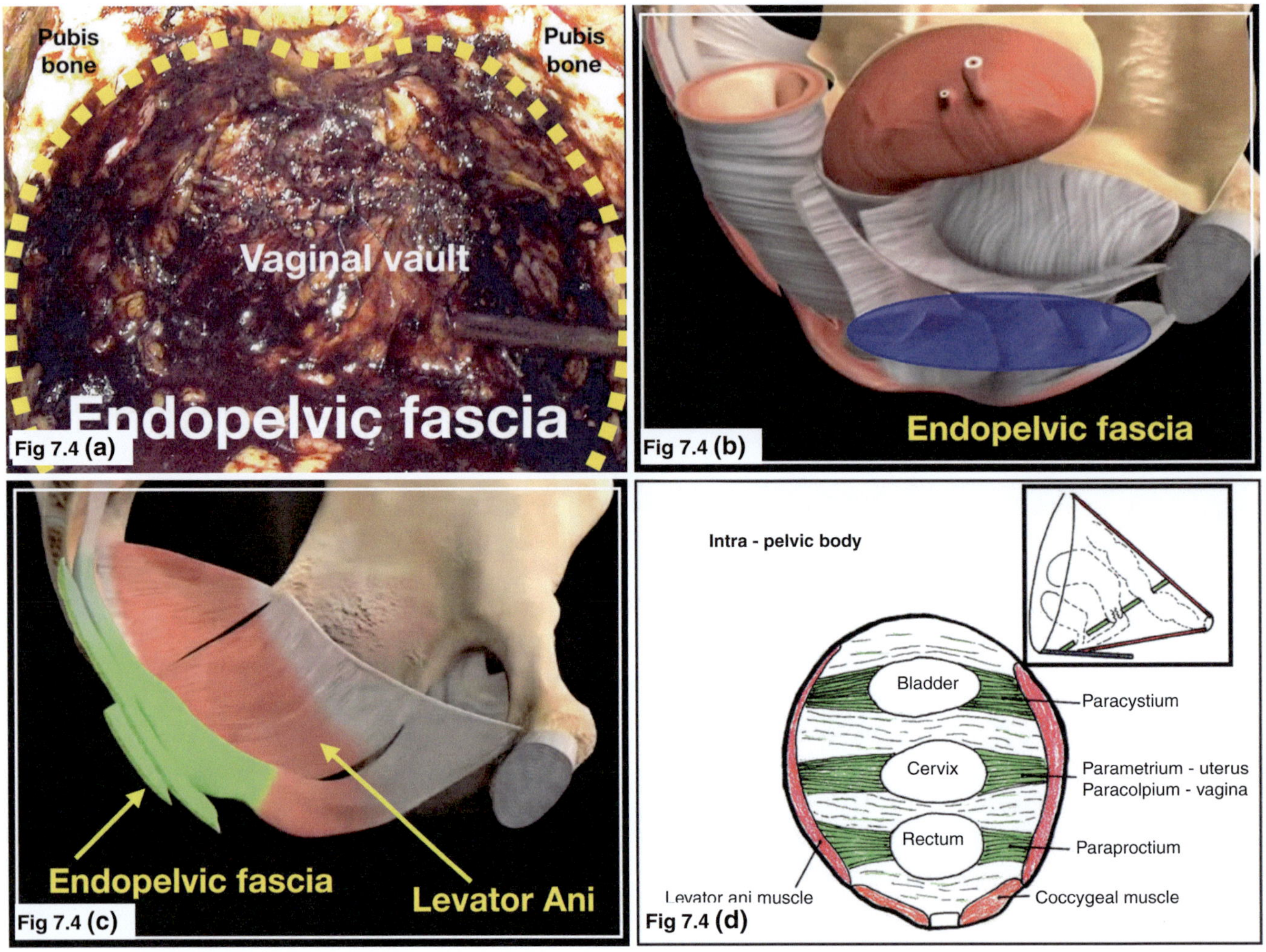

Fig. 7.4 Endopelvic fascia. (**a**) The image is taken from a case of anterior exenteration where the urethra stump is incorporated with the vault sutures. The whole area under the yellow dotted lines is the area which represents the endopelvic fascia. (**b**) Diagrammatic representation of the endopelvic fascia and their expanses across the pelvic floor as shown. Like the old saying goes, *all roads lead to Rome, all pelvic dissections end at the endopelvic fascia*. (**c**) In conditions of removing the pelvic organs, i.e. the bladder, uterus and part of the rectum. The extent of the endopelvic fascia has been demonstrated in this diagram. (**d**) The latest concept of the endoplevic fascia states that the endopelvic fascia is a complex of vesicohypogastric fascia (lateral paracystium), transverse cervical ligament (lateral parametrium) and lateral ligament of rectum (lateral paraproctium) and their relation to each other and the respective organs is explained in the schematic picture of the pelvis in the inset. (**e**) The endopelvic fascia can be traced from the level of the pubic symphysis. It covers the obturator internus muscle which is attached midway at the inner aspect of the pubic bone. Thus the endopelvic fascia can be seen there. The image has been taken from a case of anterior exenteration after anterior mobilisation of the bladder and after dissecting the prevesical space. (**f**) The endopelvic fascia can be seen covering the urethra and the vagina as well anteriorly. Underneath the endopelvic fascia lies the vaginal veins. Later posteriorly the vagina is covered with the Denonvilliers' fascia which communicates with the endopelvic fascia at the base. (**g**) As previously discussed, the end point of dissection of the paravesical and the pararectal space is the levator ani (endopelvic fascia) as shown in the image. The image has been taken from a routine laparoscopic radical hysterectomy. (**h**) The image is from the anterior exenteration where the paracolpium is resected completely making the floor of pararectal and paravesical space as a common floor of endopelvic fascia. (**i**) In the case of anterior exenteration the paravesical space dissection is extended cranially and communicated with the prevesical space after mobilisation of the bladder and the floor here is also made common, covered with endopelvic fascia. The central column of tissue is the vagina and the urethra. (**j**) This image shows the endopelvic fascia being present commonly under the pararectal, paravesical and prevesical space on one side of the pelvis. (**k**) Similar dissection on the opposite side has also been done. The endopelvic fascia communicates with each other across the dissection of the Denonvilliers' fascia which meets the endopelvic fascia at midline behind the uterus. Thus the uterus along with the paracolpium and bladder can be resected en bloc. (**l**) Final view of anterior exenteration seen. The vaginal vault closed with polyglactin sutures. The Foley's catheter is seen through the remnant urethra stump. The entire visible floor is covered with the endopelvic fascia. (**m**) Diagrammatic representation of the endopelvic fascia shaded in yellow. The urogenital and rectal hiatus have been labelled. (**n**) In certain cases the endopelvic fascia appears more translucent making the underlying levator ani muscle visible as shown in the image. Posteriorly the coccyges and the levator ani muscles are partly covered by endopelvic fascia and the Waldeyer's fascia (discussed later). (**o**) Dissection below the level of the endopelvic fascia often injures the vaginal veins which causes torrential haemorrhage. Secondly after directing through the levator ani fat exposed is the fat of ischiorectal fossa. Ischiorectal fossa is not a part of the pelvic cavity. It is the part of perineum. Hence the limit of pelvic floor dissection is at the level of the endopelvic fascia

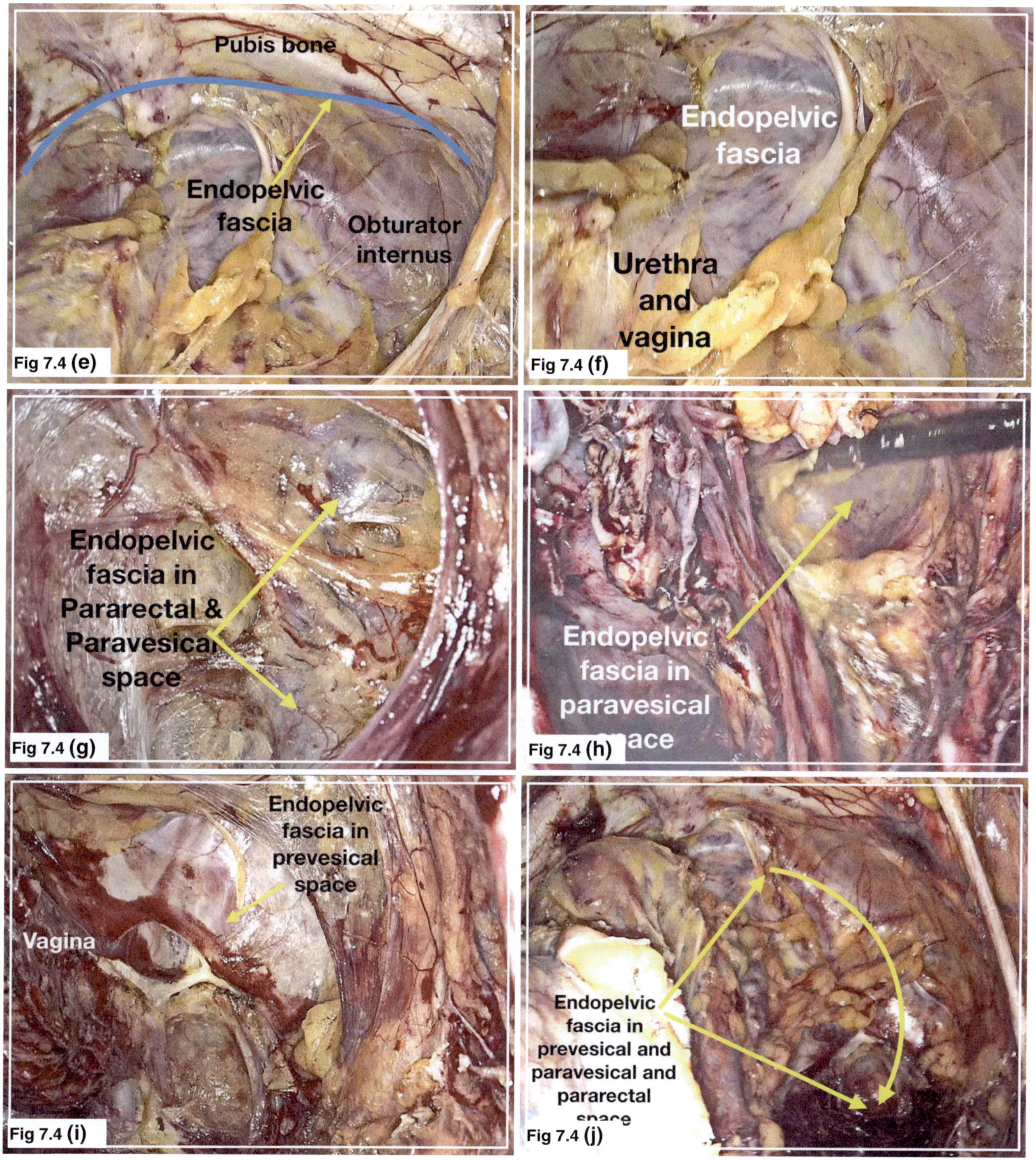

Fig. 7.4 (continued)

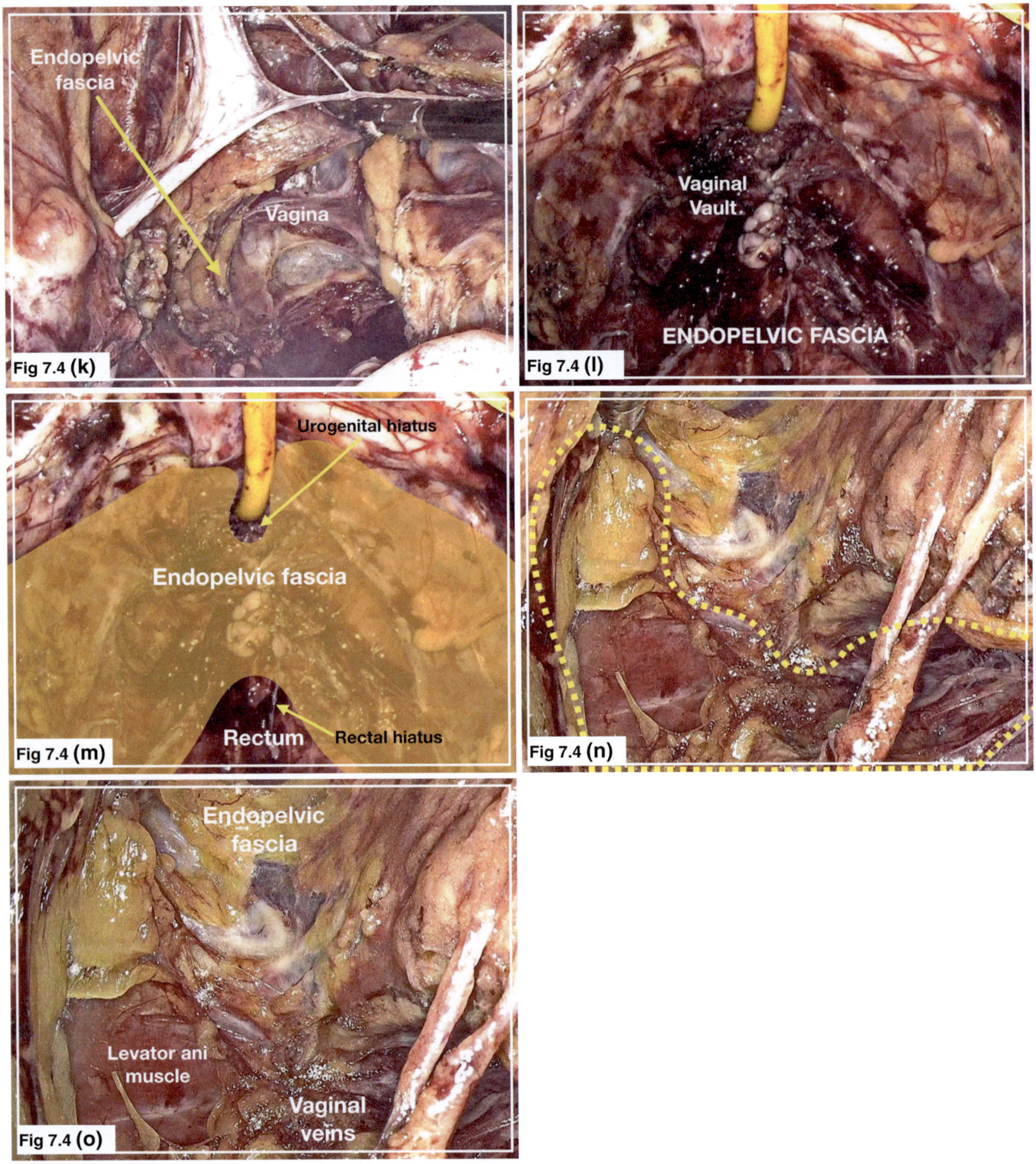

Fig. 7.4 (continued)

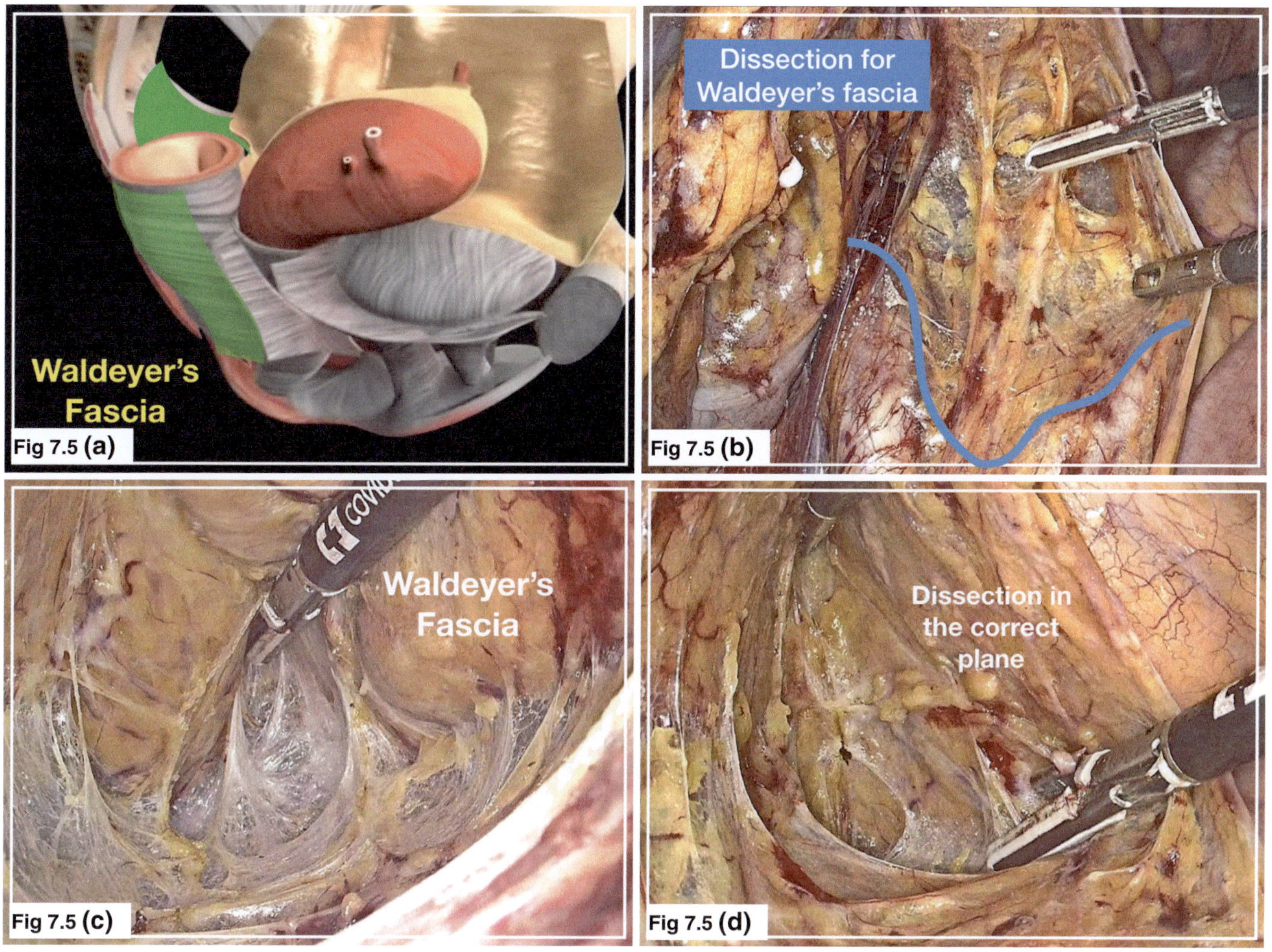

Fig. 7.5 Waldeyer's fascia. (**a**) Diagrammatic representation of the Waldeyer's fascia. The avascular fascia behind the rectum. Like previously discussed rule, the rectum is covered by avascular fascia of the Denonvilliers' fascia anteriorly and the Waldeyer's fascia posteriorly. (**b**) Real-time image of the beginning of the Waldeyer's fascia at the level of pelvic brim near sacral promontory. The Waldeyer's fascia is dissected in cases of posterior exenteration during mobilisation of the sigmoid or rectum in the retrorectal or presacral space. The light blue line denotes the beginning of the Waldeyer's fascia. (**c**) As explained in the previous chapter on presacral space, the Waldeyer's fascia lies over the sacral region. Under the Waldeyer's fascia lie the important (vital) presacral veins which tend to bleed torrentially when injured. Hence it is important to always remain anterior and above the Waldeyer's fascia. (**d**) *Fat belongs to rectum*. Thus here in this fascia own goal is to remain below the fat as the rectum is above. The avascular plane of dissection lies below the fat always. (**e**) Often the Waldeyer's fascia is adherent in the midline as shown in the image. The dissection here is to be done with caution as forceful dissection would lead to injury to the presacral veins. (**f**) The concept of the veins under the fascia has been demonstrated here as well. Dissection in the wrong plane leads to injury to the branches of the rectal veins as seen here. Presacral veins bleed excessively and hence are not demonstrated on them. The presacral veins lie underneath the Waldeyer's fascia and the rectal veins lie anterior to the fascia. (**g**) Rectal veins are smaller veins for which haemostats can be achieved with energy sources itself. But it is to be kept in mind that the coagulation is done on the fascia and not on the vein, with the fascia being a mechanical support to the veins. Superficial coagulation of fascia transmits the energy to the veins needed to coagulate. (**h**) The internal iliac vein can be faintly seen under the Waldeyer's fascia. This is the second reason why dissection is to be done with caution. The presacral vein drains into the internal iliac vein. Thus injury to the presacral vein leads to indirect bleeding from the internal iliac vein. (**i**) The communication of the presacral veins with the internal iliac veins can be seen. The presacral veins can be seen under the Waldeyer's fascia. The mobilised rectum appears as a characteristic "*buttocks of infant*" appearance. (**j**) *Buttocks of infant* appearance as seen in the image. (**k**) As previously mentioned the rectum is covered by the Denonvilliers' fascia anteriorly and its dissection up to the endopelvic fascia helps separate the rectum anteriorly. However for the posterior dissection similar dissection up to the endopelvic fascia is done at the Waldeyer's fascia side. (**l**) Posteriorly the Waldeyer's fascia is seen communicating with the endoplevic fascia and thus the rectum is mobilised from all sides. (**m**) The Waldeyer's fascia is also seen present on the floor of the pararectal space as seen in the image. The internal iliac artery can be identified. (**n**) Diagrammatic representation of the two spaces sharing a common fascia. (**o**) Similarly in a case of laparoscopic radical hysterectomy the Waldeyer's fascia can be identified as a separate avascular plane at the floor near its cranial end. (**p**) Similar dissection of the fascias can be seen on the left side of the same case of laparoscopic radical hysterectomy explained in the previous image. (**q**) Diagrammatic representation of the communication between the two fascias has been explained with the help of the image

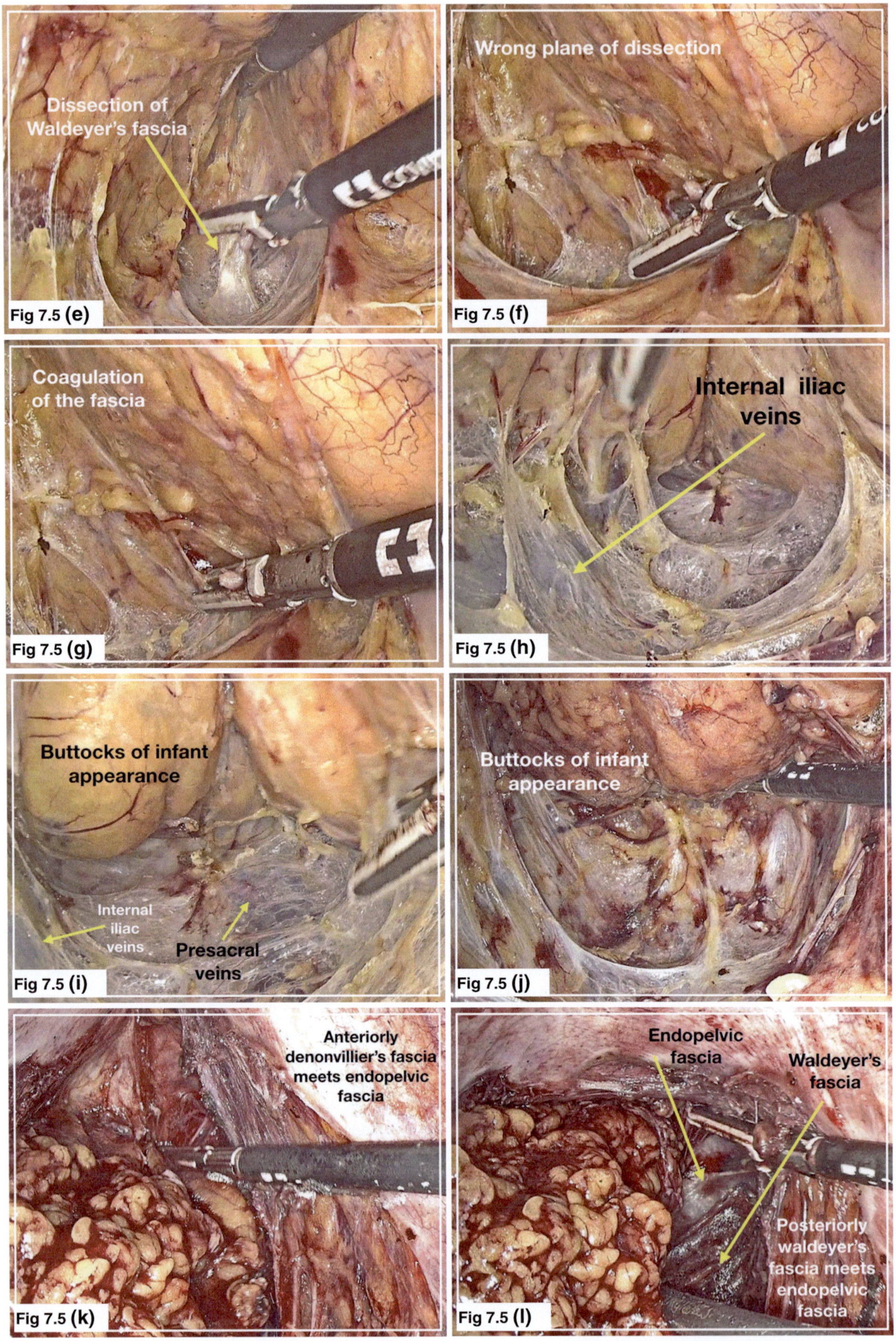

Fig. 7.5 (continued)

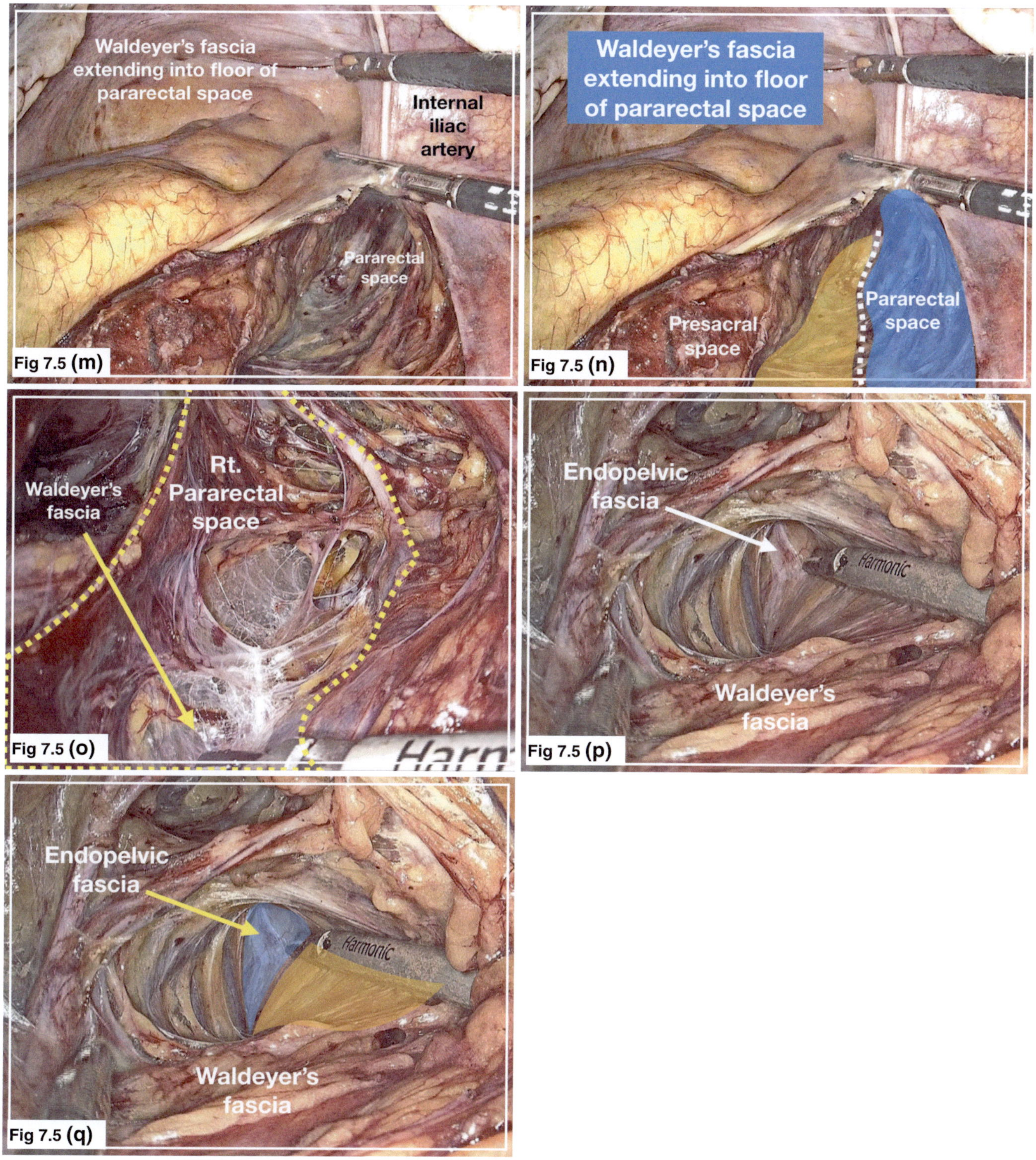

Fig. 7.5 (continued)

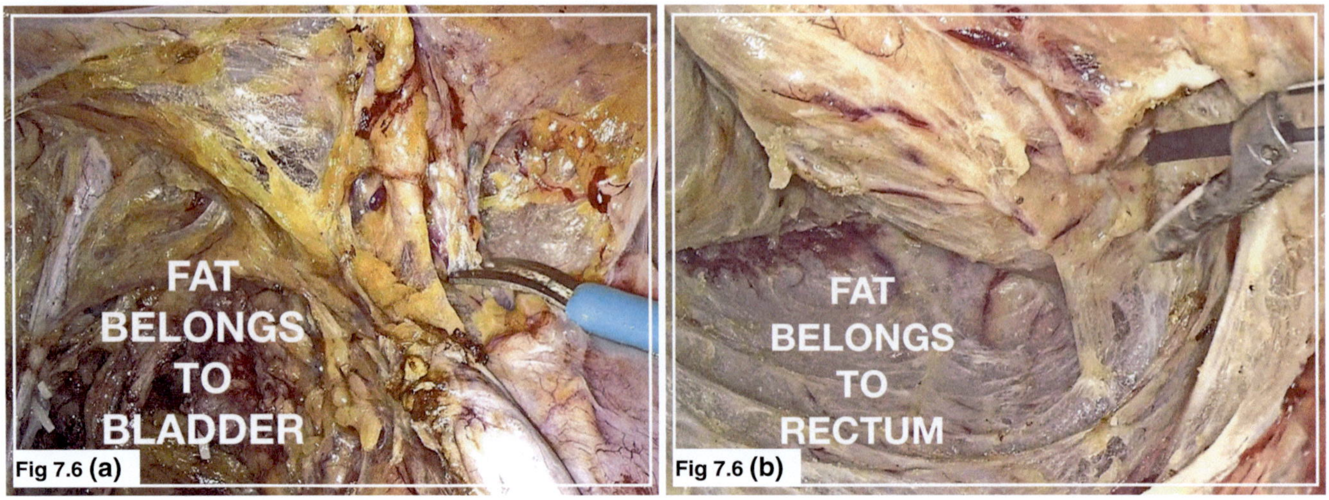

Fig. 7.6 (**a**) "Fat belongs to the bladder". (**b**) "Fat belongs to the rectum"

8 Anatomy of the Ureter

The ureteric anatomy is probably the most important consideration in pelvic surgery (Figs. 8.1, 8.2, 8.3, 8.4, 8.5, 8.6, 8.7, 8.8, and 8.9).

The ureter crosses the common iliac at the level of sacral promontory from lateral to medial side (Figs. 8.10, 8.11, 8.12, 8.13, 8.14, 8.15, 8.16, 8.17, and 8.18).

The ureter travels in its own endopelvic fascia (Figs. 8.19, 8.20, 8.21, 8.22, 8.23, and 8.24).

It travels in between the fork of the uterine artery and the uterine vein (Figs. 8.25, 8.26, 8.27, 8.28, 8.29, 8.30, 8.31, 8.32, 8.33, 8.34, 8.35, 8.36, 8.37, 8.38, 8.39, 8.40, 8.41, 8.42, 8.43, 8.44, and 8.45).

Classically called "water under the bridge". This anatomy is important when there is haemorrhage; if there is venous bleeding, the ureter should be lifted anteriorly and the bleeding should be controlled while if there is arterial bleeding it comes from the top (Figs. 8.46, 8.47, and 8.48).

It then turns medially and anteriorly to pass on the anterolateral aspect of the upper third of the vagina towards the bladder in its own "tunnel" of the endopelvic fascia. This commonly known ureteric tunnel is actually the uterovesical ligament. This ligament consistently contains two veins. The ureters enter the bladder at the corners of the trigone approximately 2.5 cm apart.

The ureter is always lateral to the uterosacrals (Figs. 8.49, 8.50, 8.51, 8.52, and 8.53).

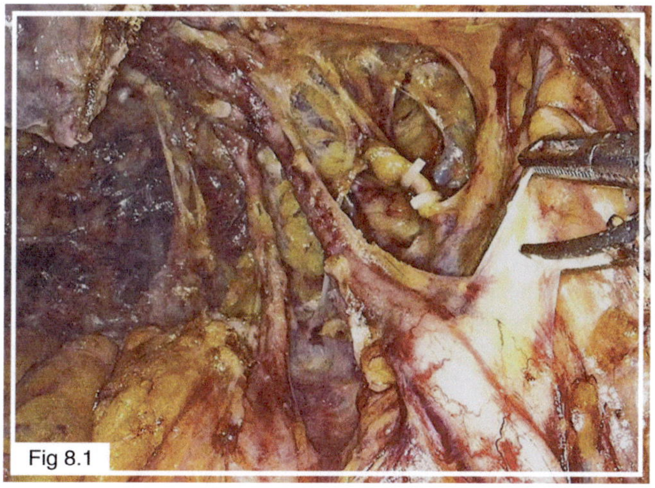

Fig. 8.1 Ureter: The ureter is the most encountered vital structure in the pelvis, in males and females alike. The ureter traverses a complex course where it comes in relation to almost every important structure in the pelvis. Thus knowing the detailed anatomy becomes of paramount importance. As shown in this image the ureter can be seen from the sacral promontory travelling deeper into the depths of the pelvis

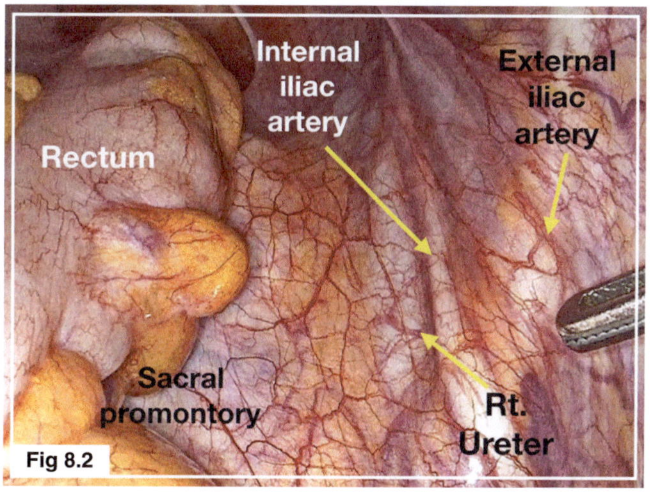

Fig. 8.2 Ureter: Often the ureters can be seen through the peritoneal layer lateral to the sacral promontory. The peristalsis is often used as a marker for identification. However it is important to understand its normal anatomical lie and its course to have more reassurance for identification than relying on its peristalsis. This chapter deals with the various anatomical relations of the ureter with other vital structures. This should help the viewers identify ureters in still images than relying on peristalsis for identification

S. Puntambekar et al., *Laparoscopic Pelvic Anatomy in Females*, https://doi.org/10.1007/978-981-13-8653-4_8

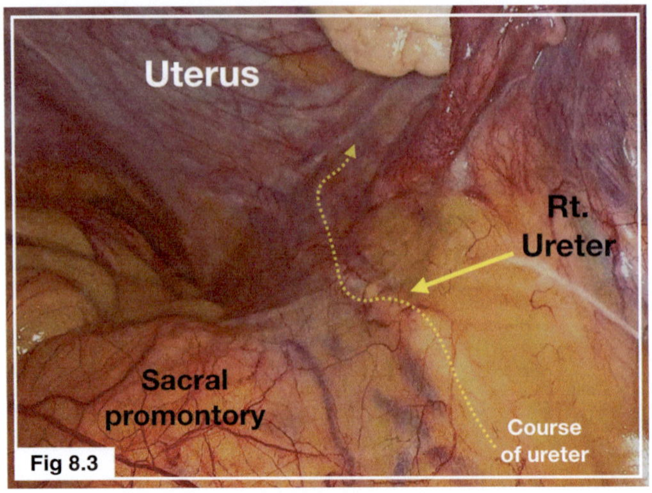

Fig. 8.3 Ureter: The ureter can be traced up to its origin in the dotted yellow lines. These are visible on careful visualisation but often lose their visibility during operative intervention due to energy sources or blood or connective tissue dissection. Thus it is of paramount importance to have alternative means of identification of the ureter along its entire course. Terms of anatomy and relation to various structures

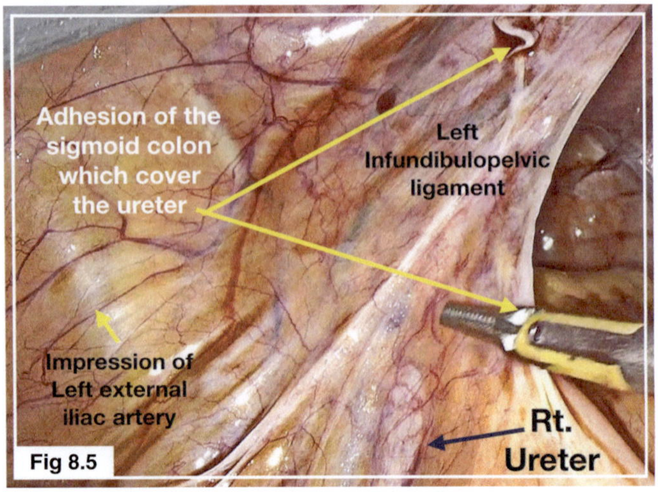

Fig. 8.5 Ureter: The left ureter is often difficult to trace at the level of sacral promontory due to congenital adhesion of the sigmoid colon to the lateral pelvic wall. Secondly due to left-side rotation of the colon the fat deposition in the retroperitoneum is higher on the left side

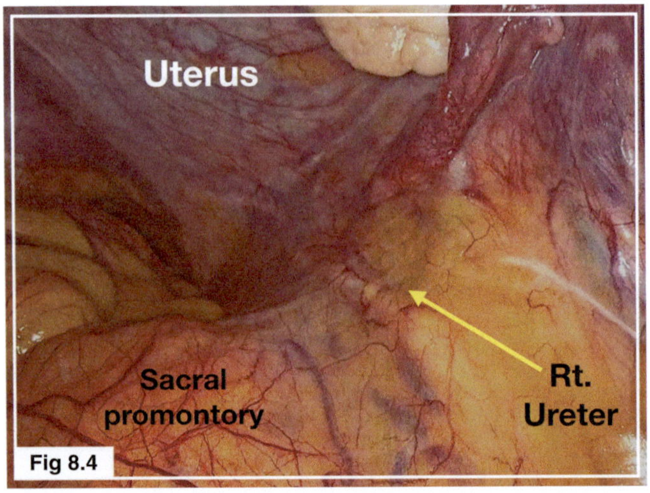

Fig. 8.4 Ureter: Variable amount of retroperitoneal fat can often obscure the view of the ureter through the ureters and can be viewed by gentle stroke on the lateral side of the sacral promontory and look for peristalsis. In the condition of uncertainty gentle strokes on the ureter can initiate peristalsis which distinguishes the ureter from the external iliac vessels

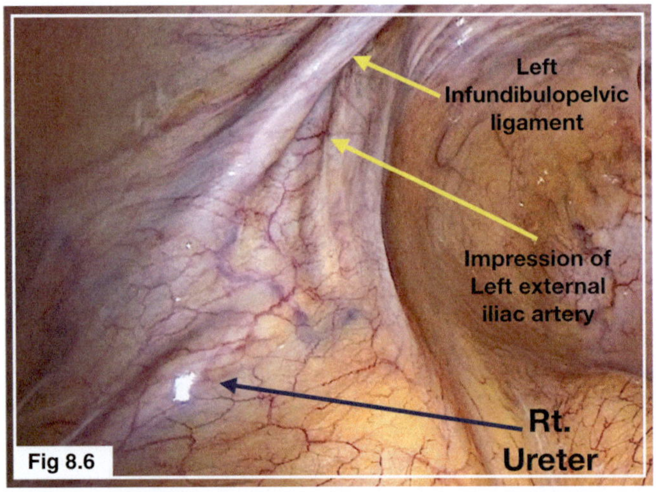

Fig. 8.6 Ureter: The left ureter is difficult to see through the translucent peritoneum layer. However the lateral approach of parental space dissection can easily reveal the ureter. The ureter always remains medial to the infundibulopelvic ligament. A part of ureter is covered with fat which makes it look like it disappears just below the infundibulopelvic ligament

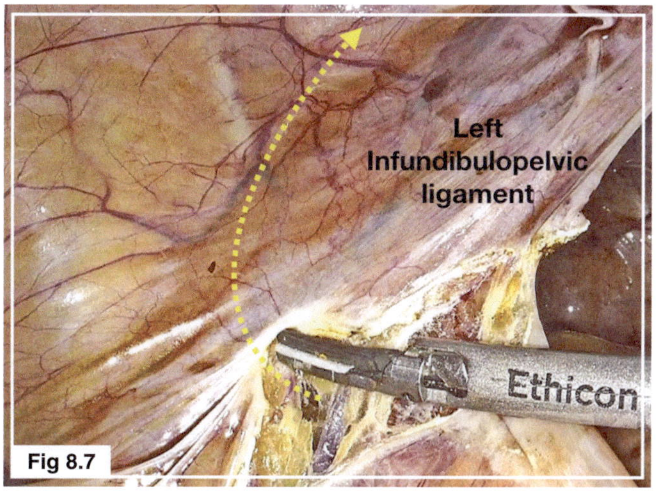

Fig. 8.7 Ureter: Irrespective of the amount of retroperitoneal fat, the left ureter can be easily visualised by dissecting the peritoneum lateral to the infundibulopelvic ligament (by lateral approach). As shown in subsequent images the ureter appears to be present and in continuity of the impression previously seen through the translucent peritoneum

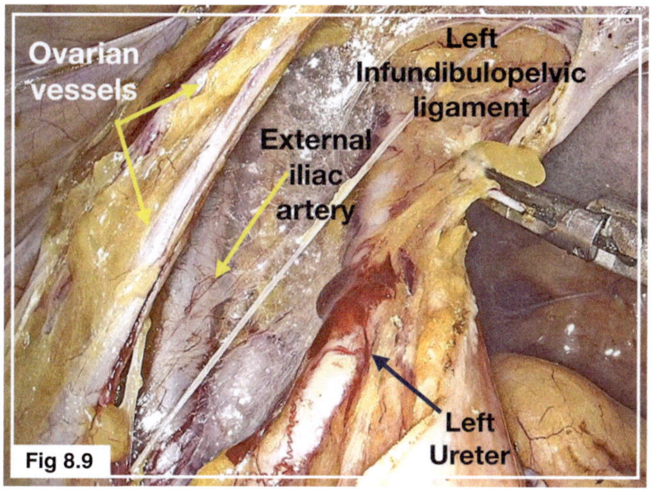

Fig. 8.9 Ureter: After identification of the ureter on the lateral side the peritoneum is dissected on the medial side. The medial approach is the most definitive way of identifying the ureter. The infundibulopelvic ligament can be given traction laterally so as to expose the medial surface. The first structure to appear on dissecting the peritoneum is the ureter. As shown in the image the course of the ureter can be seen up to the external iliac vessels

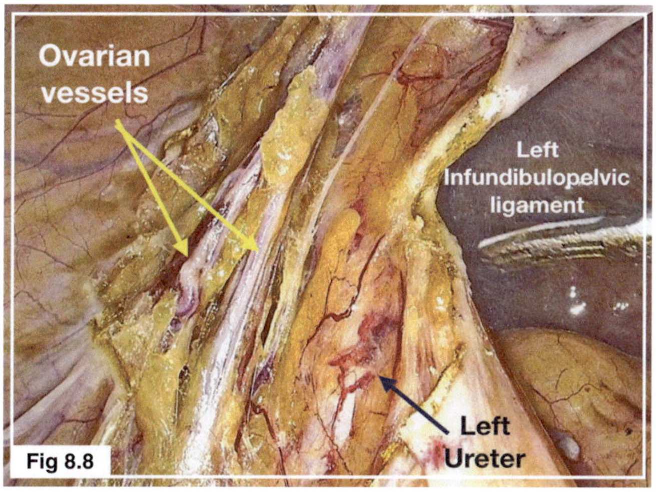

Fig. 8.8 Ureter: The ureter can be seen medial to the ovarian vessels or medial to the infundibulopelvic ligament on dissection of the peritoneum. It is considered that the ureter carries its own mesentery. This is discussed later in the chapter

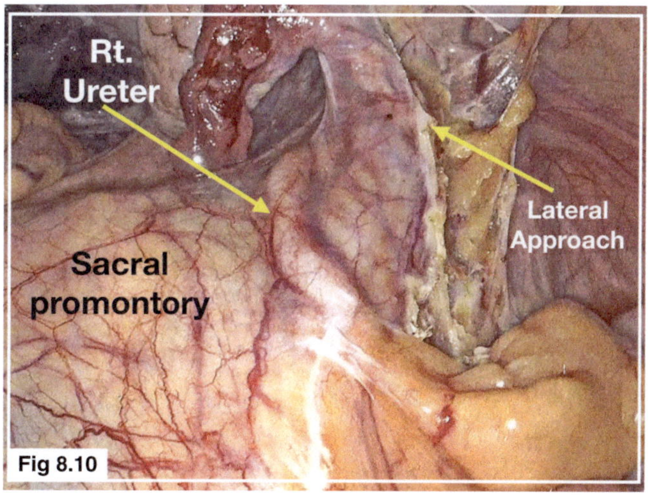

Fig. 8.10 Ureter: The right ureter impressions can be seen on the peritoneum. However its course cannot be seen completely as it dips deeper into the pelvis. The peritoneum has been incised by the lateral approach as it can be seen in the image. Now the medial edge of the peritoneum is retracted medially to expose the pararectal space and visualise the ureter

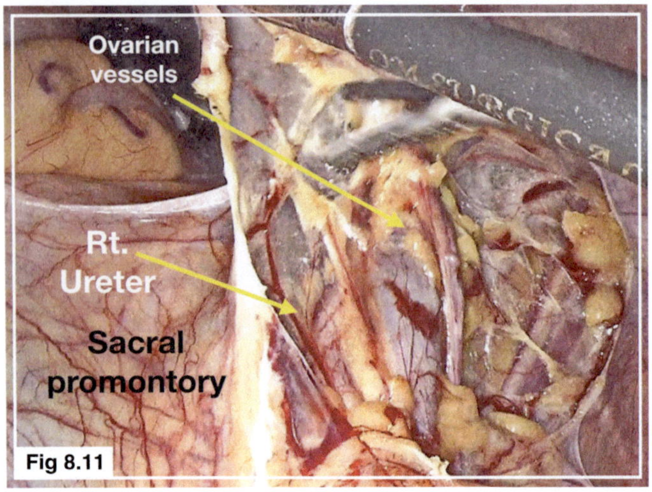

Fig. 8.11 Ureter: As the medial edge of the incision is retracted towards midline, the ureter has been seen in a meandering course around the ovarian vessels; hence it was seen only in a short segment from above the peritoneum. This dissection of the peritoneum can help understand and confirm the course of ureter during any pelvic surgery. Although often confusing the ovarian vessels can remain lateral or medial to the ureter depending upon the traction provided onto the vessels indirectly but the infundibulopelvic ligament. However *they do not remain in the same plane*

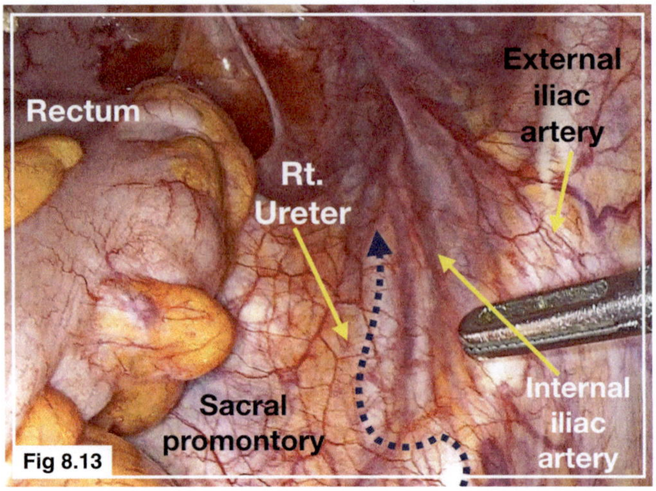

Fig. 8.13 Ureter: At sacral promontory: The right ureter here is clearly seen to cross over the external and internal iliac artery. It crosses at the bifurcation of the common iliac artery at the level of sacral promontory. This can be further confirmed on dissection of the peritoneum covering the ureter at that level. The blue dotted line denotes the course of ureter

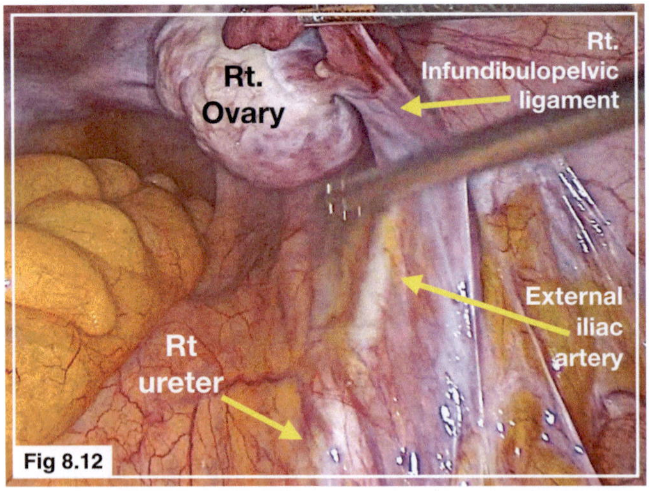

Fig. 8.12 Ureter: At sacral promontory: The right ureter is seen crossing over the external iliac vessel onto the lateral side. However in the next image the presence of internal iliac can also be confusing while identifying structures. Thus it is best to dissect the peritoneum and confirm

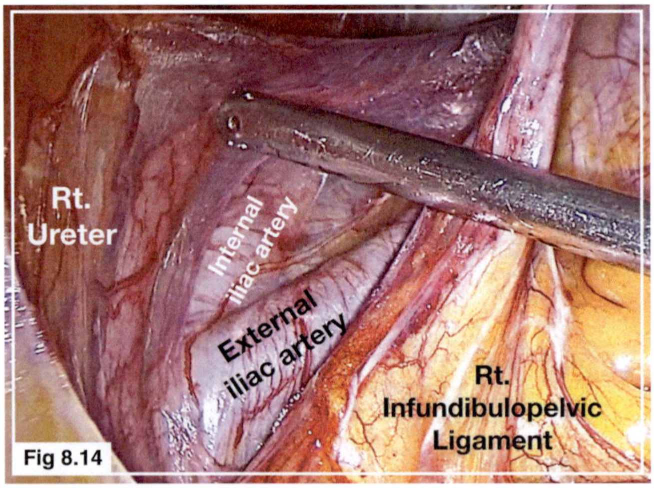

Fig. 8.14 Ureter: On dissecting the peritoneum the bifurcation of the common iliac artery is seen. The ureter thus travels over the origin of external and internal iliac artery at the level of sacral promontory

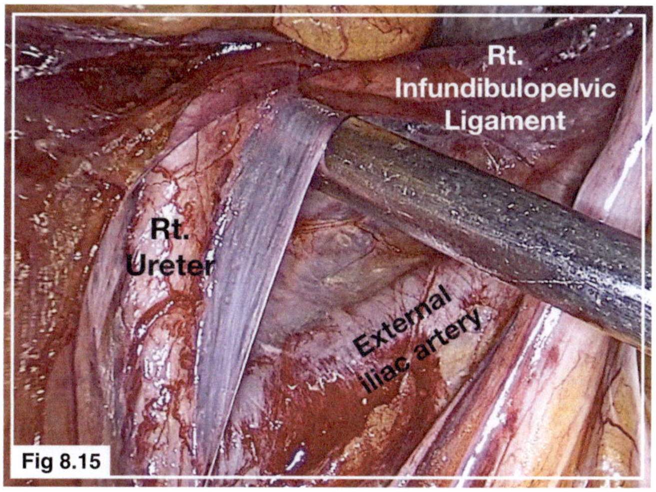

Fig. 8.15 Ureter: At sacral promontory: The ureter lies above the iliac vessels but it has its separate fascia plane and is significantly mobile and free of attachments. To assess the bifurcation of the common iliac vessels, the medial approach of the retroperitoneum can be extended cranially to expose the psoas muscle and the common iliac artery easily

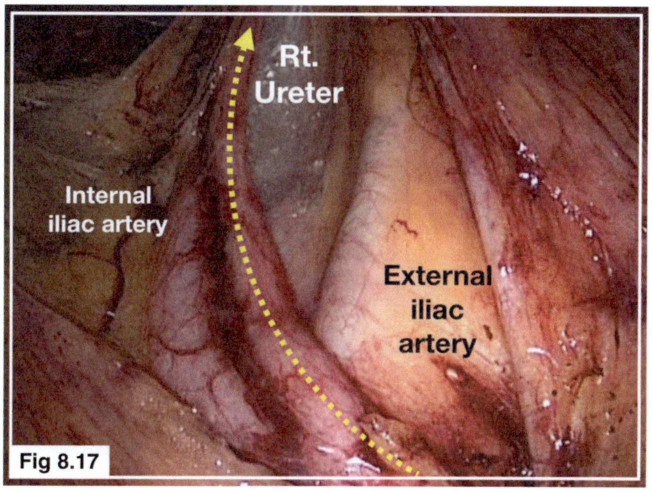

Fig. 8.17 Ureter: At Sacral promontory: Final view of the ureter at the level of sacral promontory with the ureter voyaging over the bifurcation of the iliac vessels. This image has been taken from another case of laparoscopic radical hysterectomy for a case of Ca cervix

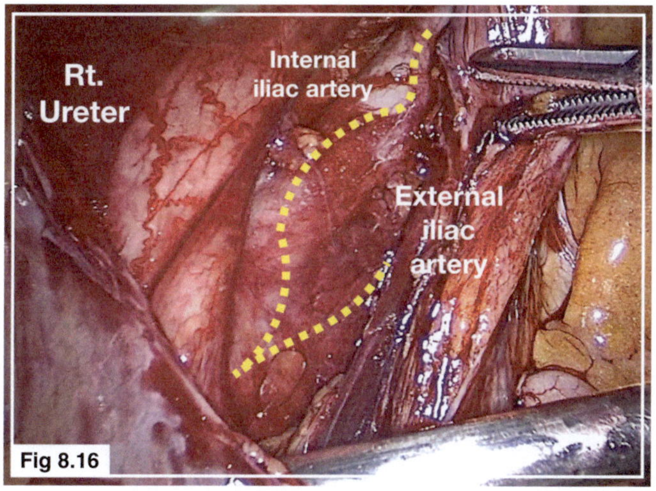

Fig. 8.16 Ureter: At sacral promontory: The minor capillary blood vessels on the peritoneal surface can be damaged during forceful dissection of the retroperitoneal spaces and can often lead to haemorrhagic fields. Thus it is advised to handle the fat tissue with gentle caution and not force dissection through fat to search for fascial planes. A misleading fold of peritoneum can be seen under the ureter that has been created by the traction provided by the instrument underneath it. The yellow dotted line denotes the course of the iliac vessels

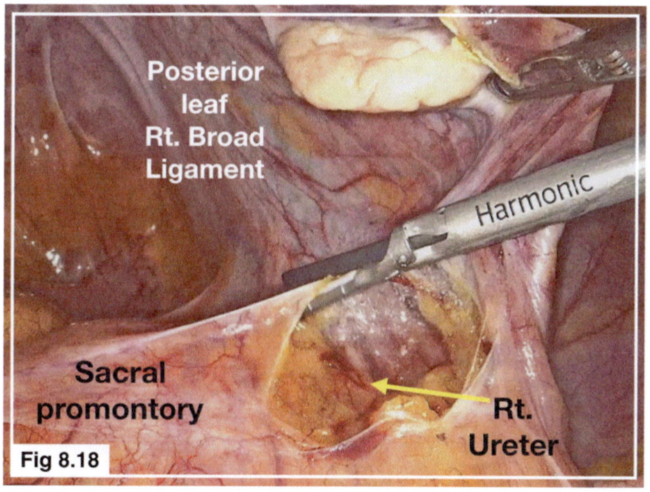

Fig. 8.18 Ureter and its own mesentery: In a case of laparoscopic radical hysterectomy the retroperitoneum is opened medial to the infundibulopelvic ligament. The ureter is the first structure visualised. The ureter is concealed by the retroperitoneal fat. Gentle strokes over the ureter help increase its visibility by separating the fat and by stimulating the peristalsis as well

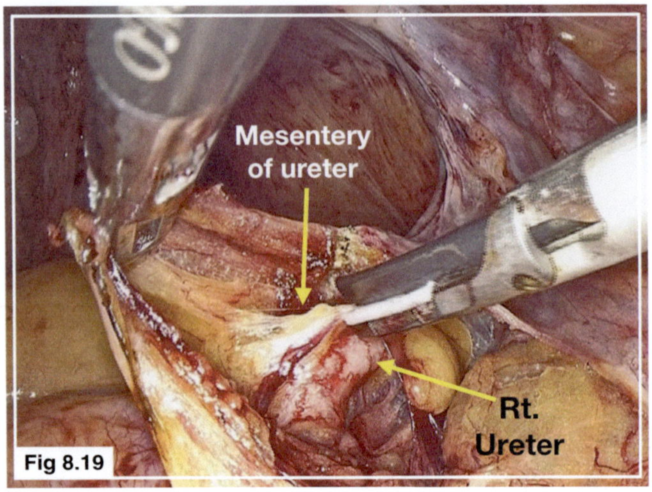

Fig. 8.19 Ureter and its own mesentery: On close dissection it is seen that a layer of fat is closely attached to the ureter interpreted with minor capillary vessels. This brings us to the concept of *ureter having its own mesentery*

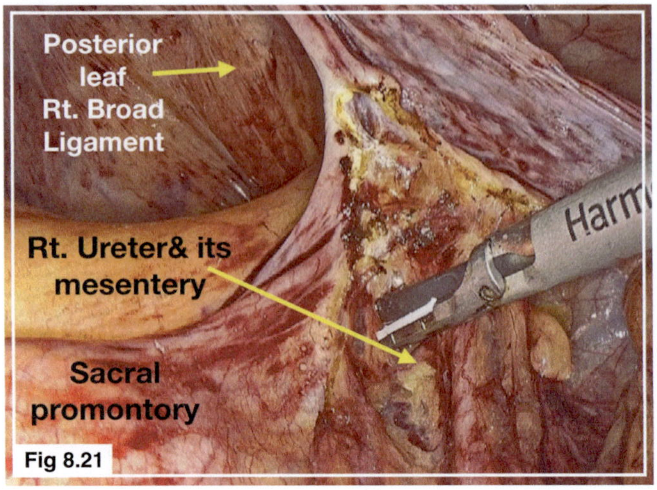

Fig. 8.21 Ureter and its own mesentery: The mobilisation of ureter from the medial or the lateral side is done keeping its mesentery in consideration at all times. The ureter is initially mobilised from the lateral side like routinely seen in all images above. Mobilisation of the ureter from its medial side is done to separate the ureter from the posterior leaf of broad ligament

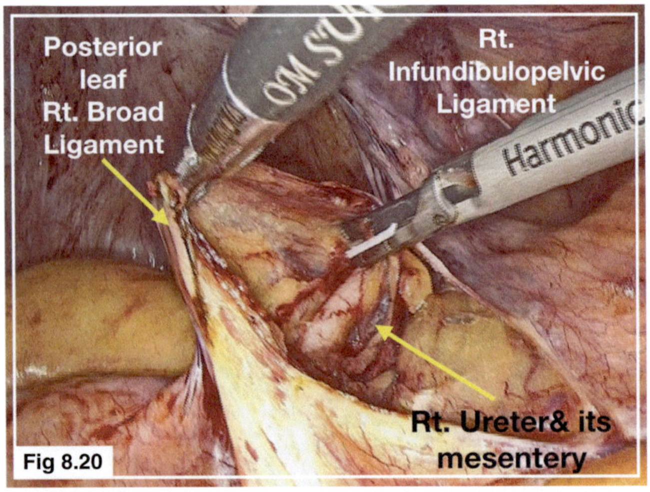

Fig. 8.20 Ureter and its own mesentery: The ureter along with its mesentery should be stripped off the posterior leaf of broad ligament in the manner of the ureter exfoliating from the peritoneum

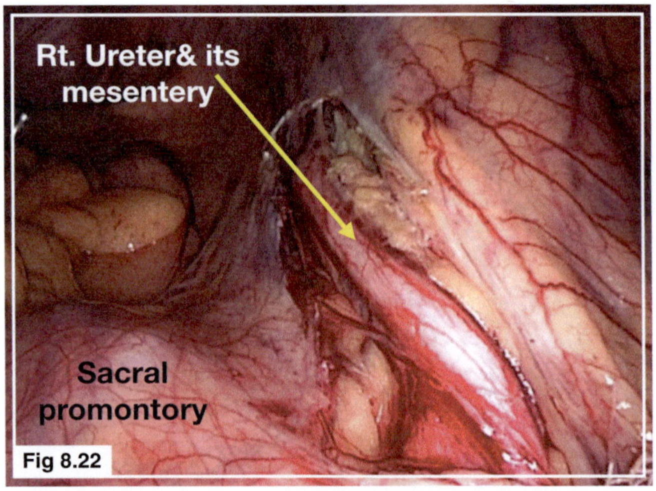

Fig. 8.22 Ureter and its own mesentery: The capillary-like network of vessel wrapped around the ureter forms the mesentery. However they are prone to rupture during forceful dissection leading to significant haemorrhage and inability to appreciate the mesentery as a whole. Such finer dissections can be achieved more easily with laparoscopy owing to its higher magnification definer and accurate surgical instruments

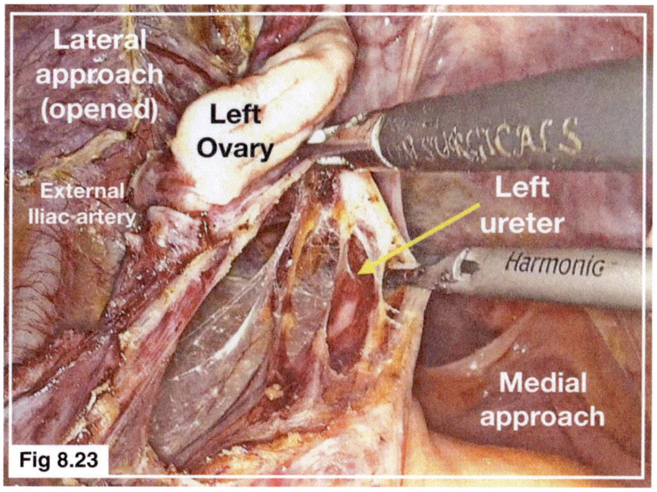

Fig. 8.23 Ureter and its own mesentery: Similar dissections can be seen on the left side as well, owing to the congenital adhesions of the sigmoid colon on the left side. It is easiest to open via the lateral approach. Following this once the ureter is visualised, the leaf of the broad ligament can be dissected from medial side with a high assurance of not injuring any structure underneath the peritoneum

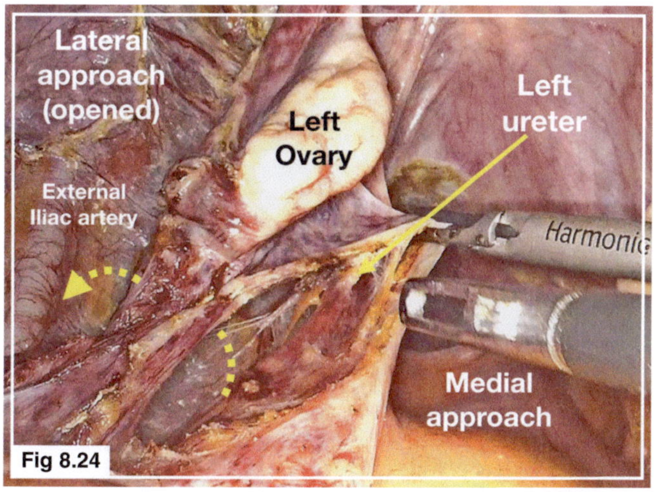

Fig. 8.24 Ureter and its own mesentery: After opening the peritoneum from both sides, the ovarian vessels can be easily dissected from the connective tissue underneath it. The rest of the dissection of the ureter is continued in routine manner of medial approach. The yellow dotted arrow indicates the area cleared by blunt dissection

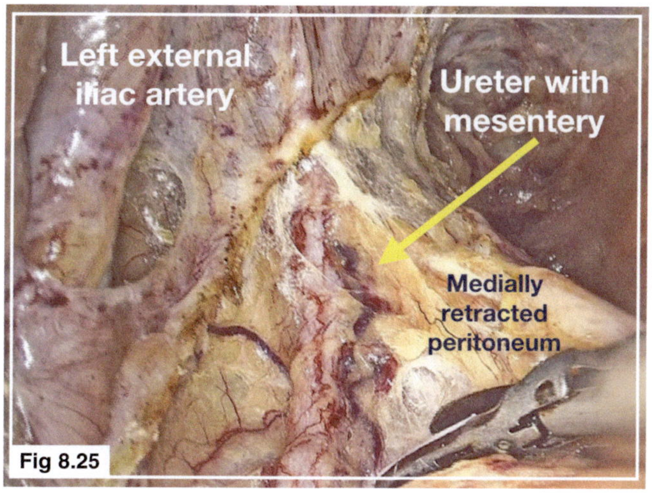

Fig. 8.25 Ureter and its relations: On establishing the orientation of the ureter at the level of sacral promontory, the course along the pararectal space needs to be established. At all times the external iliac artery remains lateral to the ureter. The pararectal space is best examined with the posterior leaf of broad ligament retracted medially, thus opening the space

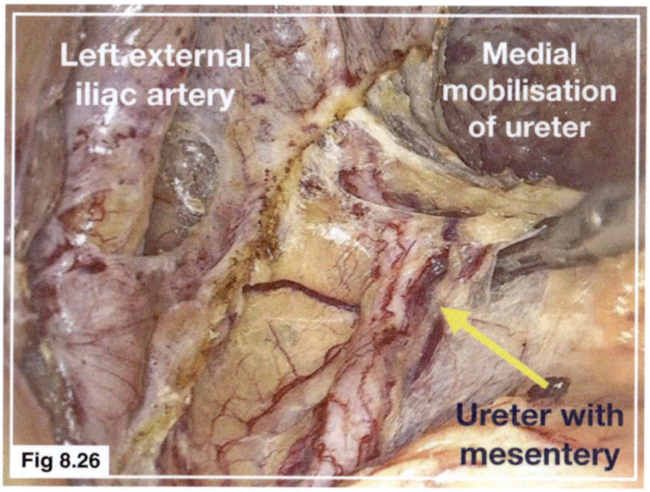

Fig. 8.26 Ureter and its relations: The ureter is always dissected along with its mesentery. Thus to free the ureter completely from the posterior leaf of broad ligament it is first mobilised medially. As we dissect deeper into the pelvis the ureter comes closer to the uterus; thus freeing the ureter medially makes it fall away from the ligament and thus providing a conducive field to cut the peritoneum

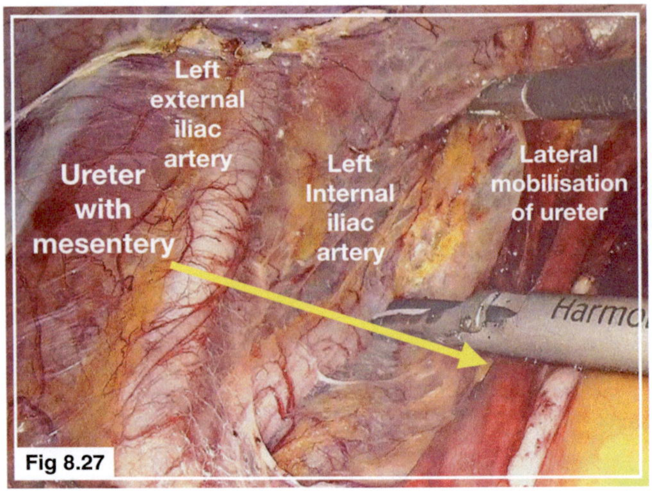

Fig. 8.27 Ureter and its relations: The ureter is mobilised from the lateral side for dissecting the space of vessels. The ureter is retracted gently towards the midline, and internal iliac artery lies on the immediate lateral side of the ureter. The dissection is done in a parallel direction to the long axis of the ureter and in the same plane as the ureter

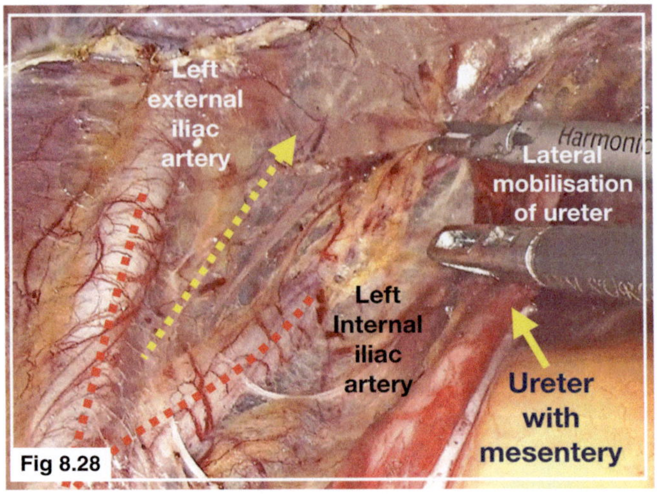

Fig. 8.28 Ureter and its relations: The internal iliac can be dissected right up to its origin, as the ureter crosses over the bifurcation of the common iliac artery. It means that the origin of both the external and internal iliac arteries lies just underneath the ureter at that point. Thus blunt dissection from the point of origin provides an advantage of being in the correct plane of dissection. The yellow dotted line signifies the direction of trisection while the red line denotes the course of the iliac vessels

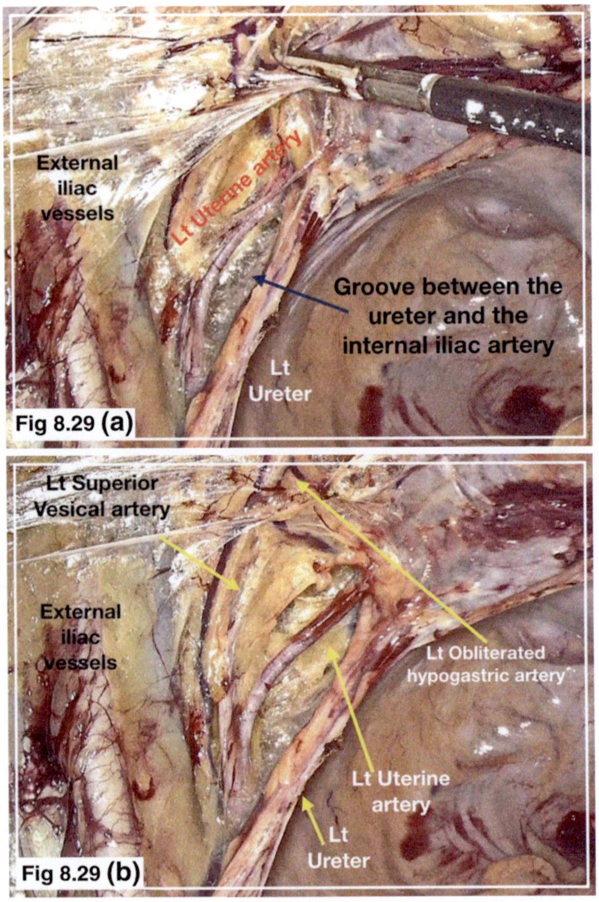

Fig. 8.29 (**a**, **b**) Ureter and its relations: On entering the groove between the ureter and the internal iliac artery, the first structure to obstruct downward separation of planes is the uterine artery. This is however confirmed only after tracing the vessel medially to see if it crosses the ureter. The superior vesical artery is also seen. The anterior division of the internal iliac artery finally terminates into the obliterated hypogastric artery

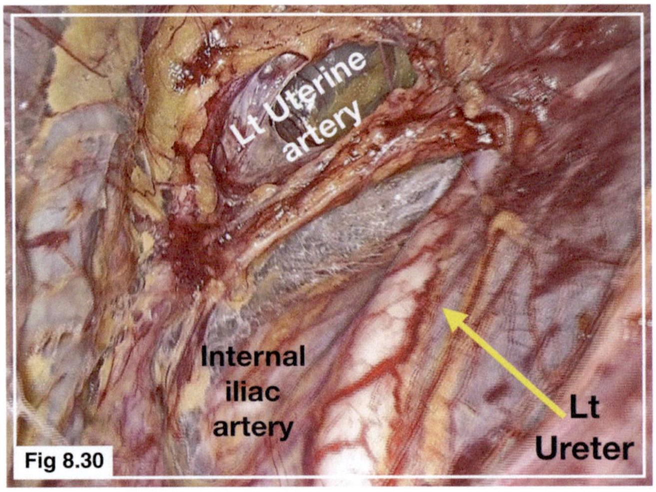

Fig. 8.30 Ureter and its relations: The uterine artery is seen as the first vessel to travel across the ureter. It follows the principle of laterality of vasculature followed by the pelvic organs and their blood supplies. *All pelvic organs are medial and their blood vessels travel from the lateral to the medial side.* Thus the first structure to obstruct downward dissection between the ureter and the internal iliac artery is the uterine artery

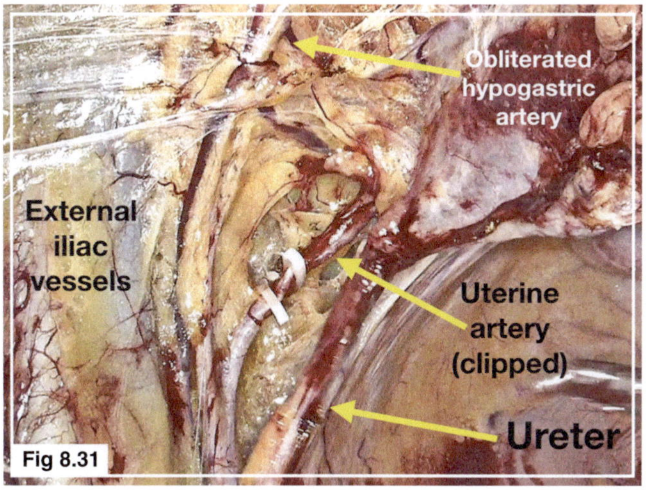

Fig. 8.31 Ureter and its relations: The uterine artery is clipped at its origin. In the condition of radical hysterectomy the uterine artery needs to be dissected, so that the uterine vein underneath can be mobilised

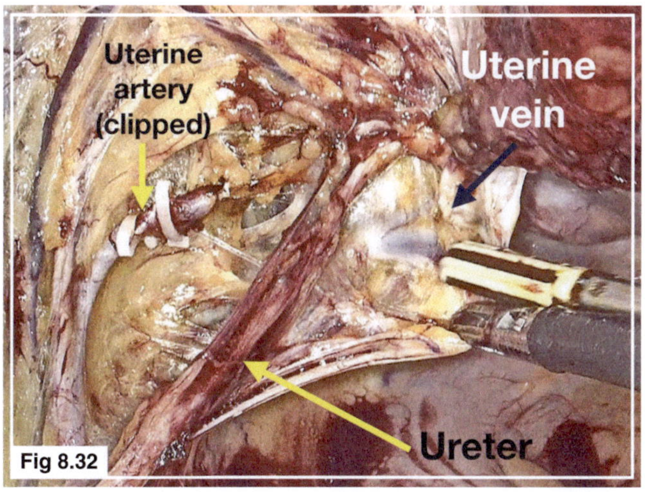

Fig. 8.32 Ureter and its relations: The uterine vein is seen under the ureter in this image. The uterine vein can also be traced under the uterine artery. Hence clipping and cutting the uterine artery is a necessary step for dissection of the uterine vein. In this case the uterine vein has specifically been dissected medial to the ureter so as to do a nerve-sparing procedure (explained later)

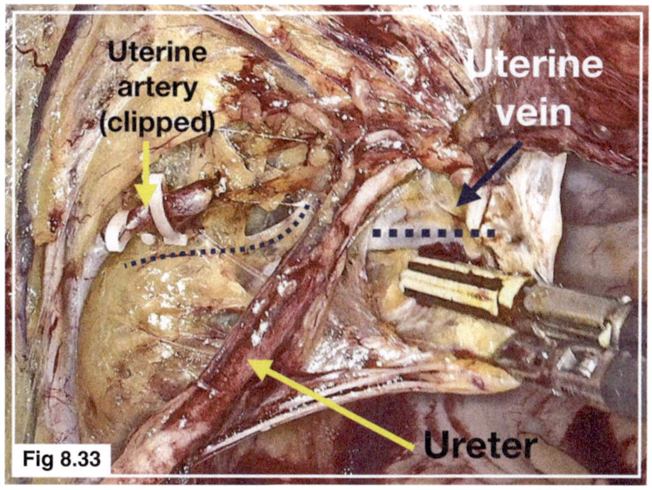

Fig. 8.33 Ureter and its relations: The blue dotted line denotes the course of the uterine vein. The uterine vein can be dissected anywhere along its course. If dissected lateral to the ureter it leads to non-nerve-sparing radical hysterectomy. This leads us to the new concept that the *ureter lies in the fork between uterine artery and vein*, unlike our previous concept of water under the bridge (artery over the ureter). More images ahead will be depicting this newer concept

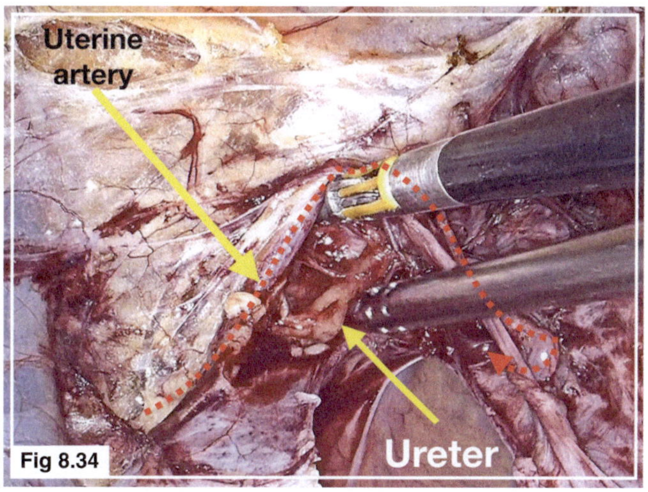

Fig. 8.34 Ureter and its relations: In a case of nerve-sparing radical hysterectomy the tortuous course of uterine artery has been identified. The ureter can be seen as a tubular structure covered in its mesentery (yellow arrows). The ureter travels from below the uterine artery. The red line denotes the course of uterine artery

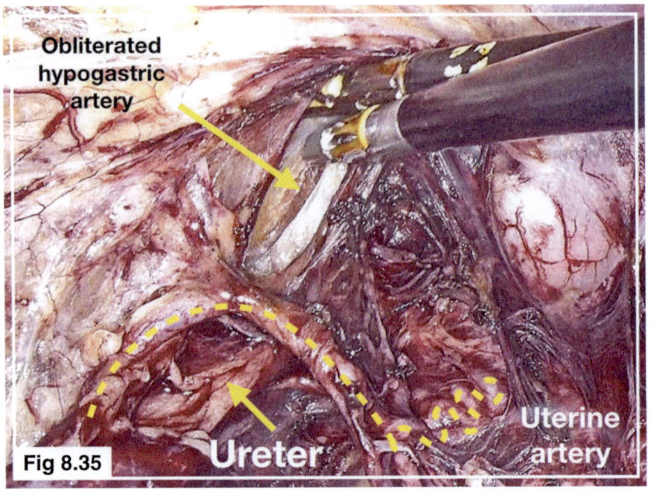

Fig. 8.35 Ureter and its relations: The ureter is seen as a thin band of tubular structure wrapped in fat under the course of the uterine artery. While the ureter travels forwards the uterine artery changes its course after it crosses over the ureter. The uterine artery is dissected anteriorly from its origin to reveal the obliterated hypogastric artery near the interior abdominal wall. The yellow dotted line shows the course of uteri artery and its tortuosity near the uterus

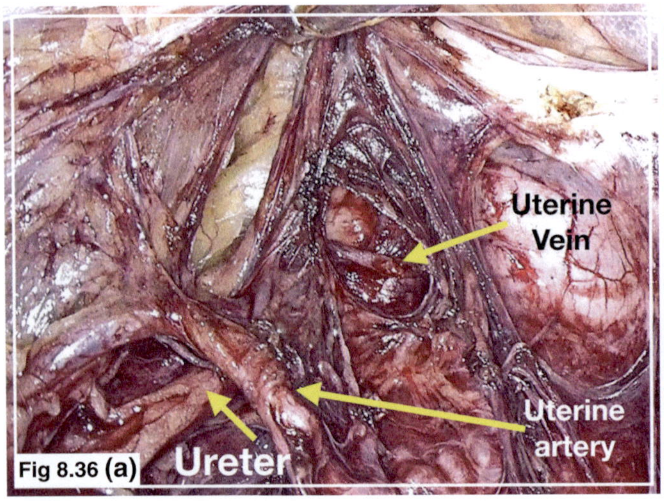

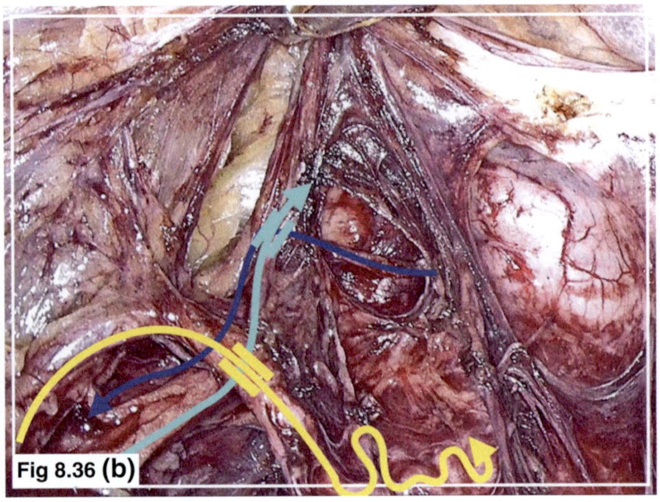

Fig. 8.36 (**a**, **b**) *Ureter lies between the fork*: The subsequent pairs of images will explain the relation of the uterine artery and vein with the ureter. This image is of the dissection of the ureter and uterine vein near the uterus near the Yabuki space. *Ureter lies in the fork between uterine artery and vein*. The (**b**) image highlights the course of the vessel and ureter with yellow being the uterine artery, light blue being the ureter and dark blue being the uterine vein. There are arrows also present which show the direction of flow so as to avoid confusion. The brackets drawn over the intersection denote the vessels which travel over the other. The colour of the bracket represents the vessel crossing over

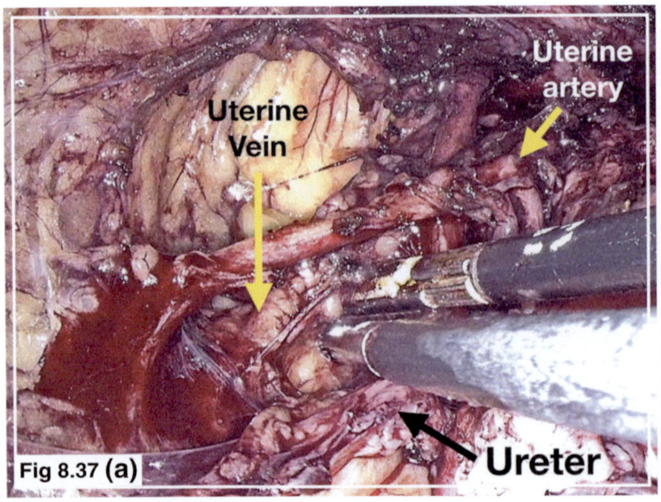

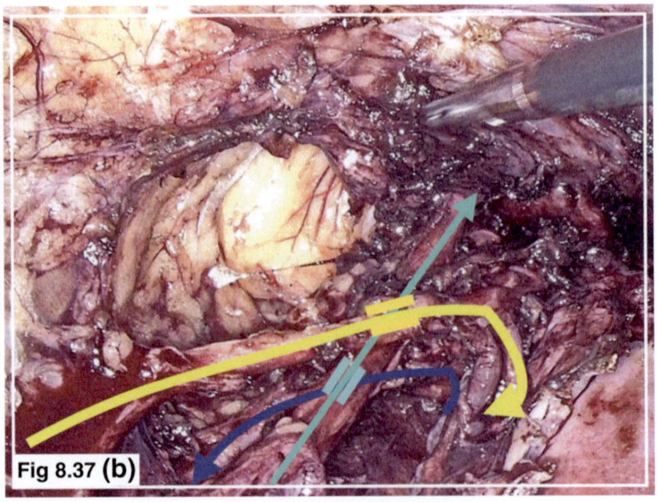

Fig. 8.37 (**a**, **b**) *Ureter lies between the fork*: While dissecting the uterine vein lateral to the ureter the relation can be seen more clearly. The uterine vein though lies almost congruent to the course of uterine artery but at a plane much below as the ureter intersects in between

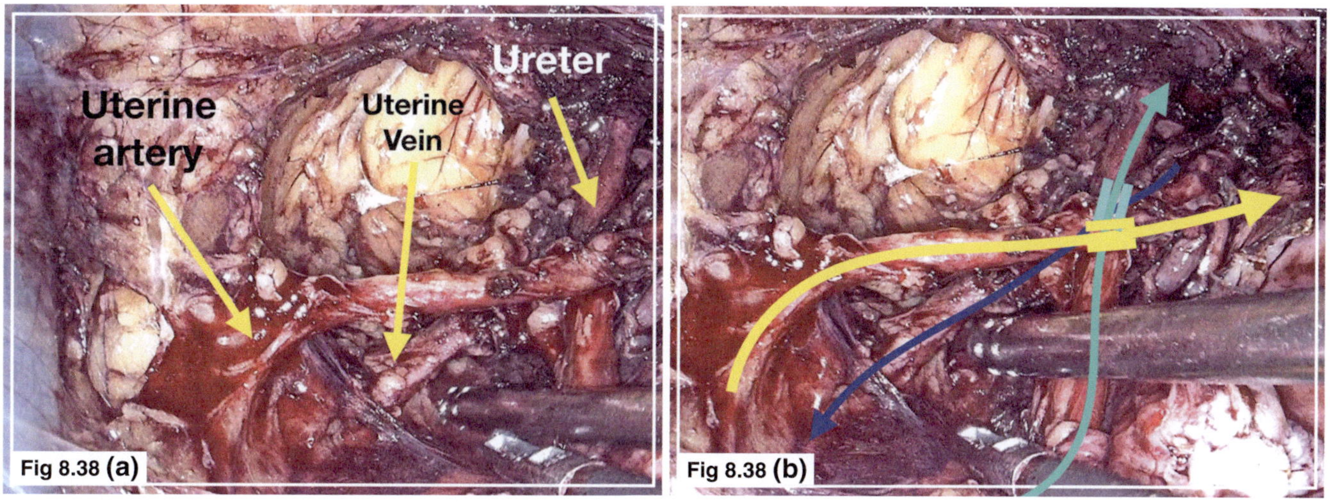

Fig. 8.38 (**a**, **b**) *Ureter lies between the fork*: All three structures and their relations to each other can be well explained with this pair of image

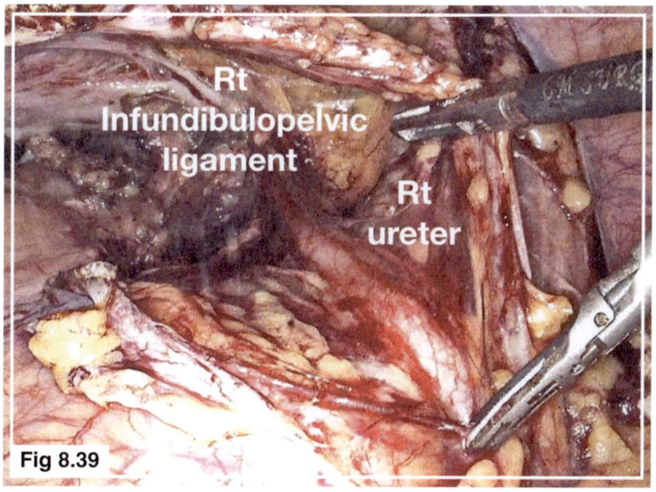

Fig. 8.39 Ureter and its relations: Similarly these concepts can be replicated on both sides. The ureter here is seen almost up to the uterus. The right infundibulopelvic ligament has been retracted laterally so as to expose the pararectal space medially and make the ureter visible more easily

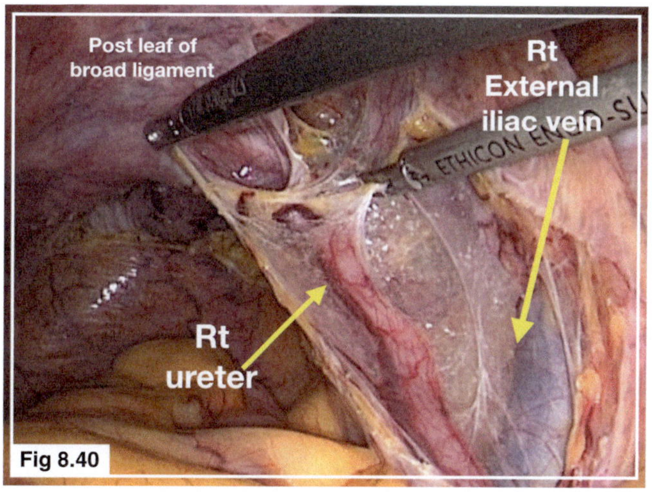

Fig. 8.40 Ureter and its relations: The initial course of the ureter can be traced up to the uterosacral ligament. There is a flimsy network of connective tissue on either side of the ureter. The dissection on the lateral side will reveal the internal iliac artery and the uterine artery while the medial side will reveal the hypogastric nerves

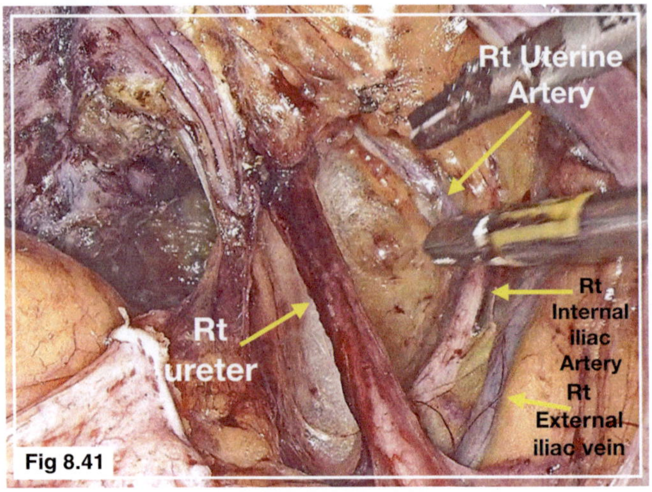

Fig. 8.41 Ureter and its relations: The uterine artery can be seen branching out from the internal iliac artery at an early stage. It can be confirmed by either tracing its origin backwards or seeing if it crosses over the ureter forwards. The uterine artery has been traced backwards to its origin in the internal iliac artery. It is the first artery to obstruct the dissection of the ureter laterally

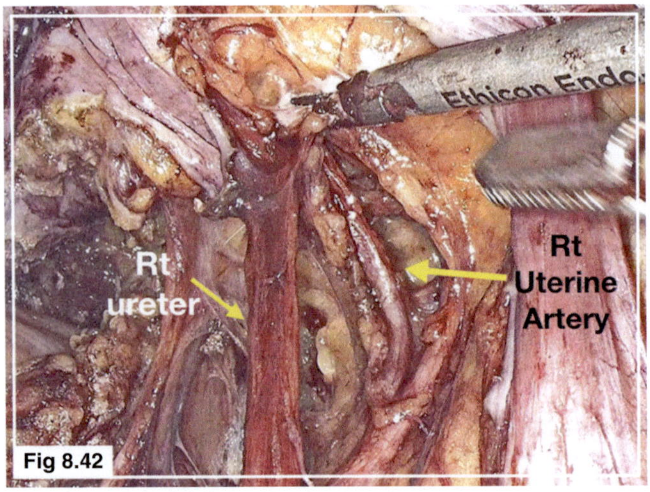

Fig. 8.42 Ureter and its relations: The paravesical space is dissected anteriorly to the uterine artery. This helps delineate the uterine artery itself and also helps dissect the uterine vein which lies underneath and parallel to the uterine artery

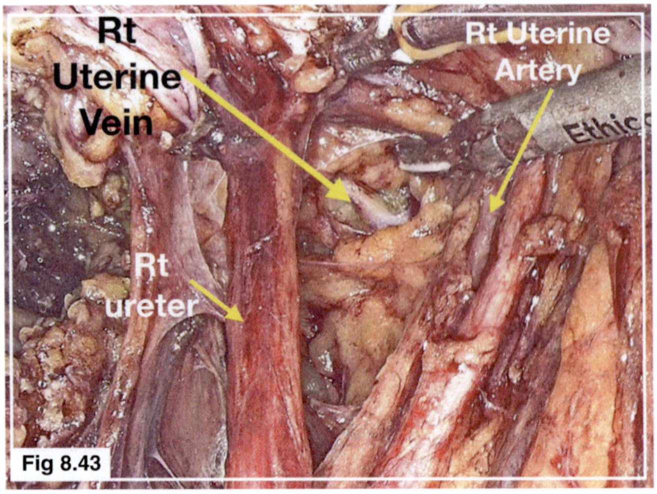

Fig. 8.43 Ureter and its relations: The segment of the uterine vein lateral to the ureter has been dissected and identified. The uterine artery along with the continuation of the internal iliac artery has been retracted laterally to expose the underlying uterine vein

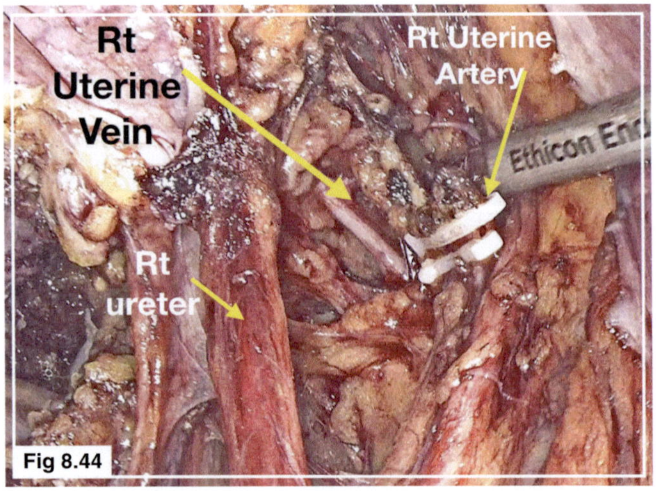

Fig. 8.44 Ureter and its relations: The uterine artery has been clipped and cut to expose the area underneath it. This helps in easy and direct visualisation of the uterine vein. The uterine vein is to be traced medially below the ureter

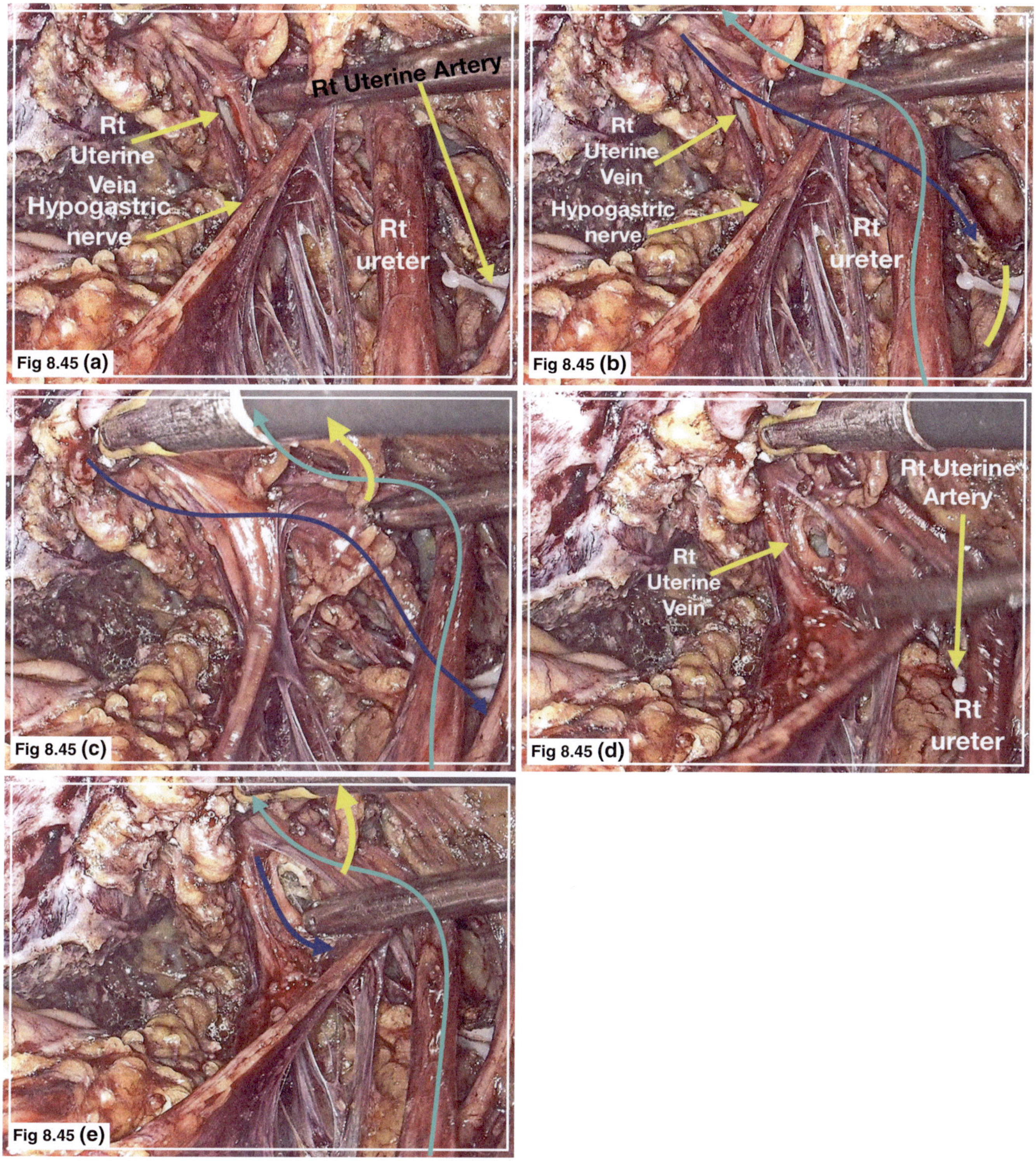

Fig. 8.45 (**a**–**e**) Ureter and its relations: (**a**, **b**) The uterine vein is dissected medially. It remains in a plane below the ureter. The uterine vein carries along with it the parasympathetic fibres or the pelvic splanchnic nerves which communicate with the hypogastric nerve and supply the uterus and bladder for their autonomic function. (**c**) The lateral segment of uterine vein is dissected in this image. (**d**, **e**) The medial segment of the uterine vein has been dissected. Thus clipping of the uterine vein is of great significance when nerve-sparing procedure is to be conducted. As seen the branch of hypogastric nerve supplying the uterus lies close to the uterine vein while the branch supplying the bladder travels straight and undeviated. The yellow, light blue and dark blue lines represent the uterine artery (clipped), ureter and uterine vein

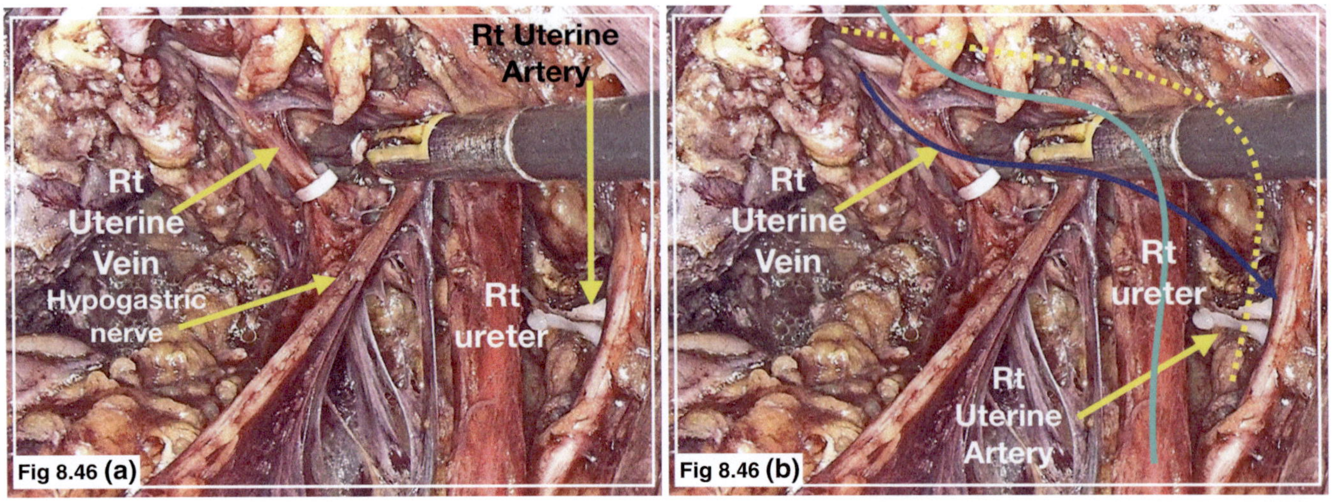

Fig. 8.46 (**a**, **b**) *Ureter lies between the fork*: The uterine vein clipped medially due to nerve-sprain procedure, the uterine artery clipped at the origin and the ureter travelling in between the two vessels

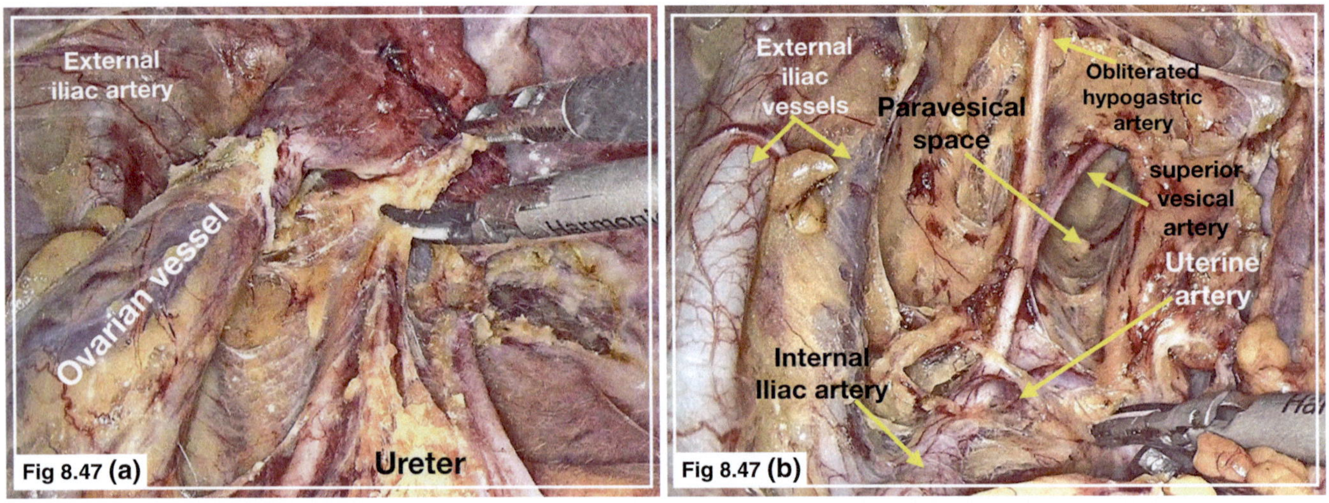

Fig. 8.47 Ureter and its relations: The following images have been taken from the donor uterus for uterine transplant. The harvested vessels here are the left uterine artery and the left uterine vein. (**a**) The initial dissection of the infundibulopelvic ligament exposing the ovarian vessels. The ovarian vessels lie lateral to the ureter but at a *higher plane*. The external iliac vessels lie lateral to the ureter but in the *same plane*. The ureter here is dissected off the peritoneum till the apex of the uterosacral ligaments. (**b**) The pararectal space has been dissected. The paravesical space is seen as a hollow space bounded by the superior vesicle artery above and the uterine artery inferiorly. The termination of the internal iliac artery is seen as the obliterated hypogastric artery. (**c**) It is seen that many fine capillary branches are present on the uterine artery which supply the mesentery of the ureter. These minor vessels need to be clipped, sealed and cut so as to prevent haemorrhage during re-anastomosis to the donor vessels. Thus many such minor branches are present all around the uterine artery supplying the ureter at multiple levels. (**d**) The diagrammatic representation of the course of the uterine artery and the ureter to understand the orientation of the structures and their relations to each other. Yellow represents the uterine artery while light blue represents ureter. (**e**) The ureter travels under the uterine artery to be inserted into the bladder. Clip applicator here has been used to clip one feeding vessel from the uterine artery to the ureter as discussed above previously. (**f**) Course of the uterine artery and ureter in the pararectal space after complete dissection of uterine artery and sealing all the feeding vessels to the ureter. It can be seen that ureter remains below the uterine artery near the uterus. (**g**) Since the uterine artery *cannot* be dissected and cut off in a case of uterine transplant, it is retracted along with the ureter towards the midline. This exposes the paravesical space and thus eases dissection of the uterine vein as seen in the image. (**h**) Diagrammatic representation of the uterine artery, veins and ureter can be seen depicting the course of the tubular structures in the pararectal space. (**i**) After complete dissection of the uterine artery and vein along with the ureter in the pararectal space, the concept of *ureter lies in the fork between uterine artery and vein* can be demonstrated. (**j**) Arrow diagram of the vessels and their course as seen in the pararectal space after dissection of vessels and the ureter. The uterus has been retracted on the opposite side. (**k**) *Ureter lies between the fork of uterine artery and the uterine vein* has been clearly demonstrated in this image. The final image of dissection of all the vessels and its minor branches and the ureter. (**l**) Arrow diagram showing the course of the uterine artery ureter and the uterine vein. The concept of ureter lies between the fork of uterine artery and vein has been explained in the image

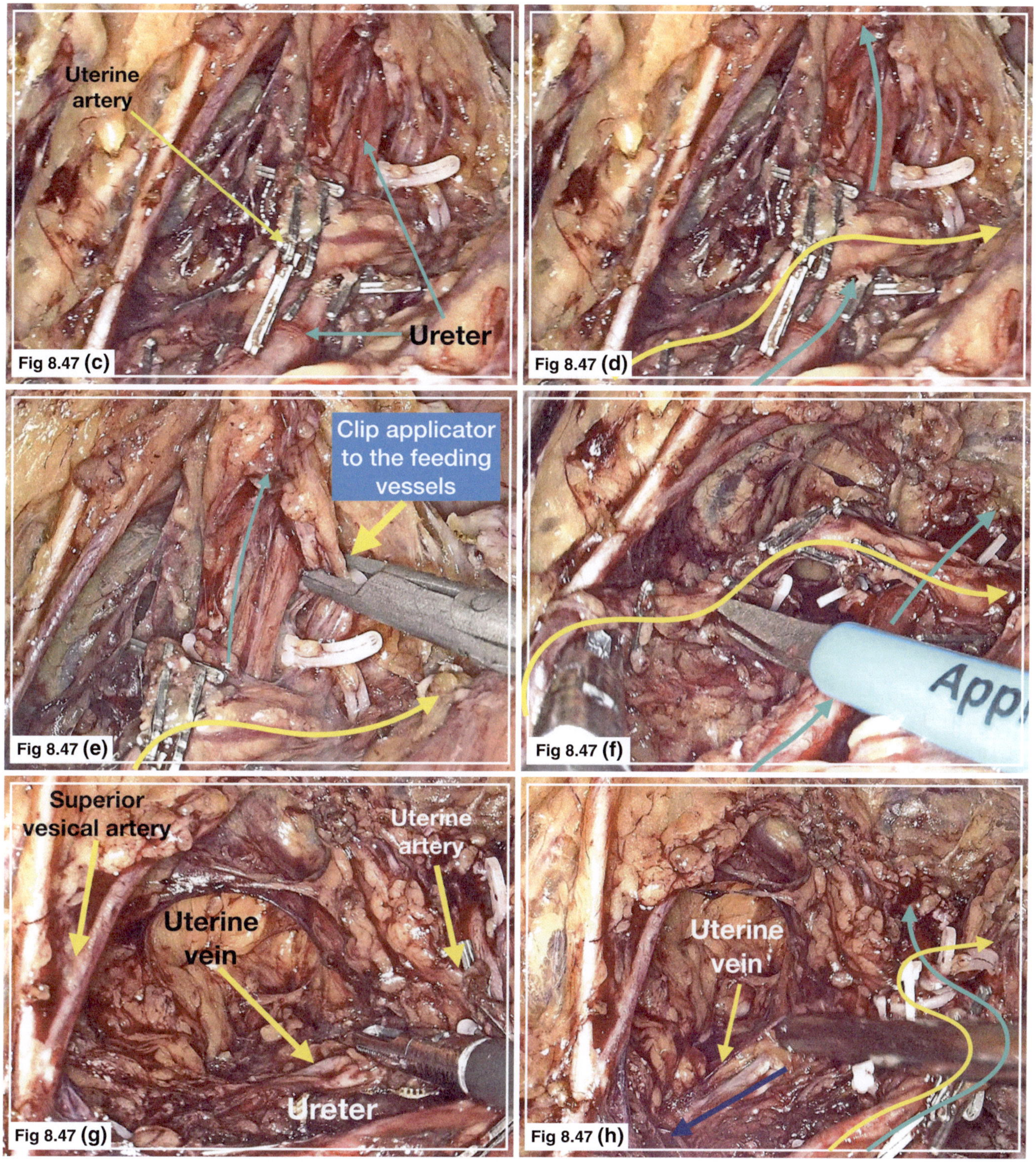

Fig. 8.47 (continued)

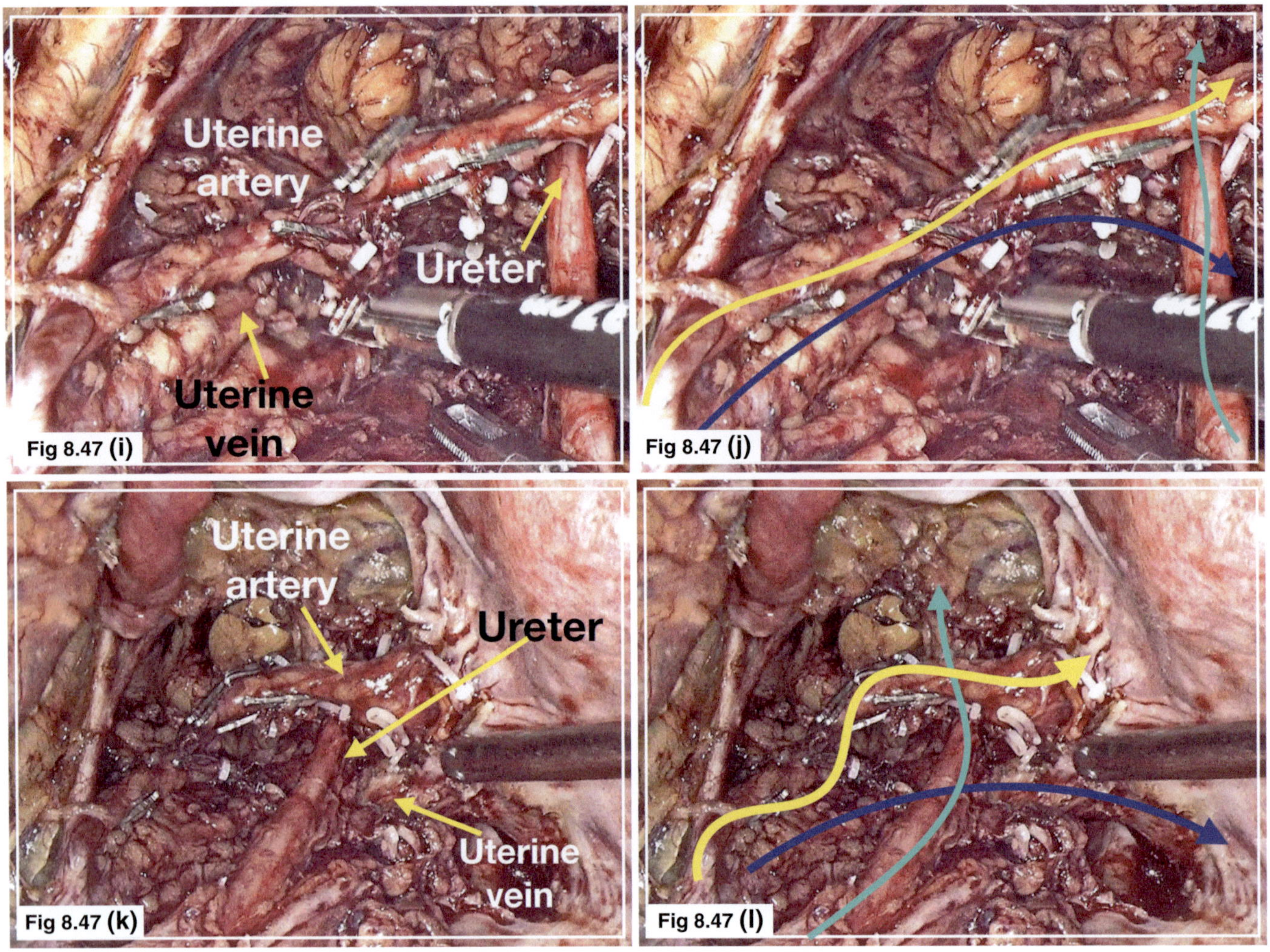

Fig. 8.47 (continued)

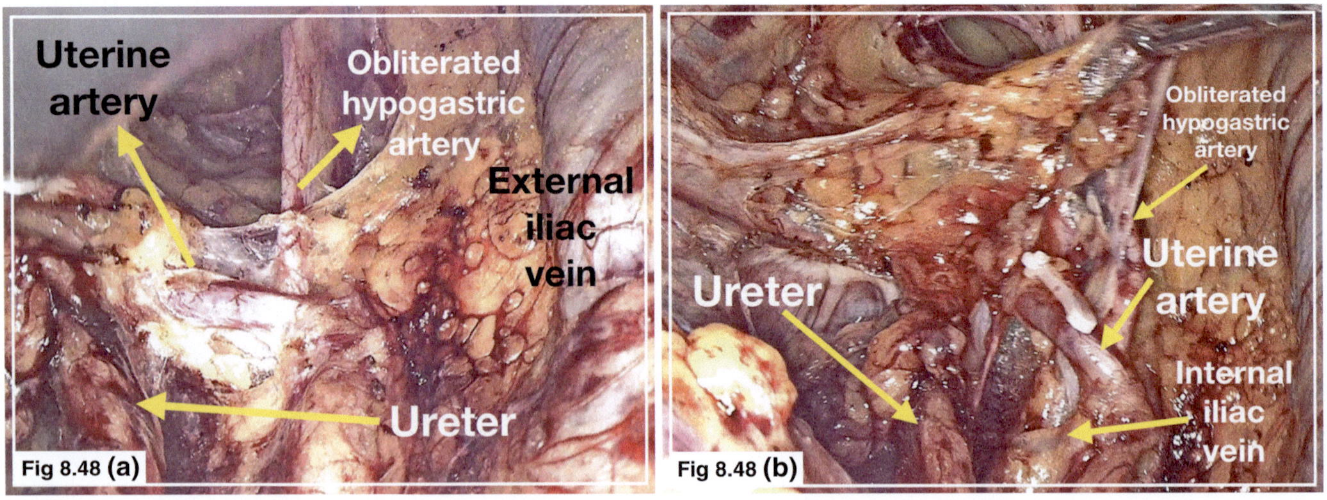

Fig. 8.48 Ureter and its relations: The right uterine artery and the right uterine vein have been harvested here for uterine transplant. The uterus is anteverted in this image. (**a**) Similar dissection of the pararectal space is done till the uterine artery is visible and separated from the ureter. The terminator of the internal iliac artery is also traced upwards. (**b**) Similar feeding vessels to the ureter have been clipped and cut. The course of the uterine artery is gently dissected. The internal iliac vein is usually deep seated. However it can be seen here under the internal iliac artery at the origin of the uterine artery as it also follows an identical course of the internal iliac artery but much deeper in most cases. (**c**) The uterine vein can be seen at its confluence with the internal iliac vein. The uterine vein is easiest to dissect at the segment lateral to ureter and parallel and below the uterine artery. (**d**) The concept of *ureter lies in the fork of uterine artery and vein* can be seen clearly in the right pararectal space in the image. (**e**) Diagrammatic representation of the course of the uterine artery and vein along with ureter and their correlation to each other can be seen

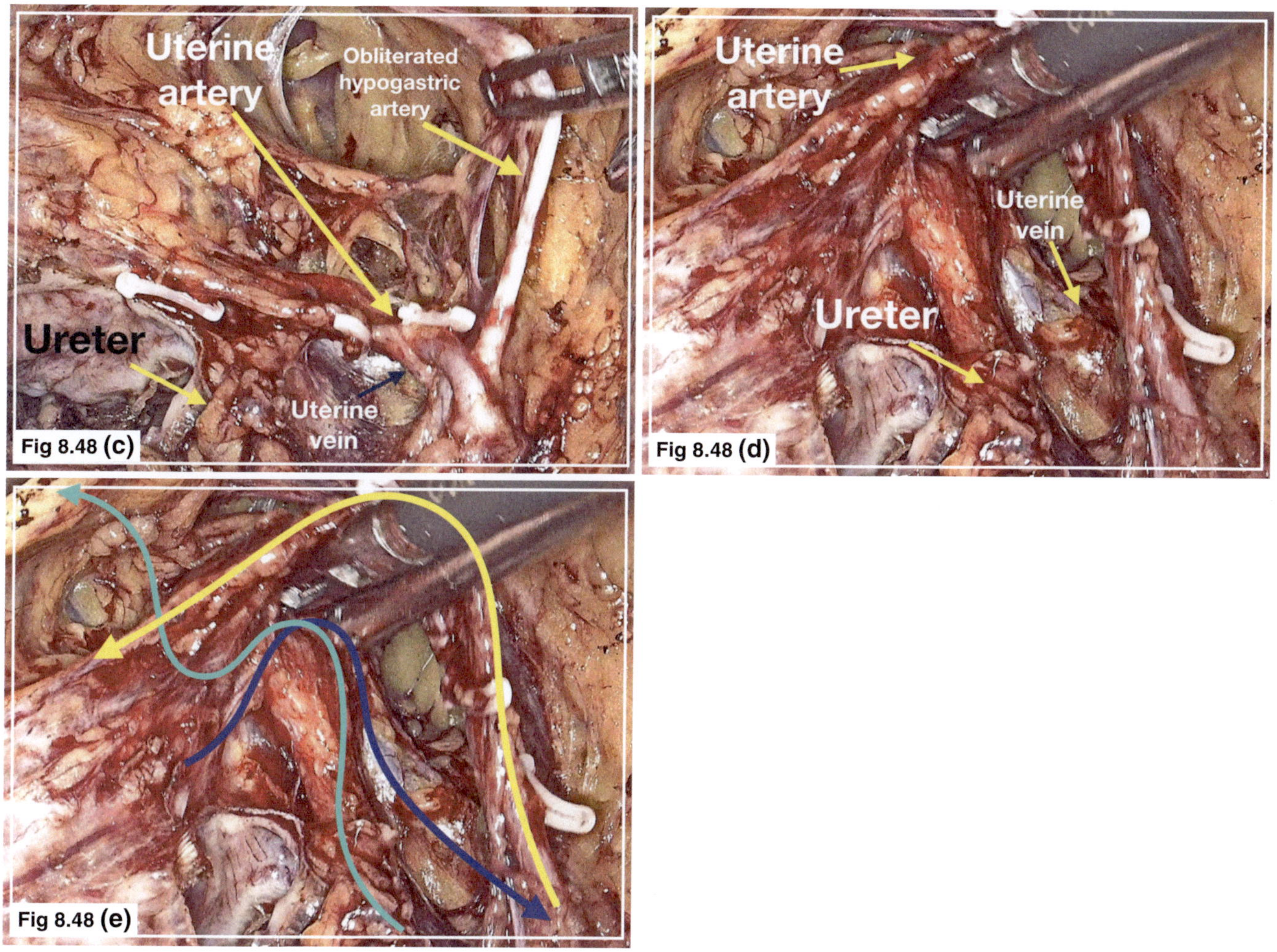

Fig. 8.48 (continued)

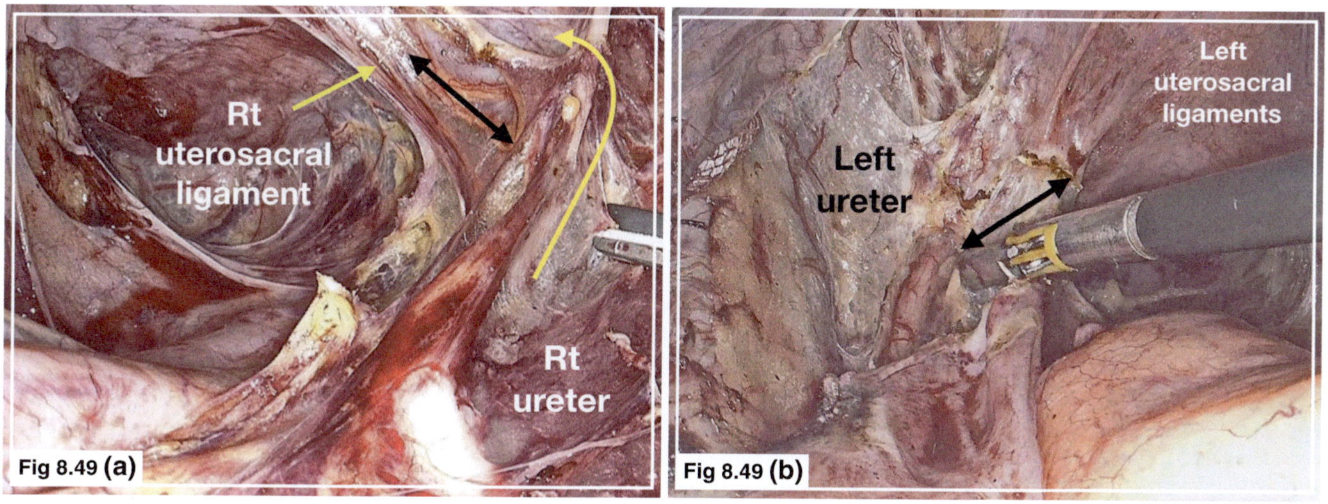

Fig. 8.49 (**a**–**e**) Ureter and the uterosacrals: The following series of images represent the distance of the ureter from the uterosacral ligaments. According to various text references the ureter is considered juxtaposed to the uterosacral ligaments. These series of images have been taken on various different hysterectomies. Each image belongs to a different patient. All images have been taken advanced to the part of ureter after crossing over the uterine artery only. Each image shows a minimum of 4–5 cm distance between the ureter and the uterosacral ligaments. The series of images have been provided to reduce the phobia of the ureter amongst the viewers

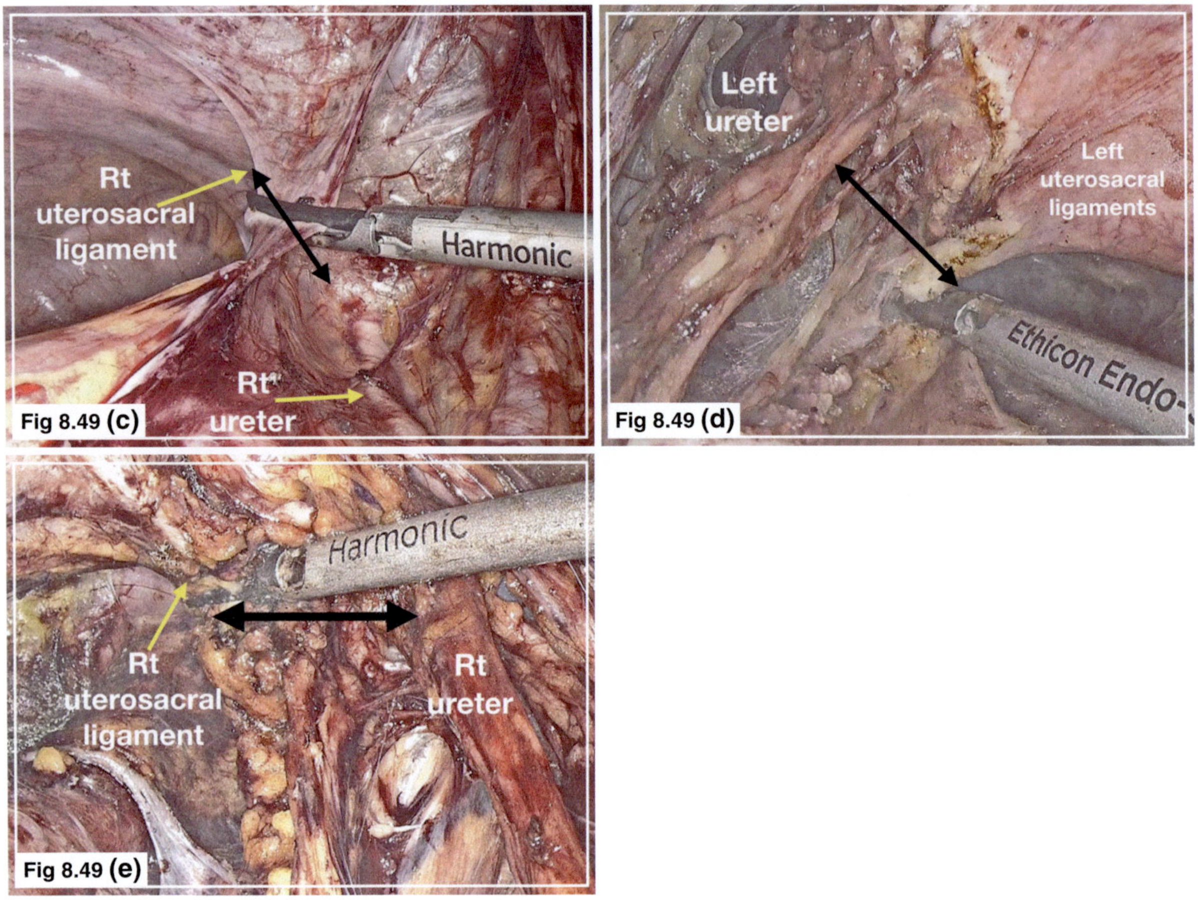

Fig. 8.49 (continued)

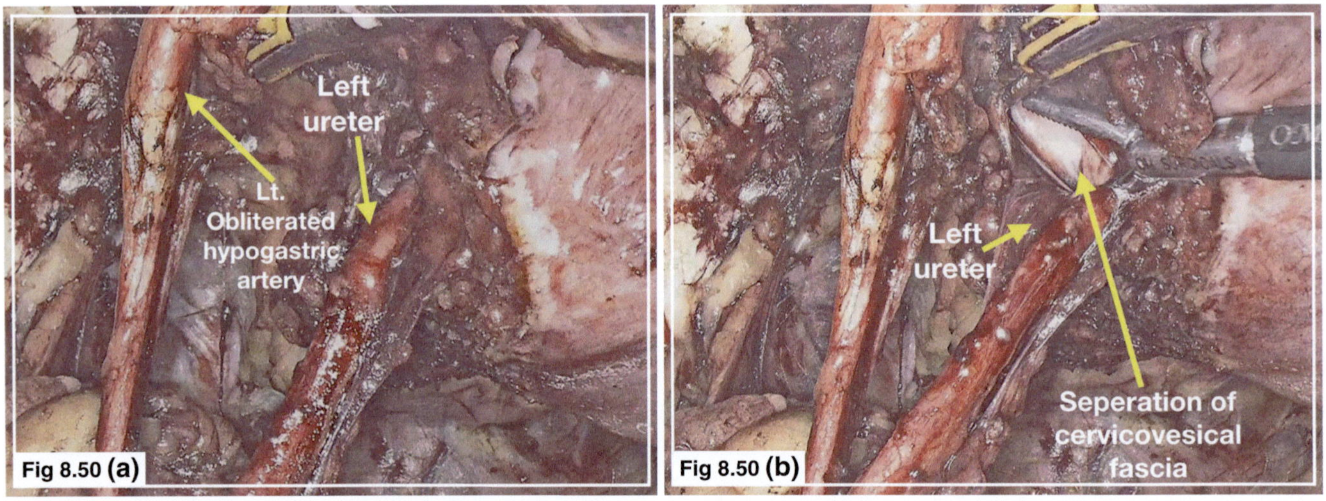

Fig. 8.50 (**a**–**h**) Ureteric tunnel: Ureteric tunnel dissection is often considered the most difficult part of tunnel dissection. These series of step-by-step images can help guide tunnel dissection as well as explain the relevant anatomy. (**a**) The ureter dissection at the end of the pararectal space dissection leads to the tunnel where the ureter lies in close proximity to the uterus and also the most common area of thermal injury. (**b**) With the help of laparoscopic Maryland forceps the anterior cervicovesical ligament is dissected and made visible in the least traumatic manner with minimal use of energy sources. (**c**) The separated anterior cervicovesical ligament is dissected with cold scissors. Energy sources are avoided as much as possible. (**d**) The anterior cervicovesical ligament contains small veins which often bleed during routine open surgery. Hence here the clips are applied prior to resecting the anterior cervicovesical ligament. (**e**) Anteriorly the ureter is now freed from its anterior surface as seen in the image. (**f**, **g**) The posterior cervicovesical ligament is dissected off from the anterior surface of the uterus so as to free the ureter from all its attachments. (**h**) The posterior cervicovesical ligament is clipped and then dissected just like the anterior cervicovesical ligament keeping the vessels in consideration

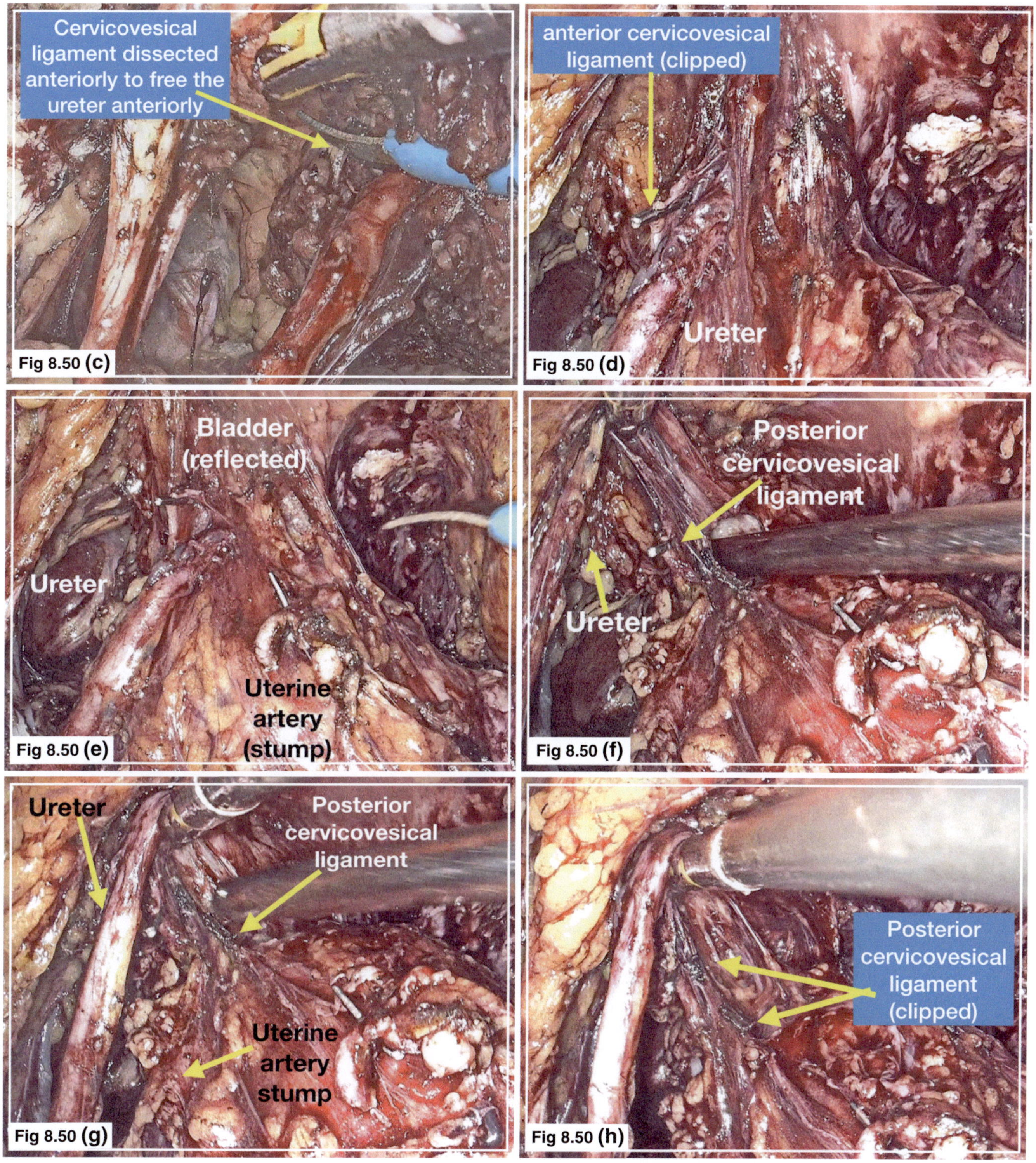

Fig. 8.50 (continued)

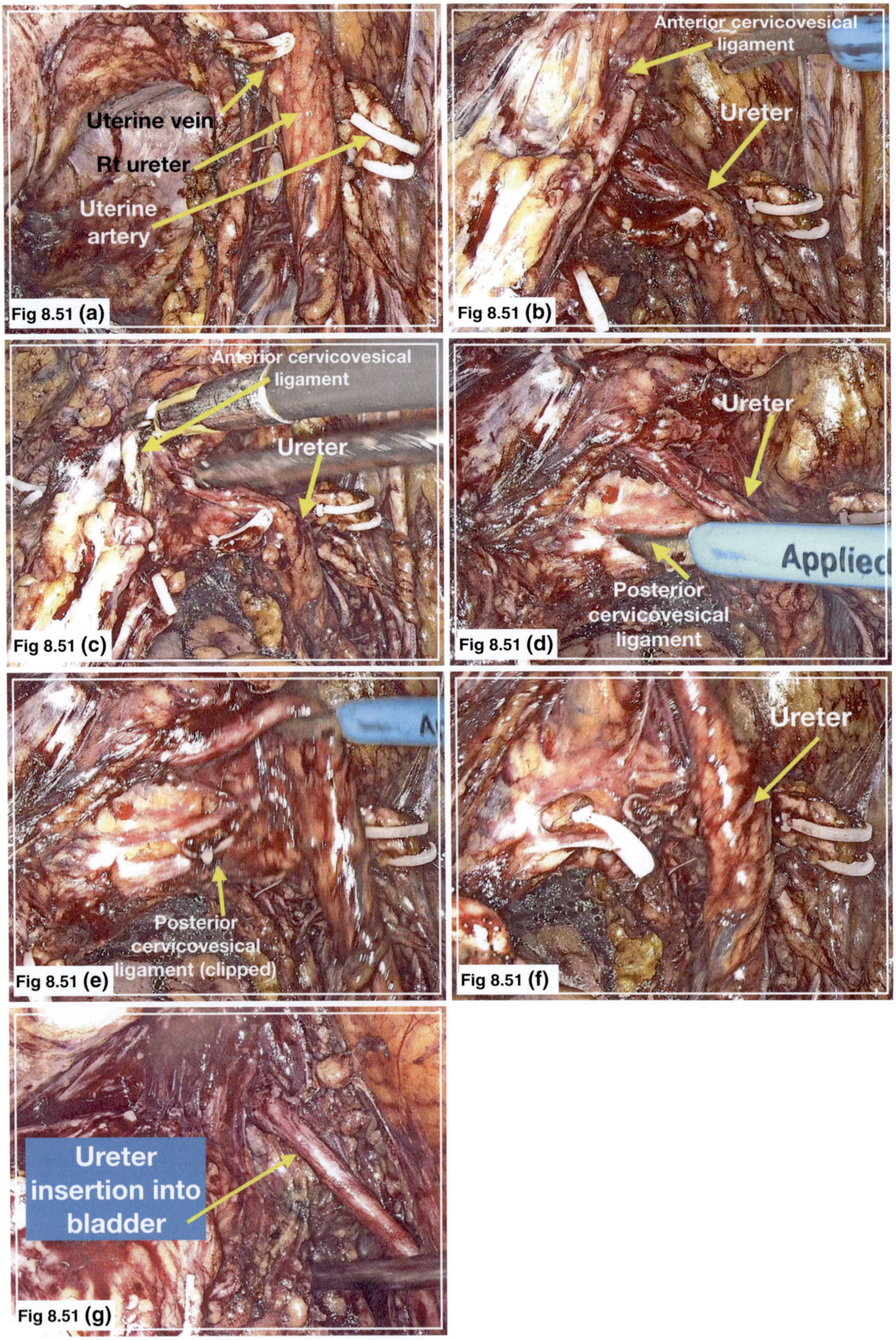

Fig. 8.51 (**a**–**g**) Ureteric tunnel: Ureteric tunnel dissection has been done on the right ureter. (**a**) The orientation of the tunnel; the ureter is seen between the uterine vein and artery which have already been clipped and cut. The clip medial and below the ureter is the uterine vein and further lateral is the uterine artery. (**b**, **c**) Dissection of the anterior cervicovesical ligament. (**d**, **e**) Dissection of the posterior cervicovesical ligament. (**f**, **g**) Final end point of the tunnel dissection. Right ureter is seen free from attachments from all sides

Fig. 8.52 End point: The end point of hysterectomy with specimen retrieval and appearance of the vault has been demonstrated in this image. The vagina contains a small tampon-like structure made out of gauze pieces stuffed in a surgical glove to create a snuggly fitting tampon to maintain an air-sealed compartment

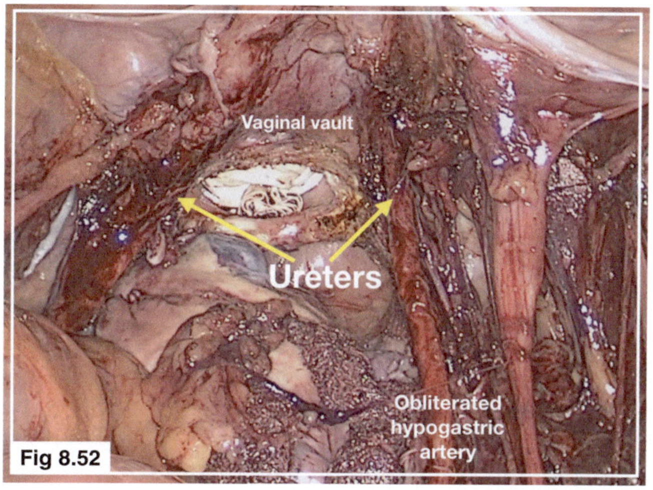

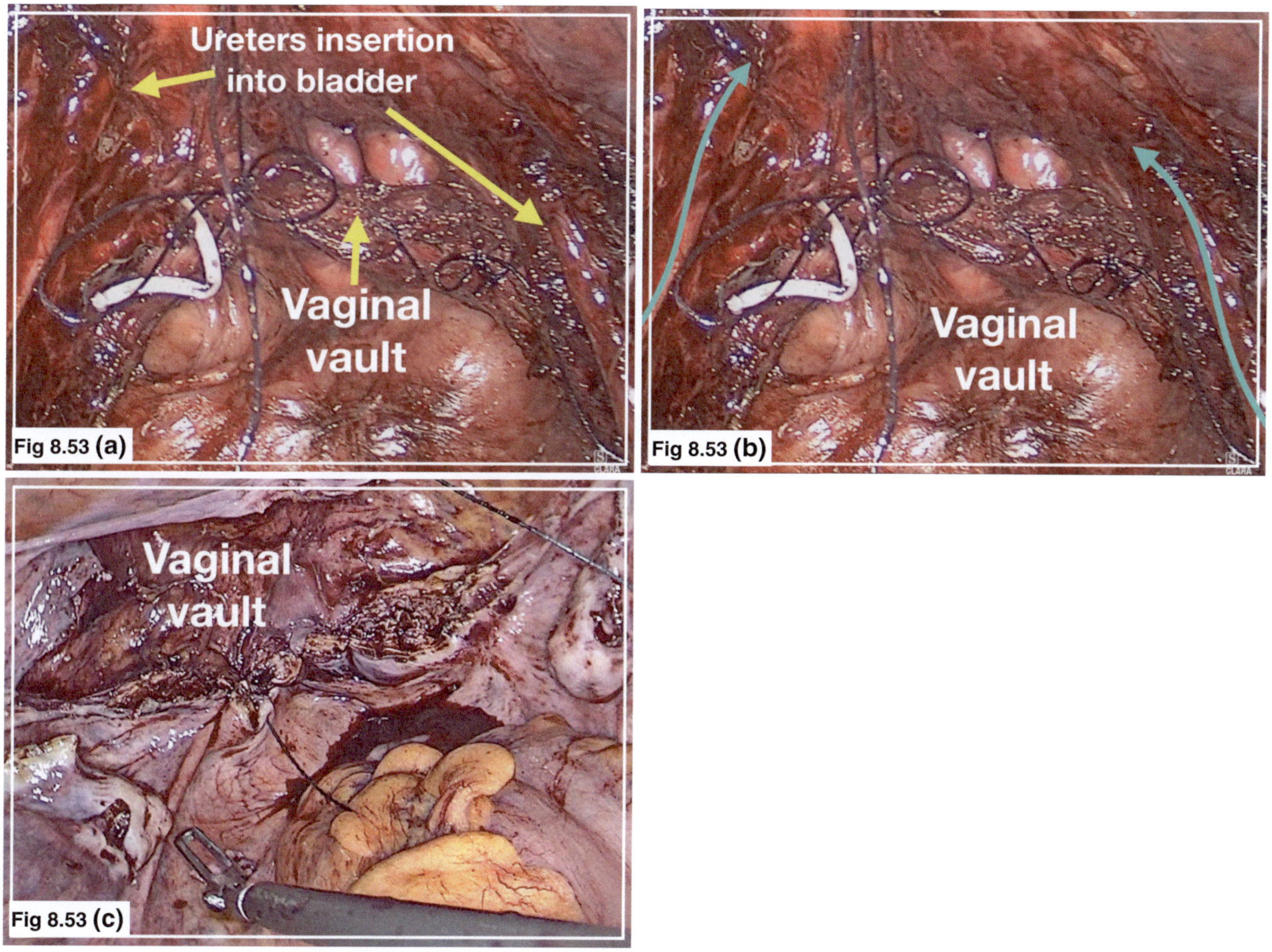

Fig. 8.53 (**a**–**c**) End point: The final image of the vault can be seen. (**a**, **b**) Radical hysterectomy with ureteric tunnel dissection leading to exposure of the ureter till its insertion into the bladder can be clearly seen and appreciated. (**c**) Image of the vault in case of the intrafascial hysterectomy for a benign condition (fibroid/AUB) with the ureter completely concealed under the peritoneum demonstrates that the amount of dissection is done in a case of tunnel dissection

8.1 Blood Supply

The blood supply of the ureter is divided into upper third, middle third and lower third.

(a) The upper segment is supplied by branches of the renal, gonadal or adrenal arteries.
(b) The middle portion receives from the internal iliac artery, small peritoneal twigs and branches from the arteries of the posterior abdominal wall.
(c) The lower segment is the pelvic ureter, which is supplied by branches of common iliac artery or internal iliac artery and its branches (Figs. 8.54, 8.55, 8.56, 8.57, 8.58, 8.59, and 8.60).

All these vessels run up and down the ureter to form an anastomotic plexus in the adventitial coat of the ureter. This anastomosis is deficient in some individuals; hence excessive mobilisation of the ureter can lead to necrosis.

Remember

The blood supply of the ureter is parallel to its course. This can be seen as a separate mesentery. This ureteric mobilisation when done should be done along with its mesentery. This avoids the ureteric denudation and avascular fistula at a later date. The presence of mesentery also allows the complete ureteric mobilisation from the sacral promontory up to the uterovesical junction, thus allowing type III radical hysterectomy to be performed (Figs. 8.61, 8.62, 8.63, 8.64, and 8.65).

The ureter is vulnerable for injury at the entry into the bladder which is the narrowest part of the ureter, and at the point where the uterine artery crosses the ureter (Figs. 8.66 and 8.67).

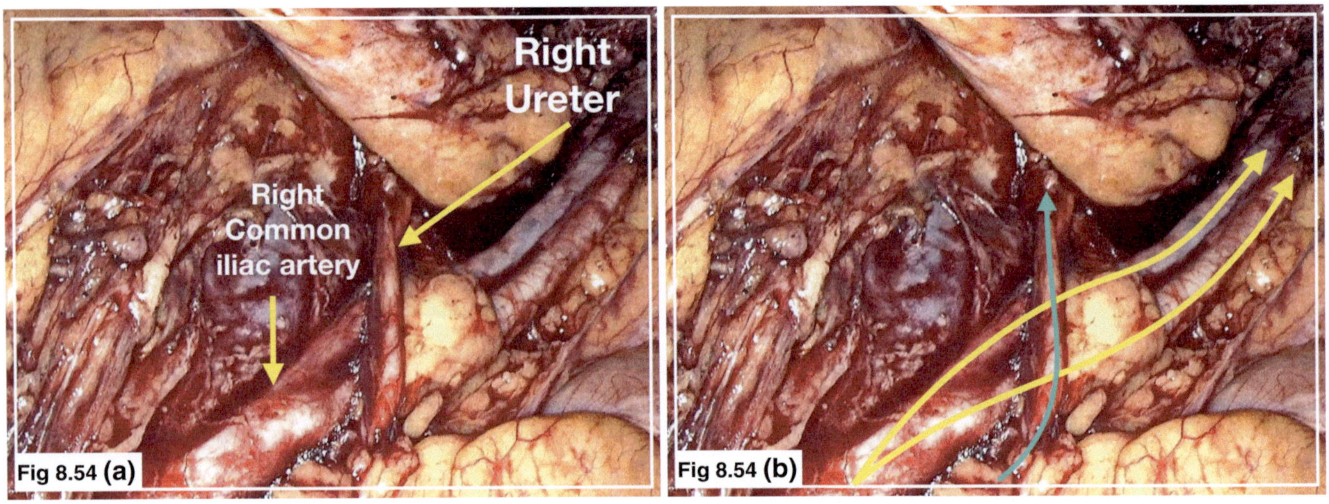

Fig. 8.54 (**a**, **b**) Abdominal ureter: The external iliac artery is traced and dissected upwards towards its origin at the bifurcation of the common iliac artery and further up to the abdominal aorta for para-aortic lymph node dissection. The right ureter is seen crossing over the bifurcation of common iliac artery

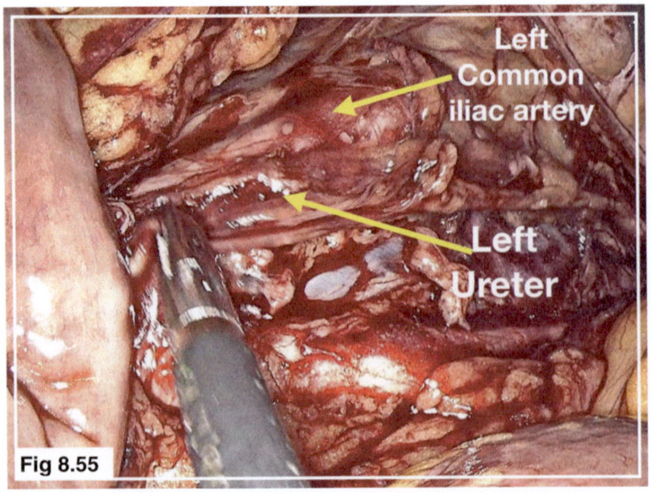

Fig. 8.55 Contralateral ureter: The left common iliac artery can be seen and the ureter is seen in its course travelling medial to the vessels after crossing over

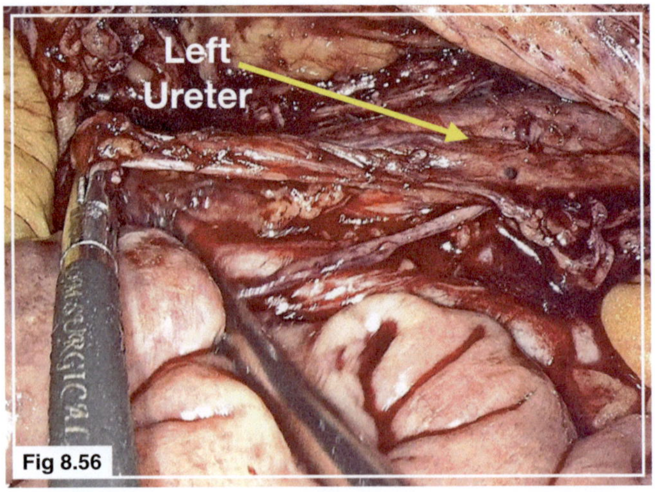

Fig. 8.56 Contralateral ureter: The left ureter is seen from the right side during para-aortic lymph node dissection. The left ureter is raised and the fat is extracted for complete clearance of lymph nodes

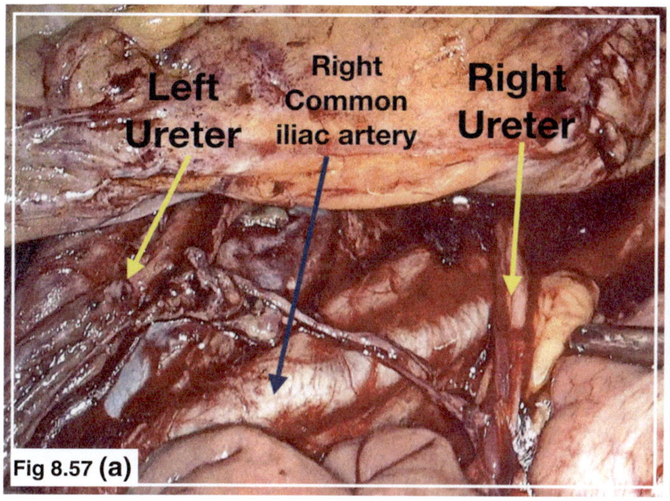

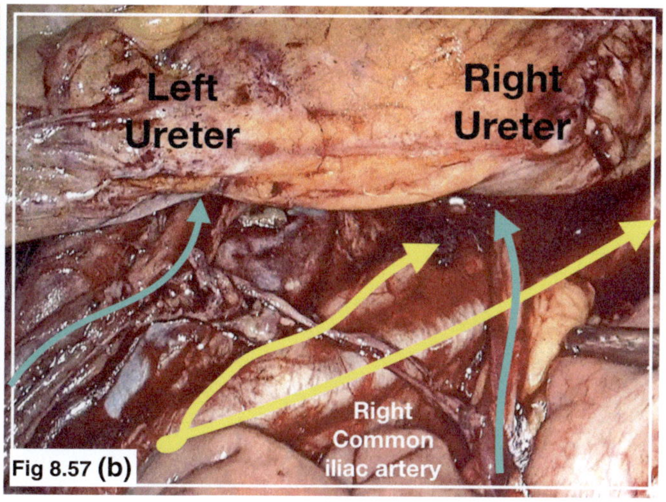

Fig. 8.57 (**a**, **b**) Bilateral ureters: During transperitoneal para-aortic lymph node dissection the common iliac arteries are traced and dissected and thus bilateral ureters are visualized in this same field of vision adjacently

Fig. 8.58 Contralateral ureter: The image demonstrates the visibility of the left ureter during mobilisation of the colon during a case of posterior exenteration

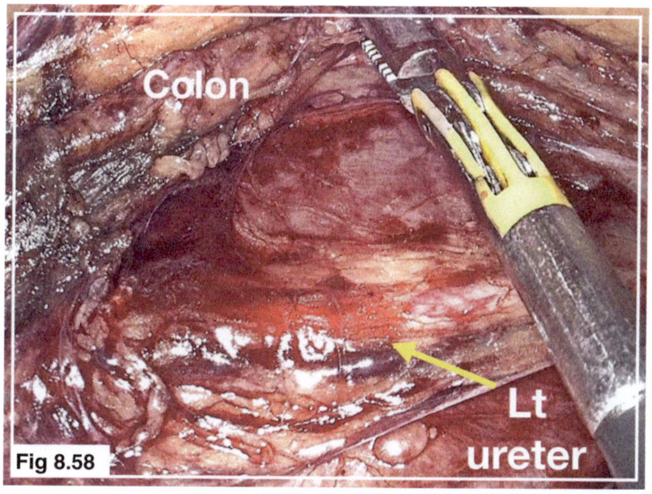

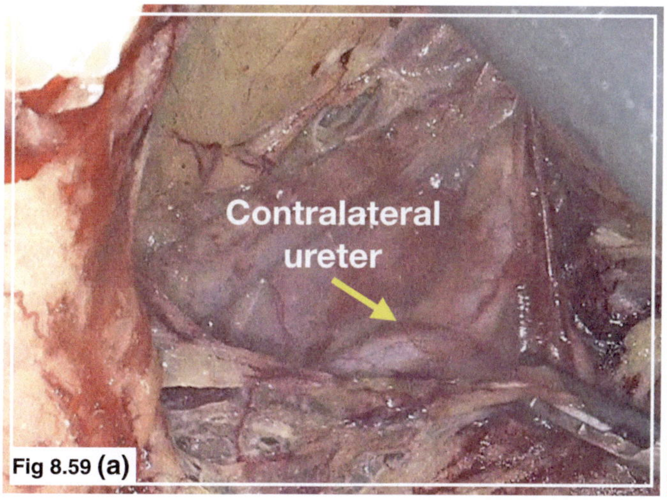

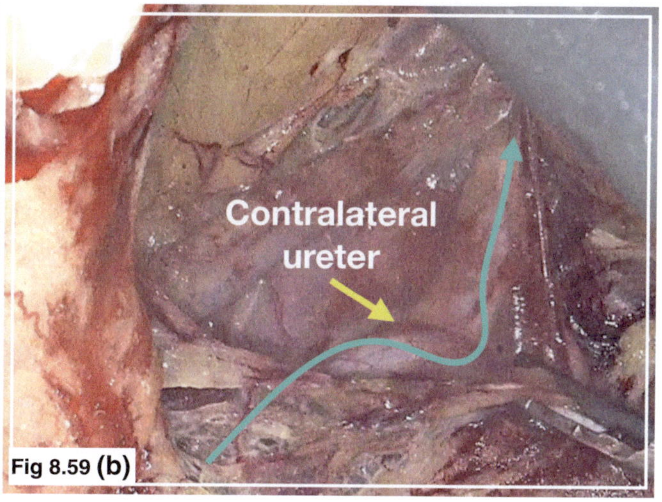

Fig. 8.59 (**a**, **b**) Contralateral ureter: The left ureter can be viewed clearly form the right side in condition of para-aortic dissection during mobilisation of the bowel during posterior exenteration. This image has been taken from a case of post-exenteration during mobilisation of the sigmoid colon

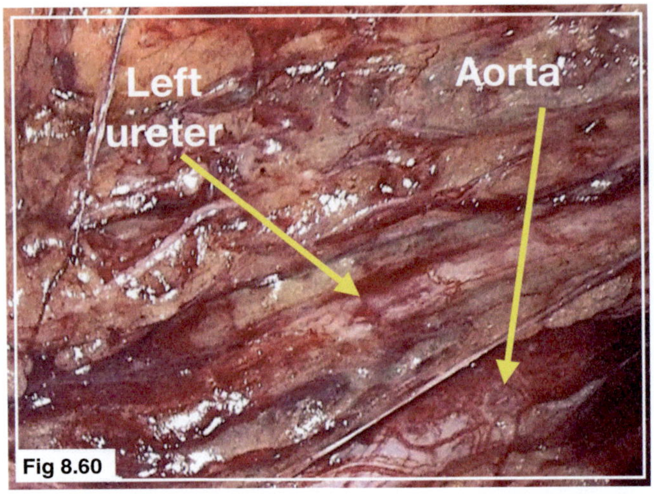

Fig. 8.60 Contralateral ureter: The left ureter is seen alongside the abdominal aorta during para-aortic lymph node dissection from the right side which is why the ureter appears at a higher plane than aorta; otherwise on the ipsilateral side the ureter is lateral/paramedian and below the level of aorta

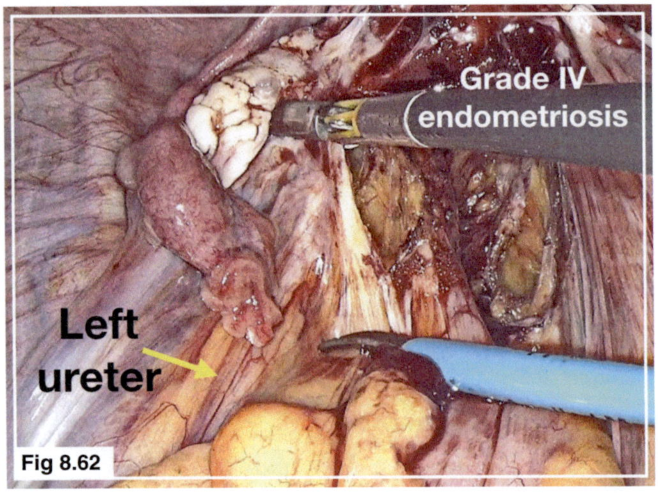

Fig. 8.62 Endometriosis: In conditions of severe grade IV endometriosis where the pouch of Douglas is obliterated. The ureter can be used as a guide to navigate deeper into the pelvis owing to its long course. On identification of the ureter the retroperitoneal dissection can be initiated and thus other vital structures can be traced

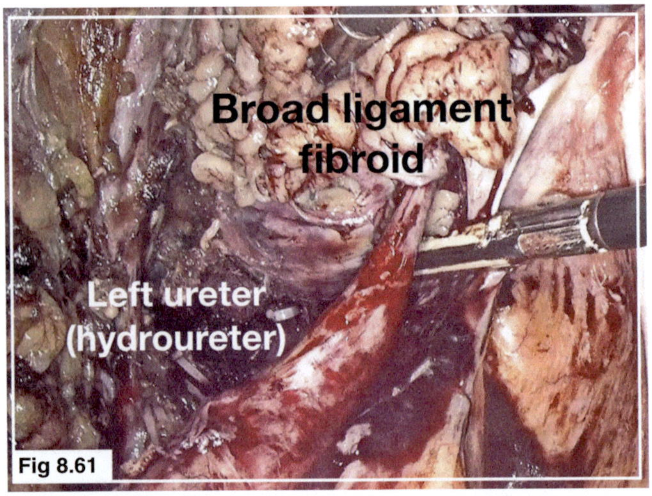

Fig. 8.61 Broad ligament fibroid: In a rare case of broad ligament fibroid it was seen that the ureter can be completely encased/engulfed by the tumour in all sides. This leads to significant hydrometer

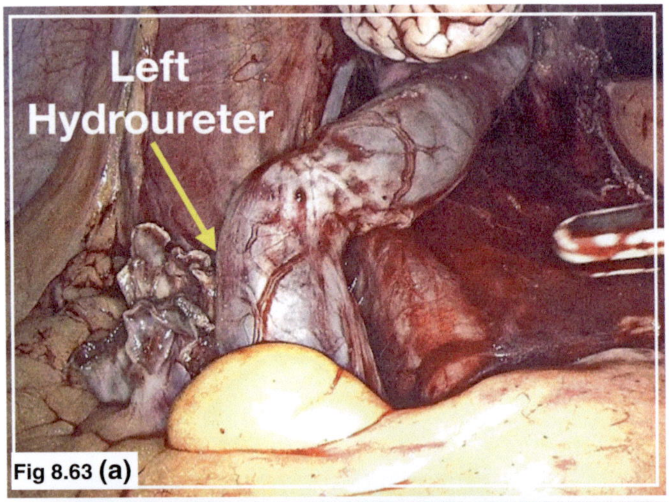

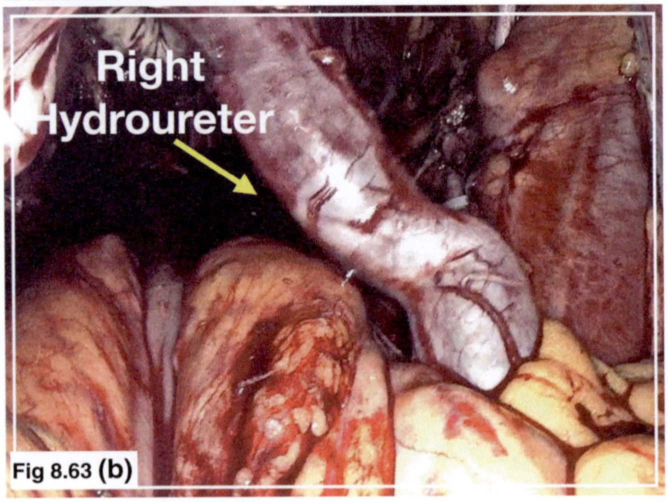

Fig. 8.63 (**a**, **b**) Hydronephrosis: These images have been taken in a case of bilateral hydronephrosis caused by an obstruction by a locally aggressive cervical cancer invading the bladder on the trigonal region

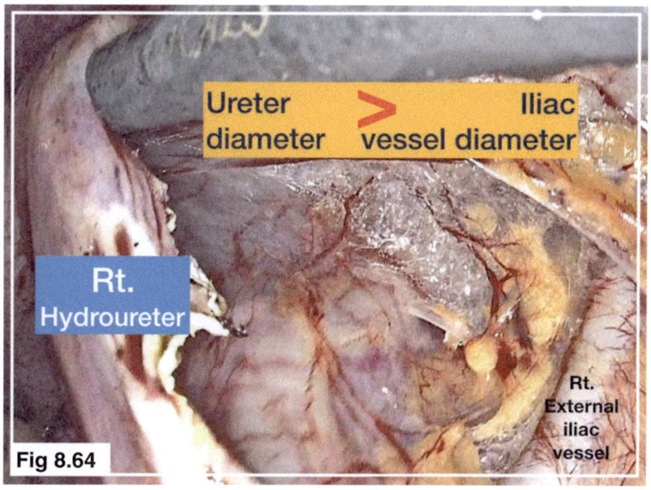

Fig. 8.64 Hydronephrosis: In comparison to the above two images this image has been taken for comparison with surrounding tubular structures. The image clearly shows abnormally larger diameter of the ureter as compared to the external iliac artery. It is for the viewer not to confuse with the size of the tubular structure with external iliac vessels. It is best to trace such structures when in doubt. The ureter seems to be attached to the paracolpos by small fibrous bands, which have to be cut to reach the uterovesical junction

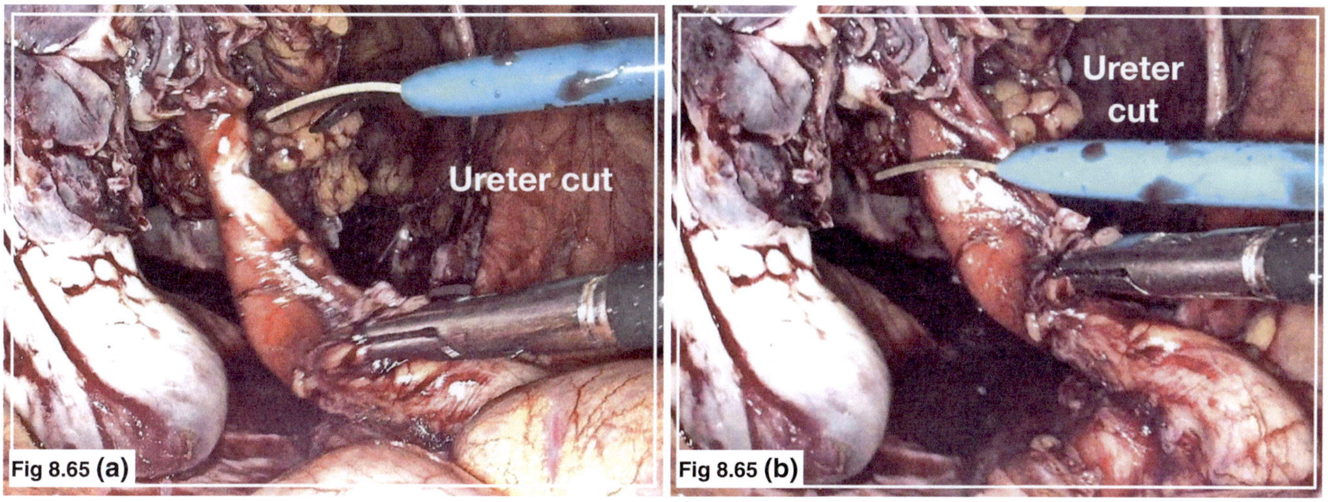

Fig. 8.65 (**a**, **b**) Anterior exenteration: In a case of locally advanced cervical cancer the patient underwent anterior exenteration where the ureters were deposited. These images demonstrate cutting of the ureter near the bladder with in situ DJ stents

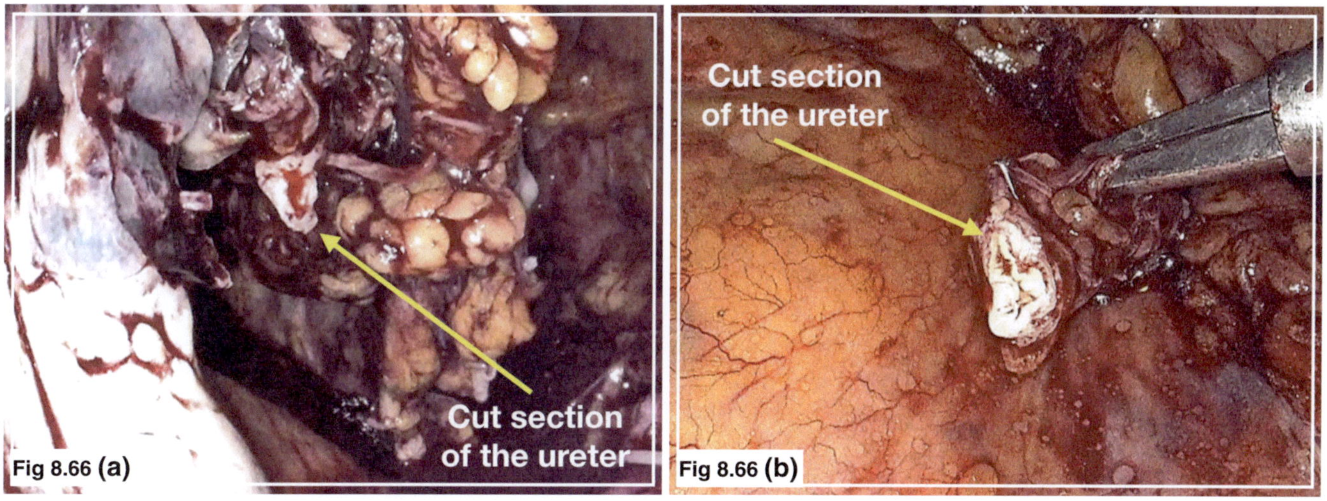

Fig. 8.66 (**a**, **b**) Ureter cut section: Here two images demonstrate the star-shaped lumen of the cut-out ureter. These images have been taken from two different patients who underwent anterior exenteration for locally advanced disease mentioned above

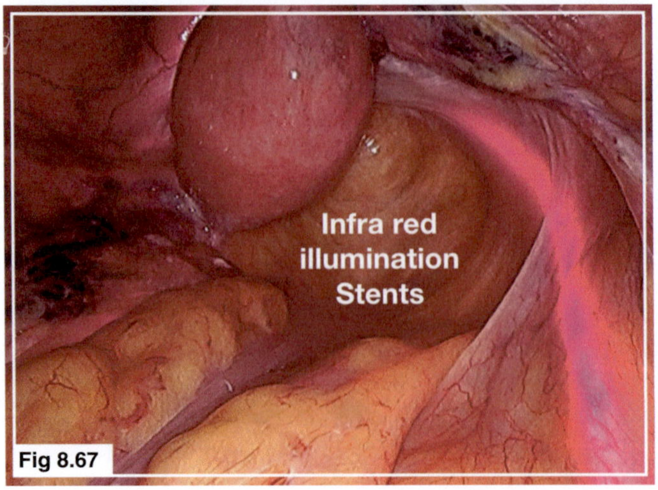

Fig. 8.67 Ureter innovations: The latest innovation in handling ureter is the development of infrared illuminating stent. These stents are inserted preoperatively and with an infrared pulse camera and light source the stents can be illuminated for dissection purposes

9 Nerves

9.1 The Genitofemoral Nerve (Fig. 9.1)

It lies lateral to the external iliac artery on the psoas muscle. The nerve should be protected during pelvic lymphadenectomy. It runs parallel till it dips down into the psoas muscle. The injury to this nerve can lead to parenthesis in the medial side of the thigh (Figs. 9.2, 9.3, 9.4, 9.5, 9.6, 9.7, 9.8, 9.9, 9.10, 9.11, 9.12, 9.13, 9.14, 9.15, 9.16, 9.17, and 9.18).

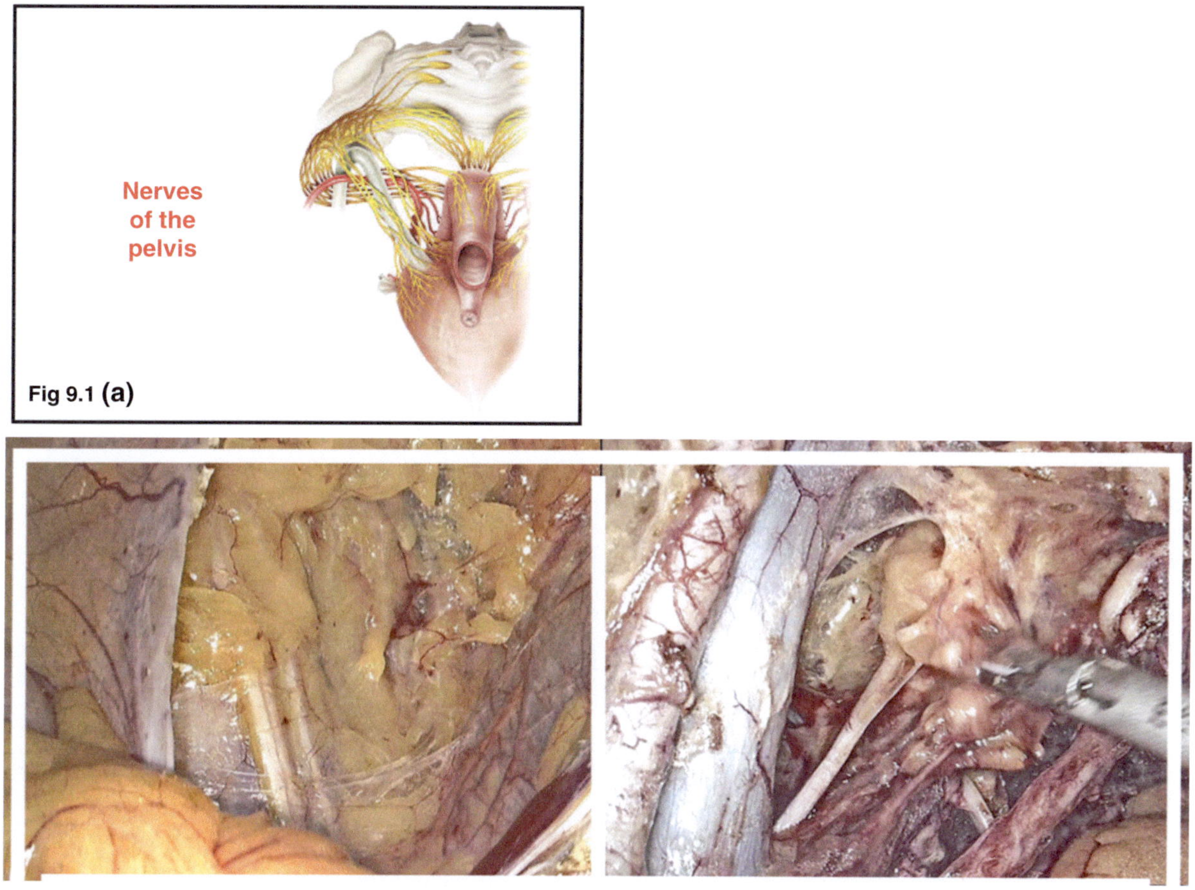

Fig. 9.1 (**a**) The nerves of the pelvis. (**b**) All four nerves: The following nerves have been shown in the image. The genitofemoral nerve on the top left corner, the obturator nerve in the top right corner, the hypogastric nerves on the bottom right corner and the pelvic splanchnic nerves on the bottom left corner. In this chapter there will be multiple number of images of each nerve shown with variable amounts of surrounding fat. Considering that the nerves are retroperitoneal in location, their appearances in variable amount of interspersed fat will help in understanding the location, normal lie and course and hence the dissection of the nerves

S. Puntambekar et al., *Laparoscopic Pelvic Anatomy in Females*, https://doi.org/10.1007/978-981-13-8653-4_9

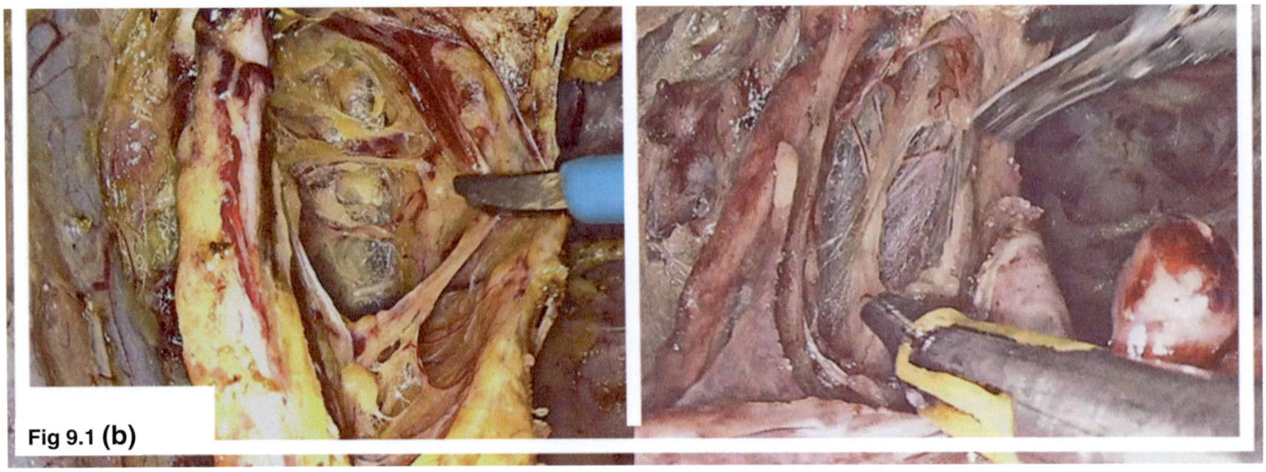

Fig. 9.1 (continued)

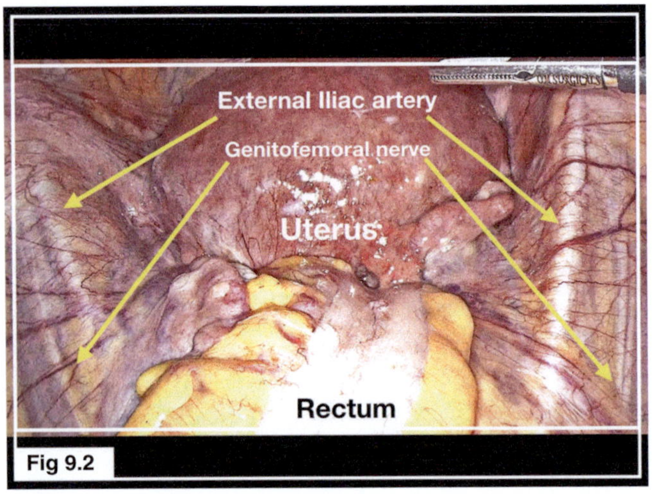

Fig. 9.2 Genitofemoral nerve: This is a case of grade IV endometriosis where the uterus and the rectum are adherent to each other and impacted/obliterated the pouch of Douglas. Genitofemoral nerves are seldom seen through the peritoneum owing to the fat present in the retroperitoneal region. However as seen here through the peritoneum they lie lateral to the external iliac artery and run parallel to it as well. They rest upon the psoas muscle

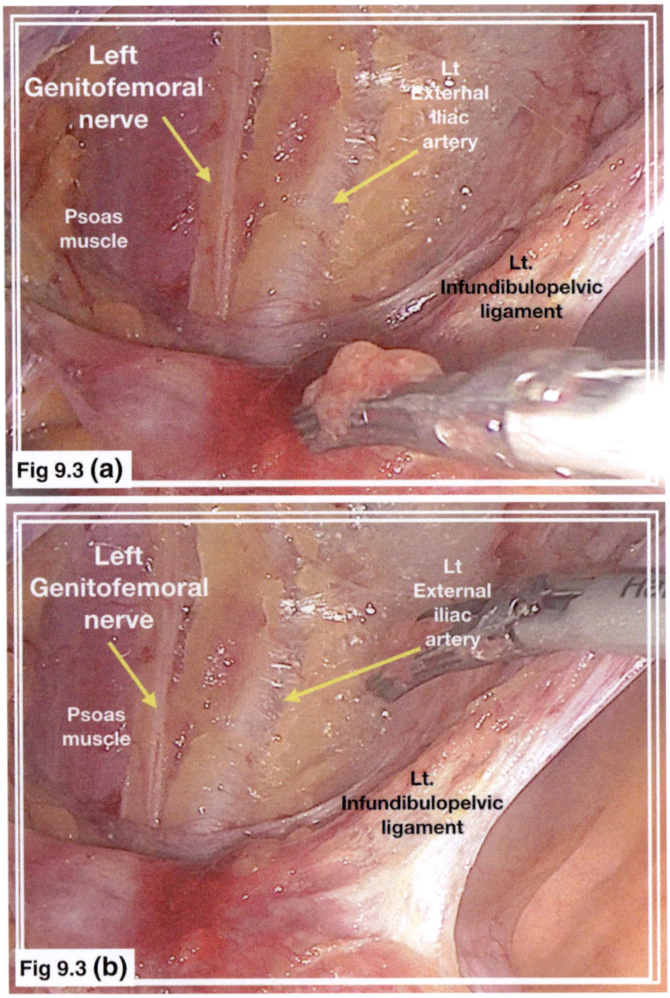

Fig. 9.3 (**a**, **b**) Genitofemoral nerve: The genitofemoral nerve is best appreciated into lateral approach of the pararectal space dissection discussed later in Chap. 11

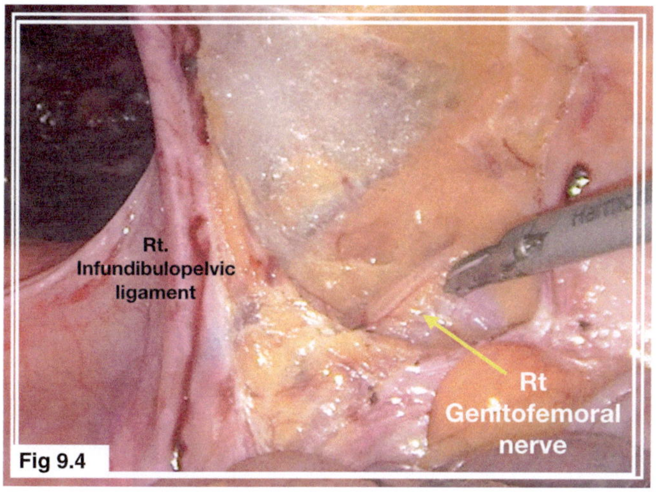

Fig. 9.4 Genitofemoral nerve: Often the nerve is interspersed in retroperitoneal fat which is why it can be difficult to dissect and appreciate. Gentle traction on the infundibulopelvic ligament medially opens the pararectal space more widely, thereby either enabling the psoas muscle to be seen with the genitofemoral nerve or helping in the dissection of the external iliac artery to later identify the nerves

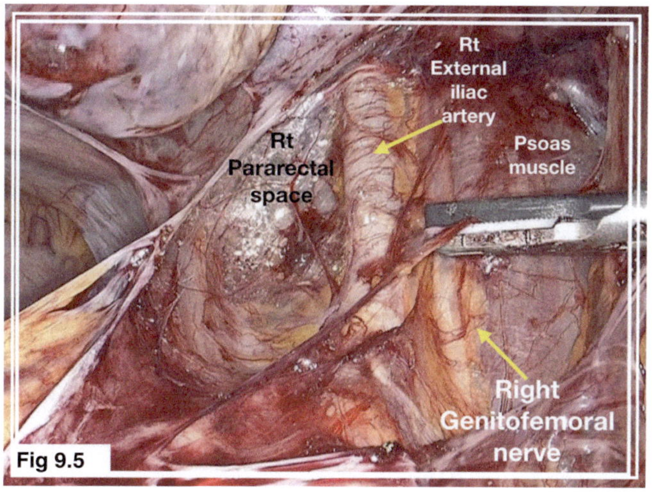

Fig. 9.5 Genitofemoral nerve: Dissecting the infundibulopelvic ligament in case of planned oophorectomy exposes the pararectal space for dissection. This is seen in the image where the infundibulopelvic ligament has been excised

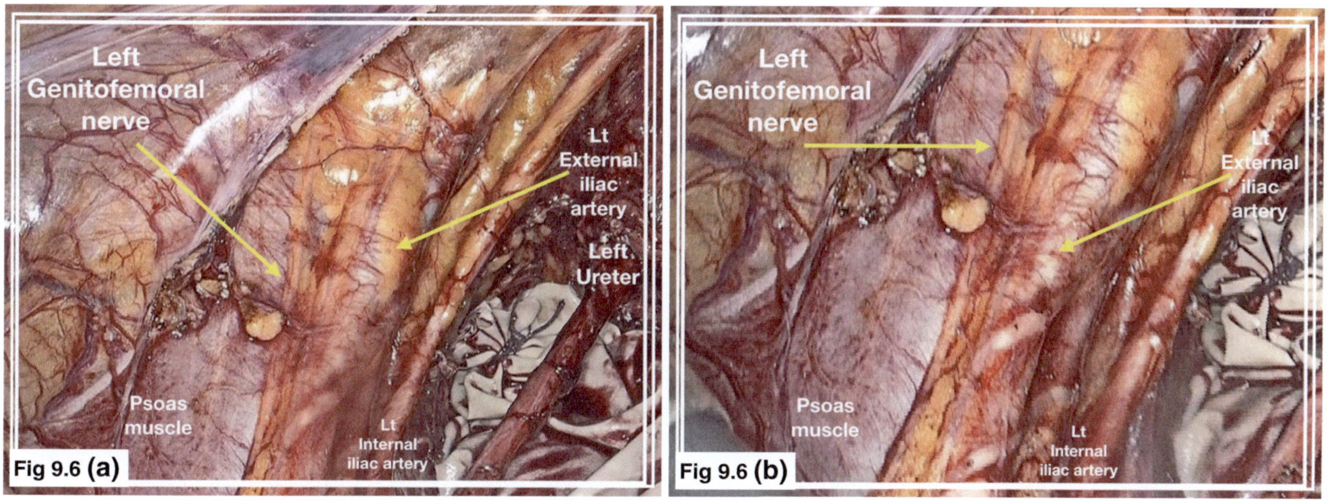

Fig. 9.6 (**a**, **b**) Genitofemoral nerve: Since the fat distribution in the retroperitoneal area is not uniform, mirror images of both sides are not possible. The genitofemoral nerve of the same patient of the above image on the left side shows varied length and thickness. Blunt dissection in the form of gentle strokes can expose the nerves

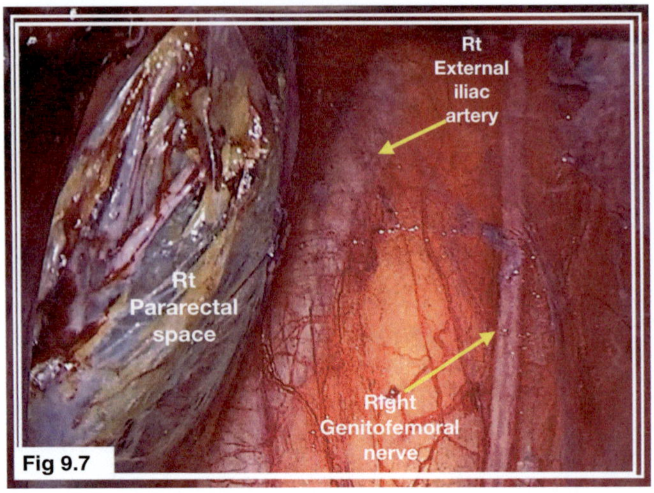

Fig. 9.7 Genitofemoral nerve: Often inflammation on the peritoneal surfaces due to iatrogenic (previous surgery) reasons or infection may cause adherent peritoneum leading to the haemorrhagic fields. However careful dissection can help the nerves stand out from the fat more easily then

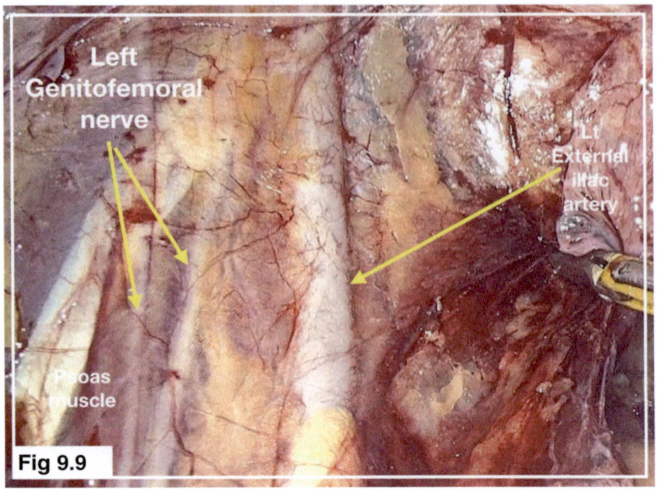

Fig. 9.9 Genitofemoral nerve: Dissection of the connective tissue with blunt instrument can also help in visualising the structures more clearly. The genital and femoral heads of the genitofemoral nerve can be seen separately here. The tendon of psoas muscle can also be seen lateral to the nerves; they can often be confused or hidden with the nerves. But they always remain lateral to the external iliac artery

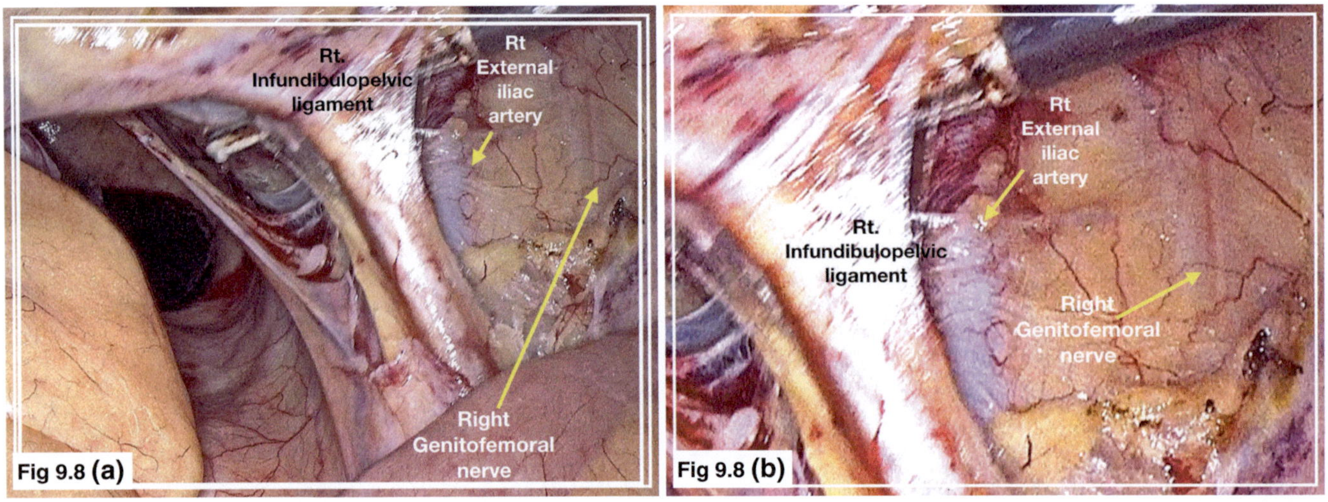

Fig. 9.8 (**a**, **b**) Genitofemoral nerve: The nerve can be seen interspersed with the retroperitnoneal fat which can be seen on a more magnified view

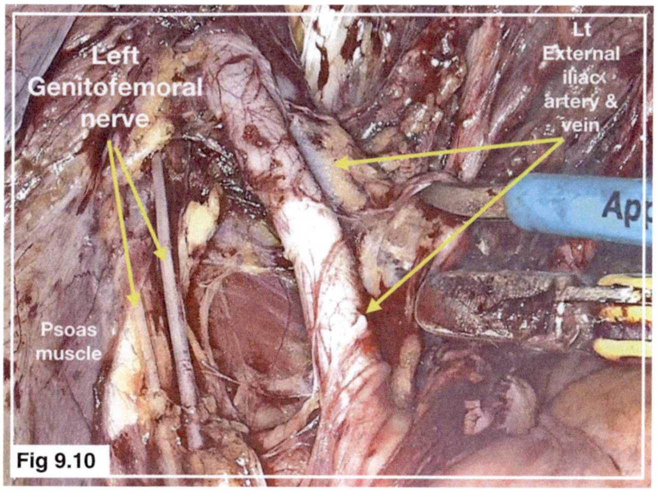

Fig. 9.10 Genitofemoral nerve: The nerves can be seen clearly after lymph node dissection in case of minimal haemorrhage like seeing this image. Post-lymphadenectomy the nerves are easily appreciated

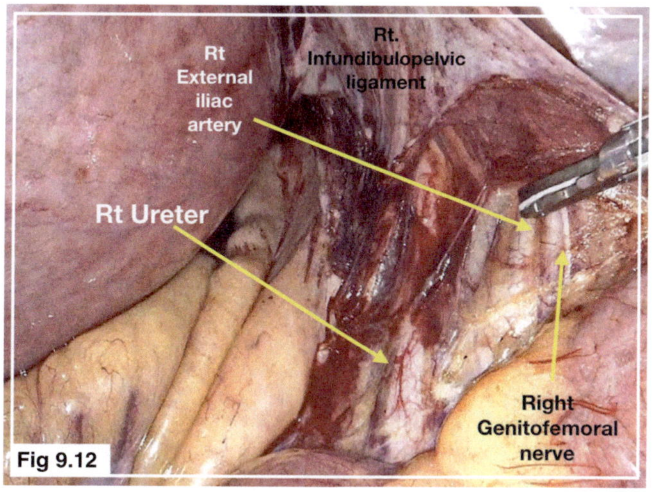

Fig. 9.12 Genitofemoral nerve: The external iliac artery lies between the genitofemoral nerve and the ureter or the ureter lies most medial to the nerve. The nerve can be approached from the medial side with certain amount of difficulty by retracting the infundibulopelvic ligament upwards and medially and tracing the eternal iliac artery

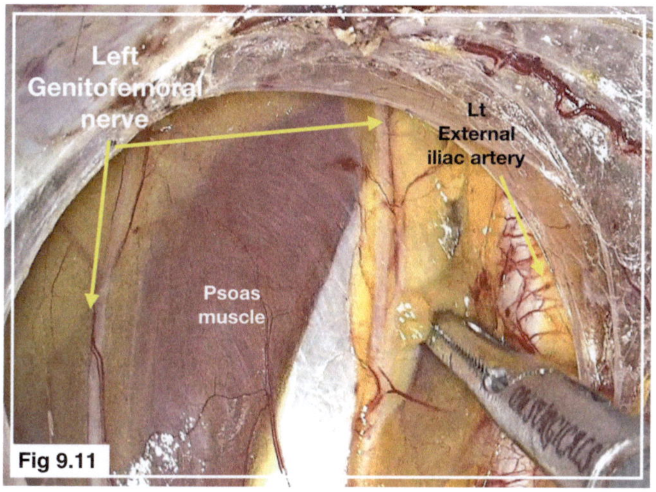

Fig. 9.11 Genitofemoral nerve: The two heads of genitofemoral nerve, the genital branch and the femoral branch, can be seen splayed and separated early at the psoas muscle

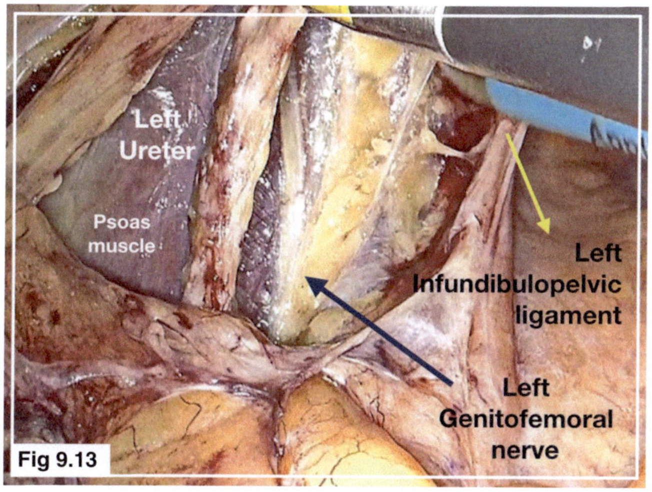

Fig. 9.13 Genitofemoral nerve: Gentle traction onto the ureter may also help dissect the connective tissue over the psoas muscle, thus revealing the genitofemoral nerve

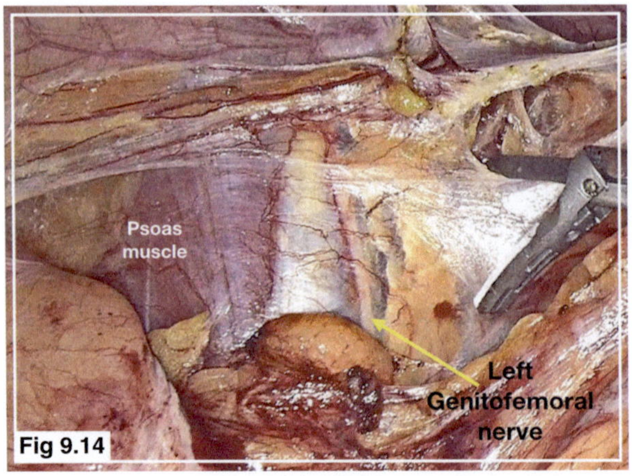

Fig. 9.14 Genitofemoral nerve: The genitofemoral nerve here appears on the medial or anterior side of the external iliac nerve. The traction onto its connective tissue superficially causes this appearance and dissection of these tissues can be done with blunt instruments

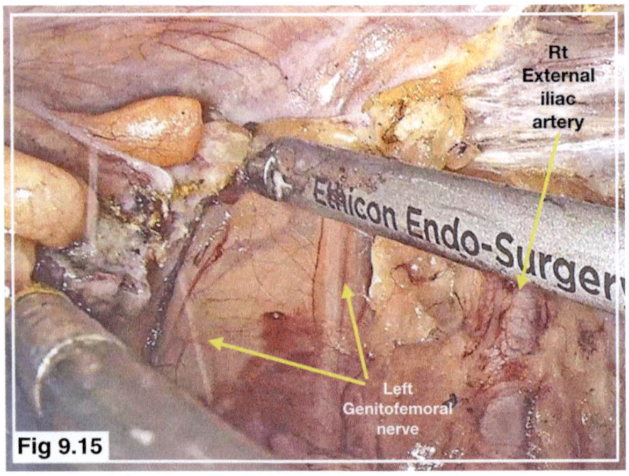

Fig. 9.15 Genitofemoral nerve: Lateral dissection of the peritoneum helps open the retroperitoneal space and thus visualise the psoas muscle as well as the genitofemoral nerves

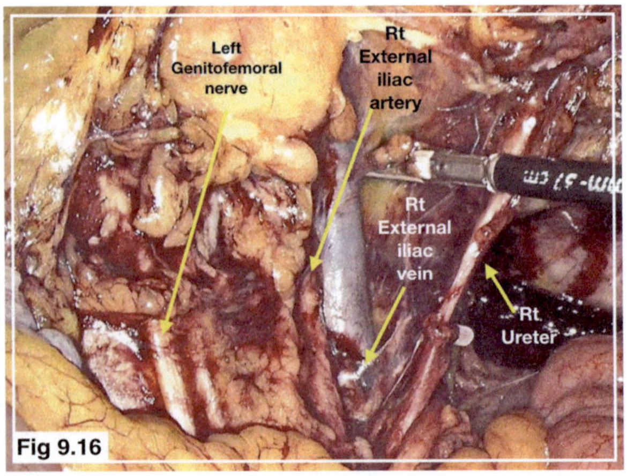

Fig. 9.16 Genitofemoral nerve: Genitofemoral nerve seen post-lymphadenectomy and its relations with the vital structures appreciated. From lateral to medial—genitofemoral nerve—external iliac artery—external iliac vein—ureter. The internal iliac artery lies at a plane lower than the ureter

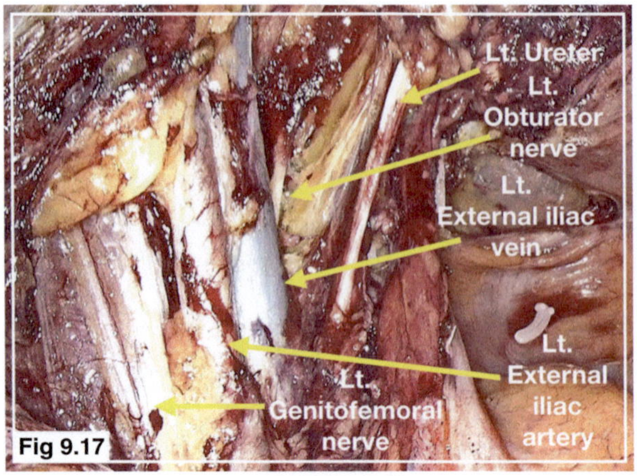

Fig. 9.17 Genitofemoral nerve: Relation to the obturator nerve/completed pararectal space dissection. The genitofemoral nerve lies superior and lateral to the external iliac artery over the psoas muscle, while the obturator nerve lies medial and below the level of the external iliac artery

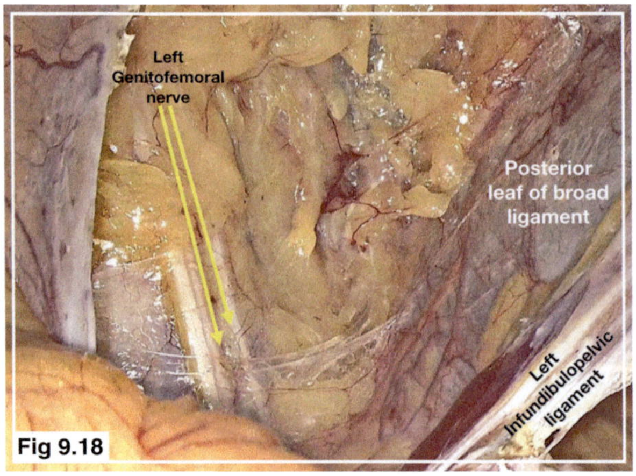

Fig. 9.18 Genitofemoral nerve: Most commonly seen view of the genitofemoral nerve

9.2 The Obturator Nerve

Lies in the bifurcation between the iliac arteries. The obturator artery and the veins run parallel and posterior to the nerve in its entire course. The vein drains directly into the presacral veins. Thus the plane of dissection during obturator lymphadenectomy should be superficial to the nerve. The nerve lies at a deeper level than the external iliac artery and the vein (Figs. 9.19, 9.20, 9.21, 9.22, 9.23, 9.24, 9.25, 9.26, 9.27, 9.28, 9.29, 9.30, 9.31, 9.32, 9.33, 9.34, 9.35, 9.36, and 9.37).

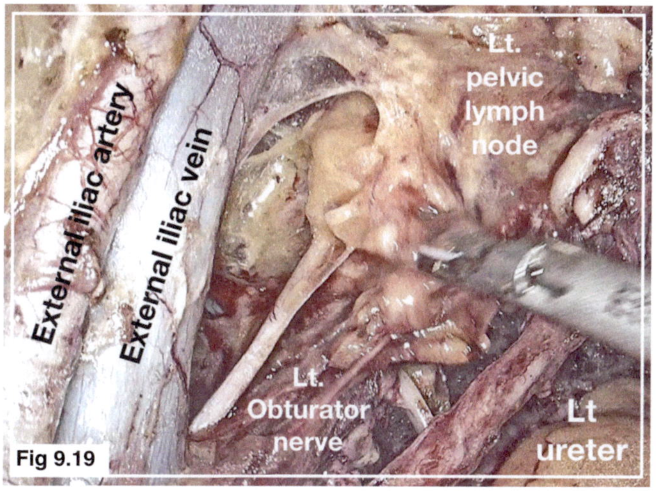

Fig. 9.19 Obturator nerve: The obturator is the most commonly encountered nerve in radical hysterectomy as it forms one of the boundaries of pelvic lymph node dissection. It is mandatory to dissect lymph node till the visualisation of the obturator nerve and not any further. The nerve forms visual confirmation of complete lymph node dissection

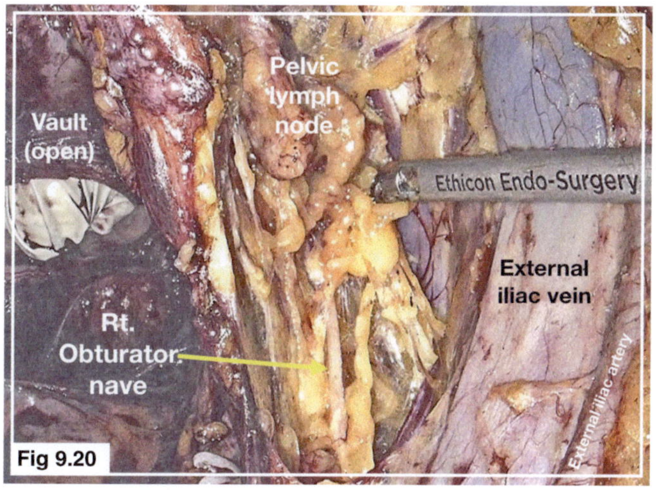

Fig. 9.20 Obturator nerve: Lymph node dissections are considered as a more morbid procedure as it involves manipulation of vital structures like the external iliac vessels. The external iliac vein is often pressed so as to extract maximum fat from the retroperitoneal space during lymph node dissection. The obturator nerve is seen to appear at the cranial region, underneath the external iliac vessels

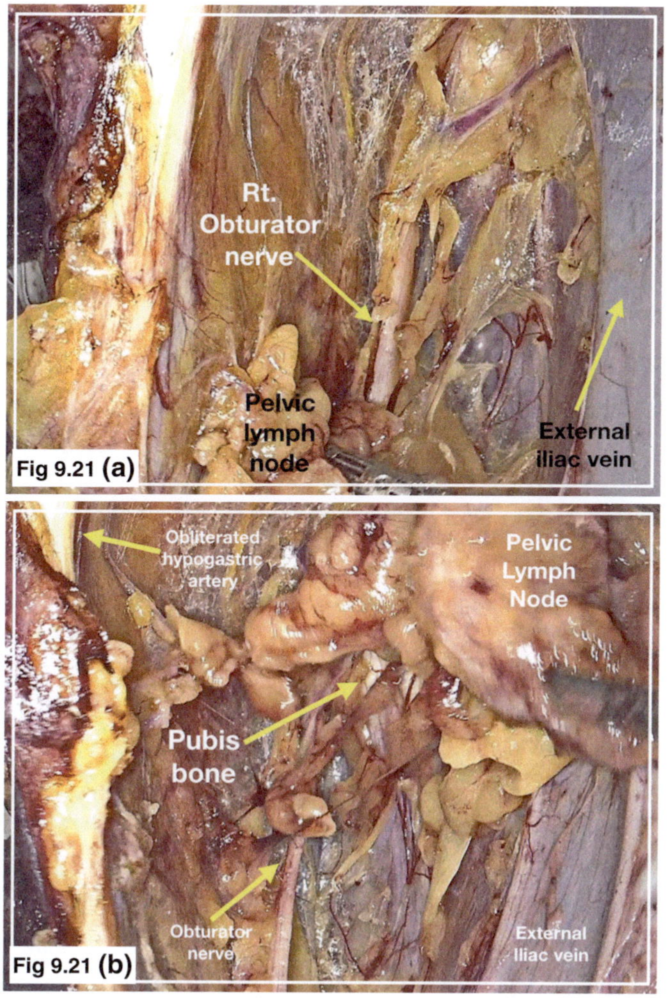

Fig. 9.21 (**a**, **b**) Obturator nerve: The image here shows exposed Rt obturator nave with incomplete lymph node dissection. Exposure of the pubis bone suggests complete lymph node dissection with exposed obturator nerve. The obturator nerve always lies lateral to the obliterated hypogastric artery

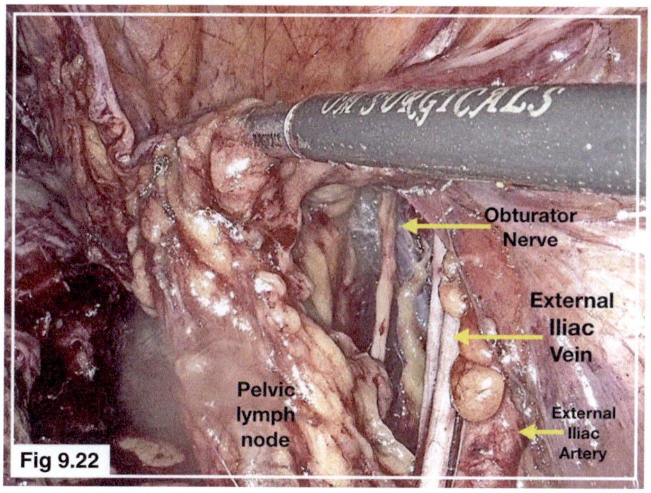

Fig. 9.22 Obturator nerve: The direction of extraction of lymph nodes is lateral to medial along the curve of the external iliac vein and pubis bone to allow maximum lymph node yield. The obturator nerve forms the barrier/lower limit of dissection

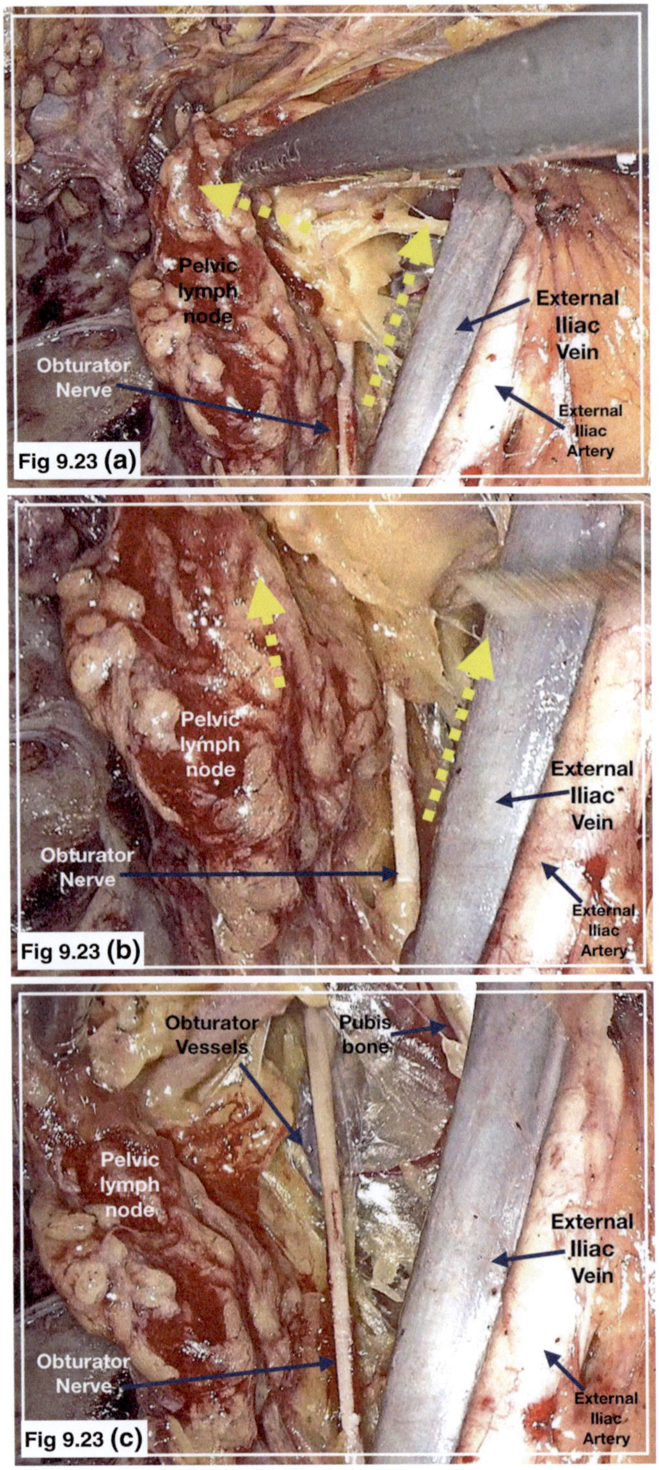

Fig. 9.23 (**a**–**c**) Obturator nerve: Step-by-step categorical lymph node dissection on the inferior surface, exposing the obturator nerve. All dissection should begin from the cranial to caudal direction and medial traction applied to the lymph node mass and thus the obturator nerve becomes visible from the sacral region first (yellow arrows). (**b**) Later the direction of traction on lymph node mass is cranial towards the abdominal wall. (**c**) On final dissection the complete obturator nerve is exposed with the obturator vessels seen underneath occasionally. The pubic bone is exposed and the lymph nodes are removed en bloc

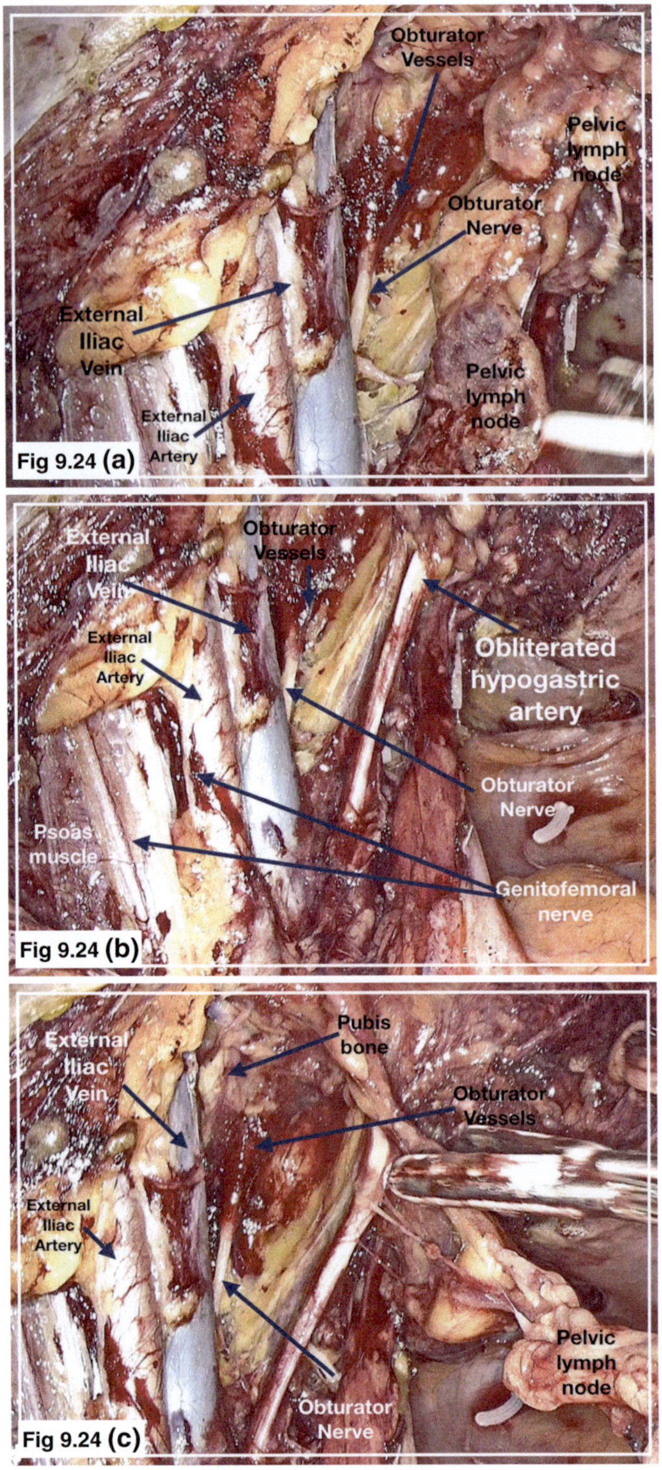

Fig. 9.24 (**a**–**c**) Obturator nerve: Step-by-step dissection of lymph nodes, thus exposing the left obturator nerve

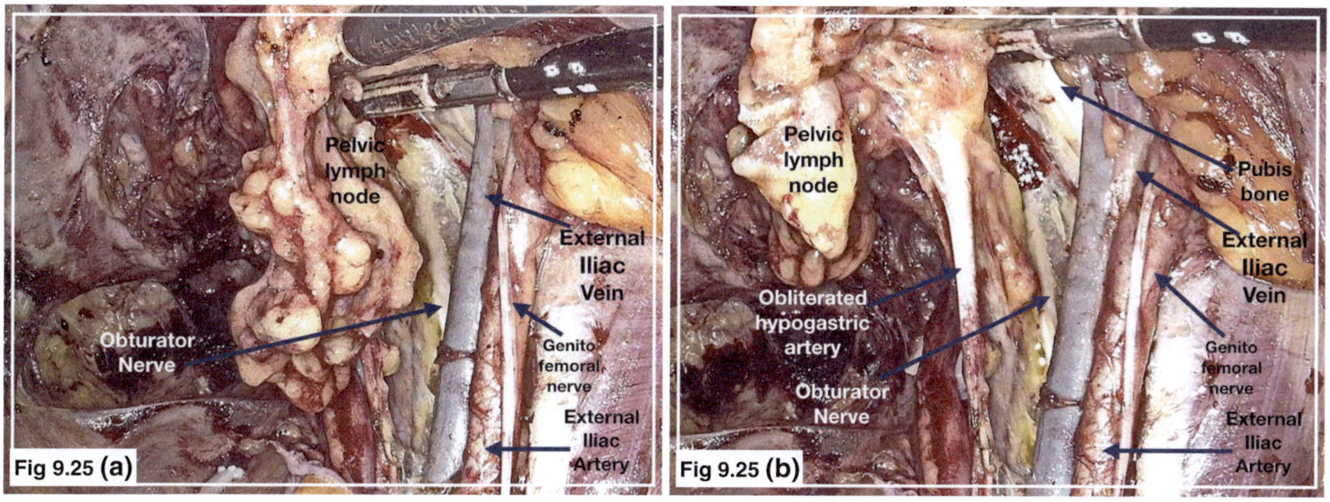

Fig. 9.25 (**a**, **b**) Obturator nerve: Relations between the obturator nerve with the obliterated hypogastric artery and the genitofemoral nerve have been explained

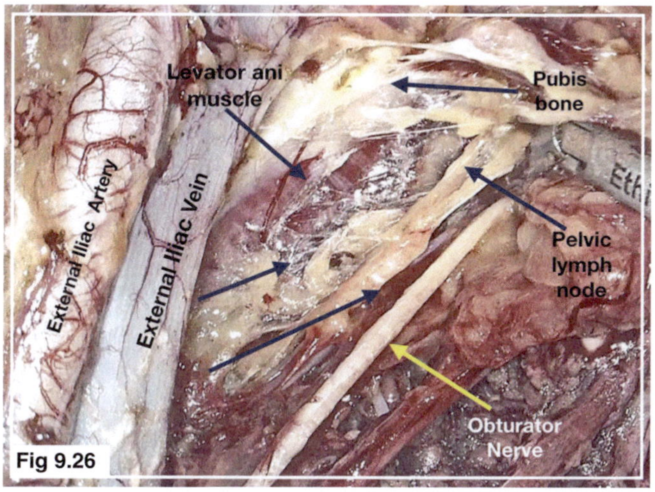

Fig. 9.26 Obturator nerve: En bloc lymph node dissection revealing the left obturator nerve, the pubis bone and the lector ani muscle covered by endopelvic fascia

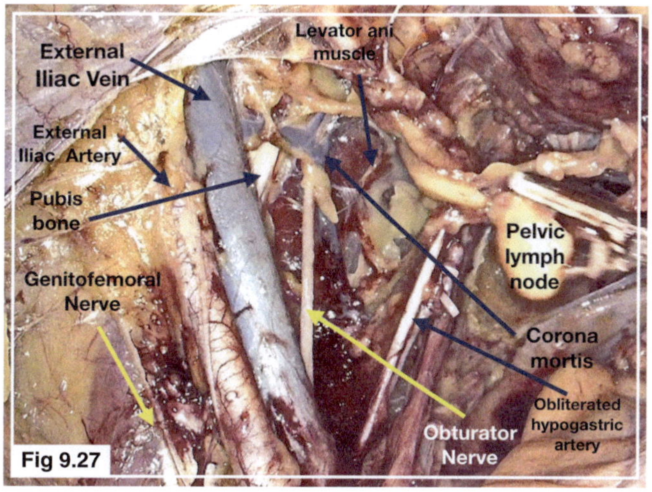

Fig. 9.27 Obturator nerve: Corona mortis is the only vessel communicating the external iliac vein to the internal iliac vein via the obturator nerve. This is often seen as an arch-shaped structure on the pubis bone. Injury to this vessel leads to torrential haemorrhage

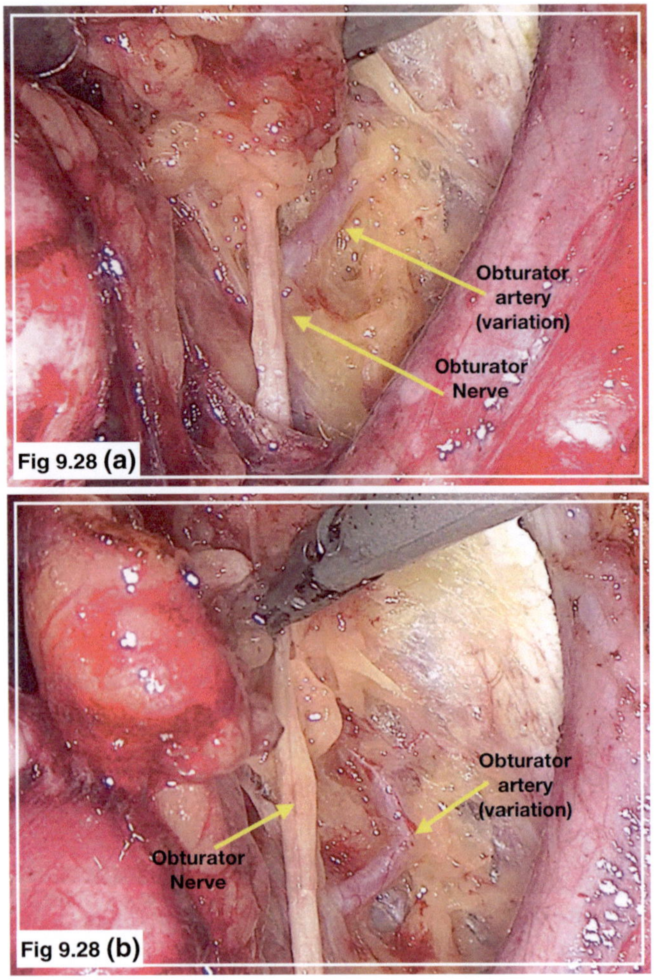

Fig. 9.28 (**a**, **b**) Obturator nerve: This is a variation in the course of obturator artery observed in a case of laparoscopic nerve-sparing radical hysterectomy for a case of Ca endometrium. The obturator artery usually follows an identical course as the obturator nerve. Here however it was seen as a zigzag structure under the obturator nerve. The obturator artery is the only branch of the internal iliac artery which travels laterally outwards unlike other branches

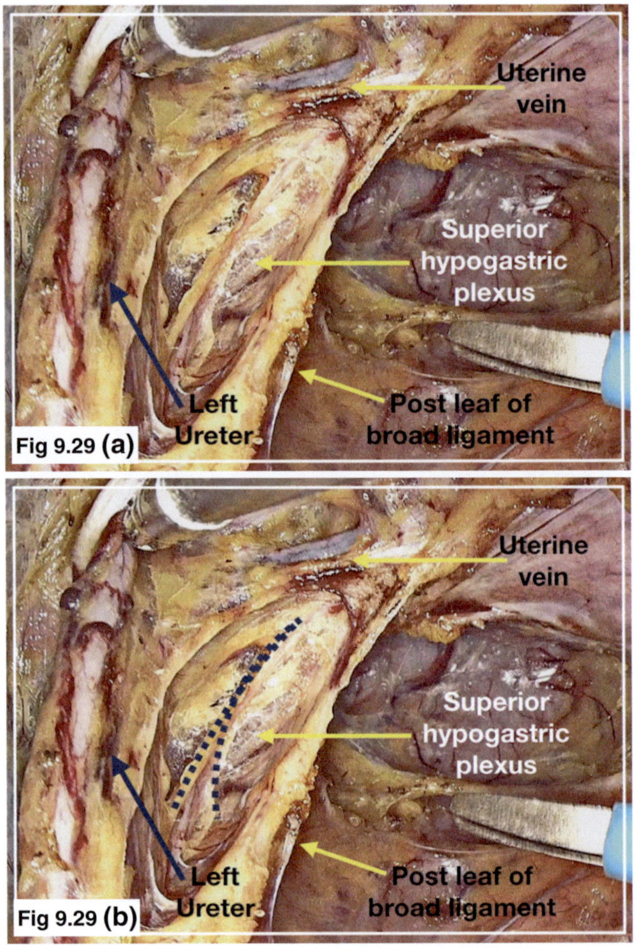

Fig. 9.29 (**a**, **b**) Hypogastric nerve: This image is from a case of nerve-sparing radical hysterectomy. The left ureter has been retracted upwards and laterally to expose the medial pararectal space for fine identification and dissection of the hypogastric nerve plexus. (**b**) The hypogastric plexus lies interspersed with fat and fibrous connective tissue of the uterosacral ligament. Hence it is often difficult to distinguish. The nerve has been labelled with blue dotted lines to identify its course with the previous image

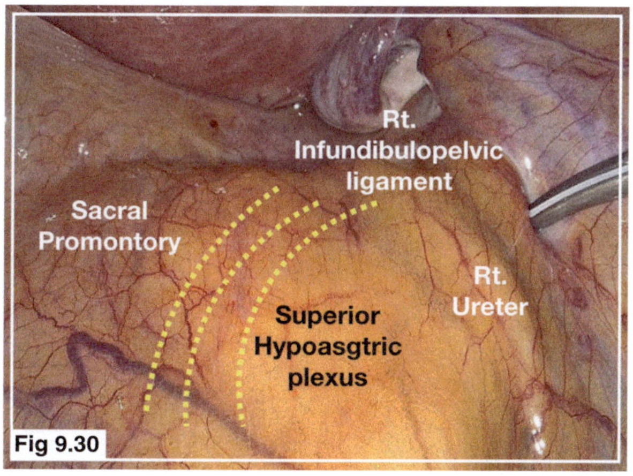

Fig. 9.30 Superior hypogastric plexus: The hypogastric nerve arises from superior hypogastric plexus which lies above the level of sacral promontory. They can be identified at the level of sacral promontory and traced downwards as the plexus coalesces to form hypogastric nerve supplying the bladder and the uterus

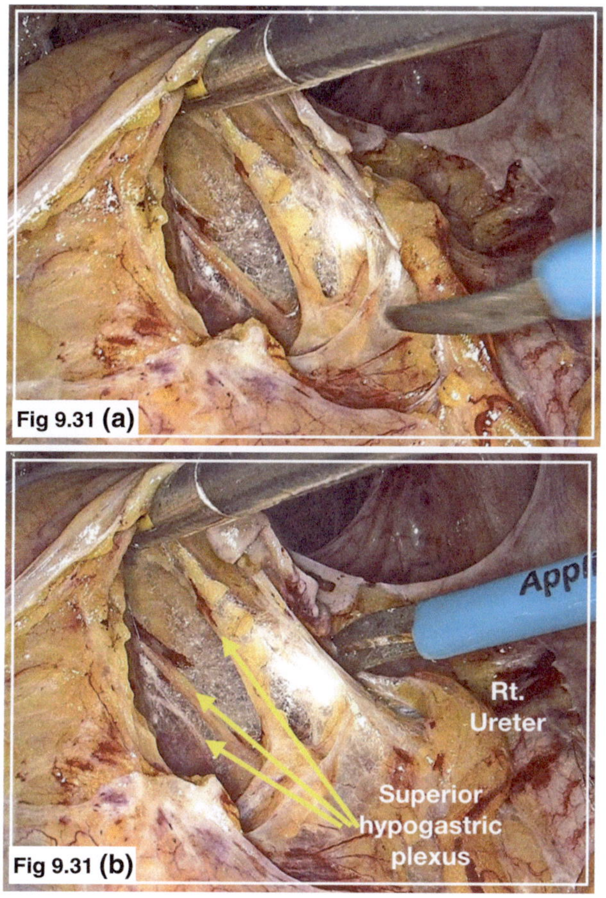

Fig. 9.31 (**a**, **b**) Superior hypogastric plexus: Nerves are often difficult to distinguish. They are interspersed with fat and within the folds of peritoneum. They appear as thin slender white strands surrounded by small amount of fat. The (**b**) image has been labelled to appreciate the nerves in their natural form on laparoscopy seen in the previous image

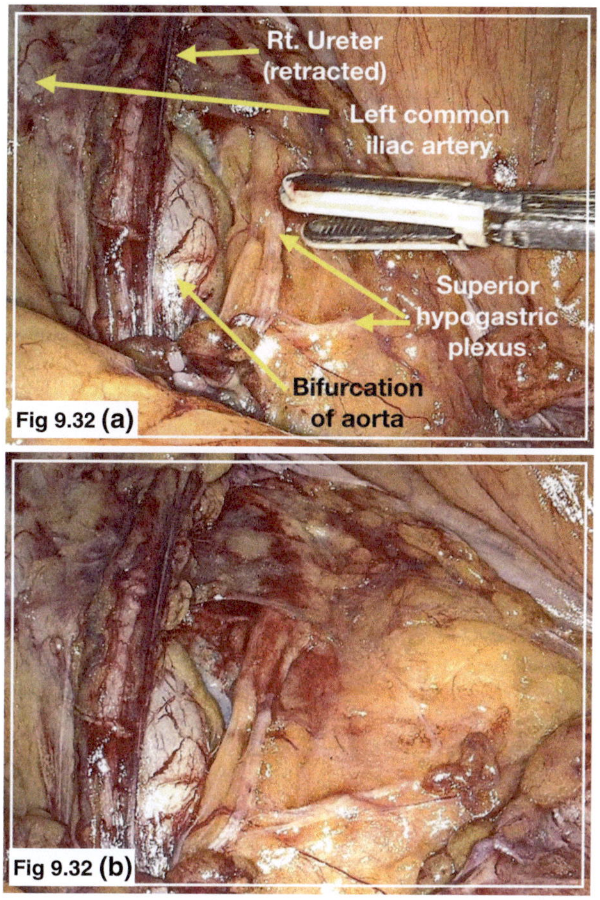

Fig. 9.32 (**a**, **b**) Superior hypogastric plexus: The superior hypogastric plexus lies above the sacral promontory and lateral to the bifurcation of the aorta and continues to remain lateral to the common iliac vessels. They change course at the level of sacral promontory as they enter the pelvis. This is a case of posterior exenteration where the bowel had to be mobilised prior to resection

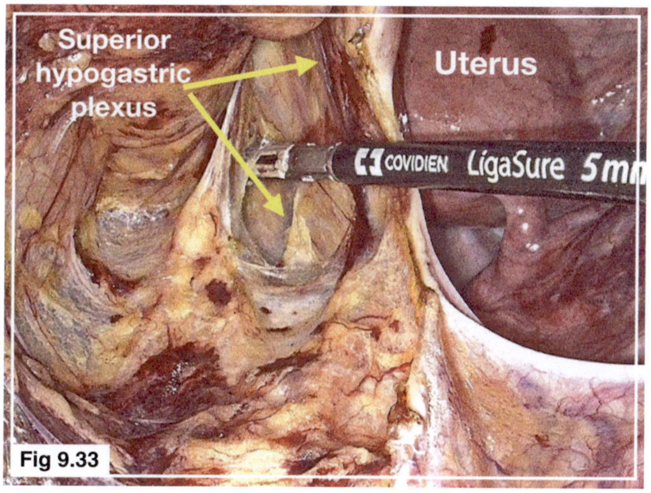

Fig. 9.33 Superior hypogastric plexus: This is the medicine view of the segment bowel that is mobilised for posterior exenteration with the uterus seen on the rear end. The superior hypogastric plexus has been labelled at certain regions

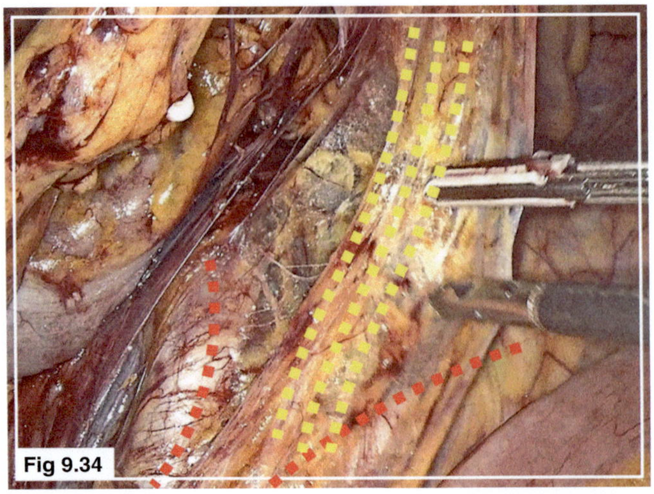

Fig. 9.34 Superior hypogastric plexus: The red dotted lines denote the course of the common iliac artery which diverges from the midline while the yellow dotted lines denote the course of the superhypogastric plexus which travels parallel and converges below the sacral promontory to form the hypogastric nerve. At this point onwards the nerves are oriented medial to the iliac vessels

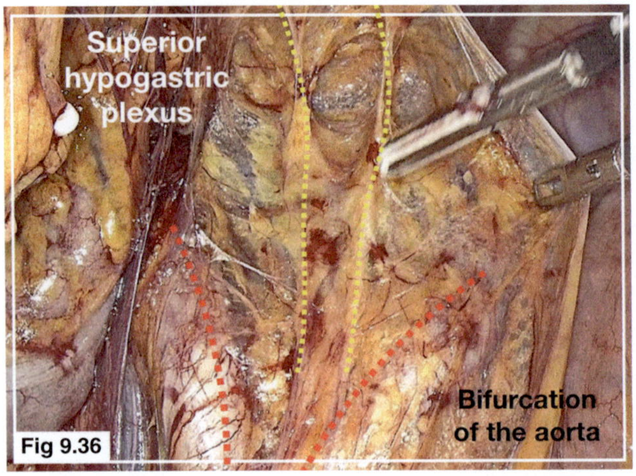

Fig. 9.36 Superior hypogastric plexus: The yellow dotted line of the superior hypogastric plexus travels along the mesentery of the bowel and thus remains paramedic and is later seen on the medial side of the uterosacral ligament

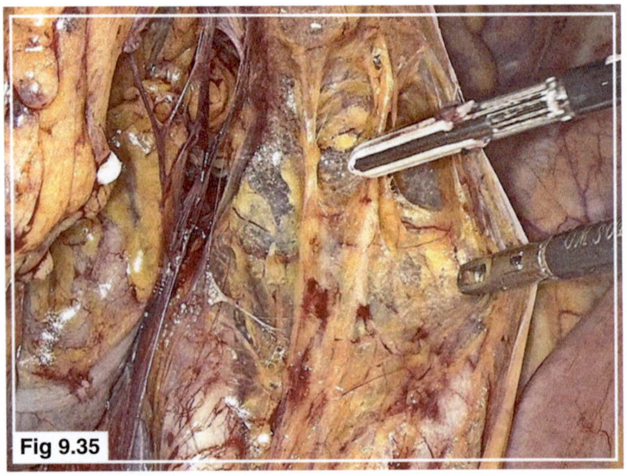

Fig. 9.35 Superior hypogastric plexus: Unlabelled diagram of the superior hypogastric plexus and its course into the pelvis

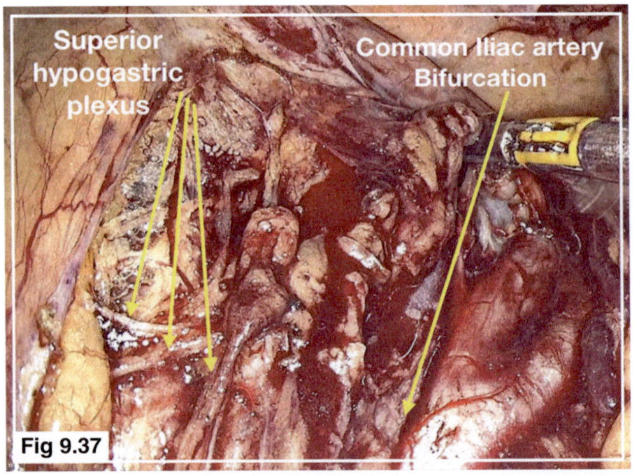

Fig. 9.37 Superior hypogastric plexus: In this image we progress towards para-aortic lymph node dissection. The peritoneal dissection is extended up to the level of abdominal aorta and inferior vena cava (IVC). The IVC can be seen below and to the right of the aorta

9.3 The Hypogastric Nerve

Arises from the superior hypogastric plexus which lies at the bifurcation of the aorta. They carry the post-ganglionic sympathetic fibres from L1, 2 and 3. The hypogastric nerves then traverse posterolaterally on either side of the rectum on their way to the bladder and the pelvic floor. These nerves lie in the Okabayashi space or the medial pararectal space (described above). At the level of the uterine vein this is joined by pelvic splanchnic nerves S2, 3 and 4. These carry the parasympathetic supply. The hypogastric nerve is identified medial to the ureter at the level of the uterosacral. It lies in the space between the ureter and the uterosacral. The branches of these nerves arise medially and supply the rectum, uterus and part of cervix. These branches have to be sacrificed to achieve a nerve-sparing radical hysterectomy (Figs. 9.38, 9.39, 9.40, 9.41, 9.42, 9.43, 9.44, 9.45, 9.46, 9.47, 9.48, 9.49, 9.50, 9.51, 9.52, 9.53, 9.54, 9.55, 9.56, 9.57, 9.58, 9.59, 9.60, 9.61, 9.62, 9.63, 9.64, 9.65, 9.66, and 9.67).

Rules

1. The key to nerve-sparing surgery is identification of the Okabayashi space.
2. The identification of the deep uterine veins.
3. The identification of the Yabuki space.

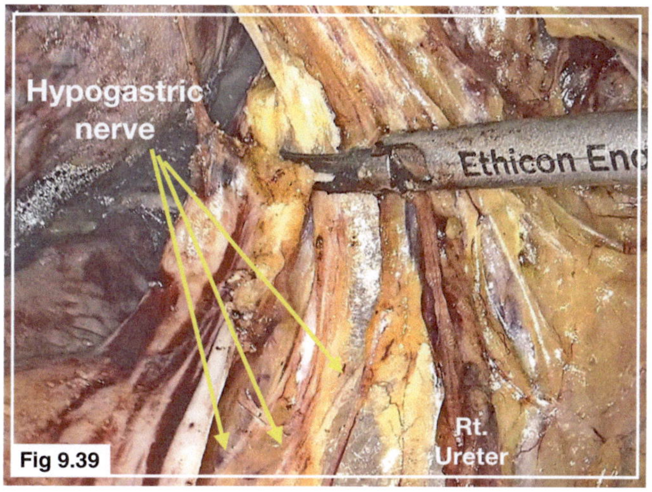

Fig. 9.39 Hypogastric nerve: In routine radical hysterectomy these nerves are cut due to resection of the uterosacral ligament which is done after distal clamping of the uterine veins followed by resection of the ligaments from lateral to medial and thus it is important to save in nerve-sparing radical hysterectomy

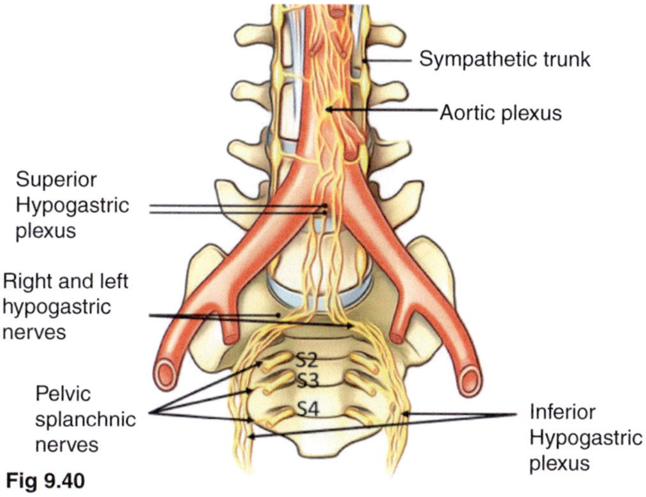

Fig. 9.40 Hypogastric nerve: Graphical and diagrammatic representation of the entire superior hypogastric plexus forming the hypogastric nerve and then communicating with the inferior hypogastric plexus

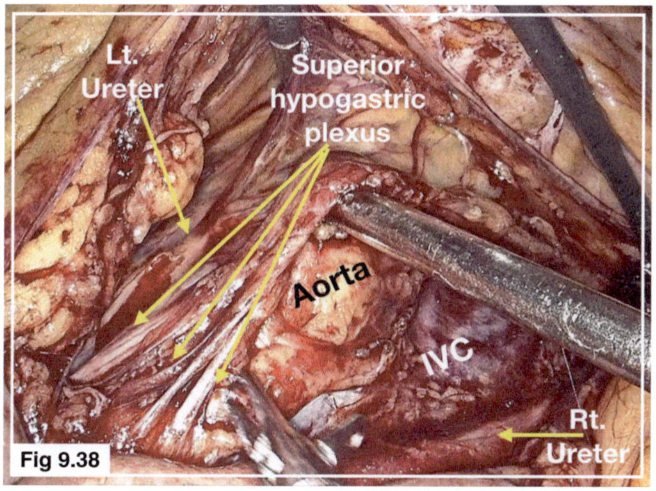

Fig. 9.38 Superior hypogastric plexus: At the level of abdominal aorta and inferior vena cava, the superior hypogastric plexus lies parallel and paramedian (lateral) to the great vessels. The superhypogastric nerves are post-ganglionic nerve fibres of L1, 2 and 3. Thus they cannot be dissected higher up. At this level bilateral ureters are visible

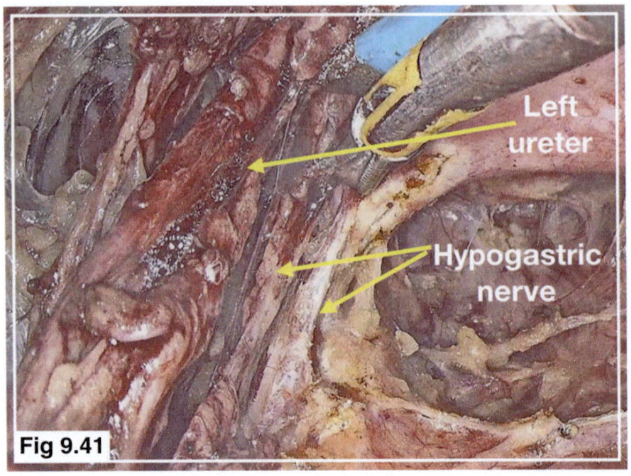

Fig. 9.41 Hypogastric nerve: Subsequent images have been displayed to show step-by-step dissection of the hypogastric nerve from their origin at the level of the superior hypogastric plexus to their two branches, one supplying the uterus immediate medially and the second continuing to supply the bladder

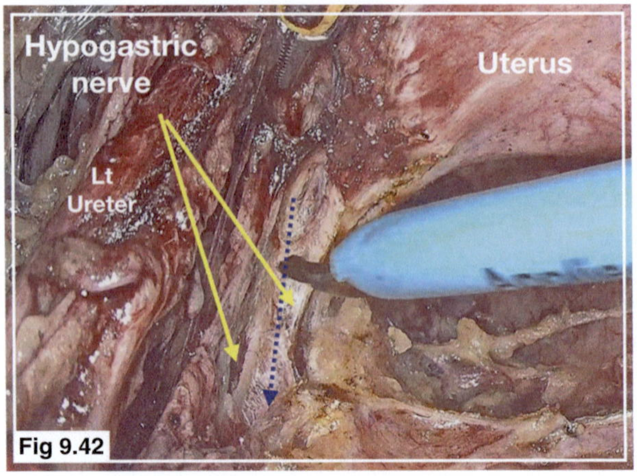

Fig. 9.42 Hypogastric nerve: The blue dotted line denotes the space, plane and direction of dissection to identify the nerves. The ureter remains lateral by traction or by natural lie. The nerves travel in longitudinal axis in a vertical, cranial-to-caudal direction

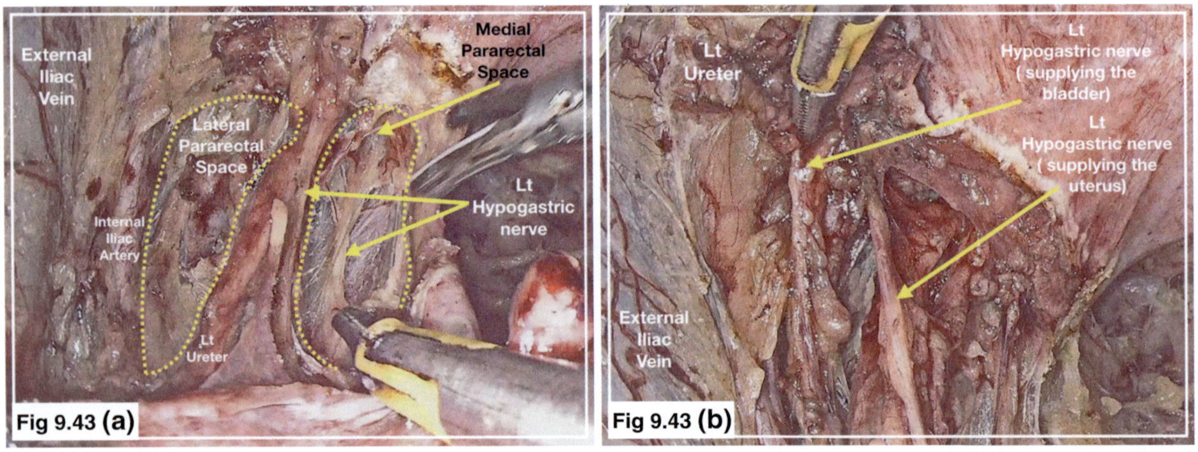

Fig. 9.43 (a, b) Hypogastric nerve: The relation of hypogastric nerve with other vascular structures has been shown in a more panoramic view. Their relation with the retroperitoneal spaces has also been shown. (b) is a magnified image of the dissected hypogastric nerves that run parallel

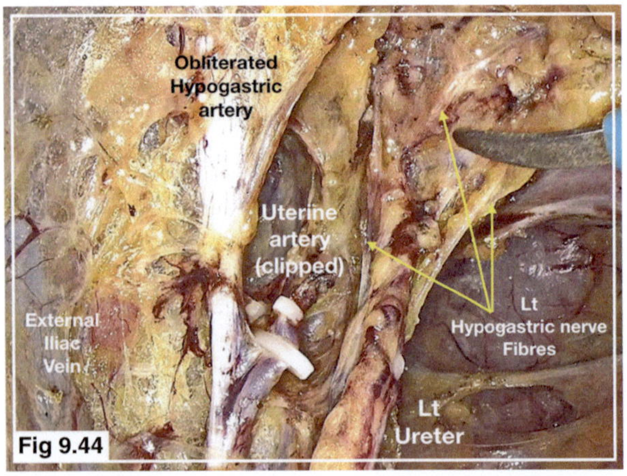

Fig. 9.44 Hypogastric nerve: Some of the nerve fibres are seen travelling with the ureter. They are dissected and brought separate. They are preserved as they travel with the ureter to supply the bladder. The ureter is retracted literally and the nerve fibres are dissected off the ureter and preserved before clipping the uterine vein. The uterine artery however has already been clipped and dissected so as to open the pararectal space and help dissect the nerves

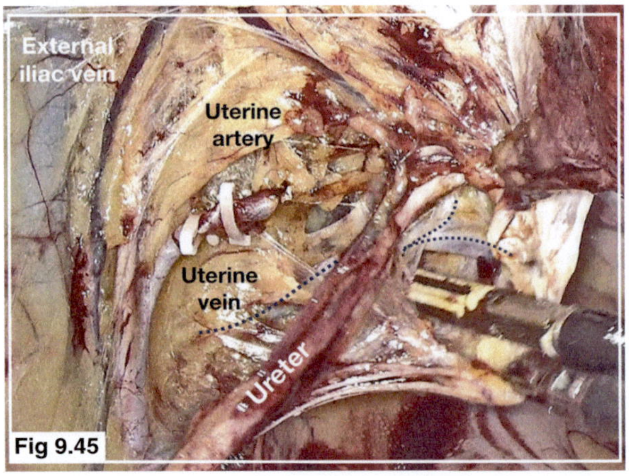

Fig. 9.45 Hypogastric nerve: The entire length of the uterine vein can be dissected up to its outflow into the internal iliac vein after clipping and cutting the uterine artery. The uterine vein lies parallel and under the uterine artery. The ureter lies above the uterine vein. The *ureter lies in the fork of the uterine artery and vein*

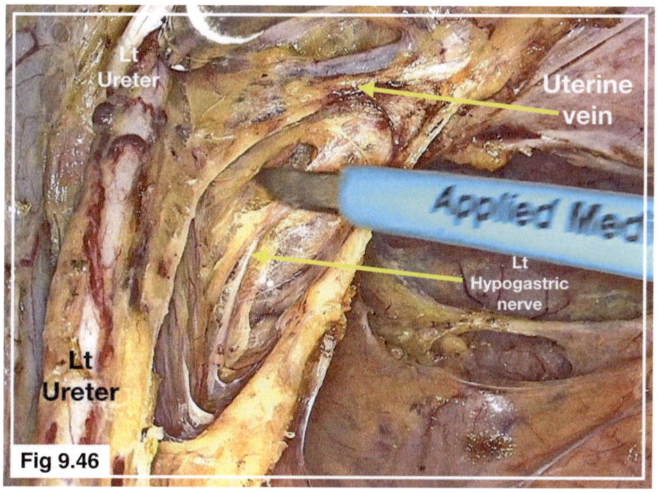

Fig. 9.46 Hypogastric nerve: After clipping the uterine artery, uterine vein lies below and parallel to the uterine artery. Dissection of the uterine vein is the most important step in nerve-sparing radical hysterectomy. Location of the clipping of the vein is the deciding step if the procedure can be nerve sparing or not

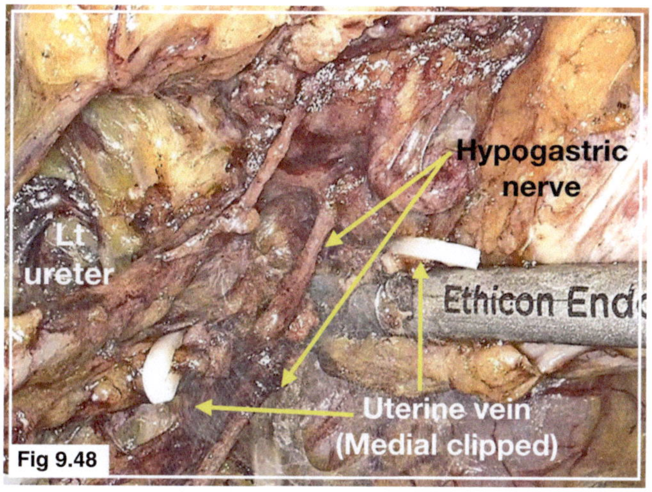

Fig. 9.48 Hypogastric nerve: Medial clipping of the uterine vein preserves the hypogastric nerve as shown in the image. The medial branch supplying the uterus can be easily transected as shown by the Harmonic in the image. In routine/non-nerve-sparing radical hysterectomy lateral clipping of the uterine would lead to severing of the hypogastric nerve, detached along with the specimen (uterus)

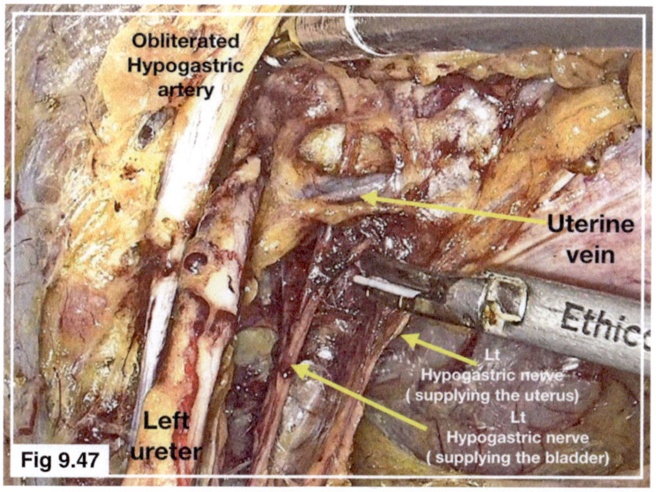

Fig. 9.47 Hypogastric nerve: In a case of nerve-sparing laparoscopic radical hysterectomy the reaction of the uterine vein with the hypogastric nerve has been displayed. In routine laparoscopic radical hysterectomy the uterine vein is clamped near its root at the internal iliac vein, as far from the uterus as possible, *lateral to the ureter* at all times. However in nerve-sparing hysterectomy, the uterine vein needs to be clipped close to the uterus, *medial to the ureter*, so as to preserve the nerve supplying the bladder

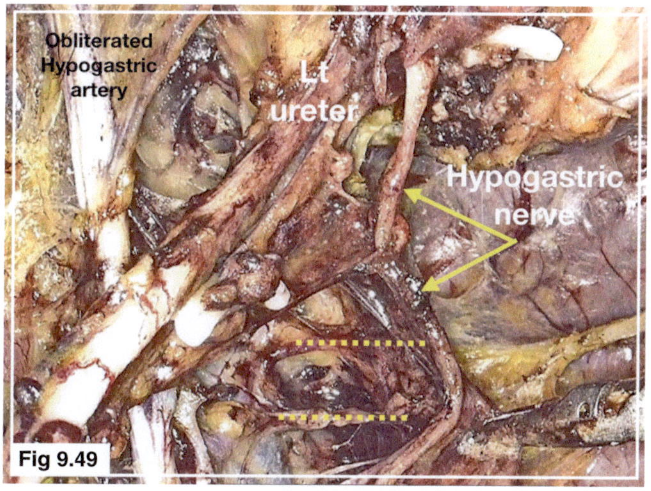

Fig. 9.49 Hypogastric nerve: The individual nerve that preserved supply to the bladder can be seen clearly in the image. It can be seen as a separate structure from the uterus and thus after hysterectomy the nerve is preserved and thus the bladder function is preserved. The yellow dotted lines indicate pelvic splanchnic nerves which supply the uterus and the bladder

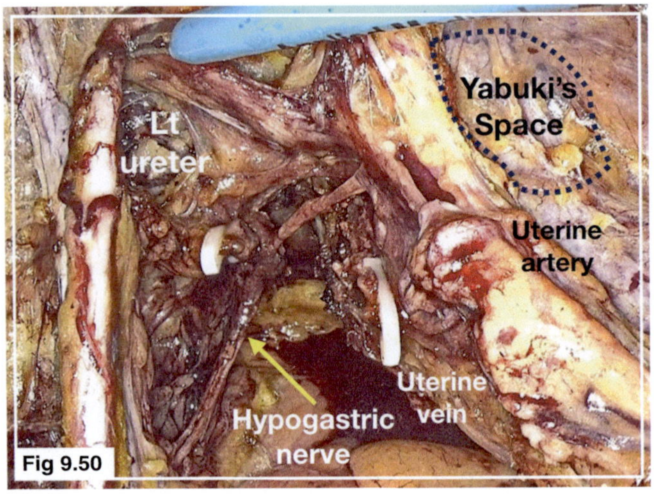

Fig. 9.50 Hypogastric nerve: After freeing the hypogastric nerve from the uterine vein, the nerve travels parallel with the ureter to supply the bladder. Hence the nerves need to be dissected at the Yabuki space as well, as shown in the figure. This area completely frees the ureter from all the attachments with uterus

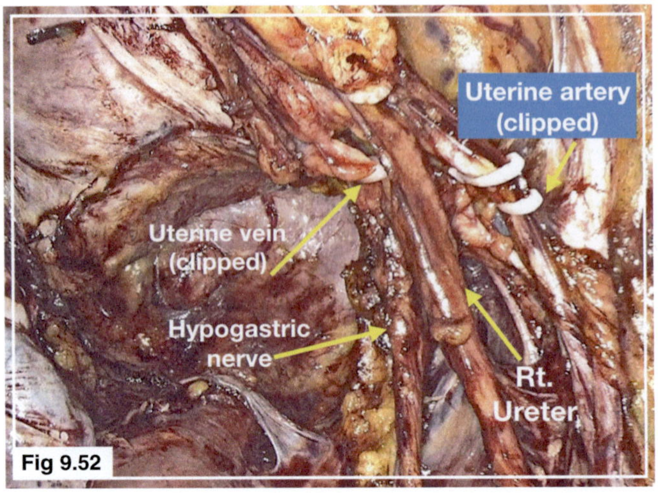

Fig. 9.52 Hypogastric nerve: Similar procedure can be done on the right side too as shown in the image. The uterine artery is clipped lateral to the ureter while the uterine vein under the ureter is clipped medial to the ureter. The hypogastric nerve is seen travelling parallel to the ureter but lateral and under the uterine vein clip. However if nerves are spared on one of the uteruses the bladder can still maintain its function post-operatively. Bilateral nerve sparing is not necessary in all cases

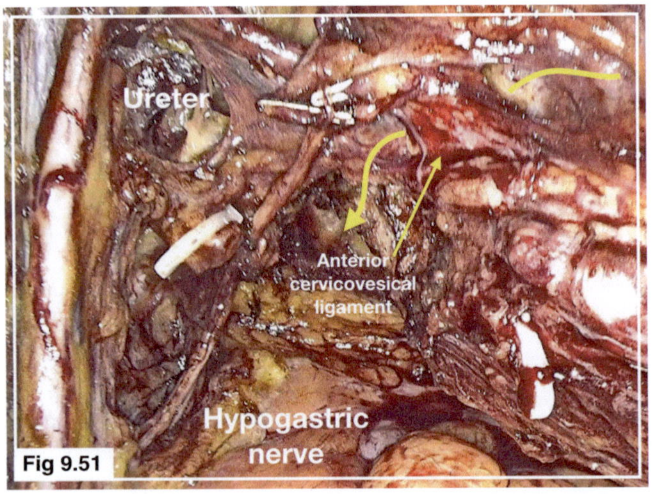

Fig. 9.51 Hypogastric nerve: In the above image the arrow mark shows the passage of nerves and ureter in the Yabuki space under the anterior cervicovesical ligament. Resection of the anterior cervicovesical ligament completely frees the ureter and the hypogastric nerve from the uterus, thus preserving its integrity and bladder function

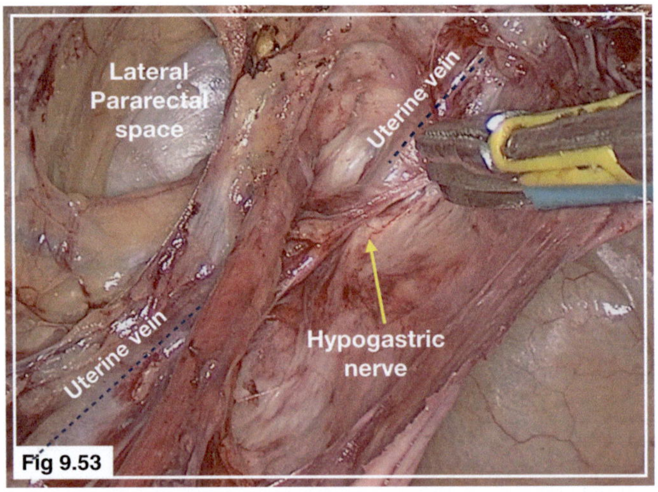

Fig. 9.53 Hypogastric nerve: In another case of Ca endometrium in an elderly postmenopausal patient, nerve-sparing laparoscopic radical hysterectomy was done. Due to old age a relatively less vascular space can be appreciated which would help in identifying the nerves more easily. In the image, the medial pararectal space has been dissected and the hypogastric nerve has been identified. Further dissection is shown in later images to show individual branches. The blue dotted lines denote the entire course of uterine vein, under the ureter. Their close relation to the hypogastric nerve has also been shown

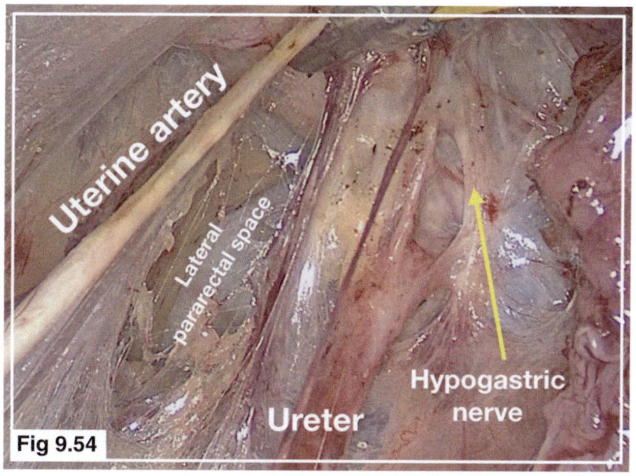

Fig. 9.54 Hypogastric nerve: Due to postmenopausal status the uterus artery appears reduced in calibre and relatively less vascular and tortuous. The ureter lies medial and under the uterine artery and nerve fibres can be seen being carried by the ureter. The uterine artery has been given an upward traction to clear more area for dissecting the ureter

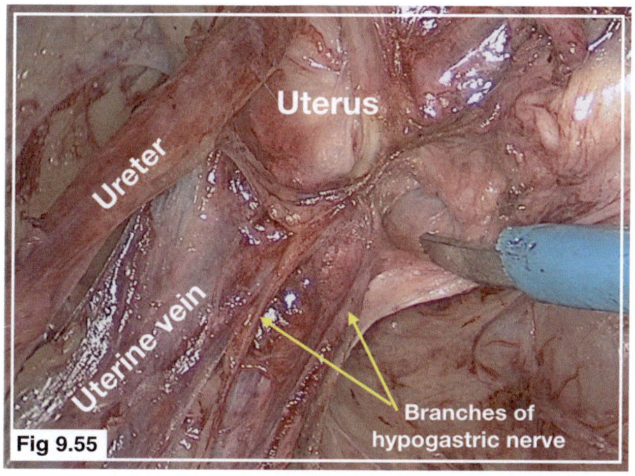

Fig. 9.55 Hypogastric nerve: Branches of the hypogastric nerve have been separated as individual branches. The ureter lies lateral to the nerves and the uterine vein close yet lateral to the nerves as well

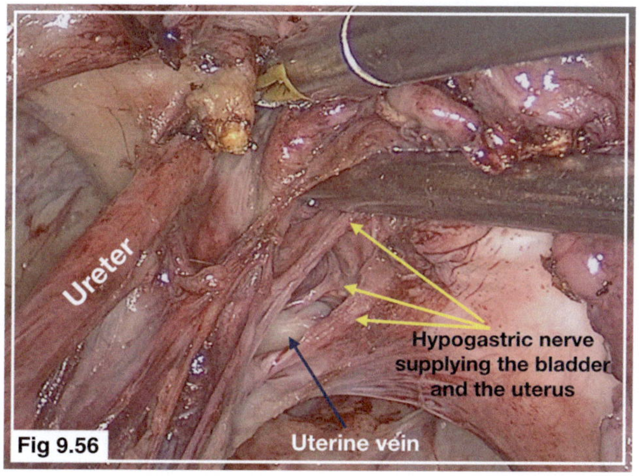

Fig. 9.56 Hypogastric nerve: The uterine vein is seen close and underneath the nerve fibres. The ureter lies lateral to the nerves and travels parallel to the uterus

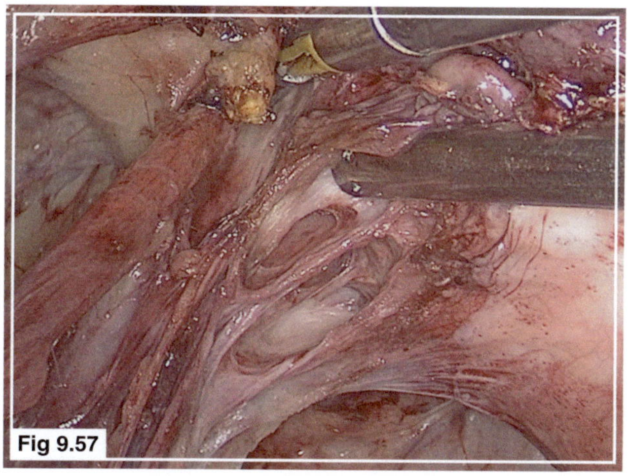

Fig. 9.57 Hypogastric nerve: The final picture (unlabelled) of dissected nerves and the structures surrounding them

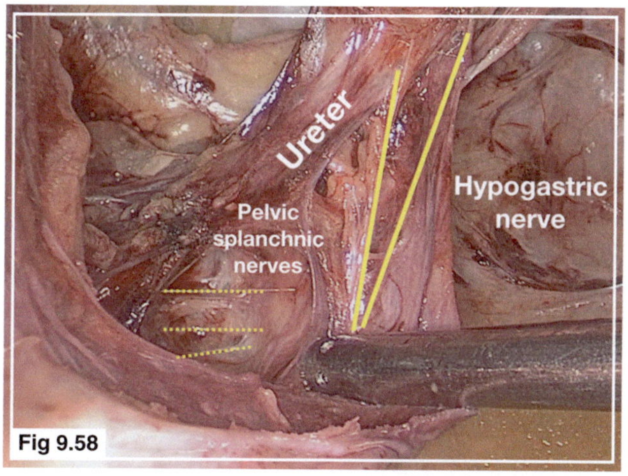

Fig. 9.58 Hypogastric nerve: While doing the dissection below distal to the uterus and near the sacral region the horizontal lines are the pelvic splanchnic nerve. They are discussed later. They communicate with the hypogastric nerve and innervate the bladder and uterus alike

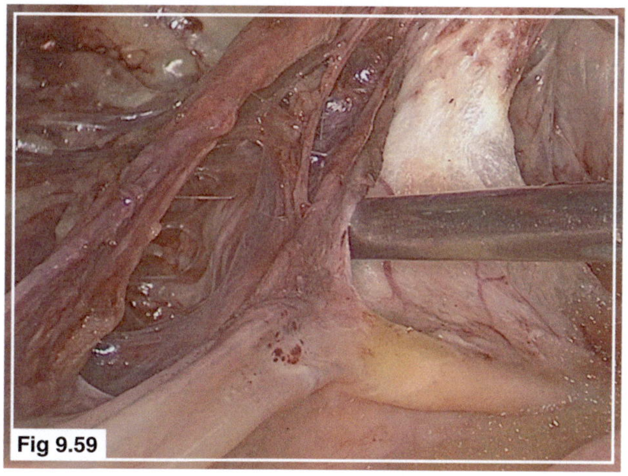

Fig. 9.59 Hypogastric nerve: Unlabelled image of the hypogastric nerve dissection with both branches supplying the uterus and bladder, respectively. The pelvic splanchnic nerve in parallel horizontal nerves

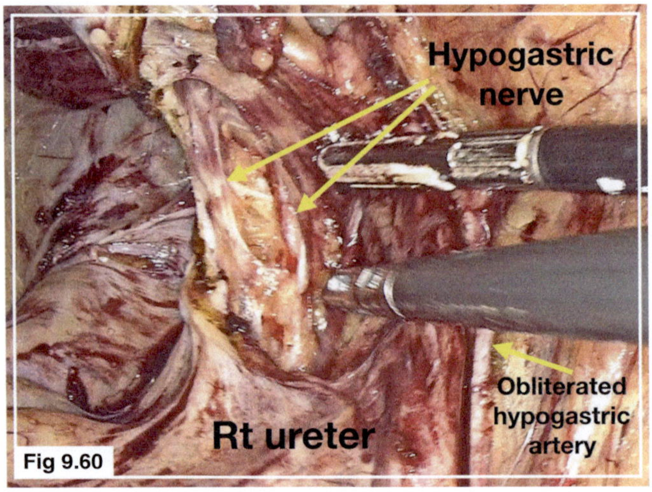

Fig. 9.60 Hypogastric nerve: In a case of laparoscopic nerve-sparing radical hysterectomy dissection is done medial to the ureter along the posterior leaf of broad ligament and the nerve fibres are identified

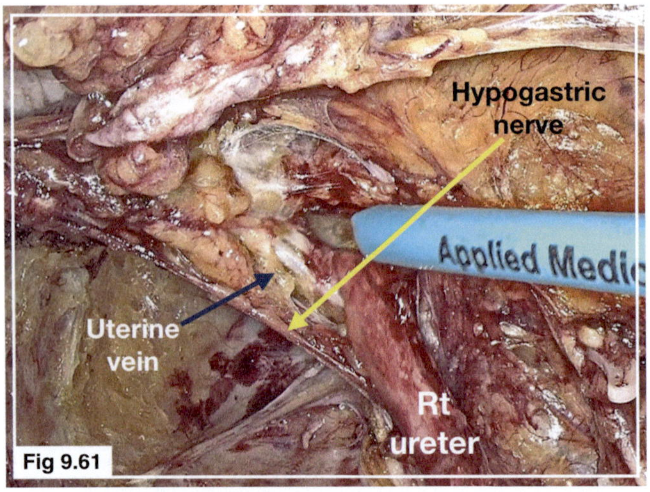

Fig. 9.61 Hypogastric nerve: After identifying the peritoneum, they are separated from the peritoneum and traced upwards towards the uterus where they are dissected from medial to the ureter. The uterine vein is also identified and dissected medial to the ureter

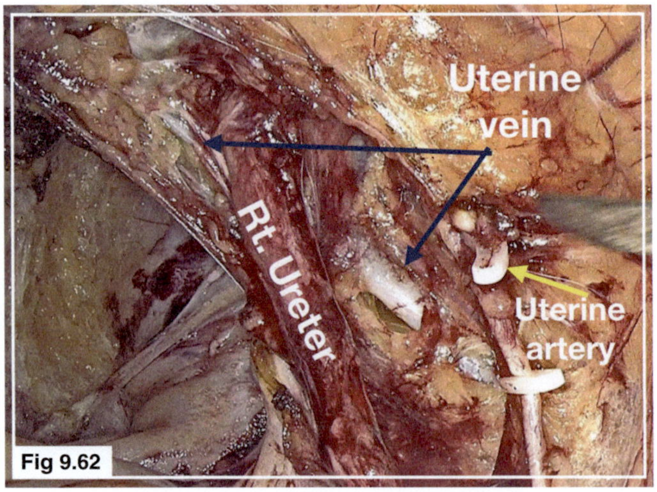

Fig. 9.62 Hypogastric nerve: The lateral part of the uterine vein is dissected so as to trace the entire course of the uterine vein. The clip if applied lateral to the uterine vein would lead to the nerves getting severed and taken up in the specimen for hysterectomy. This leads to significant loss of bladder function. It can be avoided and if indicated to clip the uterine vein medial to ureter. It is not indicated in advanced tumour as medial clipping of uterine vein would lead to reduced parametric tissue extraction/incomplete resection of the paracolpium

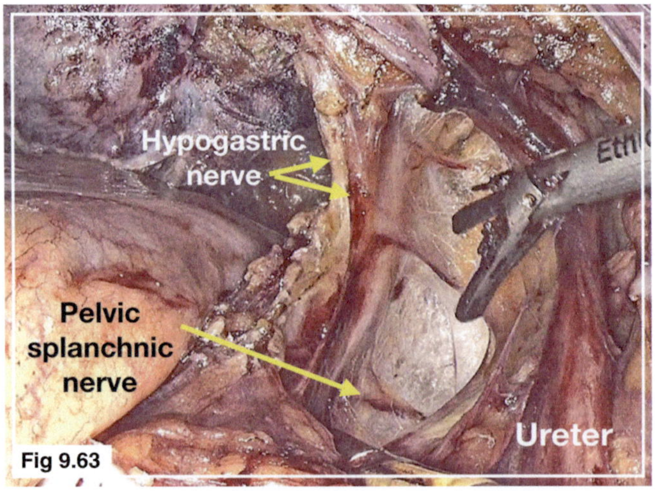

Fig. 9.63 Hypogastric nerve and pelvic splanchnic nerves: From the lateral pelvic wall parallel nerve fibres called the pelvic splanchnic nerves pass in horizontal fashion and communicate with the hypogastric nerve. This region forms the inferior hypogastric plexus

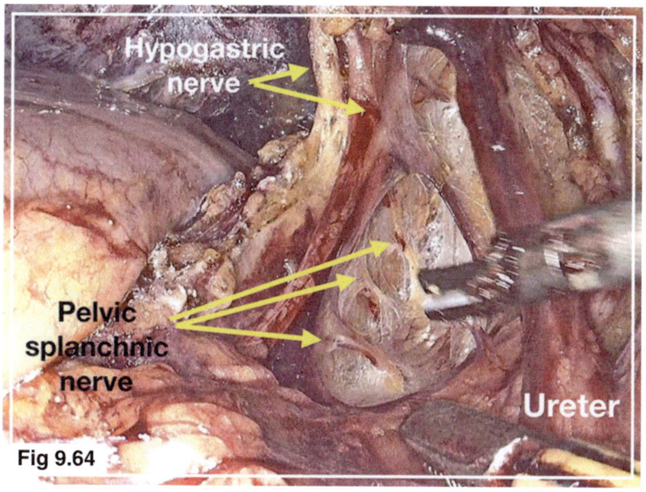

Fig. 9.64 Hypogastric nerve and pelvic splanchnic nerves: The pelvic splanchnic nerves are S2, 3 and 4 and they are often difficult to dissect. They are discussed in detail later in the chapter

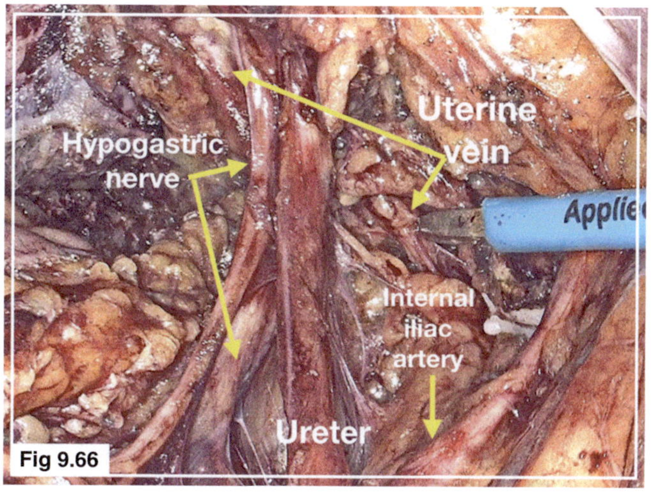

Fig. 9.66 Hypogastric nerve: The final view after dissection the branches of hypogastric nerves, the uterine vein dissected along its complete course and the ureter dividing the uterine vein into medial and lateral halves

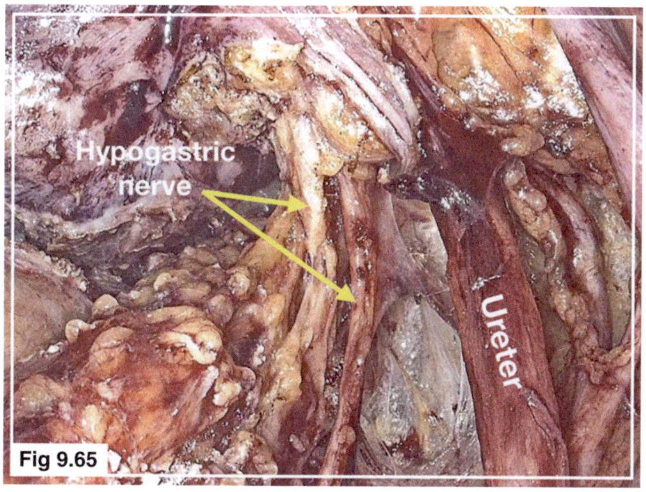

Fig. 9.65 Hypogastric nerve: The hypogastric nerve is divided into its branches supplying the uterus and the bladder, respectively. This is an important step in nerve-sparing radical hysterectomy

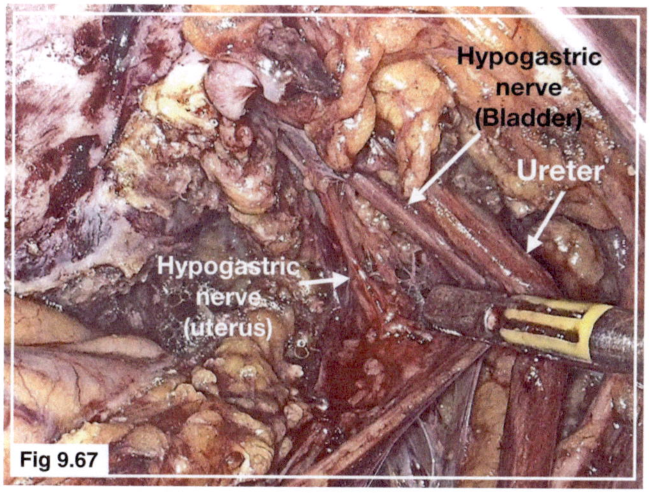

Fig. 9.67 Hypogastric nerve: Gentle traction is applied onto the branch of hypogastric nerve supplying the bladder. This branch is lateralised as it needs to be preserved

9.4 Pelvic Splanchnic Nerve

They arise from S2, 3 and 4 sacral nerves; they run parallel to the uterine vein on their way to join the hypogastric nerve from the lateral side. Thus, the distal part of the uterine vein becomes an important landmark to identify and preserve these nerves (Figs. 9.68, 9.69, 9.70, 9.71, 9.72, 9.73, and 9.74).

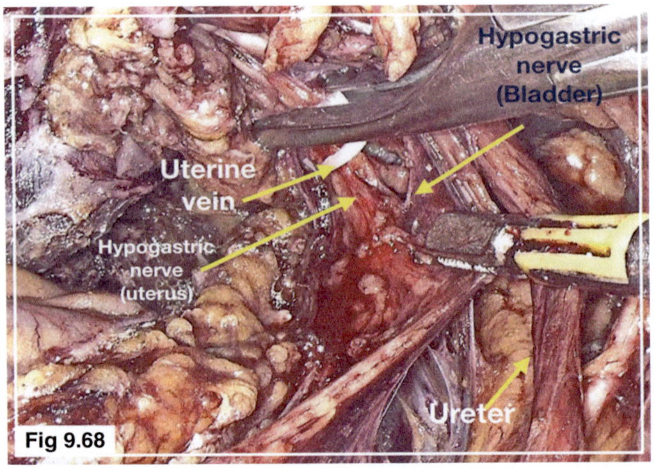

Fig. 9.68 Hypogastric nerve: Clips applied on the medial part of uterine vein incorporating the branch of hypogastric nerve supplying the uterus which is to be sacrificed. But the branch of hypogastric nerve which supplies the bladder is preserved. Thus nerve-sparing radical hysterectomy can be achieved

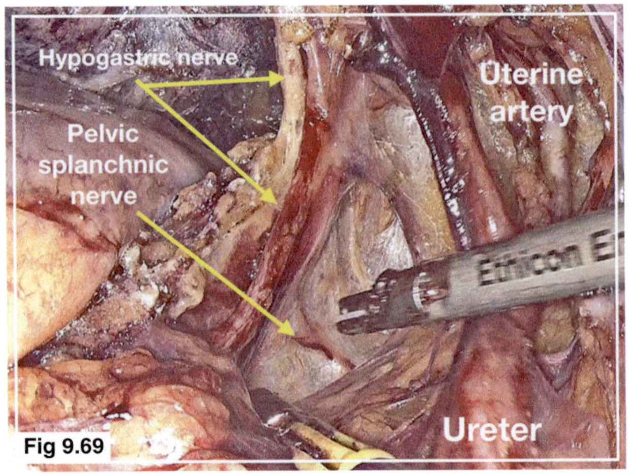

Fig. 9.69 Pelvic splanchnic nerves: S2, 3 and 4 root values of these fragile nerves are difficult to dissect as they travel horizontal to the other important structures in the pelvis which leads to severing the nerves often. They travel from the latter wall and along the uterine vein to supply the uterus and the bladder with the hypogastric nerves

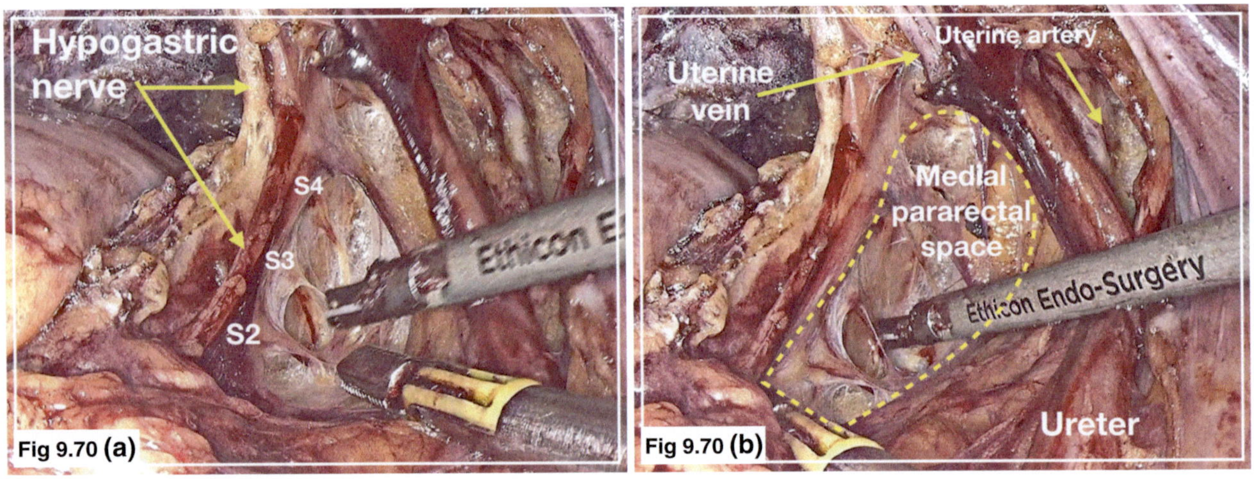

Fig. 9.70 (**a**, **b**) Pelvic splanchnic nerves: They are best seen medial to the ureter towards the sacrum. They are often seen in groups of three only. The following images will be shown in pairs and with variable obscurity by retroperitoneal fat and connective tissue

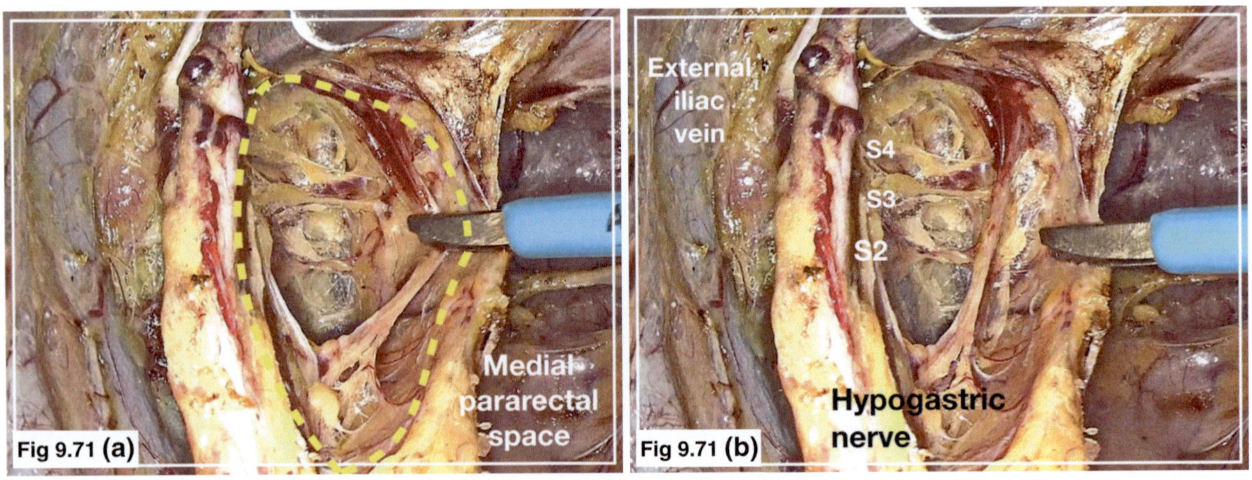

Fig. 9.71 (**a**, **b**) Pelvic splanchnic nerves: These nerves are confined to the medial pararectal space only. Panoramic view gives orientation of these nerves with other vital structures

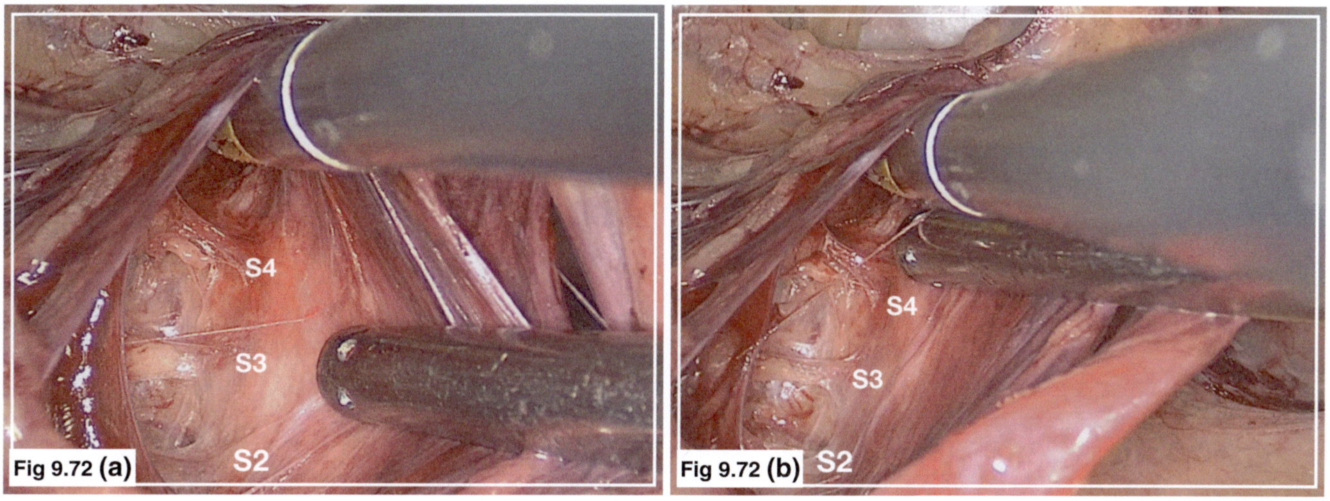

Fig. 9.72 (**a**, **b**) Pelvic splanchnic nerves: Pelvic splanchnic nerves carry parasympathetic innervation to the uterus bladder and rectum

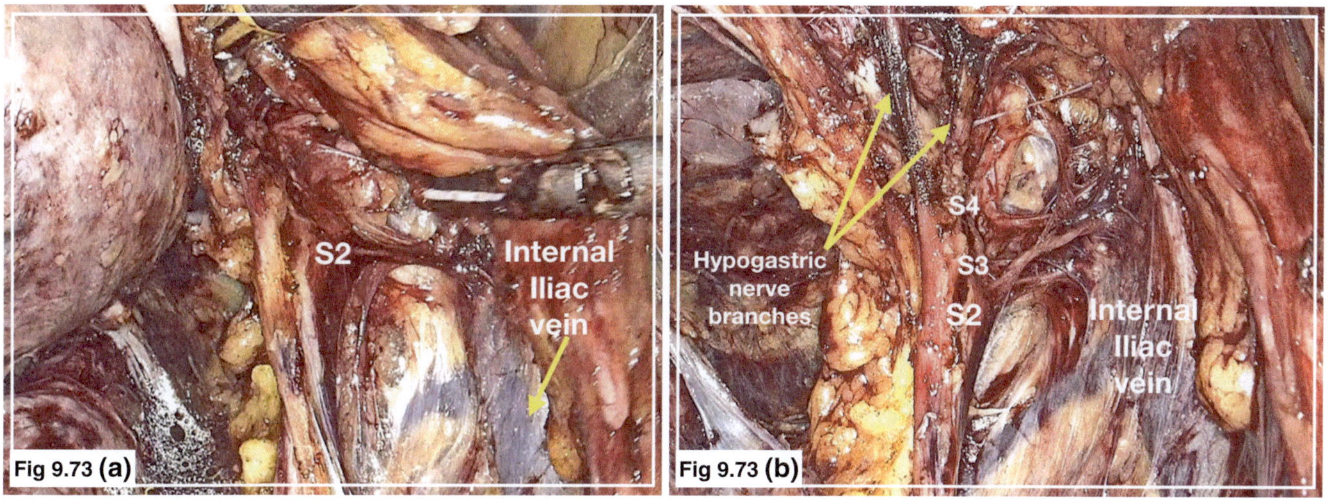

Fig. 9.73 (**a**, **b**) Pelvic splanchnic nerves: These pelvic splanchnic nerves come in close approximation to the internal iliac vein and form the structure known as *nervi erigentes*

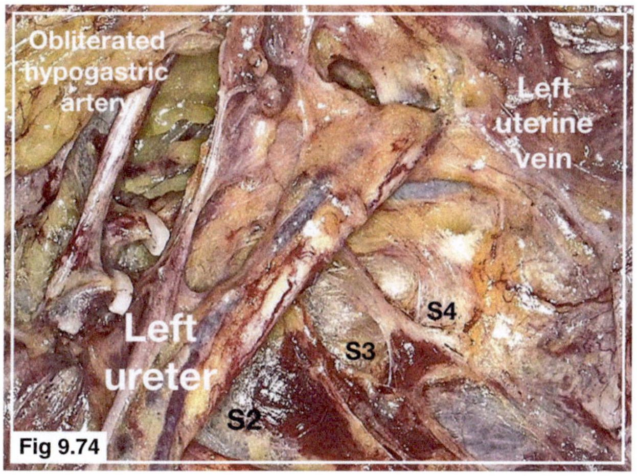

Fig. 9.74 Pelvic splanchnic nerves: Relation of pelvic splanchnic nerve with the uterine vein can be seen. The nerves lie inferior and run parallel to the uterine vein

9.5 Sciatic Nerve

Largest nerve of the body, arising from L4, 5, S1–2. It can be visualised on the floor of the pelvis at the level of the sacral promontory by retracting the common iliac vessels medially (Figs. 9.75, 9.76, 9.77, 9.78, and 9.79).

Rules

The importance of understanding the neuroanatomy is for the following procedures:

(a) Nerve-sparing surgery—radical or for endometriosis
(b) Presacral neurectomy for chronic pelvic pain
(c) Artificial stimulation of nerves for bladder and bowel incontinence

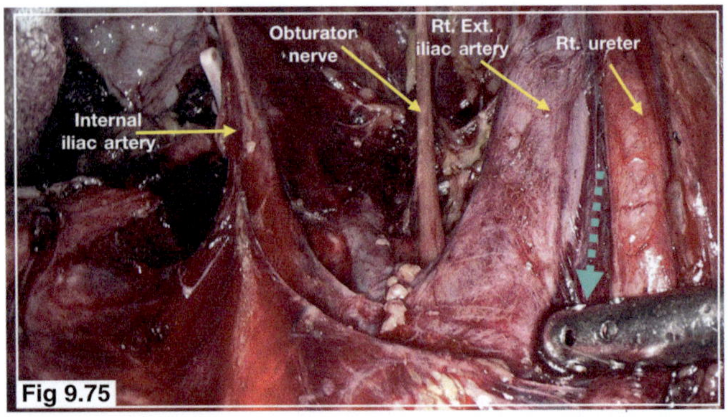

Fig. 9.75 The image has been taken form a case of Laparoscopic radical hysterectomy with bilateral pelvic lymphadenectomy. At this point after the Lymph node dissection in the pelvic region, the ureter can be seen retracted by the suction tip and placed above the external iliac artery and the obturator nerve exposed. The next step in surgery mobilisation of the external iliac artery. This is one by laterally dissecting the external iliac artery up to the entire segment of the common iliac artery. (direction iodinated in blue arrows)

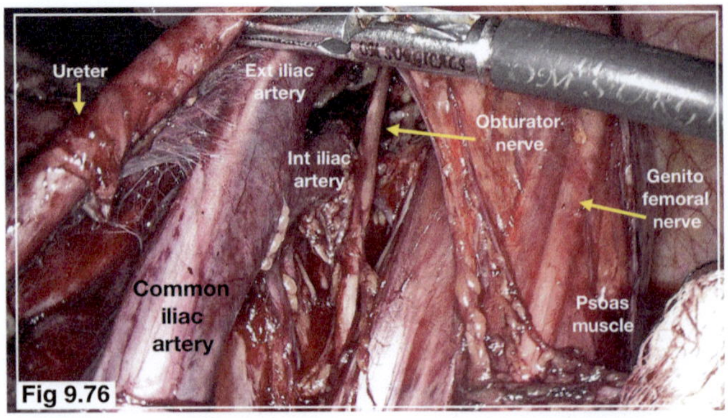

Fig. 9.76 The cranially extended dissection of the external iliac artery to at least half the segment of the common iliac artery exposes the root of the obturator nerve as seen in the image. Dissection is carried out in the plane of the iliac arteries along the medial border of the PSOAS muscle

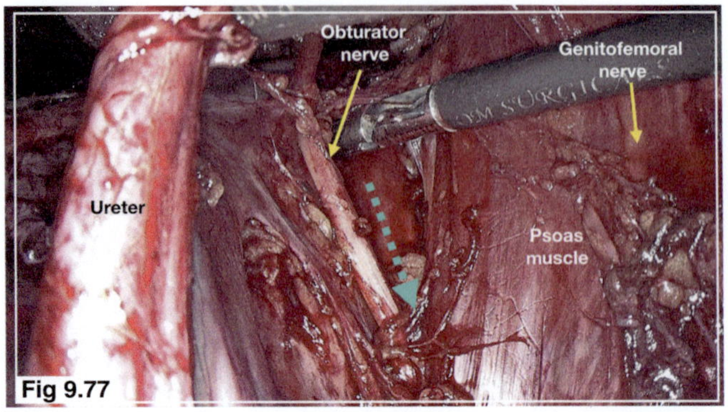

Fig. 9.77 The direction of dissection has been indicated in blue arrows tracing the obturator nerve near to its origin

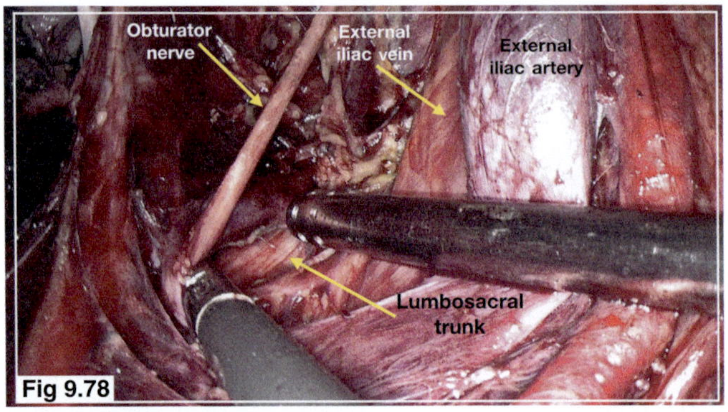

Fig. 9.78 Dissection is done near the origin of the obturator nerve. This dissection carried out along a plane perpendicular to the obturator nerve exposes the anterior division of the lumbosacral trunk of the sciatic nerve. The posterior division remain behind the pyriformis muscle. The anterior and posterior division fuse outside the pelvis to form the sciatic nerve. The poor value of obturator nerve is L2, 3, 4 while the root value of sciatic nerve is L4, 5-S1, 2, 3

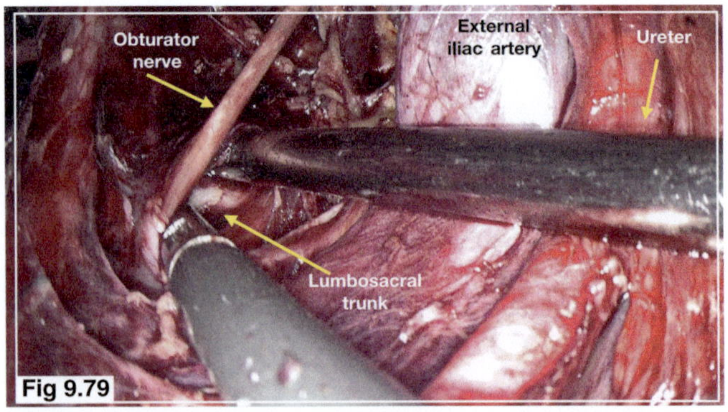

Fig. 9.79 Dissection is done near the origin of the obturator nerve. This dissection carried out along a plane perpendicular to the obturator nerve exposes the anterior division of the lumbosacral trunk of the sciatic nerve. The posterior division remain behind the pyriformis muscle. The anterior and posterior division fuse outside the pelvis to form the sciatic nerve. The poor value of obturator nerve is L2, 3, 4 while the root value of sciatic nerve is L4, 5-S1, 2, 3

Lymphatics

10

The anatomical knowledge of the lymph node location and the lymphatics is very important. The entire cancer surgery is based on the lymph nodes draining the affected part. The lymph node clearance has a huge impact on the entire overall survival. Hence the knowledge of lymphatics and lymph nodes and pattern of spread of cancers is important. The pattern of spread is related to the anatomy and there are some general rules for the lymphatic drainage in the entire body (Fig. 10.1).

The general rules are as follows:

1. Lymphatics follow the veins. Hence knowledge of the blood supply of any organ is important as this will lead to the draining lymph nodes (Figs. 10.2 and 10.3).
2. Squamous cell cancers spread by lymphatic permeation while adenocarcinomas spread by lymphatic embolisation. Therefore the lymph node dissection in squamous cancers should be en bloc. The skip metastasis is more common in adenocarcinoma (Fig. 10.4a, b).
3. Lymphovascular embolisation/spread is an independent prognostic factor. Once the lymphovascular space is involved the chances of micrometastasis increase even if the lymph nodes are showing no tutor on histopathology (Fig. 10.5).
4. The lymph node metastasis is directly proportional to the grade and depth of invasion. Anatomically the lymphatics lie in the submucosa and hence the depth of involvement

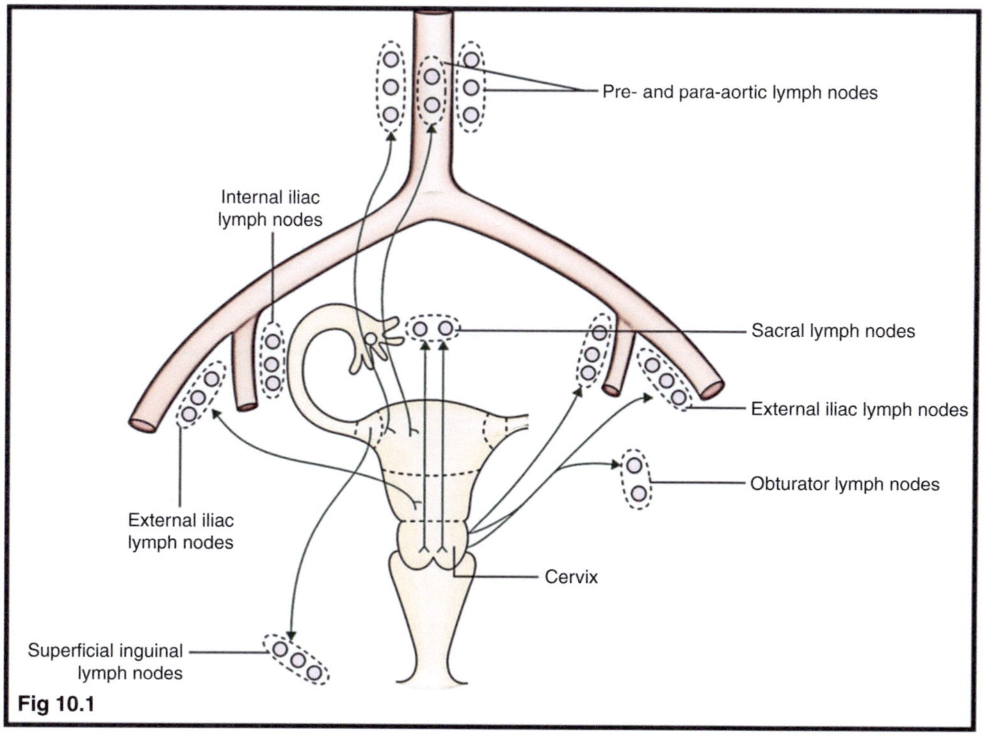

Fig. 10.1 Lymphatics: The general distribution of the female genital system and the respective lymph nodes drained by the parts of the organs

S. Puntambekar et al., *Laparoscopic Pelvic Anatomy in Females*, https://doi.org/10.1007/978-981-13-8653-4_10

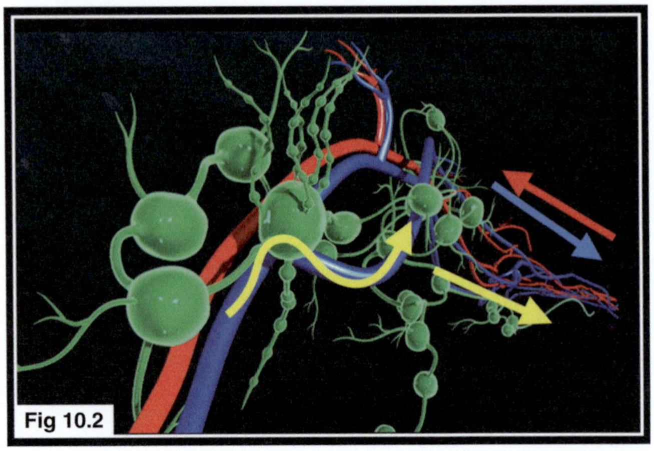

Fig. 10.2 Lymphatics rule: Diagrammatic representation of the flow of lymphatics along the vein. *Lymphatics follow the veins*

is very important to decide the adjuvant treatment in the absence of lymph node involvement (ref) (Fig. 10.6).

5. Sentinel node is a group of nodes and is the first echelon where the cancers spread. This can be identified by blue dye or indocyanine green injection.

   The basis of sentinel node is also anatomical showing that the lymph node spread takes place in a step ladder fashion and hence absence of sentinel node metastasis can avoid the further lymph node dissection (Fig. 10.7a, b).

   All the lymph nodes lie in a chain and are covered by fascia. This knowledge of anatomy is important for surgical clearance. All the lymph nodes thus can be removed en bloc (figure showing en bloc removal) (Fig. 10.8a, b).
6. The sentinel nodes can be identified only in uterine and cervical cancers (Fig. 10.9a, b)

Fig. 10.3 Lymphatics rule: *Lymphatics follow the veins*. The rule of lymphatics follows that the vein is followed universally all over the human body. The diagram represents the rule explained

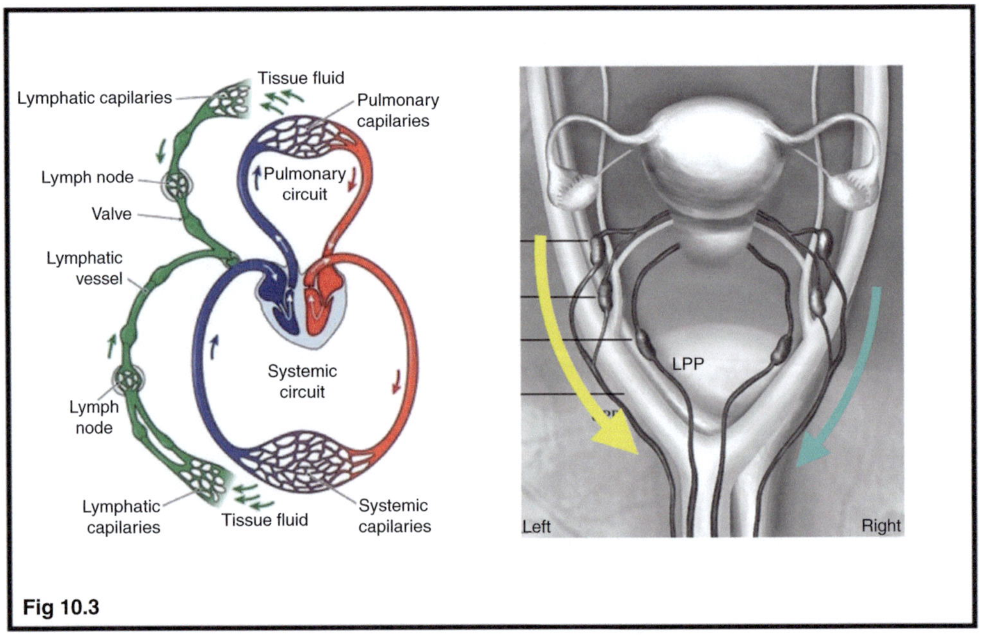

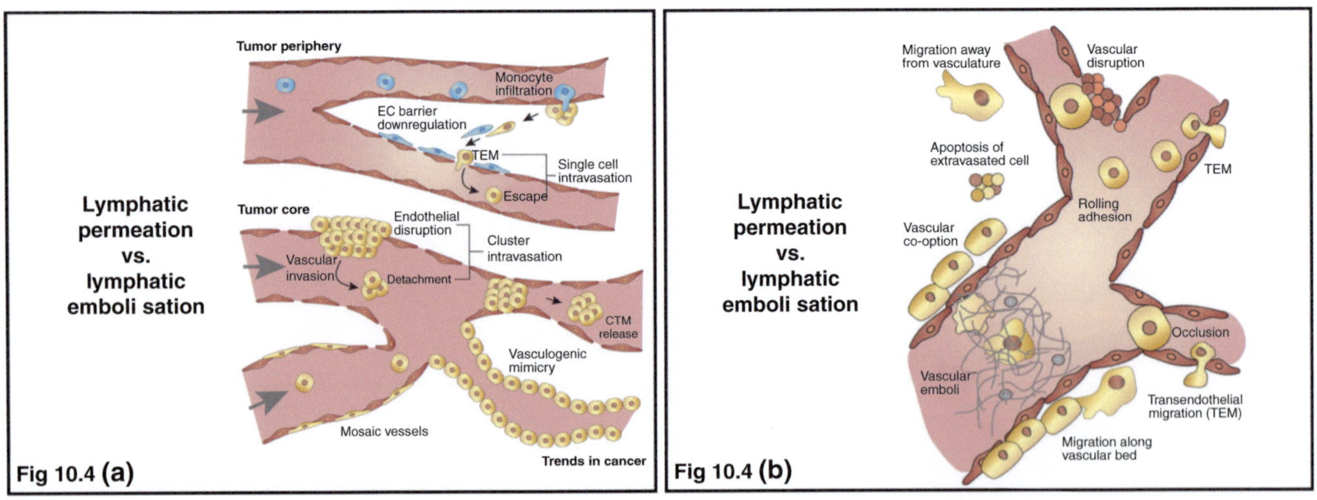

Fig. 10.4 (**a**, **b**) Lymphatics rule: Permeation vs. embolisation. The following image represents the different types of spread by lymphatics

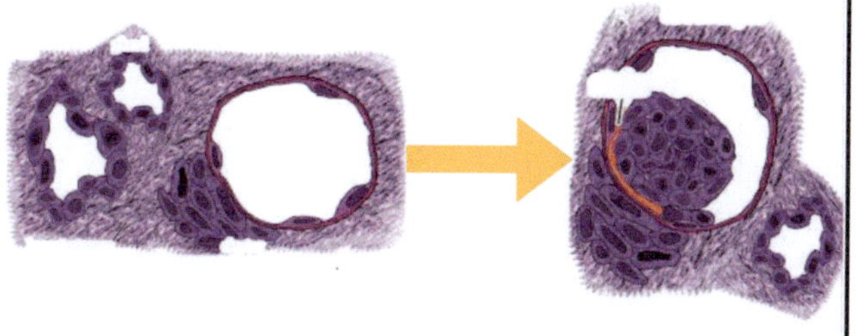

Fig 10.5

Fig. 10.5 Lymphatics rule: Lymphovascular space invasion. The image represents lymphovascular invasion of tumour cells

7. The ovarian cancer sentinel nodes cannot be identified as we cannot inject the ovaries (Fig. 10.10).

The lymph nodes draining the pelvic organs can be classified as

1. Ilio-obturator chain
2. Lumbosacral chain
3. Internal iliac chain (figure from uterine transplant)
4. Para-aortic chain (figure from extra-peritoneal para-aortic) (Fig. 10.11)

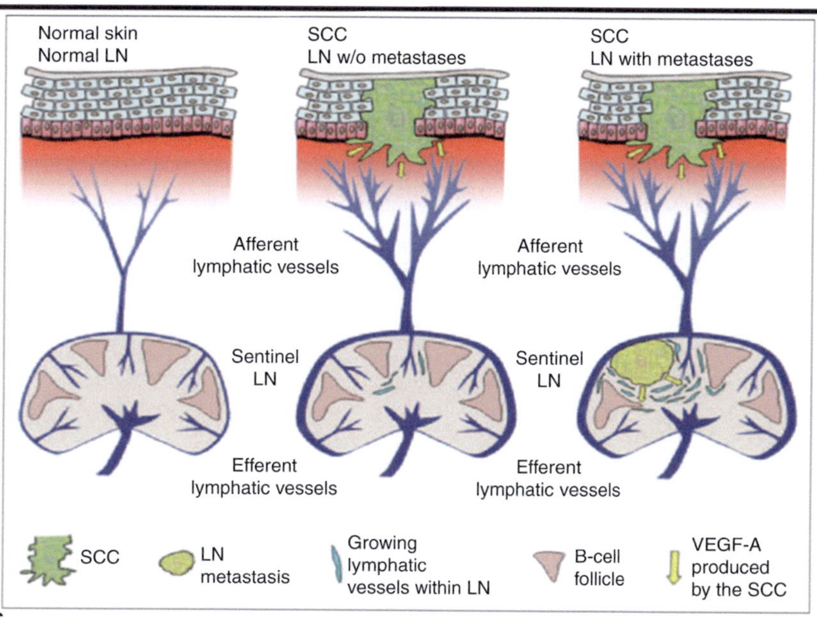

Fig 10.6

Fig. 10.6 Lymphatics rule: Depth of invasion: The image represents the rule of depth of invasion of tumour being directly proportional to the lymph node metastasis

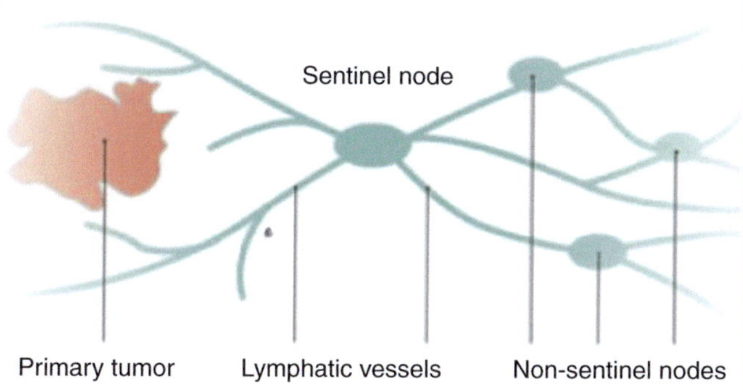

Fig 10.7 (a)

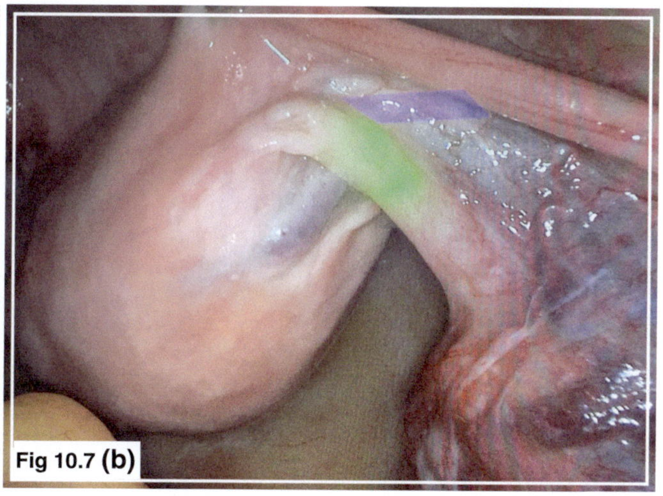

Fig 10.7 (b)

Fig. 10.7 (**a**, **b**) Lymphatics rule: Sentinel lymph nodes: The figure (**a**) shows the rule of sentinel lymph nodes and their distribution form the primary source. The figure (**b**) shows real-time images of the indocyanine green stain being taken up by the uterus. The visualisation of indocyanine green is with the help of special camera filters. These images have been taken with the help of NOVADAQ systems

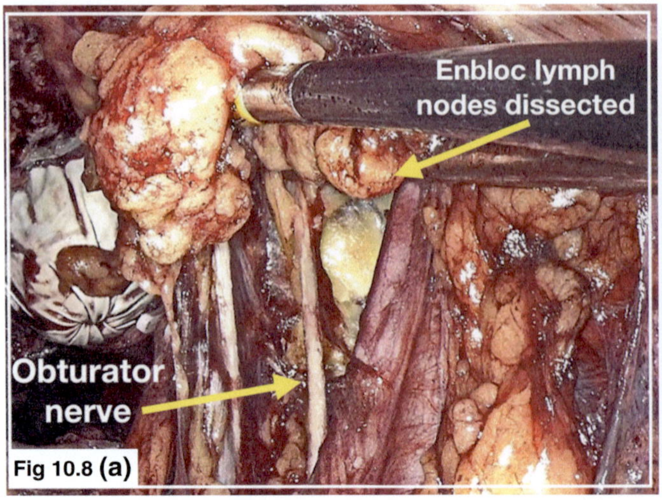

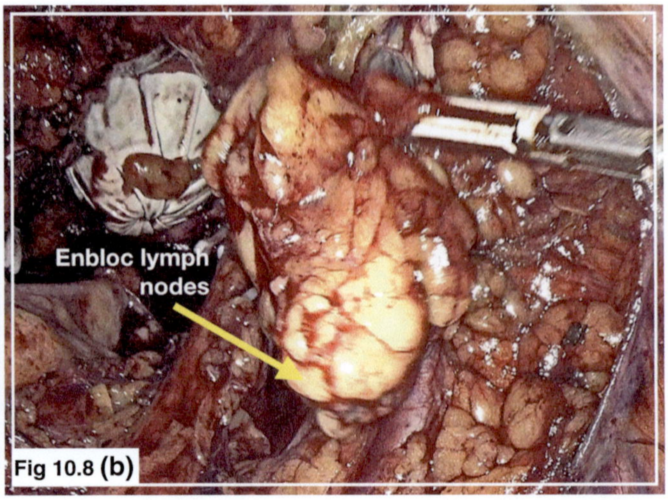

Fig. 10.8 (**a**, **b**) Lymphatics rule: En bloc dissection: The pair of images suggest that the lymph nodes are arranged in chains. There are no fascias intersecting the chain of lymph nodes which makes it easier to dissect without the use of an energy source. Thus en bloc lymph node dissection prevents bleeding in the process

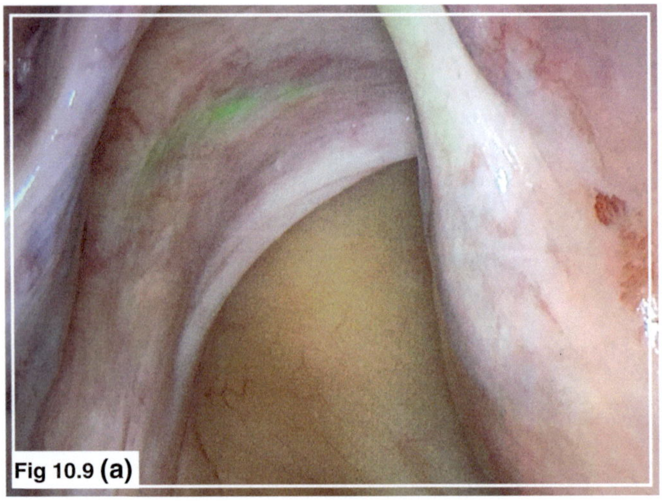

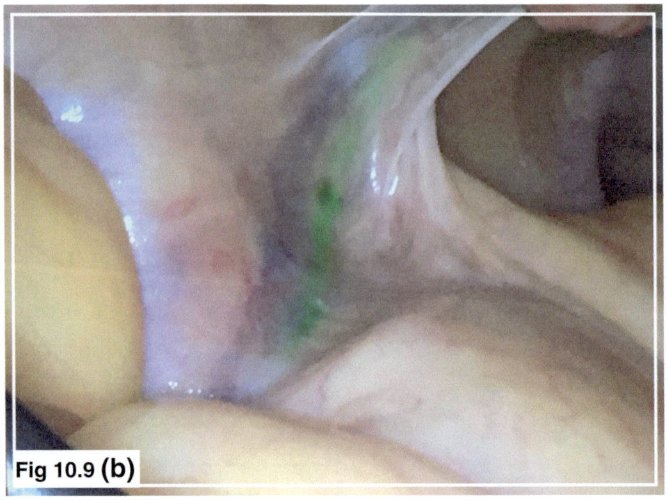

Fig. 10.9 (**a**, **b**) Lymphatics rule: The images from NOVADAQ systems show concentration of indocyanine green stain at the level of obturator lymph nodes. These images were taken from a case of cervical cancer stage IIa with visual confirmation of lymph node metastasis

Fig. 10.10 Lymphatics rule: The image is taken from a case of advanced ovarian cancer stage IIIc. Thus due to lack of infiltration to the ovary, even advanced-stage ovarian cancer cannot be detected by sentinel node biopsy. More so, the ovarian malignancies spread to para-aortic lymph nodes which makes it difficult to view the drainage of dye

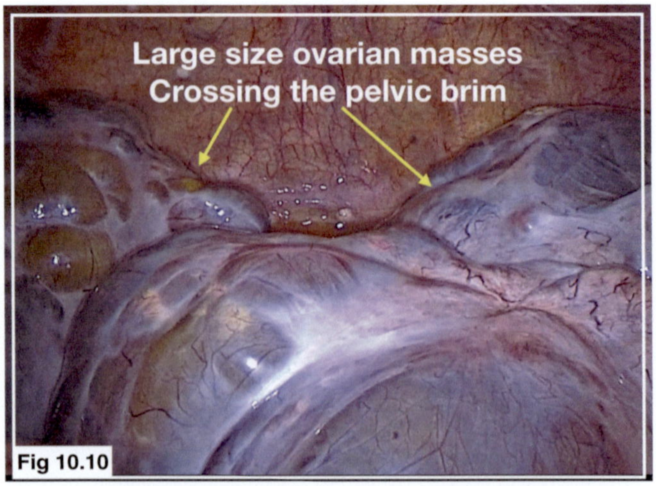

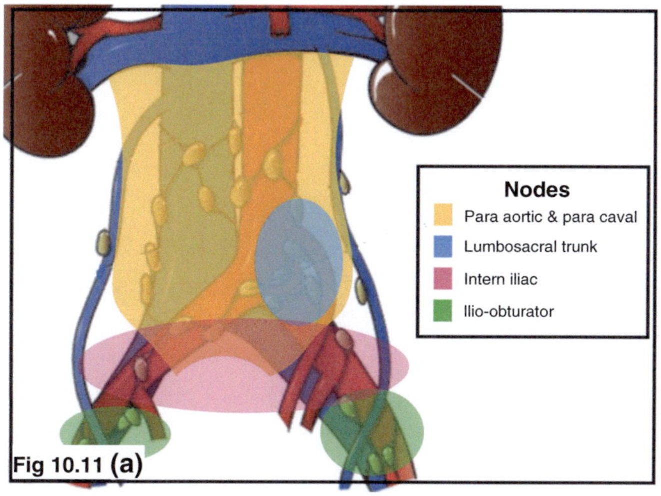

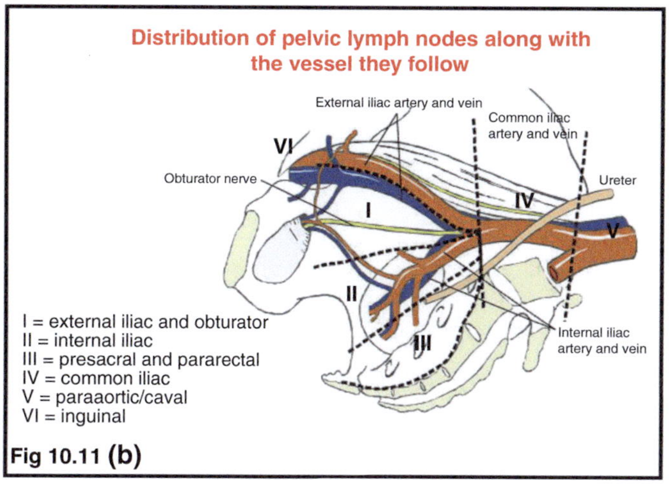

Fig. 10.11 (**a**) Lymph nodes: The image depicts a collage of the lymph nodes and their location shaded with yellow circles representing the described lymph node in detail later. (**b**) Similar distribution of pelvic lymph nodes has been demonstrated along with its venous drainage

10.1 Ilio-Obturator Nodes

1. These are situated between the external and internal iliac vessels (Figs. 10.12 and 10.13a–f).
2. The nodes are engulfed in a fascial covering and do not receive blood supply from the external or internal vessels and hence can be removed en bloc (Fig. 10.13g–j).
3. They are the first echelon/first station of spread from the cervical cancers and endocervical cancers. This is due to the anatomical venous drainage of these parts through the superficial and deep uterine veins (Fig. 10.13k–m).
4. The uterine veins travel through the Mackenrodt's ligaments and so do the lymphatic. This is the reason for lateral clearance of these ligaments in cancer surgery (Fig. 10.13n).
5. There is no anatomical continuation of the Mackenrodt's ligament beyond the internal iliac veins. This is the reason that the ilio-obturator nodes cannot be removed en bloc with uterus (figure showing lymph nodes being separately taken out) (Fig. 10.13o, p).
6. In Piver type III/Querleu CII the cardinal ligaments are transected at its lateral-most limit and hence the chances of spillage of the cancer cells from the lymphatics are less, decreasing the incidence of pelvic recurrences (Fig. 10.13q, r).
7. In the type II or C1 dissection the cardinal ligaments along with lymphatics are transected medial to the ureter and hence this type is reserved only for early cancers. Thus the basis of lymph node and lymphatic clearance is anatomy (figure of nerve sparing where the Mackenrodt's is taken medial to the ureter) (Fig. 10.13s, t).
8. The obturator nodes are anterior to the obturator nerve and vessels. Hence the plane of dissection should be anterior to the obturator nerve (Fig. 10.13u–z).

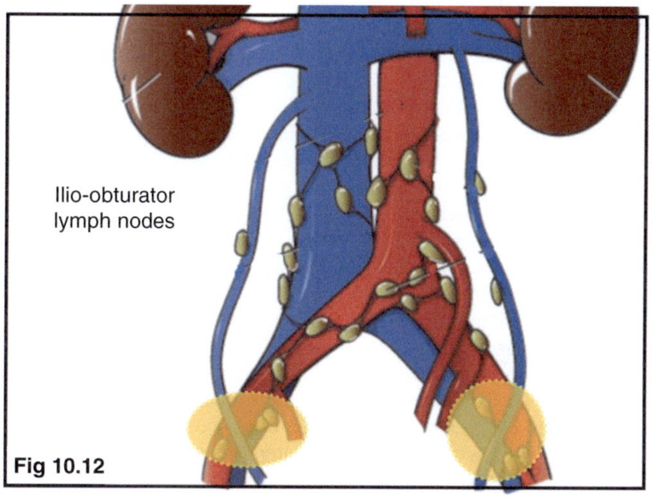

Fig. 10.12 Ilio-obturator lymph nodes: The diagrammatic representation and location of the ilio-obturator lymph nodes

9. The anatomical limits are laterally the genitofemoral nerve, medially to the anterior division of the internal iliac artery, cranially the bifurcation of the common iliac vein and caudally the corona mortis identified by the presence of superficial circumflex iliac vein crossing the pelvic bone transversely (multiple figures) (Fig. 10.14a–h).
10. Due to the fact that the entire nodes lie in one fascial covering without receiving the blood supply from the external iliac vessels the technique of dissection is always to remain parallel to the vessels (Fig. 10.14i, j).
11. Remain anterior to the obturator nerve and vessels (Fig. 10.14k, l).
12. The upper limit is the bifurcation of common iliac veins. The obturator nerve originates at the level of bifurcation (Fig. 10.14m–o).

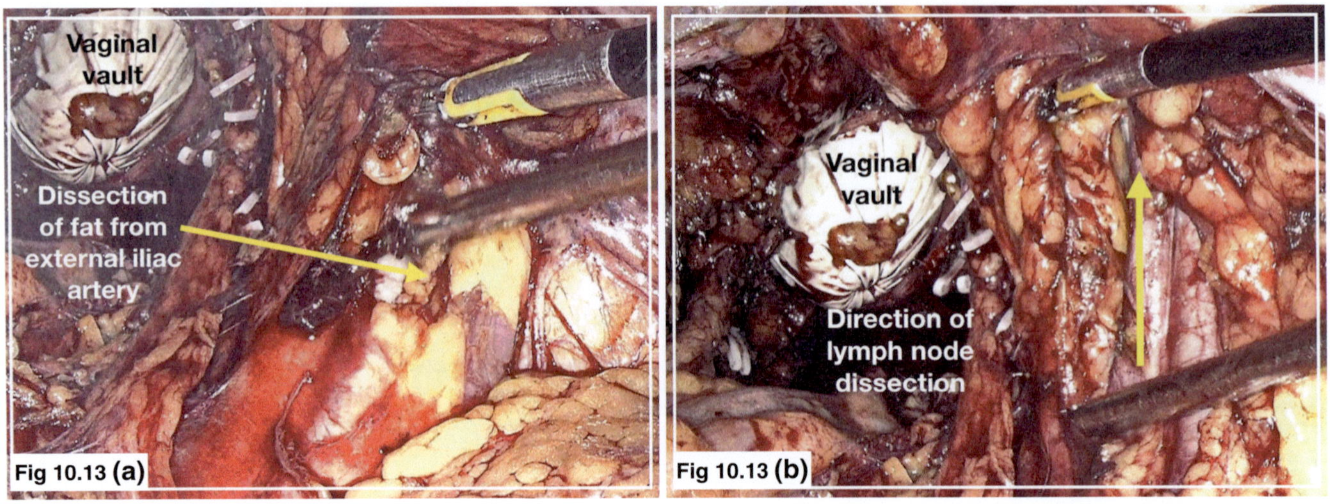

Fig. 10.13 Ilio-obturator lymph nodes: (**a**) This image has been taken from a case of Ca cervix undergoing laparoscopic radical hysterectomy with pelvic lymph node dissection. Here lymph node dissection is done after hysterectomy as more working area is provided after retrieval of the specimen. (**b**) The yellow arrow directs towards the blunt dissection done with the suction tip. The lymph nodes appear as clusters in chains as discussed previously. The principle is to develop a groove of separation between the internal and the external iliac arteries. (**c**) The plane of dissection can be traced right up to the anterior abdominal wall along the obliterated hypogastric artery. (**d**) The white line denotes the course of the internal iliac artery ultimately terminating into the obliterated hypogastric artery, thus keeping in consideration that the dissection should always be carried out lateral to the internal iliac artery and the obliterated hypogastric artery. (**e**) After creating the groove between the iliac vessel further dissection deepens the plane of dissection lymph nodes. The first structure to appear is the obturator nerve. This is the limit of dissection. No further deeper planes need to be created. (**f**) Dissection is carried along anterior to the obturator nerve and the whole group of lymph nodes are peeled off the obturator nerve as seen in the image. The internal iliac vein can be seen underneath the obturator nerve. (**g**) En bloc removal: As seen in the image merely stripping off from above and anterior to the obturator nerve peels all connected lymph nodes in chain ensuring an en bloc removal. (**h**) En bloc removal: Most dissection above obturator nerve is done from caudal to cranial direction. Sometimes the obturator needs to be dissected anterior to ensure that all lymph nodes are removed from the cave underneath the perineum near the anterior abdominal wall. (**i**) En bloc removal: The lateral limit of dissection is the lateral limit of dissection which is often seen during lymph node dissection. Sometimes by the sheer weight of the lymph nodes the later limit is exposed and thus helps easy en bloc dissection of the lymph nodes. (**j**) En bloc removal: The final picture as it appears after lymph node dissection. The obliterated hypogastric artery, obturator nerve and external iliac vein seen in medal to lateral sequence with the pubis bone anterolaterally placed and intermittently filled with empty spaces which were once covered with lymph nodes and fatty tissue. (**k**) Relation to uterine vein: One of the main reasons as to why the obturator nodes are the sentinel nodes for cervical and endocervical cancers is because of its close proximity and relation with the uterine veins. This also helps in explaining the first rule mentioned previously as lymphatics follow the veins. The ureter is seen anterior and above the uterine vein. "The fat surrounding the vein and the ureter consolidate lateral to the ureter to form the obturator lymph node. (**l**) Relation to uterine vein: In a high magnification (zoomed in) of the previous image we can see the relation of the uterine vein lying below the ureter as discussed in previous chapters and the area comprising the obturator nodes has been labelled. (**m**) Relation to uterine vein: The above-mentioned structures have been drawn with coloured lines for better understanding of the anatomy. (**n**) Relation to uterine vein: The Mackenrodt's ligament when dissected reveals vascular structures like uterine artery and vein passing across the ligament. Lateral clearance of the uterine vein is of oncological significance. The uterosacral ligament is also partly dissected to help completely open up the Mackenrodt's ligament. (**o**) Relation to uterine vein: The uterosacral ligament has been kept untouched for better understanding of the structures covered in the Mackenrodt's ligament. The internal iliac vein can be seen draing its tributaries from the uterine vein superiorly and the presacral veins inferiorly. (**p**) Relation to uterine vein: The structures described above have been labelled along with their course for a better understanding. The uterine vein which travels along a congruent course of the uterine artery going further to drain into the internal iliac vein is better understood with this image. (**q**) Relation to uterine vein: As explained in a Piver type III/Querleu CII the uterine artery being clipped laterally allows most of the fatty tissue to be directed off with the specimen. Theoretical evidence exists which states that higher lymph node yields when parametric is excised along with the specimen. (**r**) Relation to uterine vein: Another image taken from a case of laparoscopic radical hysterectomy for Ca cervix showing lateral ligation of the uterine vein to incorporate maximum Mackenrodt's ligament tissue with the specimen. Deep uterine veins can be seen separately. The deep coalesce to form the superficial thicker uterine vein which ultimately drains into the internal iliac vein. (**s**) Relation to uterine vein: Routine dissection of the uterine vein done lateral to the ureter which is later traced medially. (**t**) Relation to uterine vein: The uterine vein is traced medially and clipped. The uterine artery has already been clipped. These steps are done for Piver type II or Querleu CI hysterectomy reserved for early-stage cancers. (**u**) Relation to uterine vein: Similarly in another case of nerve-sparing laparoscopic radical hysterectomy both the uterine veins are seen clipped medial to the ureter. (**v–x**) Anterior to obturator nerve: In the past few images we had been explaining the relation of the lymph nodes to uterine vein. This area was always medial to the internal iliac artery. The following image shows lymph node dissection done lateral to the internal iliac artery. *Obturator nerve and vessels are the only structures which travel from medial to lateral onto the lateral pelvic wall.* Rest all structures travel from lateral to medial as discussed in the initial chapters. (**y, z**) Anterior to obturator nerve: The following images describe the perils of forceful dissection when done below the plane of the obturator nerve. The obturator vessel travels in a parallel direction under the nerve. They are more prone to injury with forceful dissection. Hence it is important to take caution and dissect gently as soon as the obturator nerve appears

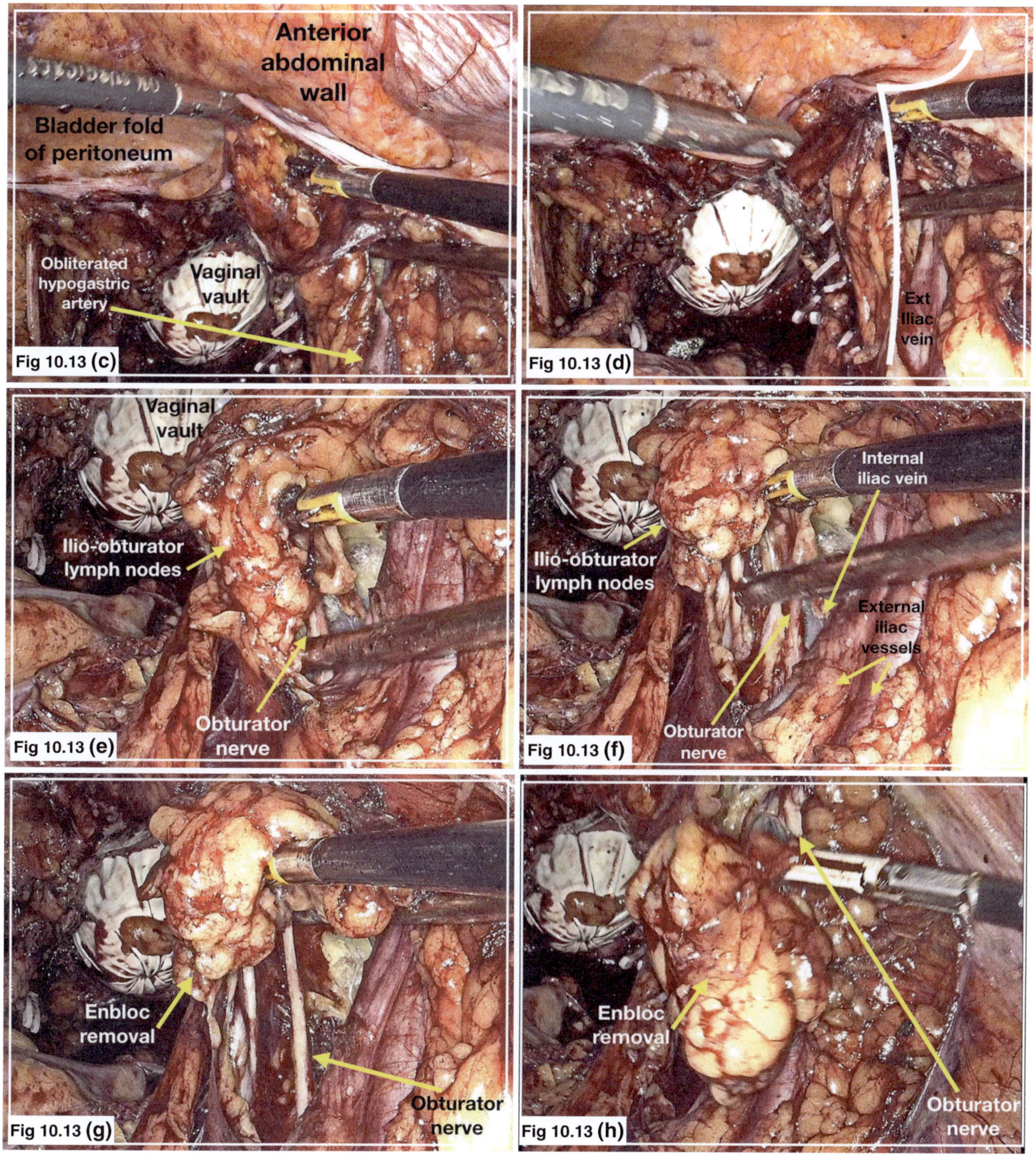

Fig. 10.13 (continued)

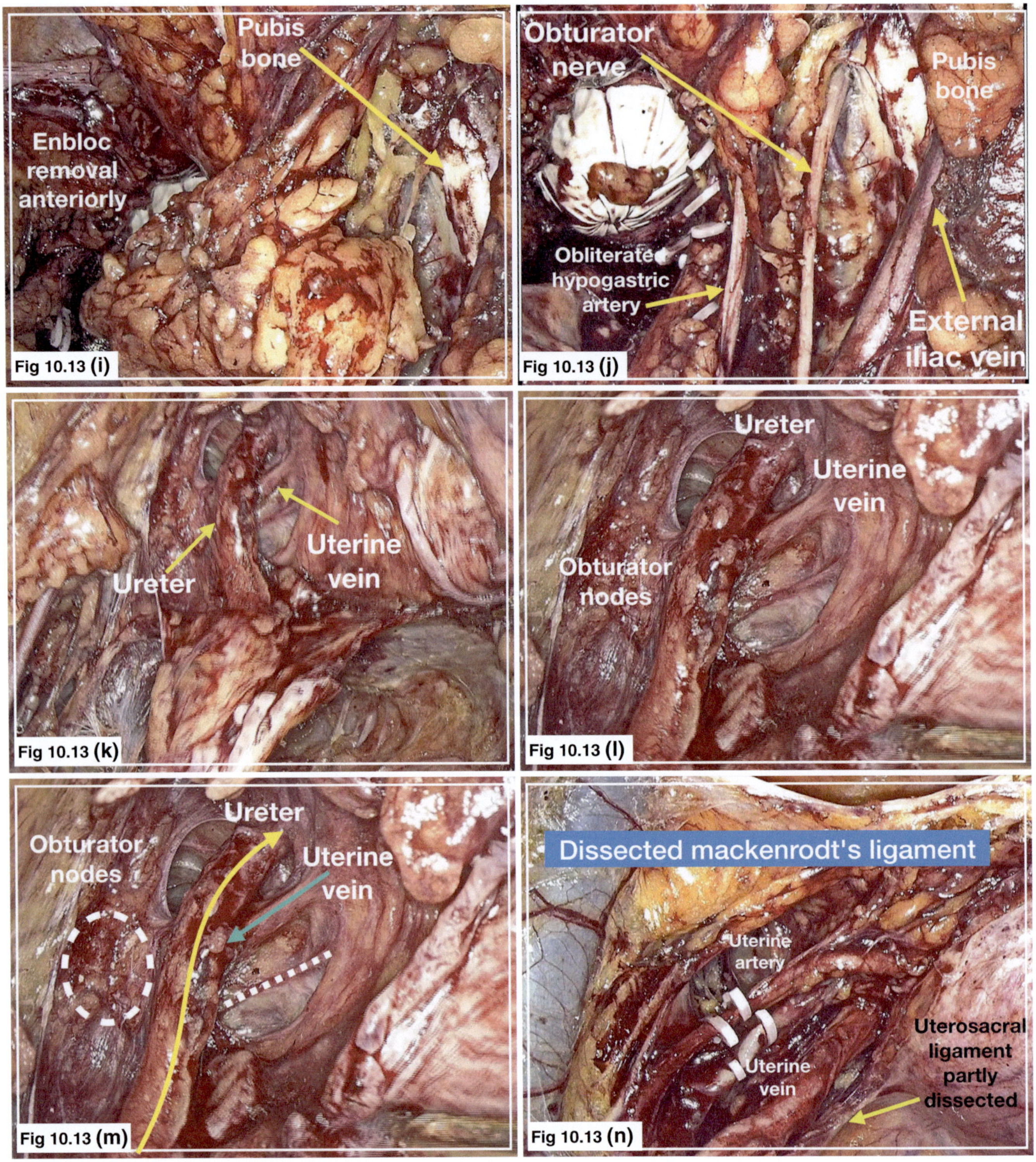

Fig. 10.13 (continued)

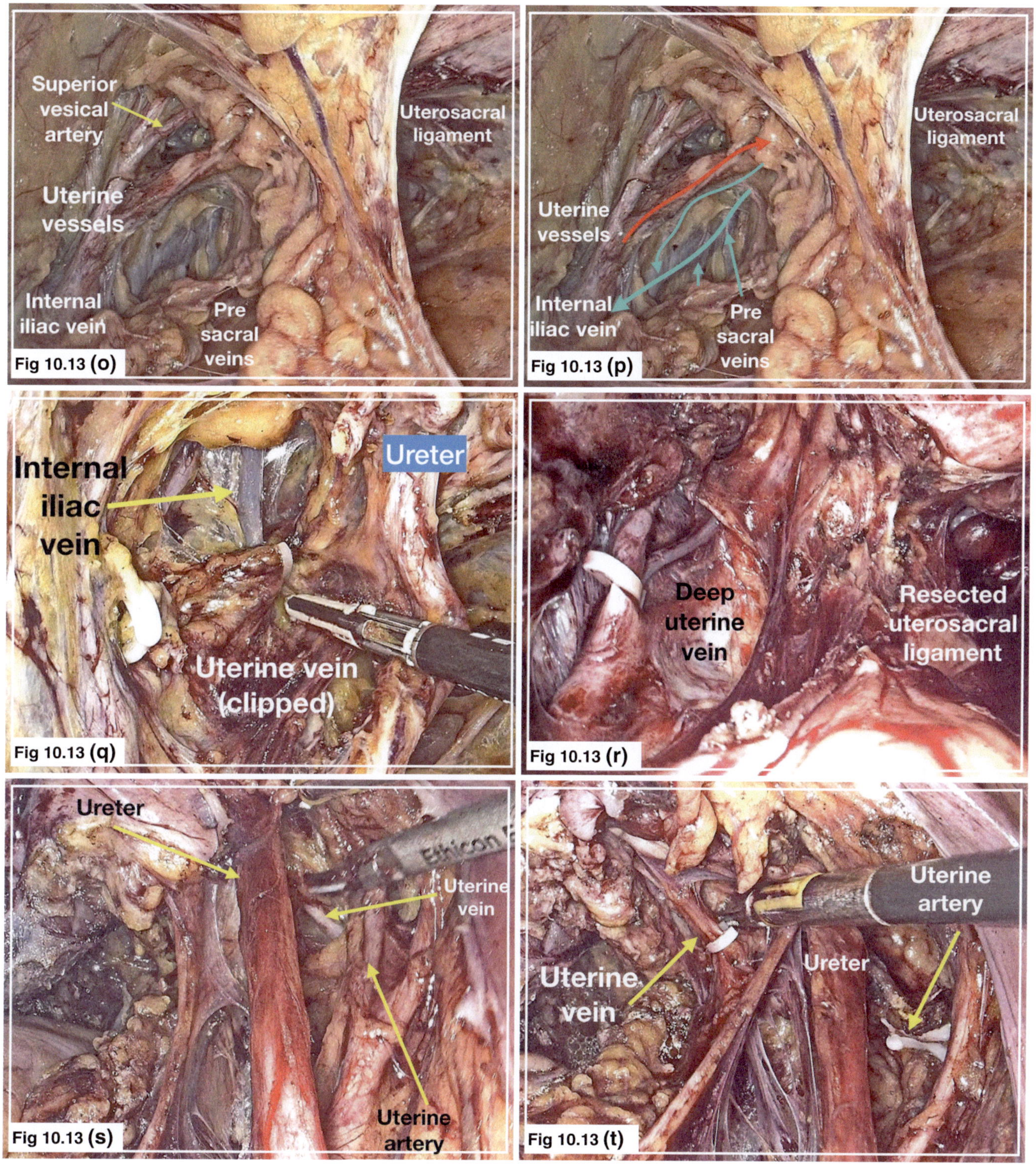

Fig. 10.13 (continued)

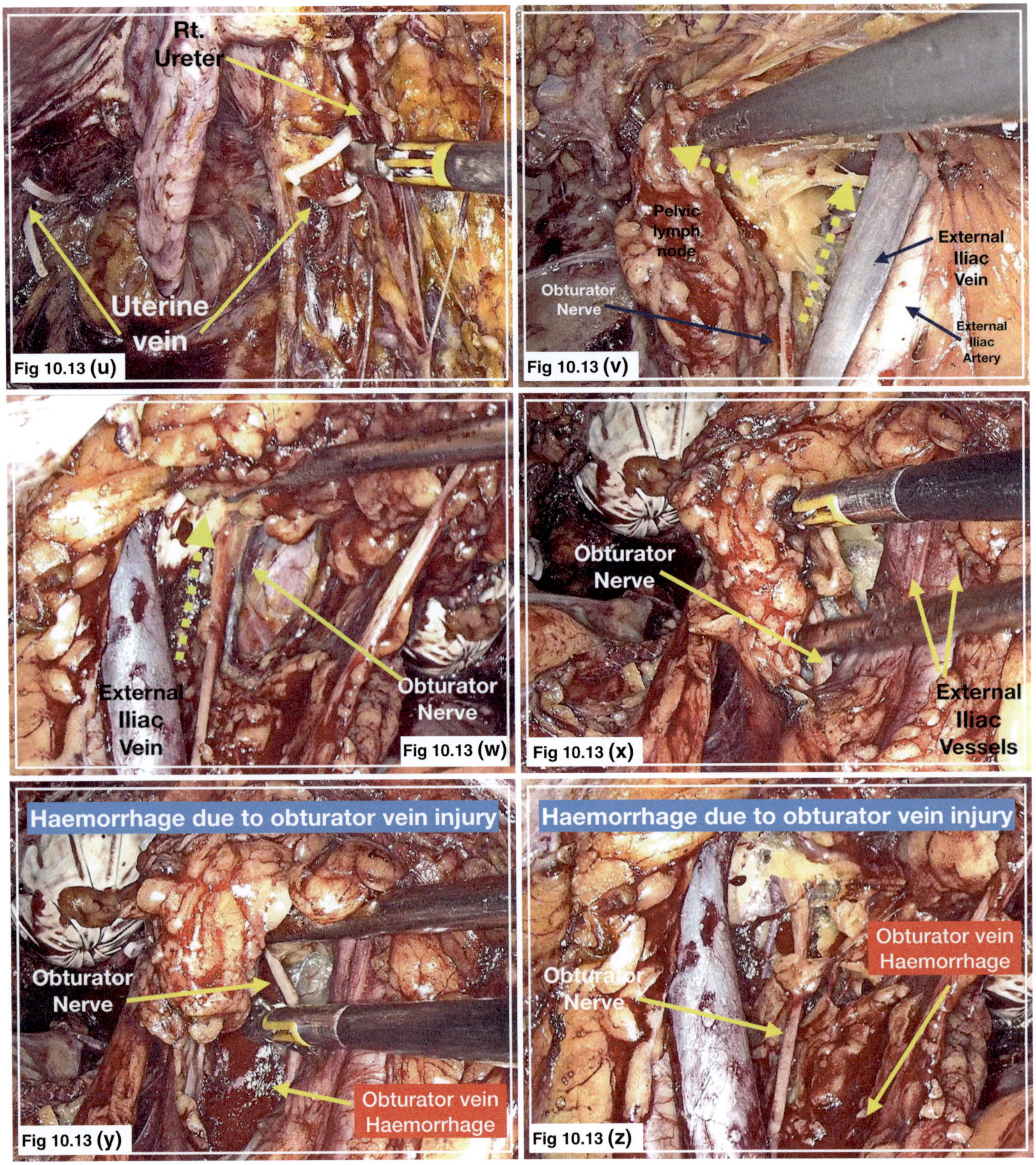

Fig. 10.13 (continued)

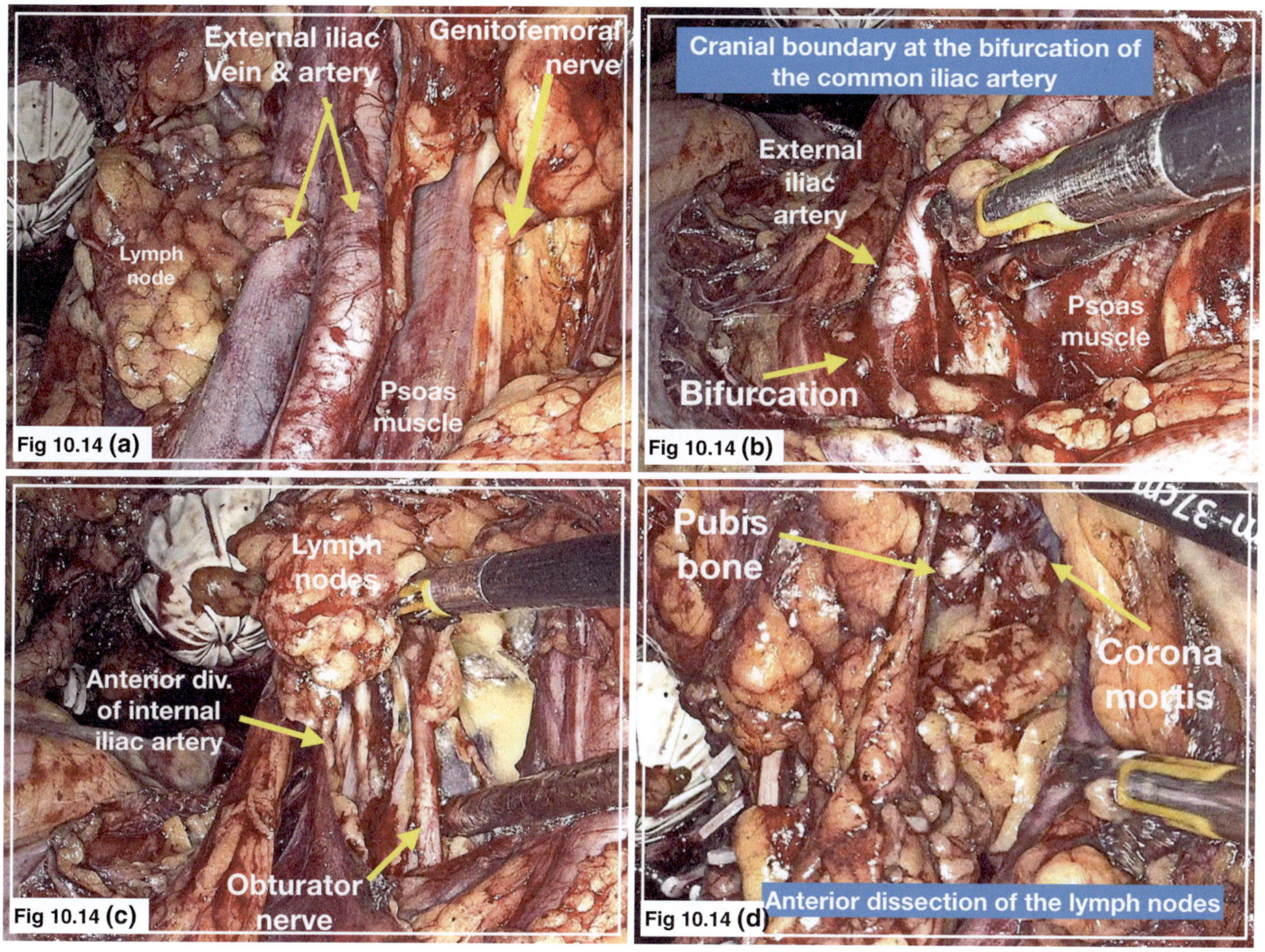

Fig. 10.14 Ilio-obturator boundaries: (**a**) The lateral boundary formed by the genitofemoral nerve can be seen in this image. Dissection of fat (for lymph node dissection) beyond this region would yield the femoral group of lymph nodes which are not beneficial for most pelvic pathologies. (**b**) The cranial limit of dissection at the bifurcation of the common iliac artery can be seen in this image. Deeper between the groove of the bifurcation the obturator can be seen. This has been shown later in subsequent images. (**c**) Always remain lateral to the anterior division of internal iliac artery (obliterated hypogastric artery) at all times while dissecting over the obturator nerve. It is the medial border of dissection. (**d**) While dissecting off from anterior surface near the anterior abdominal wall it is easy to encounter the pubis bone denoting the lateral limit of dissecting. However it is even more important to observe guarded caution due to the presence of the corona mortis or the circumflex iliac vein. (**e**) The pubis bone always appears as an extremely white and shining shimmering surface during dissection. This is due to the periosteal surface which reflects so intensely. The corona mortis is a loose tortuous course and hence further dissection to yield higher lymph node needs to be done with guarded caution. (**f**) The corona mortis can be seen clearly as a branch of the external iliac vein and it communicates with the obturator vein which is the branch of the internal iliac vein. One of the chief reasons why the corona mortis is feared is because it is the only communication between the external and the internal iliac veins. Thus injury to corona mortis would lead to bleeding from both major veins. (**g**) The clear communication between the internal and the external iliac vein can be seen in the image. The corona mortis is the bridge that communicates the external iliac vein directly with the obturator vein (internal iliac vein indirectly). (**h**) Similar dissections done on the left side and the corona mortis and obturator nerve visible on the opposite side as well. (**i, j**) Lack of intermingling fascia makes it easy for en bloc removal of lymph nodes. Simpler unidirectional strokes can help dissecting the lymph nodes. (**k**) Remaining anterior to the obturator assures bloodless dissection of the lymph nodes. The obturator nerve also appears as reflecting white tubular structures lateral to the anterior division of the internal iliac artery. (**l**) The internal iliac vein can be seen underneath the obturator nerve. It is also the reason why dissection of the lymph nodes below or beyond the obturator nerve is forbidden. (**m**) The obturator nerve can be traced up to its origin under the bifurcation of the common iliac artery. (**n**) The image is a case of laparoscopic radical hysterectomy for cervical cancer. There was an isolated calcified obturator node observed on only one side. The rest of the group of lymph nodes were matted but not calcified. (**o**) Dissection around the lymph node revealed that it was sitting around on the bifurcation of common iliac artery. The internal and external iliac artery can be seen coming from the distal end but the bifurcation is not visible

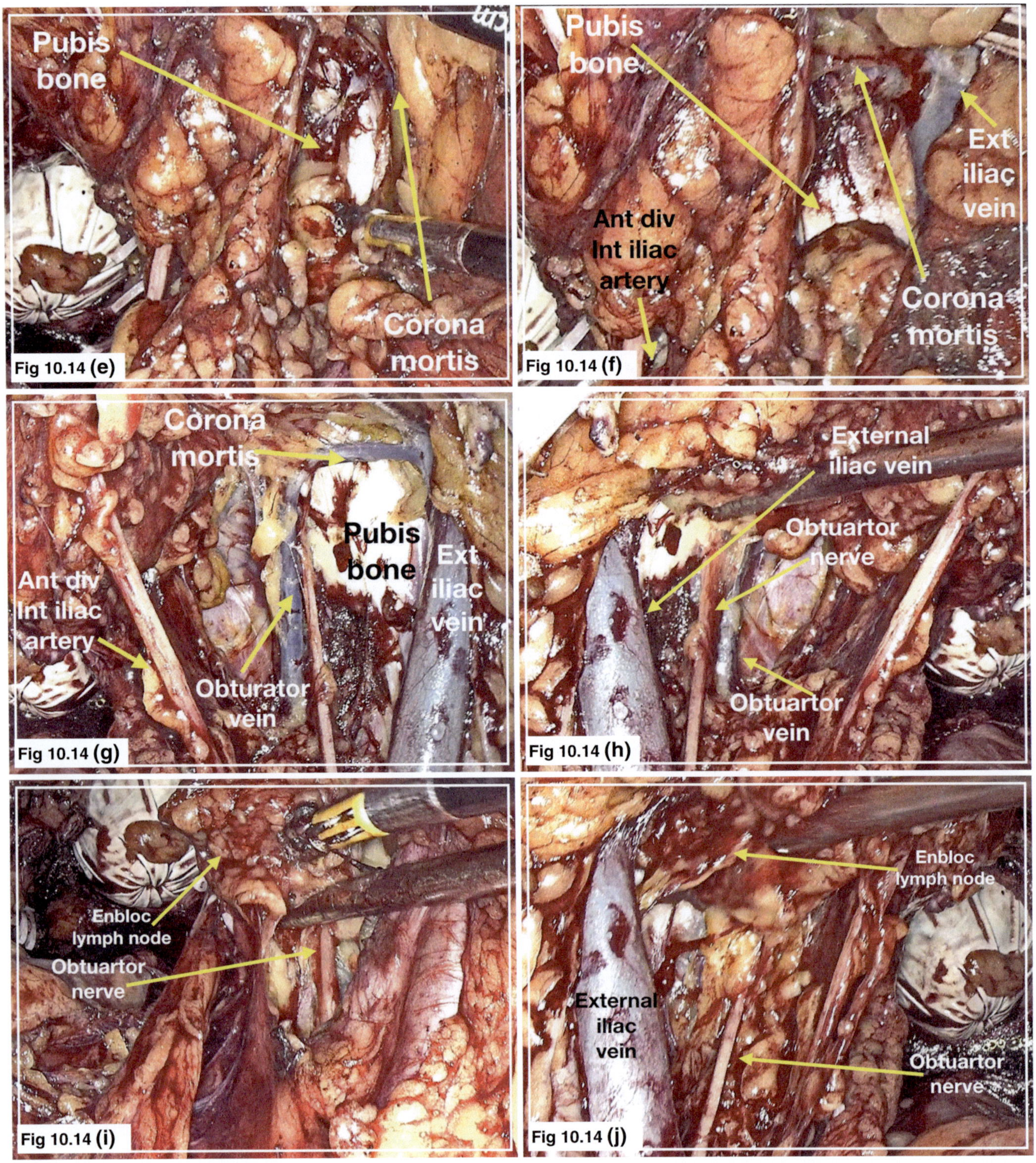

Fig. 10.14 (continued)

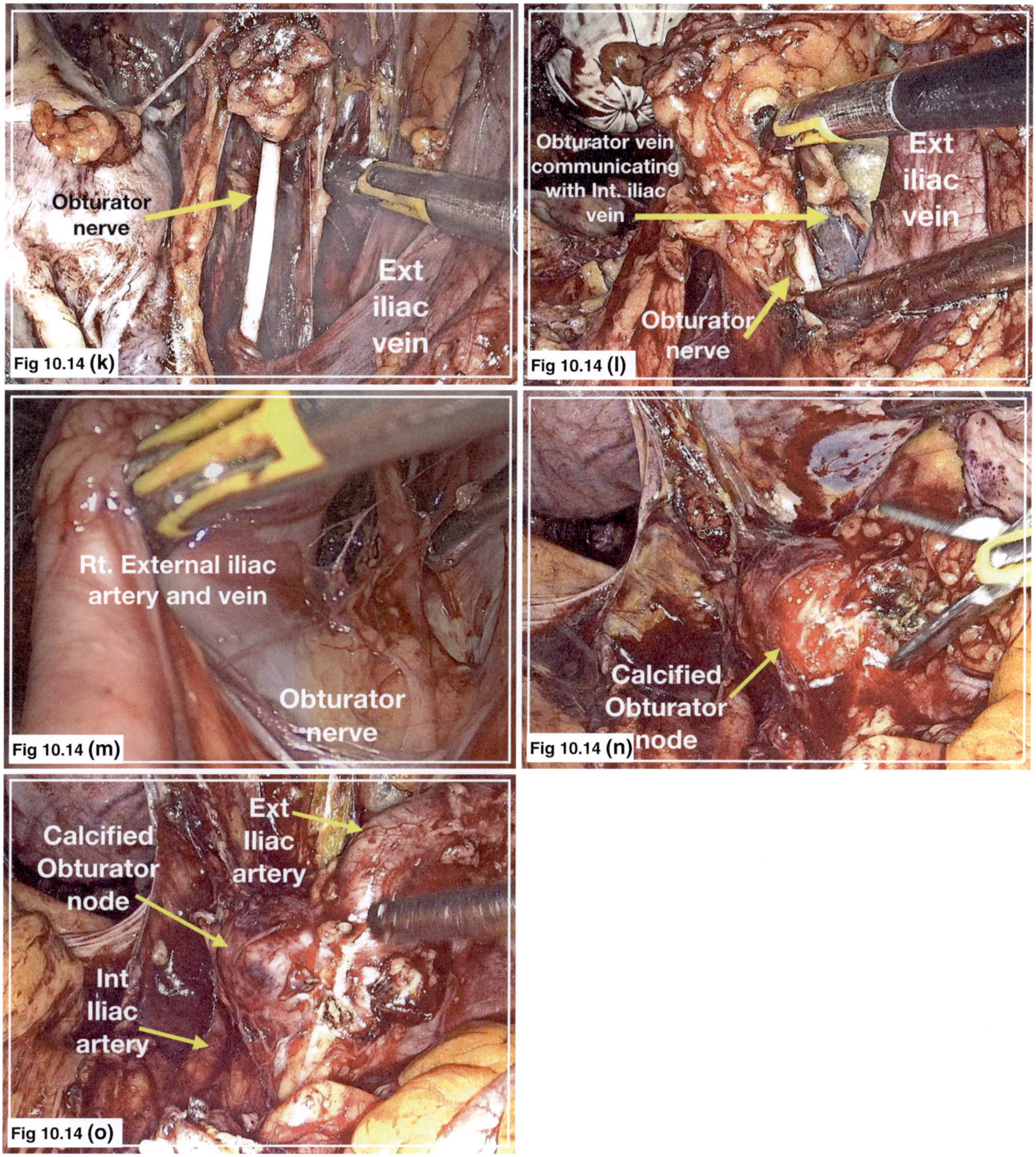

Fig. 10.14 (continued)

10.2 Internal Iliac Nodes

The anatomical location of these nodes is along the internal iliac veins.

The uterine veins drain at this level into the internal iliac vein. The urinary bladder veins all drain into the internal iliac veins through the uterine veins. This anatomy leads to these nodal involvement in large cervical cancers and also in bladder cancers. These nodes lie medial to the internal iliac artery as compared to the obturator nodes (Fig. 10.15b, c).

These nodes lie above the Waldeyer's fascia which covers the internal iliac vein. Thus the plane of dissection should lie anterior to the fascia medial to the internal iliac artery (Fig. 10.15d, e).

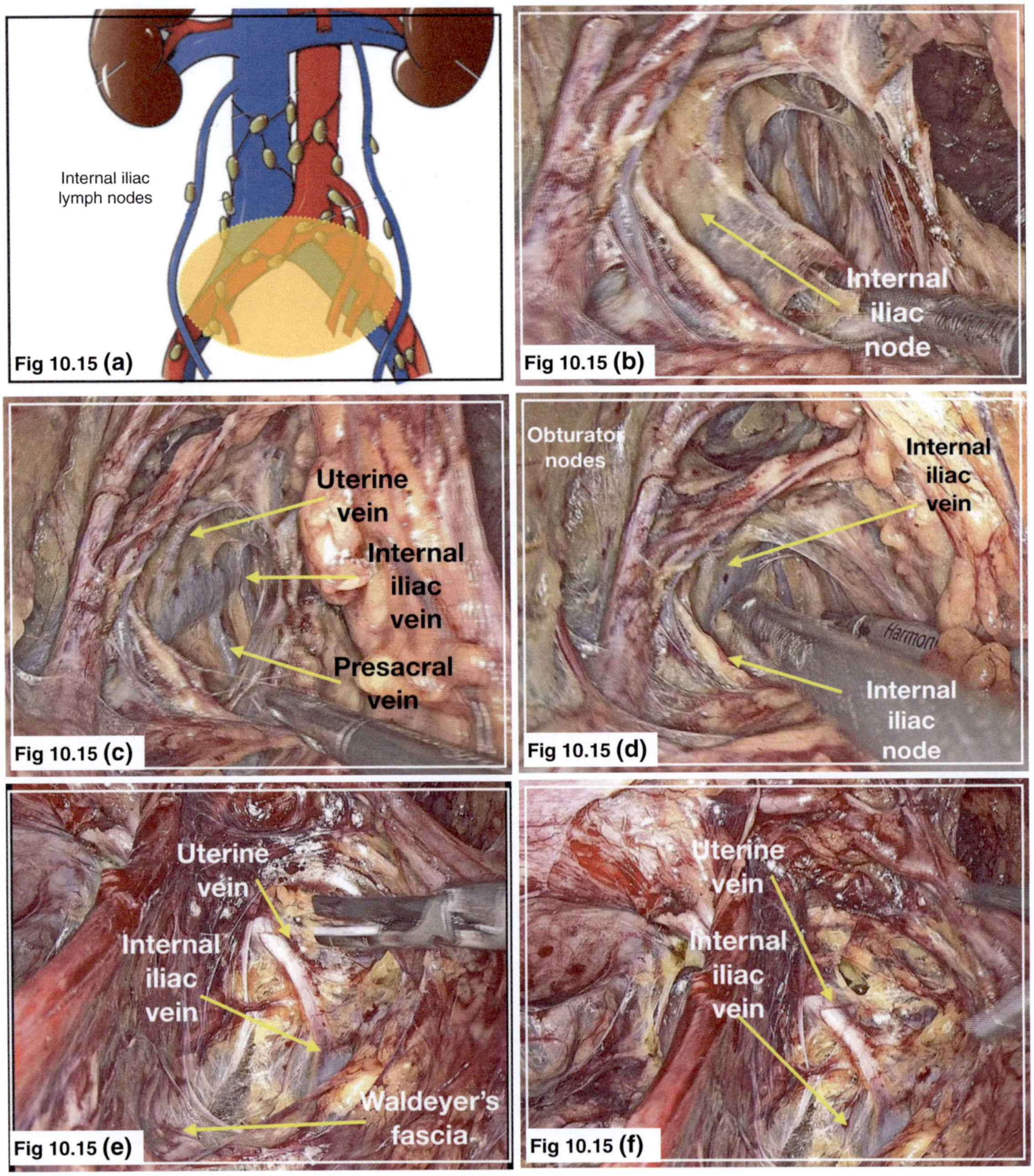

Fig. 10.15 Internal iliac nodes: (**a**) The schematic diagram and location of the internal iliac nodes have been shown in the figure. (**b**) The image shows the intact uterosacral ligament and the directed open Mackenrodt's ligament. However the area focussed here is medial to the internal iliac artery. The fat collection around the internal iliac vein is the internal iliac nodes as labelled. (**c**) Various venous tributaries drain into the internal iliac vein which is why dissection of the internal iliac node is difficult and incomplete owing to its close proximity with the great veins. (**d**) The area focussed is medial to the internal iliac artery. Area lateral to the internal iliac artery is the area for obturator lymph node dissection. (**e**) The Waldeyer's fascia can be seen at the cranial end of the internal iliac artery. The presacral veins lie underneath and thus forceful dissection is not advised at the bifurcation area. (**f**) The internal iliac vein can be clearly seen appearing from underneath the Waldeyer's fascia. The Waldeyer's fascia nearly terminates at this region where the internal iliac vein begins to appear. Thus the fascia lies more medial to the internal iliac vein and covers just the presacral veins

10.3 Lumbosacral Chain

The lumbosacral chain of nodes is posterior to the common iliac artery. They are situated along the lumbosacral trunk which then becomes the sciatic nerve (Fig. 10.16b, c).

These nodes are rarely involved except in recurrent and advanced pelvic cancers. The approach to the lymph node chain is by retracting the entire external iliac and common iliac artery medially and going from the lateral side of these vessels. The plane of dissection is anterior to the lumbosacral trunk (Fig. 10.16d–h).

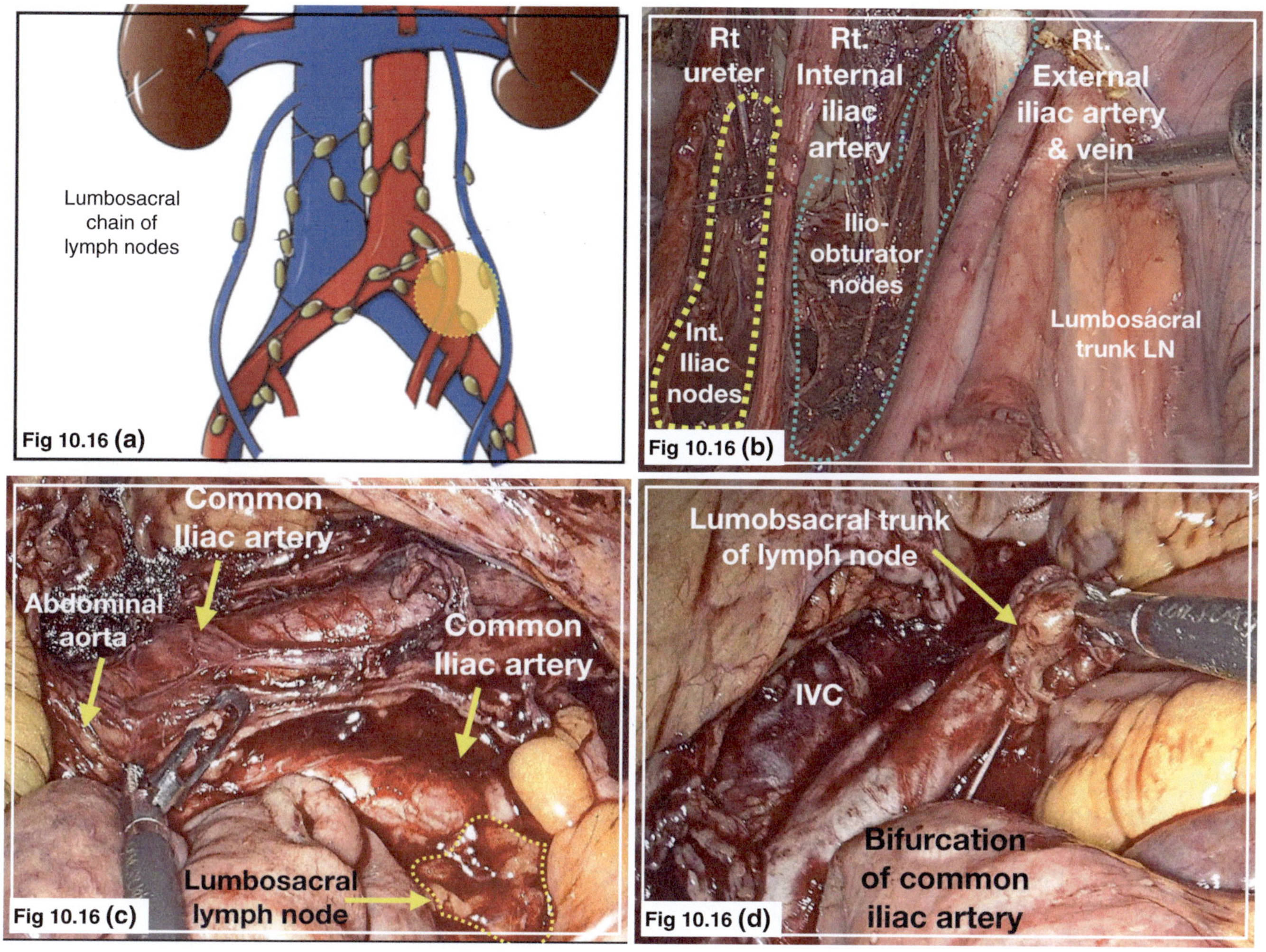

Fig. 10.16 Lumbosacral chain of lymph nodes: (**a**) The schematic diagram of the lumbosacral chain of lymph nodes has been shown in this image. (**b**) The tubular structures which run parallel have been labelled so that the location of the lymph nodes is more well defined in a comparative way. Lymph nodes lateral to the ureter are the internal iliac nodes (yellow dotted lines). Lateral to the internal iliac artery are the obturator nodes (blue dotted lines) while lymph nodes lateral to the external iliac artery are the lumbosacral chain of lymph nodes (labelled). (**c**) In conditions of transperitoneal dissection the lumbosacral lymph nodes can be traced lateral to the common iliac artery as shown in the image. (**d**) This image is taken from a case of transperitoneal approach for para-aortic lymph node dissection. Retracting the common iliac and the external iliac artery helps win better exposure of the lumbosacral trunk of lymph nodes as seen in this image. (**e**) The lymph nodes remain lateral to the common iliac artery. Minimal traction is required when lymph node dissection is combined with transperitoneal approach as shown in the figure. (**f**) In this and subsequent images the laparoscopic pelvic lymph node dissection is extended from the routine technique. Significant amount of traction is provided onto the external iliac artery to expose the area of lymph node extraction. (**g**) The principles of dissection remain the same. *All tubular structures are dissected in a direction parallel to their long axis*. These principles ensure safer dissection of lumbosacral lymph nodes. The lumbosacral trunk of nerves (not seen here) can be made visible with further higher traction at the common iliac artery and viewed laterally near the psoas muscle. (**h**) Only psoas muscle is visible at the bed at the end of dissection denoting completion of dissection. Handling of the great veins warrants the need of DVT prophylaxis in such patients

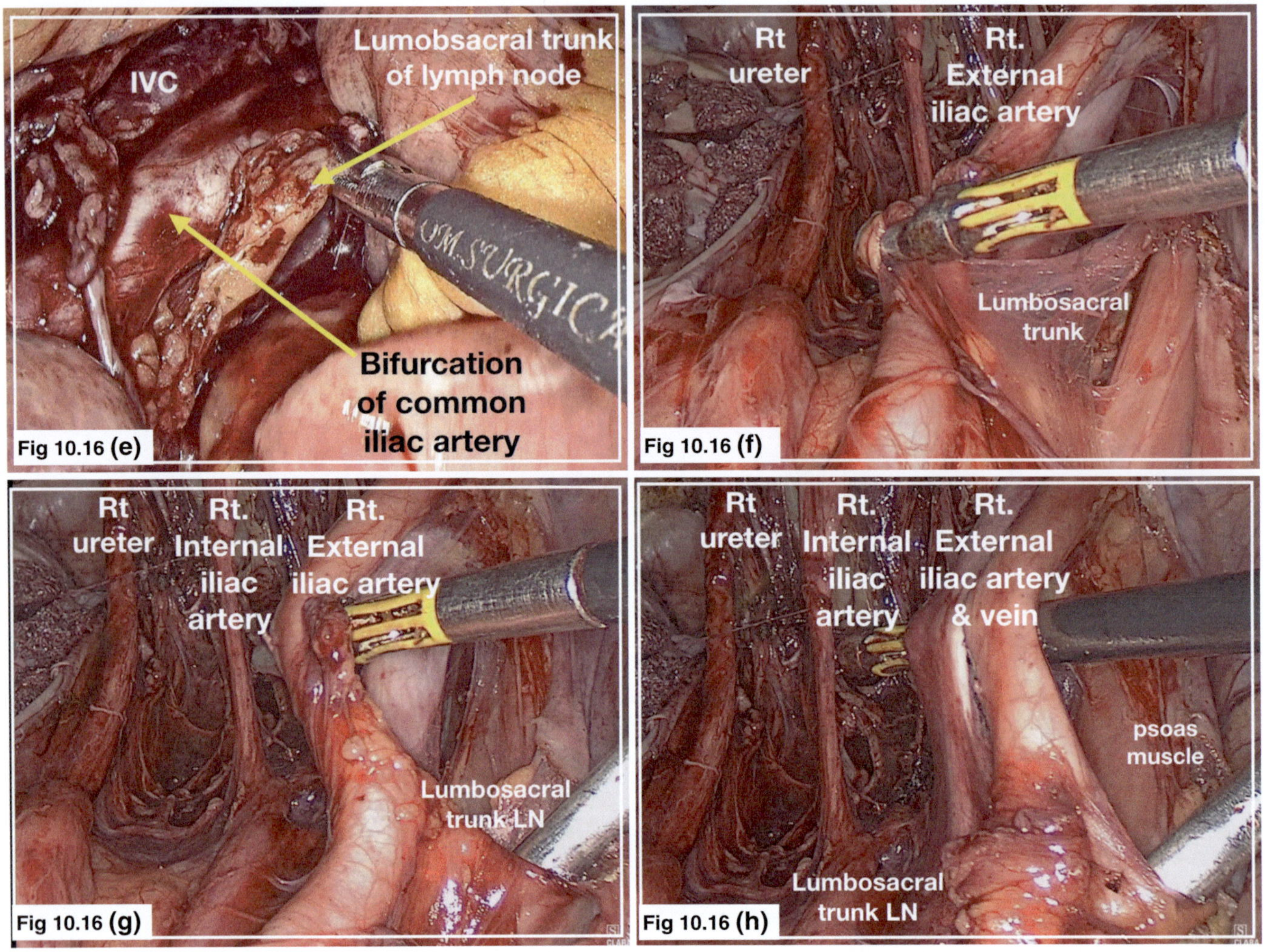

Fig. 10.16 (continued)

10.4 Para-aortic and Paracaval Nodes

The para-aortic and paracaval nodes drain the uterus, ovary, fallopian tubes, and testis in males (Fig. 10.17a).

The ovarian vein drains into the inferior vena cava at the level just below the renal veins on either side and hence the cranial limit of para-aortic nodal dissection is the left renal vein (Fig. 10.17b, c).

The lymph nodes are not in anatomical continuity and hence are divided into (1) paracaval, (2) precaval, (3) para-aortic, (4) preaortic and (5) interaortocaval (Fig. 10.17d, e)

The limits of para-aortic dissection are

1. Laterally ureter on either side
2. Cranially left renal vein
3. Caudally bifurcation of the aorta (Fig. 10.17f–h).

The inferior mesenteric vein drains into the splenic veins and hence para-aortic involvement is rare in rectal and sigmoid cancers (Fig. 10.18a).

The inferior mesenteric artery is the only branch arising from the anterior surface of the aorta (Fig. 10.18b).

There are no tributaries arising from the anterior surface of vena cava and hence the dissection of the precaval nodes can be done remaining parallel and anterior to the IVC (Fig. 10.18c).

Similarly cranial to the origin of inferior mesenteric artery there is no branch of aorta on the anterior surface. Hence the nodal dissection of the pre-aortic nodes can be done remaining parallel and anterior to the aorta (Fig. 10.18d)

On either side there are 3–4 pairs of lumbar arteries and veins (Fig. 10.19b, c).

The para-aortic and the paracaval nodes lie anterior to these lumbar vessels and hence can be easily dissected remaining parallel to the lateral border of aorta and inferior vena cava (Fig. 10.20a–h).

These are the most important group of lymph nodes for the ovarian and endometrial malignancies. Cervical malignancies are also often positive for para-aortic lymph nodes but at a very later stage.

The interaortocaval nodes also lie superficial to the lumbar vessels (Fig. 10.21a–f).

The pre-aortic and the precaval nodes lie in the plane between the postganglionic sympathetic nerves and the anterior surface of the IVC and the aorta and hence these nerves along with superior hypogastric plexus can be salvaged during the para-aortic nodal dissections (Fig. 10.22a–e).

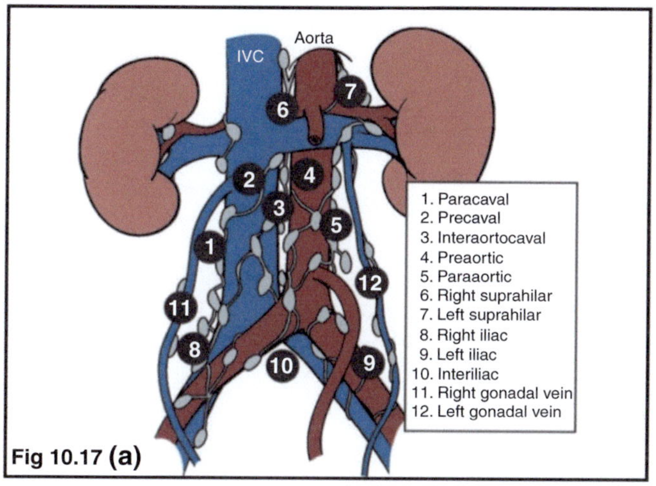

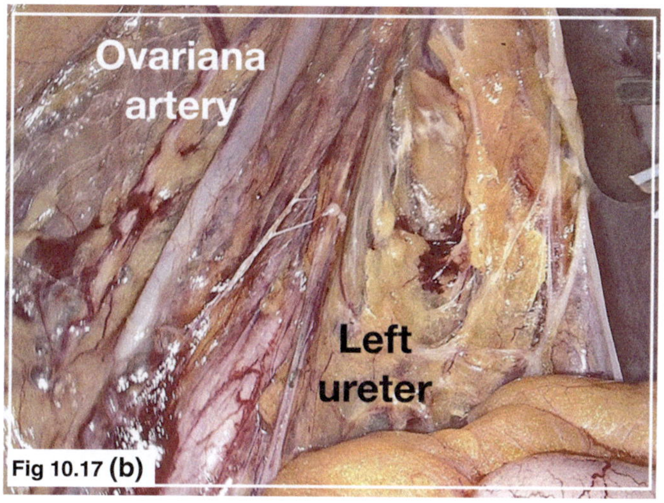

Fig. 10.17 Para-aortic and paracaval lymph nodes: (**a**) Diagrammatic representation of the cluster of para-aortic and paracaval group of lymph nodes. They are the terminal group of lymph nodes which ultimately drain from all over the visceral pelvic organs. They drain all the lymph nodes from the entire female genital system (except vulva). (**b**) Relation to ovarian vessels: Slender parallel travelling vessels parallel to the ureter can be identified as the ovarian artery. The thin muscular can also be seen in the vessel. However the ovarian veins are often more prominent and travel parallel to the ovarian artery. (**c**) Relation to ovarian vessels: The darker ovarian vein can be identified along the side of the ureter. It can be traced up to its termination where it drains into the renal vein. Thus renal vein becomes the upper limit of dissection. However seldom dissection is required till the renal vein for para-aortic lymph node dissection. (**d**) Diagrammatic representation of the various groups of para-aortic and paracaval lymph nodes and their locations highlighted with yellow circles. (**e**) Actual real-time images of the group of lymph nodes explained above in the diagram. (**f**) Boundaries: Diagrammatic representation of the boundaries for dissection of para-aortic and paracaval lymph nodes. Below the renal veins, medial to the ureter and up to the level of the bifurcation of the aorta. The ureters are labelled in light blue lines pointing downwards and medially (at the supposed position of the urinary bladder) and the areas of dissection are coloured in yellow shade. (**g**) The image shows the left ovarian vessels and ureter retracted upwards to expose the area underneath. However dissection should be carried out only medial to the ureter. (**h**) The image shows the bifurcation of the aorta. The white line denotes the border of dissection of para-aortic nodes which remain above the line. Below the line are the inter iliac nodes and the common iliac nodes on each side

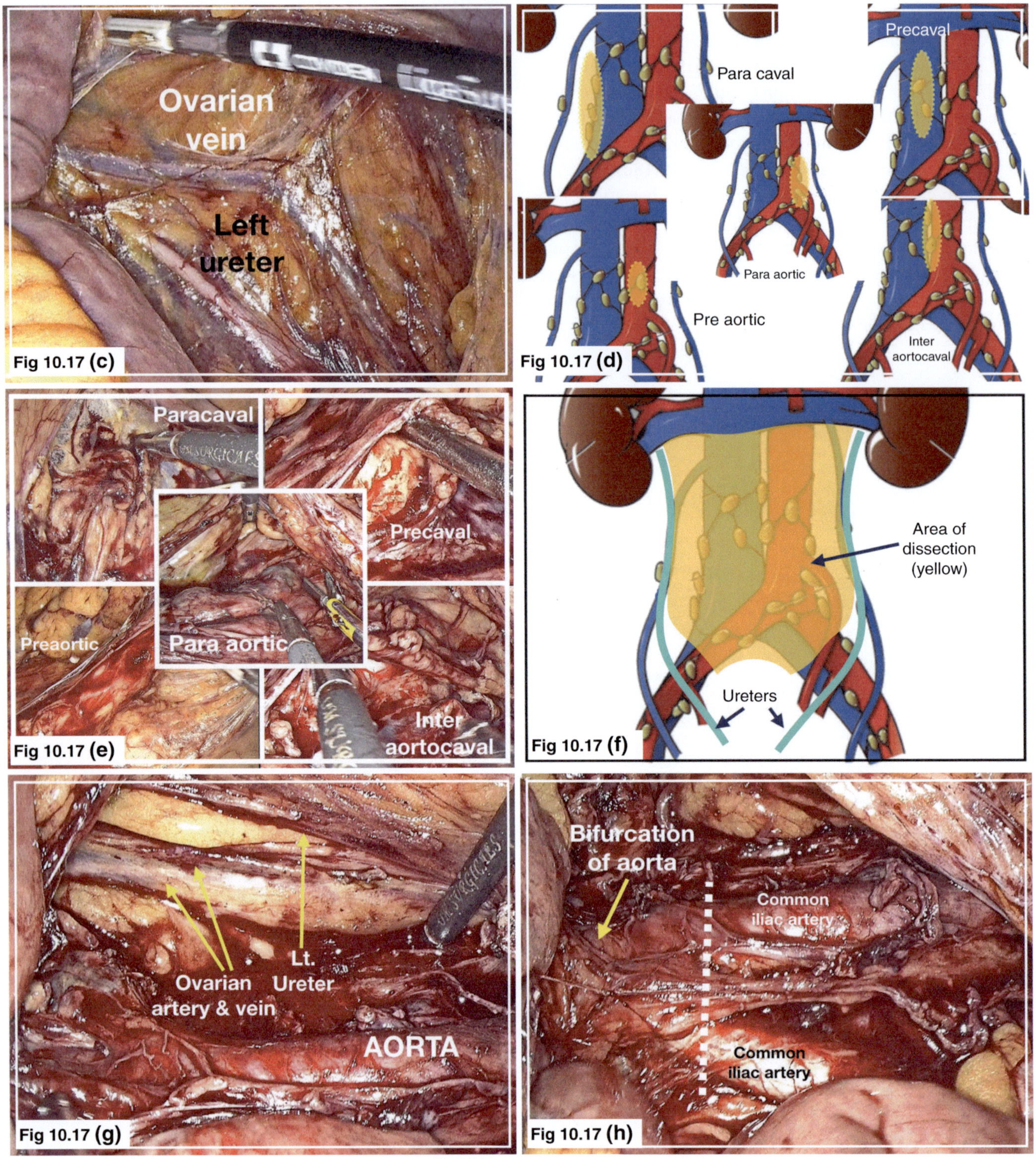

Fig. 10.17 (continued)

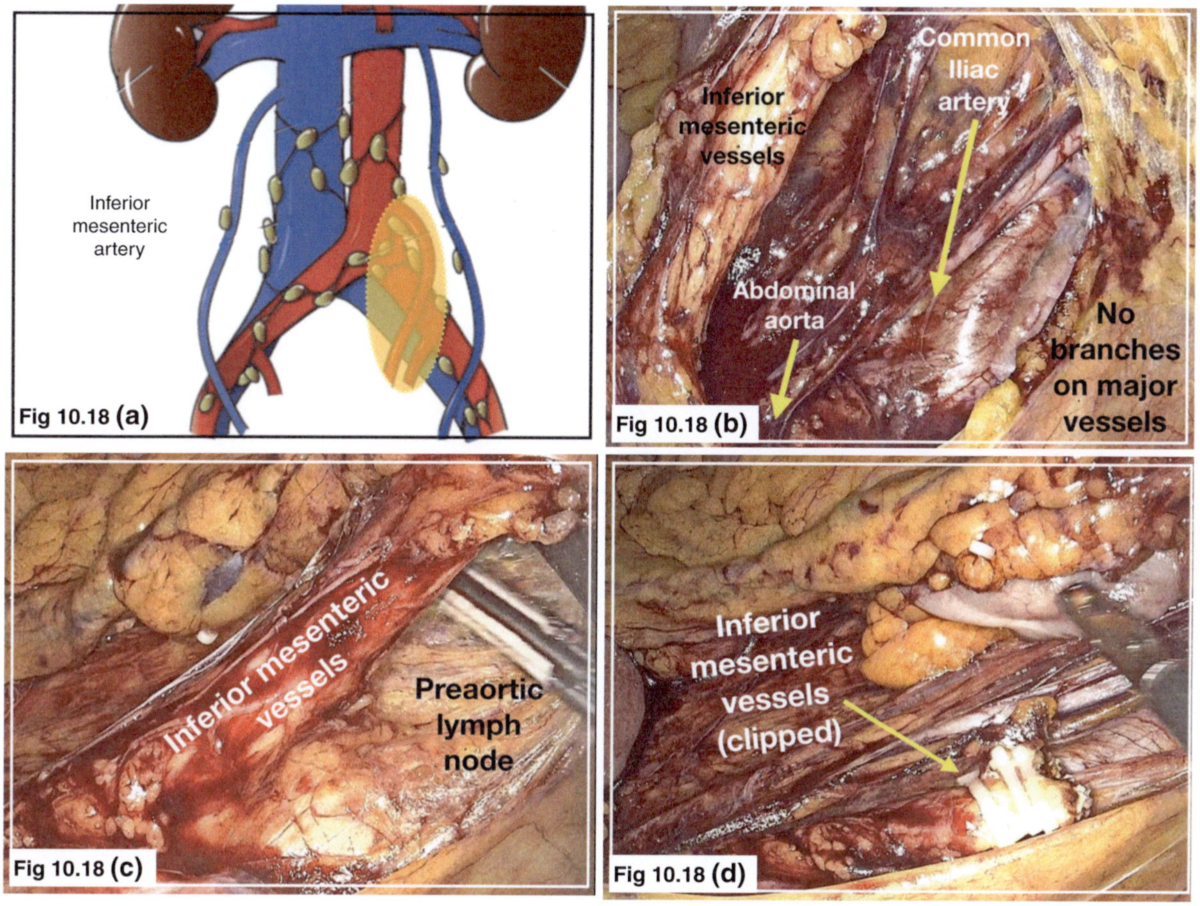

Fig. 10.18 Inferior mesenteric artery: (**a**) Diagrammatic representation of the location of inferior mesenteric group of lymph nodes. (**b**) This group of images have been taken from a case of Ca rectum undergoing laparoscopic low anterior resection. The inferior mesenteric artery is dissected and clipped and subsequent segment of colon supplied by the vessel is dissected off. The ureter, common iliac artery and bifurcation of aorta can be identified. When traced more cranially the inferior mesenteric artery can be seen arising from the anterior surface of the aorta. (**c**) The fatty tissue surrounding the inferior mesenteric artery containing the pre-aortic lymph nodes can be seen in the image. Depending upon their location they are called as pre-aortic and precaval nodes. (**d**) Clipping of the inferior mesenteric vessels helps in providing more working area for further dissection. This applies especially to the pre-aortic group of lymph nodes. The precaval group is dissected more easily than the pre-aortic group

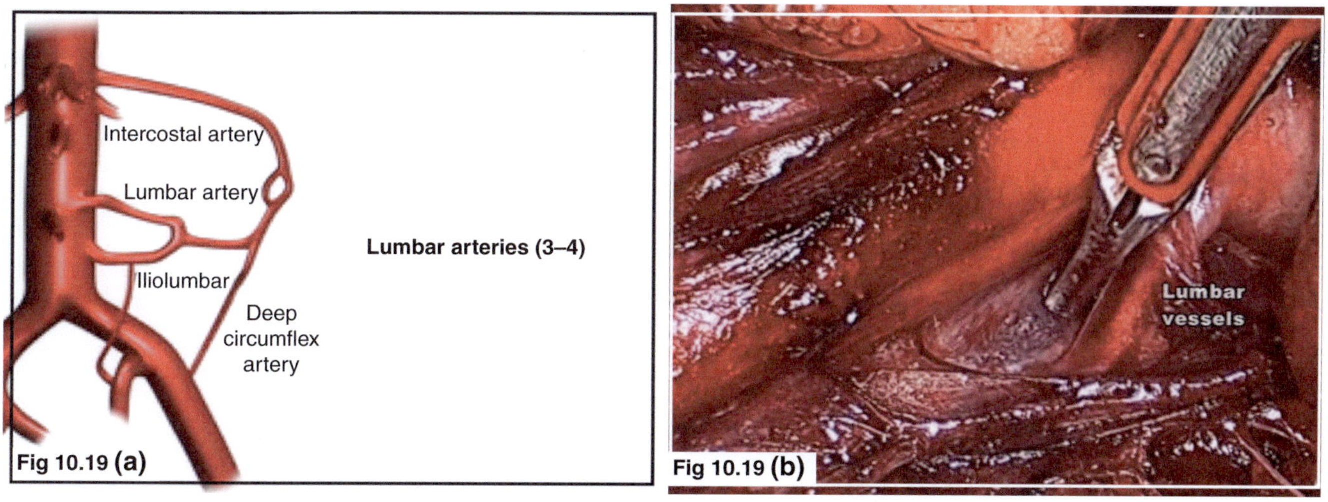

Fig. 10.19 Lumbar arteries: (**a**) The diagrammatic representation of the lumbar arteries has been demonstrated. (**b**) In a case of extraperitoneal dissection of the para-aortic lymph nodes the lumbar arteries are seen as short twig-like branches arising which often bleed on vigorous traction or dissection. (**c**) In a case of transperitoneal lymph node dissection the lumbar arteries are often seen as minor obstruction to the plane of dissection which bleed. They can be managed with energy sources

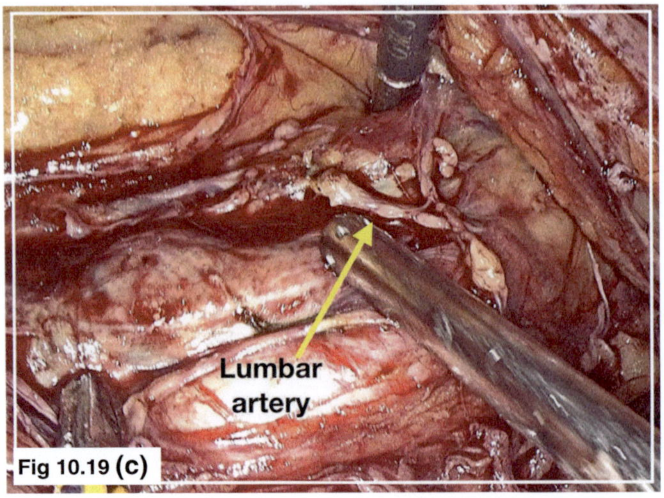

Fig. 10.19 (continued)

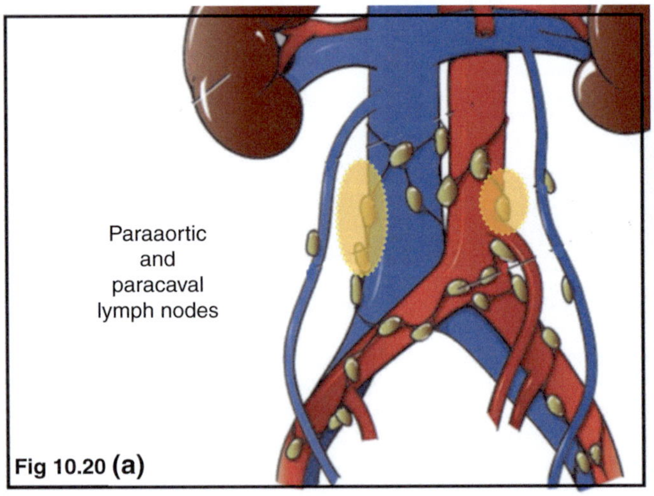

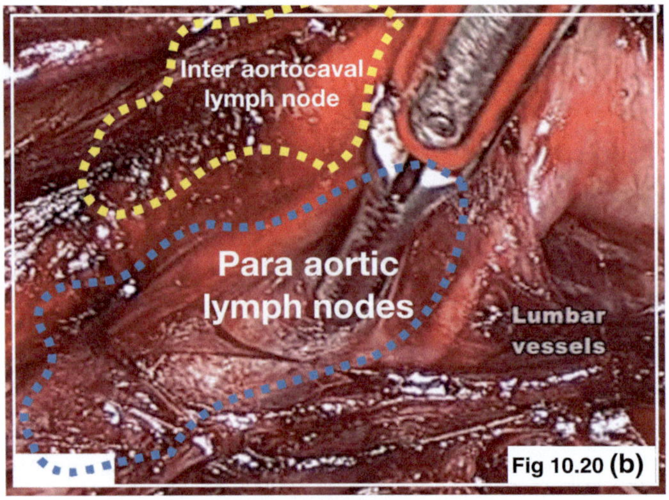

Fig. 10.20 Para-aortic and paracaval group of lymph nodes: (**a**) Diagrammatic representation of the para-aortic and the paracaval group of lymph nodes. (**b**) In a case of extra-peritoneal para-aortic lymph node dissection the group of lymph nodes can be seen demarcated by the yellow and blue doted lines. (**c**) The paracaval lymph nodes can be seen being dissected off lateral to the inferior vena cava in this case of transperitoneal lymph node dissection. (**d**) The paracaval lymph nodes are often covered by a sheath of superior hypogastric plexus of nerves which run parallel downwards to supply various visceral organs in the pelvis as discussed before. They also lie lateral to the IVC which makes their close association with the plexus common. (**e**) In a case of extra-peritoneal lymph node dissection, the para-aortic lymph nodes are dissected by clearing the fat around the great vessels as shown in the figure. (**f**) The para-aortic lymph nodes can be seen medial and exactly seated over the aorta. In this case of transperitoneal para-aortic lymph node dissection for a case of operated Ca ovary, the para-aortic lymph node had been seen to be involved on MRI. It can be confirmed visually here. (**g**) The para-aortic group of lymph nodes can be seen in small chains or cluster of lymph nodes being involved. They too can be removed in a similar manner as pelvic lymph nodes as there are no intervening fascias. (**h**) The para-aortic lymph node can be seen dissected from one end and the plane created can help in further removing more lymph nodes to improve its yield

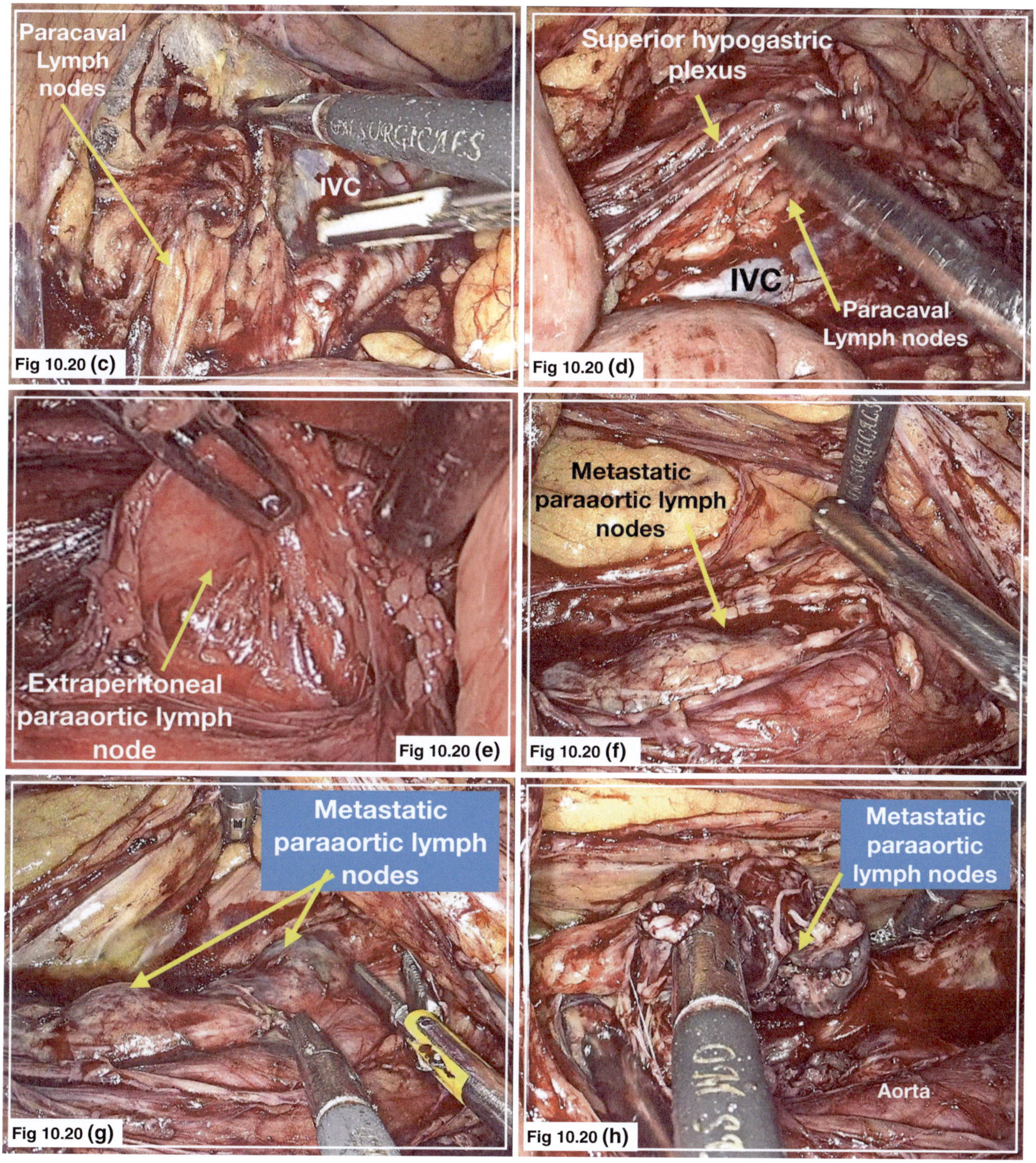

Fig. 10.20 (continued)

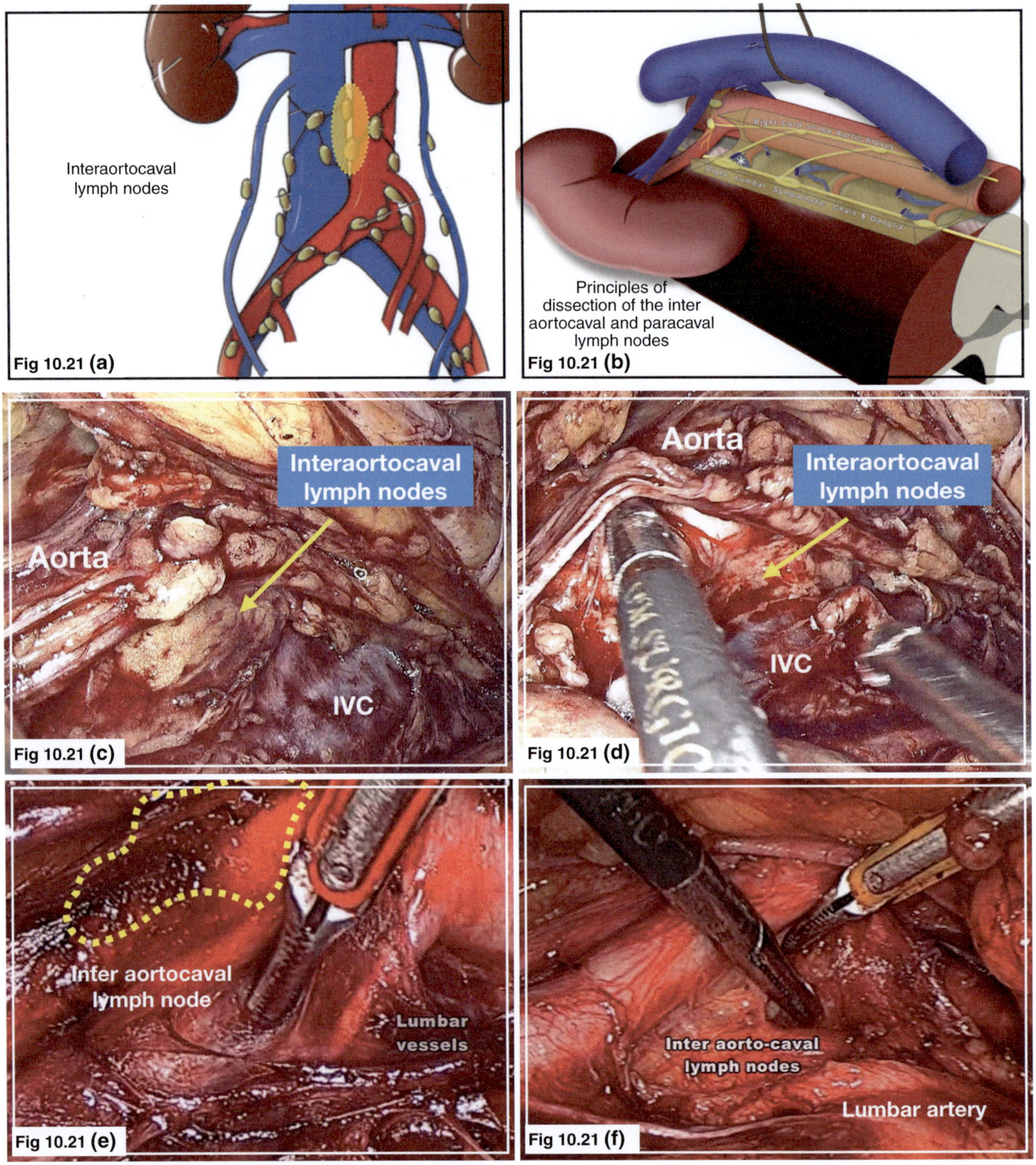

Fig. 10.21 Interaortocaval lymph nodes: (**a**) The diagrammatic representation of the interaortocaval lymph nodes and their location highlighted in yellow circles. (**b**) The principles of dissection of the interaortocaval and paracaval lymph nodes have been explained here. In open surgery it requires the mobilisation of the inferior vena cava. However it is feasible with minimal handling of the inferior vena cava in laparoscopy. (**c**) The aorta is rather more easy to mobilise as it has a muscular support which reduces post-operative morbidity as compared to mobilising the inferior vena cava. The interaortocaval lymph nodes can be seen over a clear IVC suggesting paracaval lymph node directed prior to interaortocaval node dissection. (**d**) Lifting the superhypogastric plexus often helps find the groove between the aorta and the IVC and thus find the interaortocaval lymph nodes. (**e**) In a case of extra-peritoneal lymph node dissection the location of the interaortocaval lymph nodes can be identified as yellow dotted circle. (**f**) The interaortocaval group of lymph nodes remain superficial to the lumbar arteries when traced under the IVC as shown in the image. This can be done more easily in extra-peritoneal dissection instead of transperitoneal dissection

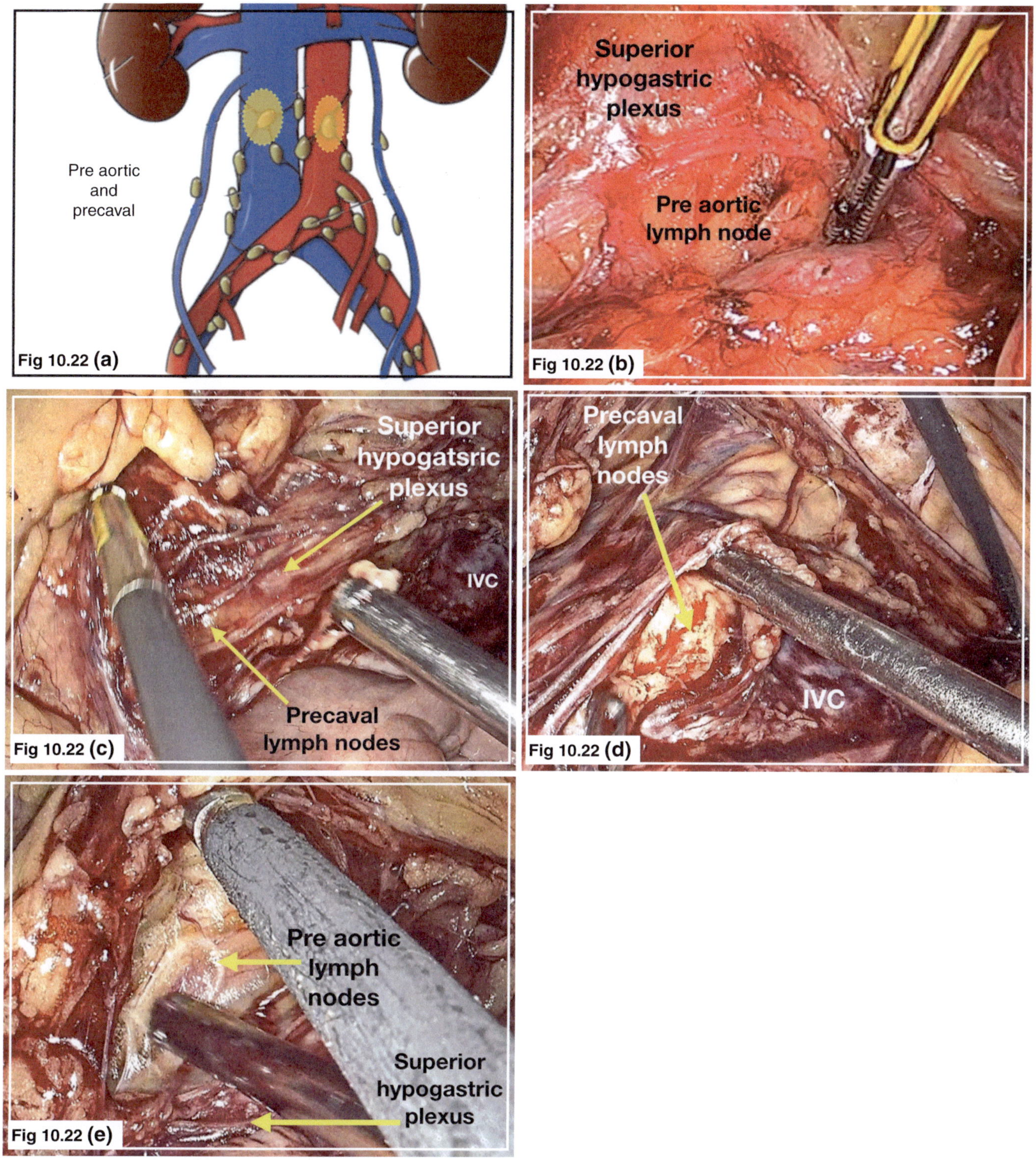

Fig. 10.22 Pre-aortic and precaval group of lymph nodes: (**a**) Diagrammatic representation of the pre-aortic and precaval lymph nodes shown in the figure. (**b**) In a case of extra-peritoneal lymph node dissection the pre-aortic and the precaval lymph nodes lie at the region where the superior hypogastric plexus arises. They lie close to the post-ganglionic fibres. (**c**) In this case of transperitoneal lymph node the origin of the superior hypogastric plexus is traced upwards and the area containing fat near the origin can be dissected to extract the precaval lymph nodes. (**d**) The postganglionic fibres of the superior hypogastric plexus can be seen retracted upwards to expose the precaval lymph nodes lying underneath it. The IVC can be seen clearly suggesting that the paracaval lymph nodes have been dissected earlier. (**e**) The pre-aortic lymph nodes can also be extracted in a similar fashion as the precaval lymph nodes. The postganglionic fibres are retracted downwards to expose the aortic region and thus remove the pre-aortic lymph nodes

11 Applications of Anatomy

11.1 Dissection of the Pararectal Space and Paravesical Space

The dissection of the pararectal space is the most important step in accessing the retroperitoneum of the pelvis for benign as well as malignant pathology in gynaecology. Access to difficult benign pathology and operability of various malignancies are some of the most important decisions which are based on the operability of the pararectal space.

1. Start the dissection at the level of sacral promontory. Cut the peritoneum medial to the infundibulopelvic ligament (Figs. 11.1b, 11.2, and 11.3).
2. Go underneath the IP ligament and expose the external iliac artery (Fig. 11.4).
3. Then remain anterior to the ureter and cut the posterior board ligament staying anterior to the ureter all the way caudally till a window is made in the anterior broad ligament (Figs. 11.5, 11.6, 11.7, 11.8, 11.9, and 11.10).
4. Then come back to the sacral promontory and retract the ureter medially. Then go parallel and lateral to the ureter from the cranial to caudal region. The level of dissection should be at the same level as the ureter. Going below the level will damage the uterine veins (Figs. 11.11 and 11.12).
5. The structure which will prevent you from going caudally is the uterine artery. The uterine artery is the only artery crossing this space transversely (Fig. 11.13).
6. Then remain parallel to the uterine artery pushing everything towards the uterus. Remain medial to the obliterated hypogastric artery. This exposes the paravesical spaces. Continue the dissection all the way till the endopelvic fascia covering the levator ani is reached (Figs. 11.14, 11.15, and 11.16).

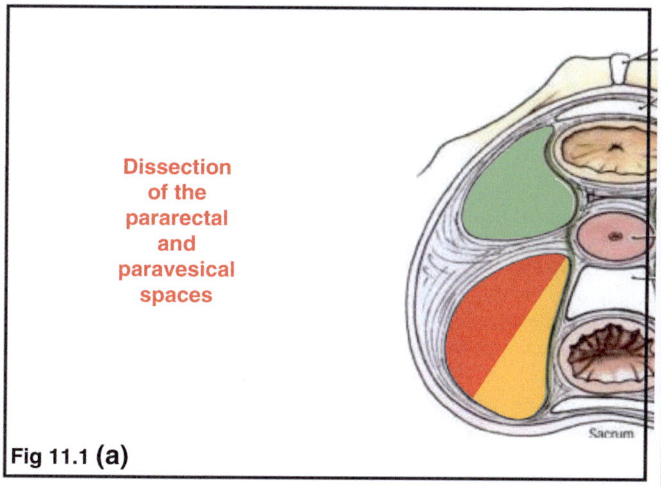

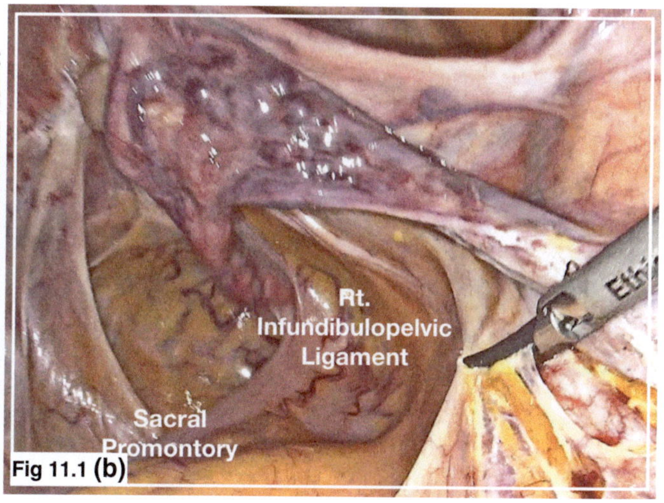

Fig. 11.1 (**a**) Dissection of pararectal and paravesical spaces. Each space has been designated with a specific colour. Green space represents the paravesical space. The red and yellow spaces comprise the pararectal space where the medial yellow space is called the Okabayashi space and the lateral red space is called the Latzko space. (**b**) Pararectal space dissection: In a case of LRH for Ca cervix, initial exposure of Rt pararectal space done from opening the retroperitoneum from medial to infundibulopelvic ligament and lateral to the sacral promontory. This is the starting point of pararectal space dissection

S. Puntambekar et al., *Laparoscopic Pelvic Anatomy in Females*, https://doi.org/10.1007/978-981-13-8653-4_11

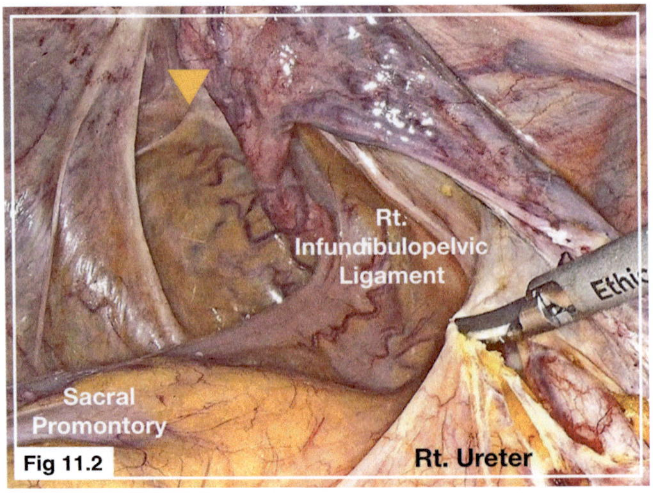

Fig. 11.2 Pararectal space dissection: While opening the pararectal space medially, the first structure to be appreciated is the *ureter*. The target area is the apex of uterosacral ligament (denoted in the yellow inverted triangle). The peritoneum is to be opened till the apex of the uterosacral ligament

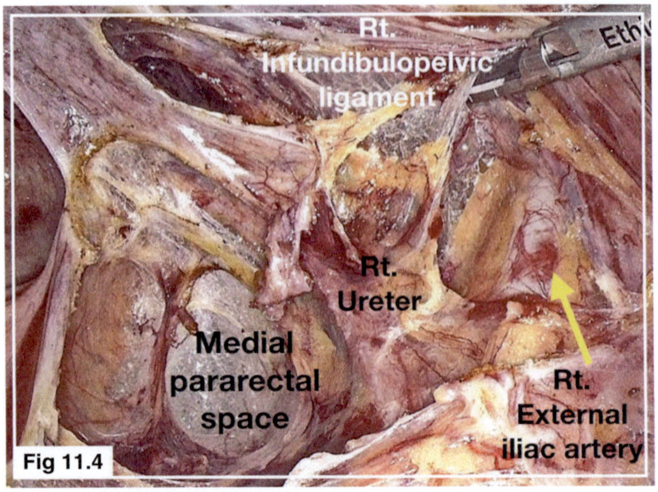

Fig. 11.4 Pararectal space dissection: Lateral traction onto the infundibulopelvic ligament exposes the pararectal space well. The external iliac artery can be visualised by going underneath the ligament. This helps in orientation of the area along with the orientation ureter and its course. The external iliac artery can be better visualised with the lateral approach discussed later

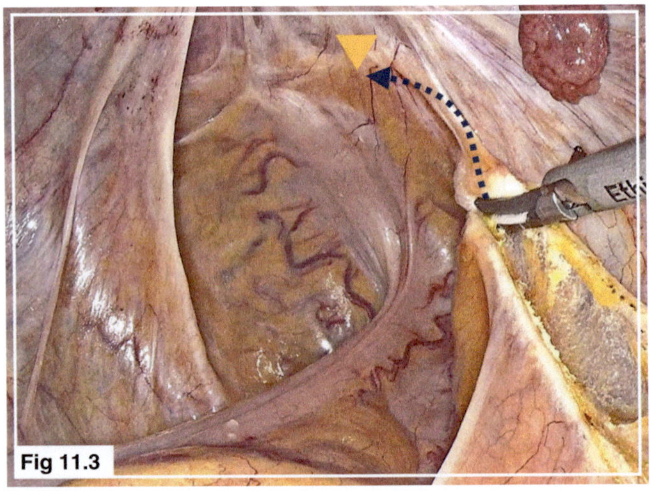

Fig. 11.3 Pararectal space dissection: It should be kept in mind that the energy source is to be kept away from the vital structures like ureter to prevent injury. Mild traction is applied on the peritoneum medially by the lower edge of the Harmonic scalpel to keep the peritoneum away from vital structures

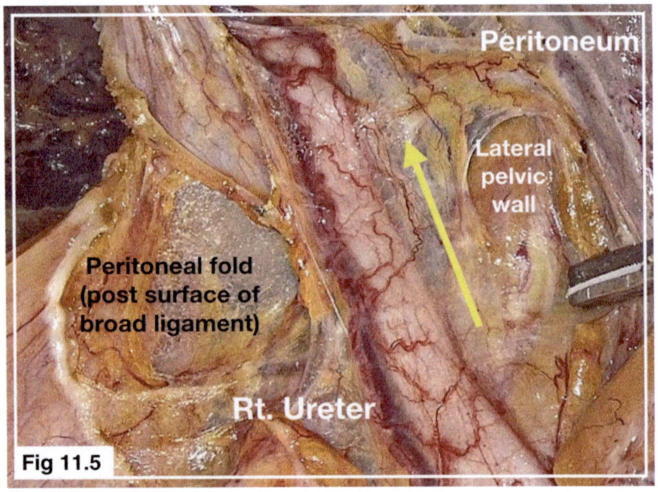

Fig. 11.5 Pararectal space dissection: Vascular structures lie superficially onto the lateral pelvic wall. The ureter can be dissected medially from the lateral pelvic, thus mobilising the ureter as well making these vascular structures more prominent. The yellow arrow shows the direction of dissection

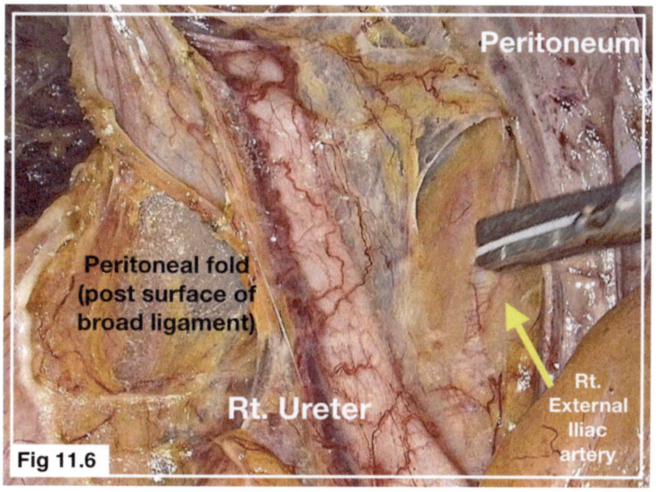

Fig. 11.6 Pararectal space dissection: The ureter is mobilised medially by blunt dissection performed laterally and parallel to the ureter. Blunt dissection follows the dictum of "tubular structures should be dissected parallel to their long axis and never perpendicular". These rules apply to all tubular structures in the pelvis, ureter arteries, veins and nerves alike

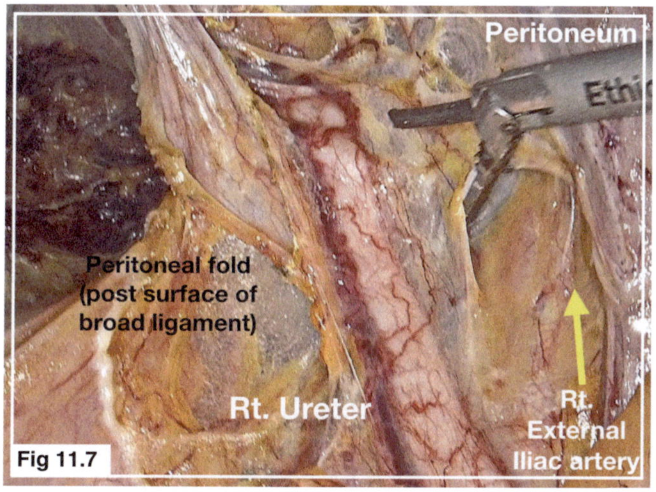

Fig. 11.7 Pararectal space dissection: Smooth blunt dissection with repeated parallel strokes lateral to the ureter reveals the superficial structures on the lateral pelvic wall, e.g. the Right external iliac artery can be seen more clearly under the peritoneum. Caution to be taken to remain *at the level* of the ureter at all times

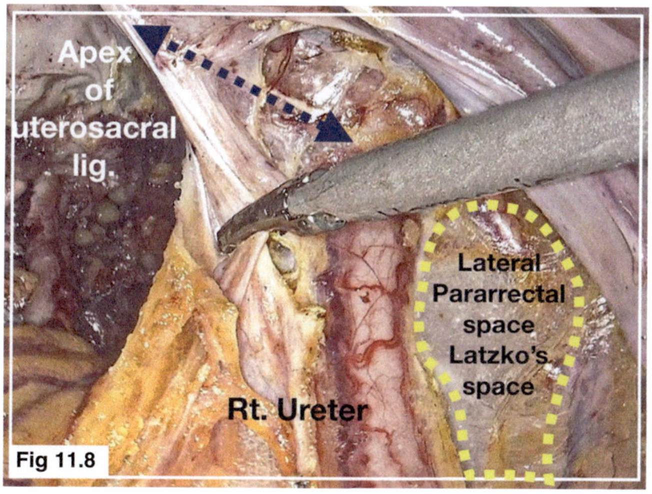

Fig. 11.8 Pararectal space dissection: The ureter is often cohesively stuck to the medial peritoneal fold or the post-leaf of broad ligament. Dissection of the peritoneum often frees the ureter and facilitates its dissection. The ureter divides the pararectal space into Okabayashi and Latzko space, i.e. medial and lateral pararectal spaces, respectively

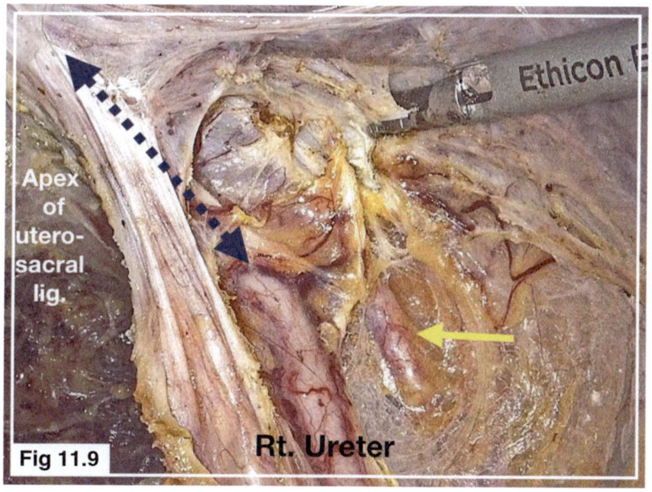

Fig. 11.9 Pararectal space dissection: At all times one must stay anterior and above the ureter. The dissection of the peritoneum for pararectal space dissection is complete only after creation of the window on the anterior leaf of broad ligament. The vascular structure (marked in yellow arrow) arising from the lateral pelvic wall is most likely uterine artery. It can be confirmed by tracing backwards to its origin or by forward to look for it to cross over the ureter

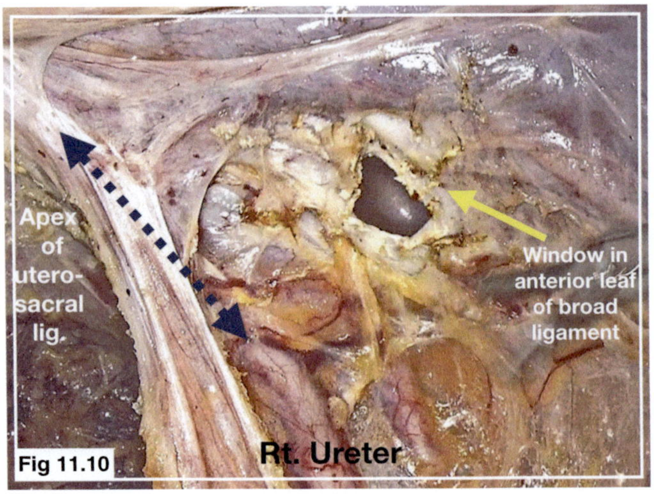

Fig. 11.10 Pararectal space dissection: Creation of window in the anterior leaf of broad ligament is seen. This creation of window follows the same principle of open surgery to ensure that no other vital structure is present before it is coagulated and dissected off

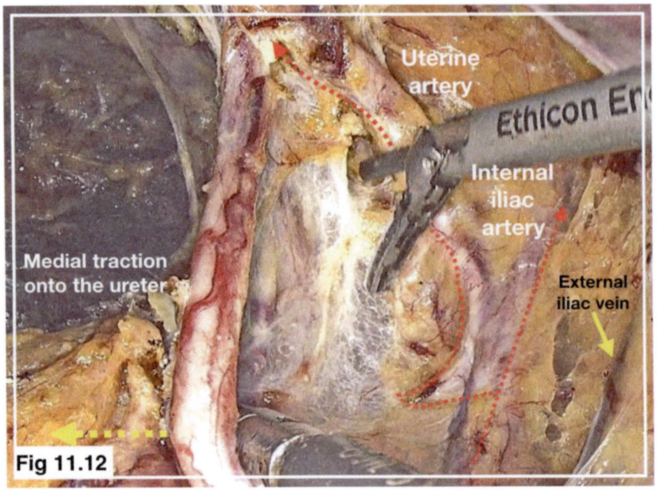

Fig. 11.12 Pararectal space dissection: Medial traction of the ureter to dissect the lateral pararectal space is best started from the level of the sacral promontory. The previously seen unidentified vascular structure is the uterine artery as its origin can be traced to the internal iliac artery. Part of the external iliac vein can be seen above the internal iliac artery helping in its identification. Secondly it is seen to travel above the ureter and cross it when traced forward

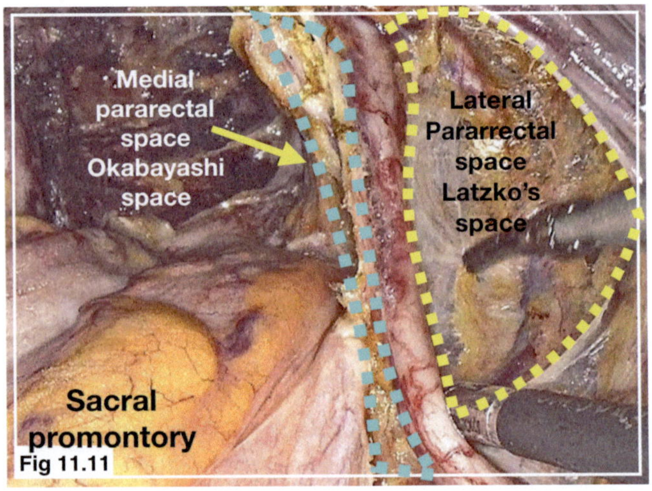

Fig. 11.11 Pararectal space dissection: The Latzko space (denoted in yellow boundaries) is best for identification of vessels and coagulating them. The Okabayashi space (denoted in blue boundaries) is a thin segment for dissection of superior hypogastric nerve plexus while conducting nerve-preserving surgeries

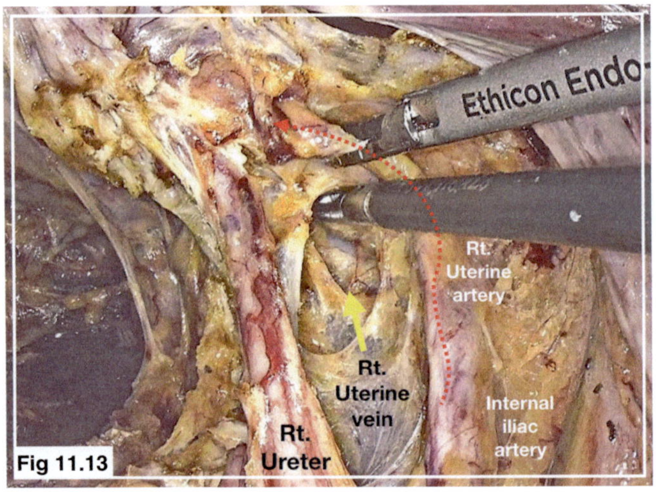

Fig. 11.13 Pararectal space dissection: As previously told, it is important to remain at the same level of ureter during dissection because the uterine vein/veins lie at a lower level to the ureter as seen in the image. Dissecting deeper increases the chances of injury to the uterine vein which leads to significant haemorrhage often difficult to control. Exposure of the uterine veins is the lower limit for pararectal space dissection. This completes the pararectal space dissection

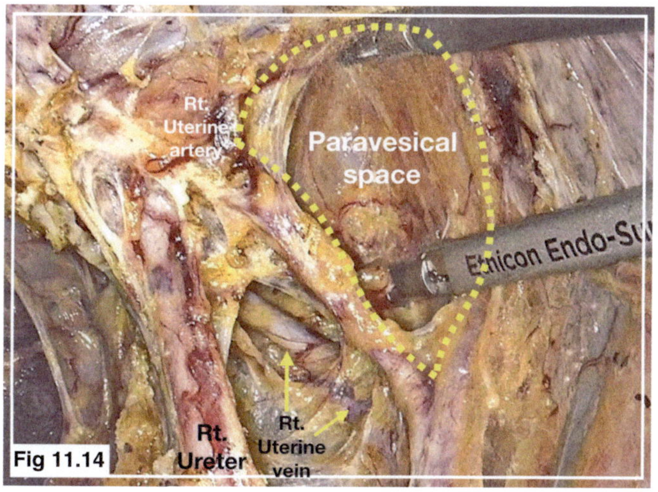

Fig. 11.14 Paravesical space dissection: After identification of the uterine artery along its entire course, dissection is done parallel, horizontal and above the uterine artery for the paravesical space dissection. All the fat in this space is pushed medially towards the uterus and go to deeper levels of dissection

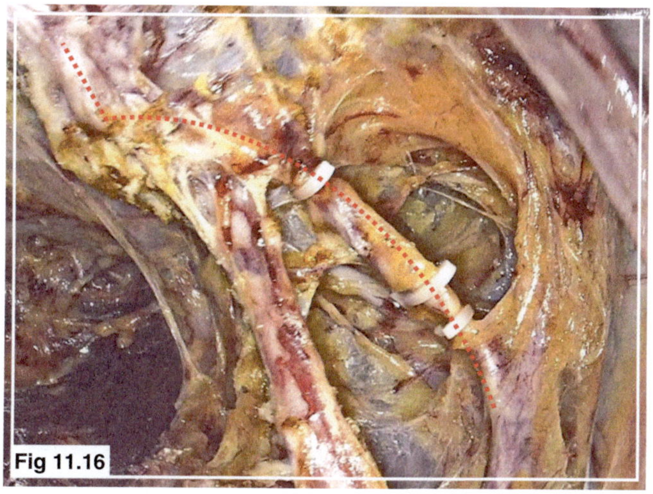

Fig. 11.16 Completed pararectal and paravesical space dissection: The ureter is identified, and uterine artery and vein are identified and clipped. The red dotted line suggests the length of the actual uterine artery and thus all the locations where the artery can be coagulated and cut

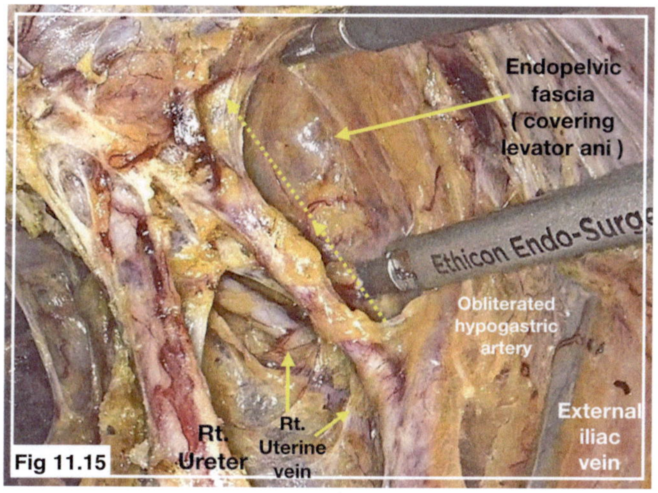

Fig. 11.15 Paravesical space dissection: The lower limit of paravesical space dissection is the levator ani. It is seen as the grey reflection of the endopelvic fascia covering it. The yellow dotted line denotes the direction of the dissection. Always remain medial to the obliterated hypogastric artery at the beginning of dissection

11.2 Medial Pararectal Space

1. Once the above steps are done retract the ureter laterally (Fig. 11.17).
2. Remain parallel and medial to the ureter. Go caudally till you reach the uterosacral ligament. This is facilitated by anteverting the uterus (Fig. 11.18).

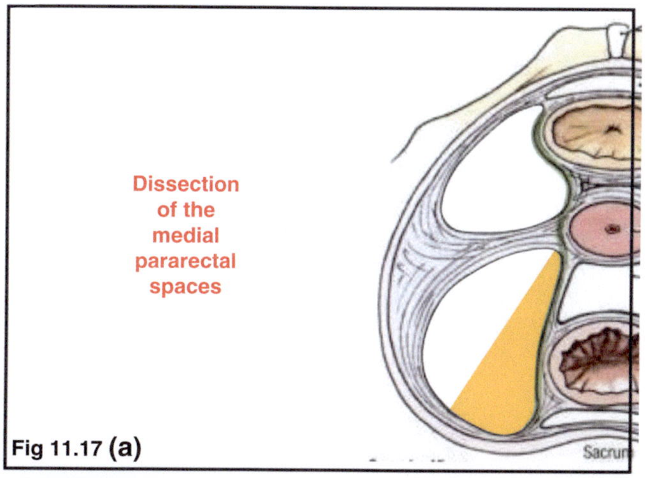

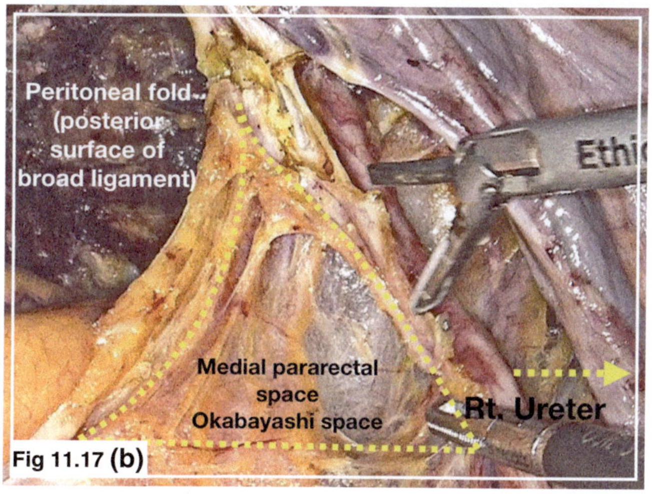

Fig. 11.17 (**a**, **b**) Medial pararectal space dissection: Lateral traction onto the ureter exposes the medial pararectal space also known as the Okabayashi space. This space is the best place to find the superior hypogastric plexus

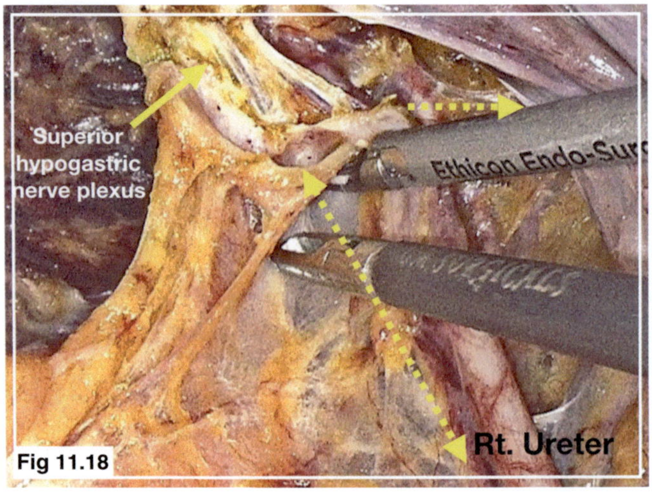

Fig. 11.18 Medial pararectal space dissection: Blunt dissection in this space is done medial and parallel to the ureter. It is done from cranial to caudal direction up to the uterosacral ligaments. The uterus seems anteverted. The lateral traction is applied from the level of sacral promontory up to the level of uterosacral ligaments as the dissection proceeds further

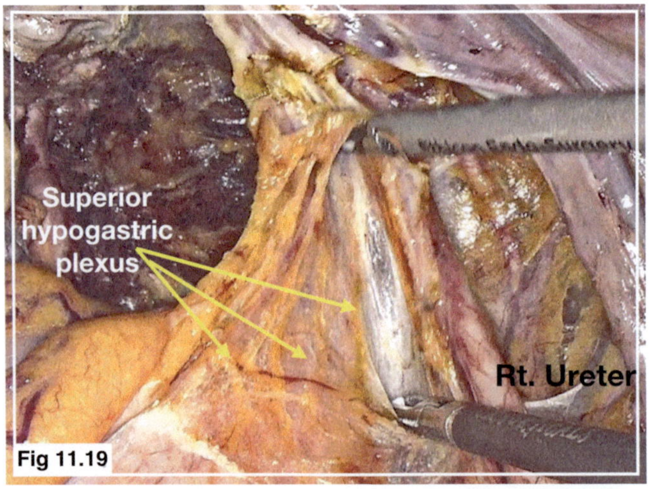

Fig. 11.19 Medial pararectal space dissection: The superior hypogastric plexus is seen as thin yellow lines radiating from the sacral region and converging at the uterosacral ligament. These fibres converge to form the superior hypogastric nerve which later blends with the parasympathetic nerve fibres S2, 3 and 4 for the hypogastric nerve and supply the uterus and the bladder

3. Remain medial to the uterosacral ligament (Fig. 11.19).
4. The hypogastric nerve can be seen running parallel to the ureter and lateral to the uterosacral ligament (Fig. 11.20).

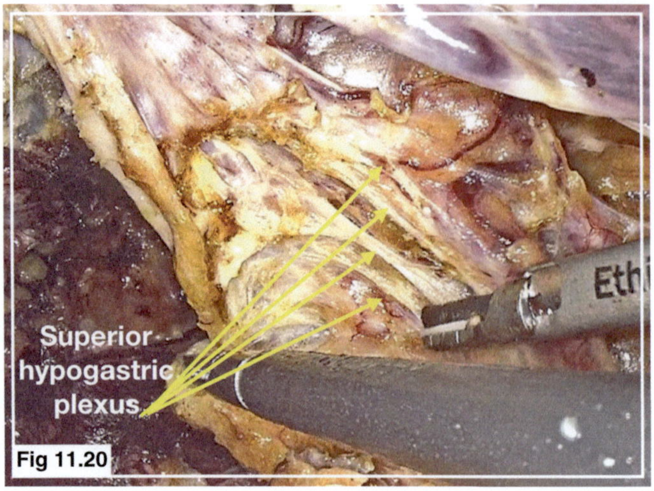

Fig. 11.20 Medial pararectal space dissection: The superior hypogastric plexus fuses to form the superior hypogastric nerve. This has two branches, one which supplies the uterus and the other which travels forward and innervates the bladder. Caution is taken during nerve-sparing surgeries to prevent damage to these fibres as they provide vital function to the urinary bladder

11.3 Exposure of the Retroperitoneum

There are two methods. One is the medial way. The steps are the same described above to open the pararectal and paravesical spaces. This is also called as the *medial* approach.

11.3.1 The Lateral Approach

1. Antevert the uterus. Open the peritoneum lateral to the IP ligament (Fig. 11.21).
2. Remain parallel to the IP ligament and cut the entire anterior part of the broad ligament all the way caudally till you reach the round ligament (Fig. 11.22).
3. Cut the round ligament. This exposes and widens the retroperitoneal space (Fig. 11.23).
4. Go laterally and expose the psoas muscle with genitofemoral nerve (Fig. 11.24).
5. Continue pushing the posterior leaf of broad ligament medially. This will expose the ureter lying closely applied to the broad ligament (Figs. 11.25, 11.26, 11.27, and 11.28).
6. Retract the ureter further medially and remain parallel and lateral to the ureter. This dissection should also go from cranial to caudal region (Fig. 11.29).
7. This will expose the lateral pararectal space. The only transverse structure crossing is the uterine artery (Fig. 11.30).

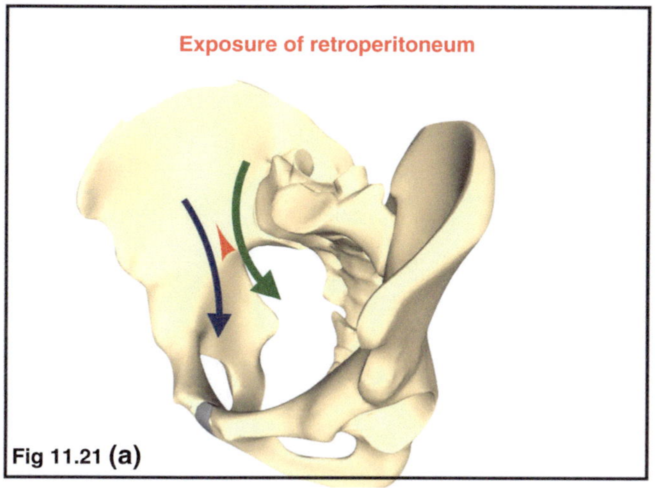

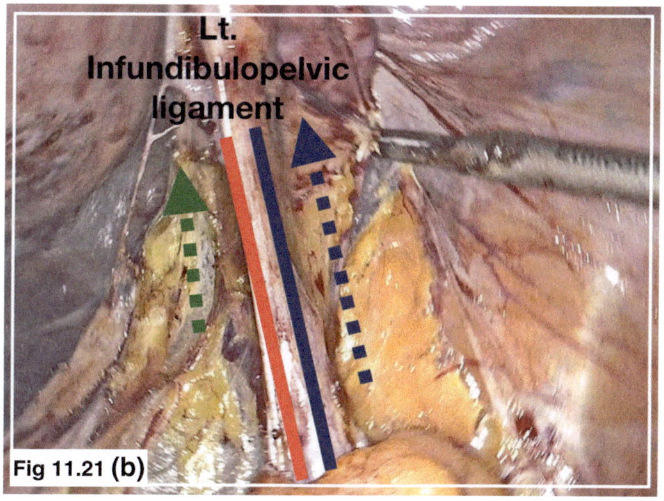

Fig. 11.21 (**a**, **b**) Lateral approach: The approach to the pararectal space can also be done from the lateral side of the infundibulopelvic ligament. This approach is also called as the oncological approach (blue arrow). And the medial approach shown previously is called as the endometriotic approach (green arrow)

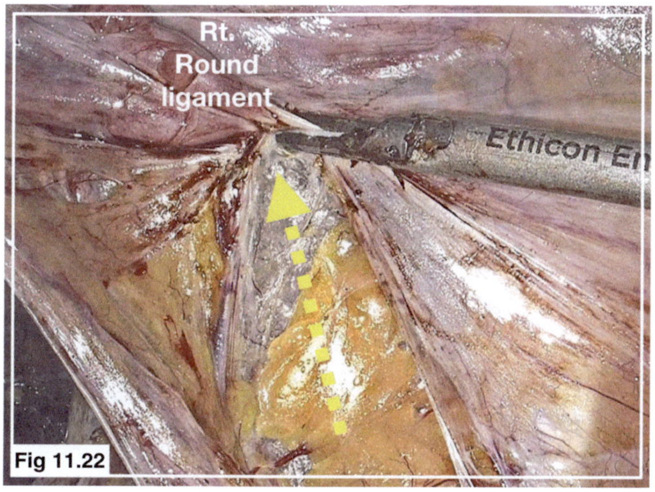

Fig. 11.22 Lateral approach: In this approach incision with Harmonic scalpel is taken from lateral to the infundibulopelvic ligament. This is done by providing medial traction to the ovary and tube and dissecting lateral to it. The incision needs to be extended beyond the round ligament. This gives better exposure to the external iliac artery underneath

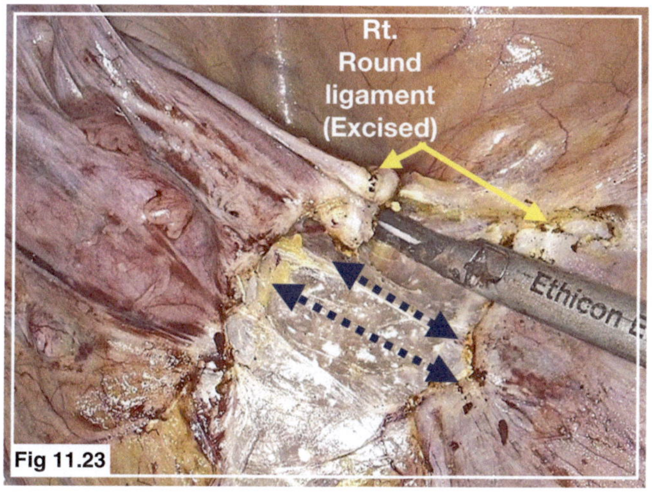

Fig. 11.23 Lateral approach: Excision of the round ligament increases the range of traction provided on the uterus and thus opens the whole pararectal space more widely

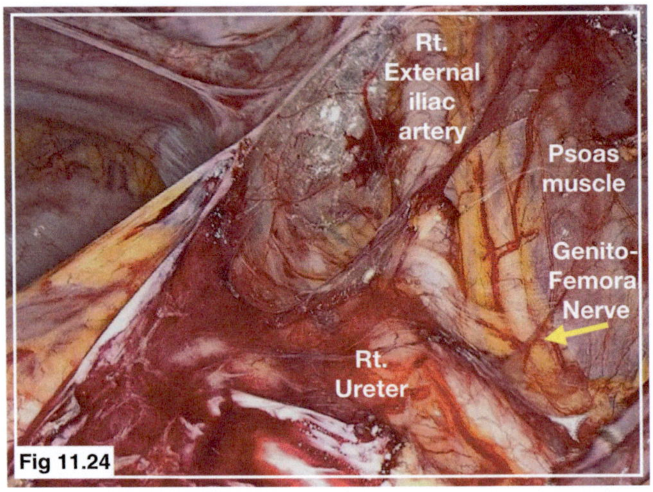

Fig. 11.24 Lateral approach: The first structure visible on the lateral approach is the external iliac vessels. Complete excision of the infundibulopelvic ligament helps reveal the ureter and the external iliac artery without any manipulations further opening the retroperitoneum and exposing the psoas muscle with the genitofemoral nerve

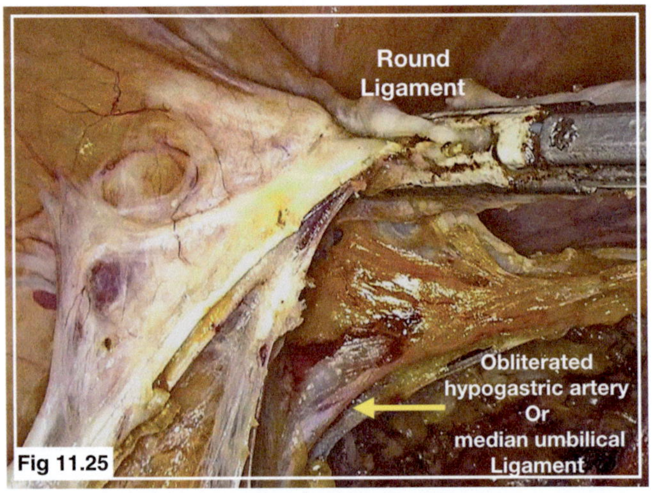

Fig. 11.25 Lateral approach: Similar steps are done on the left side as well. Peritoneum is opened laterally till the round ligament. The internal iliac artery terminates as the obliterated hypogastric artery in the pelvis in the lateral wall. It continues onto the anterior abdominal wall as the median umbilical ligament

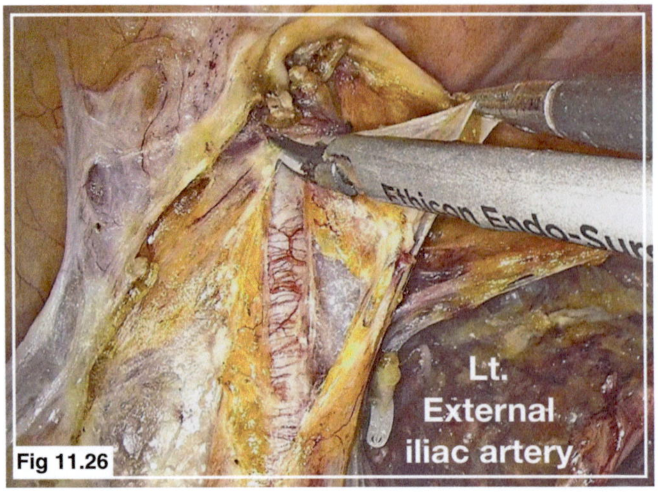

Fig. 11.26 Lateral approach: The external iliac artery can be easily visualised on the left side as well. Traction applied onto the fat covering the vessel helps in exposing the vessel clearly as well as it is primarily done in case of lymph node dissection

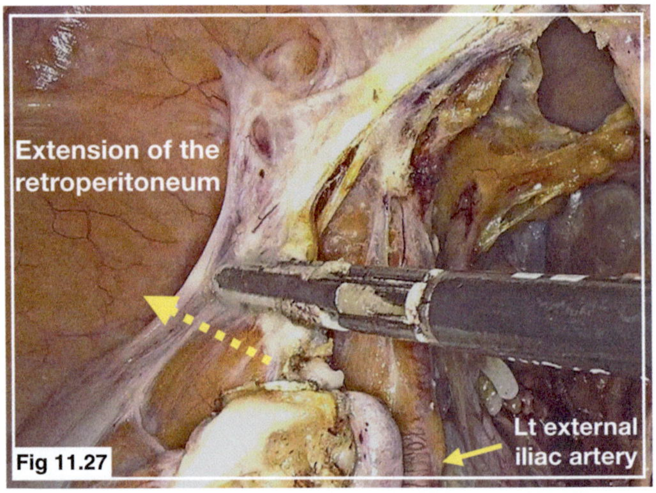

Fig. 11.27 Lateral approach: The peritoneum can be dissected further laterally at right angles to the edge of the peritoneum to widen the area and expose the underlying external iliac vessel and the psoas muscle

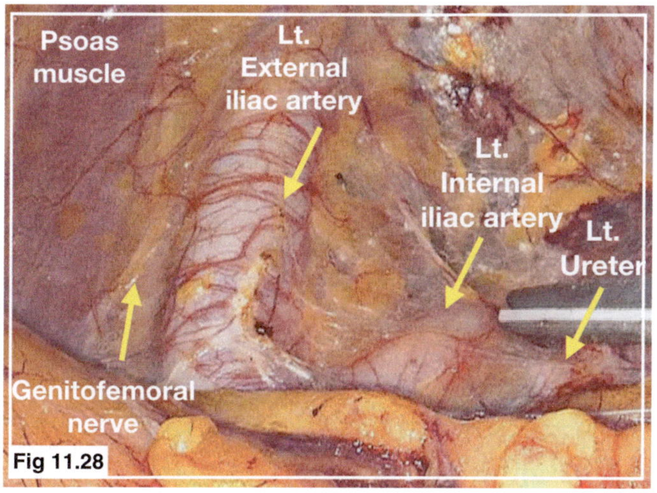

Fig. 11.28 Lateral approach: Extension of the lateral approach can be done by dissecting the peritoneum laterally and reflecting it. This exposes the psoas muscle and the genitofemoral nerve

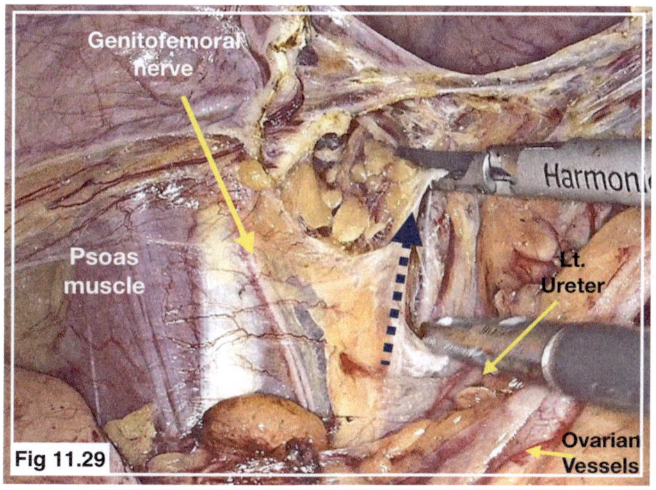

Fig. 11.29 Lateral approach: Just like the endometriotic approach blunt dissection can be carried out in direction parallel and lateral to the ureter to dissect the pararectal space. The blue arrow denotes the direction of dissection

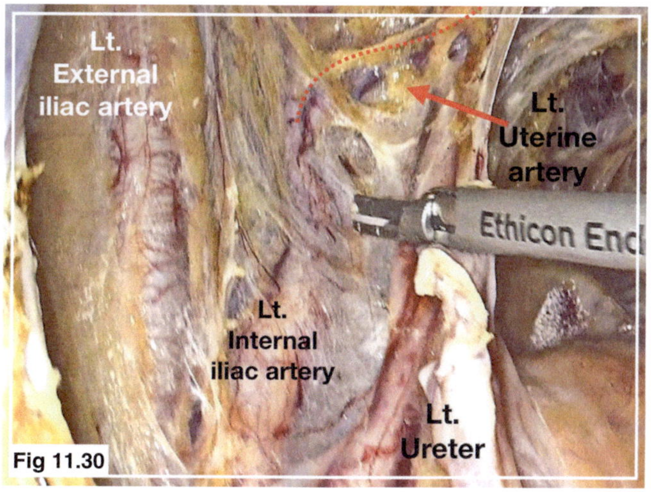

Fig. 11.30 Lateral approach: The aim of pararectal space dissection in a case of radical hysterectomy is to identify the uterine artery. The uterine artery can be seen crossing over the ureter. Thus the pararectal space dissection by lateral approach can be done with equal amount of ease as the medial or the endometriotic approach. Lateral approach of paraxial space dissection completed

11.4 Radical Hysterectomy (*Pune* Technique)

All the steps of radical hysterectomy step by step to be depicted. This means all the six baby steps (Figs. 11.31, 11.32, 11.33, 11.34, 11.35, 11.36, 11.37, 11.38, 11.39, 11.40, 11.41, 11.42, 11.43, 11.44, 11.45, 11.46, 11.47, 11.48, 11.49, 11.50, 11.51, 11.52, 11.53, 11.54, 11.55, 11.56, 11.57, 11.58, 11.59, 11.60, and 11.61).

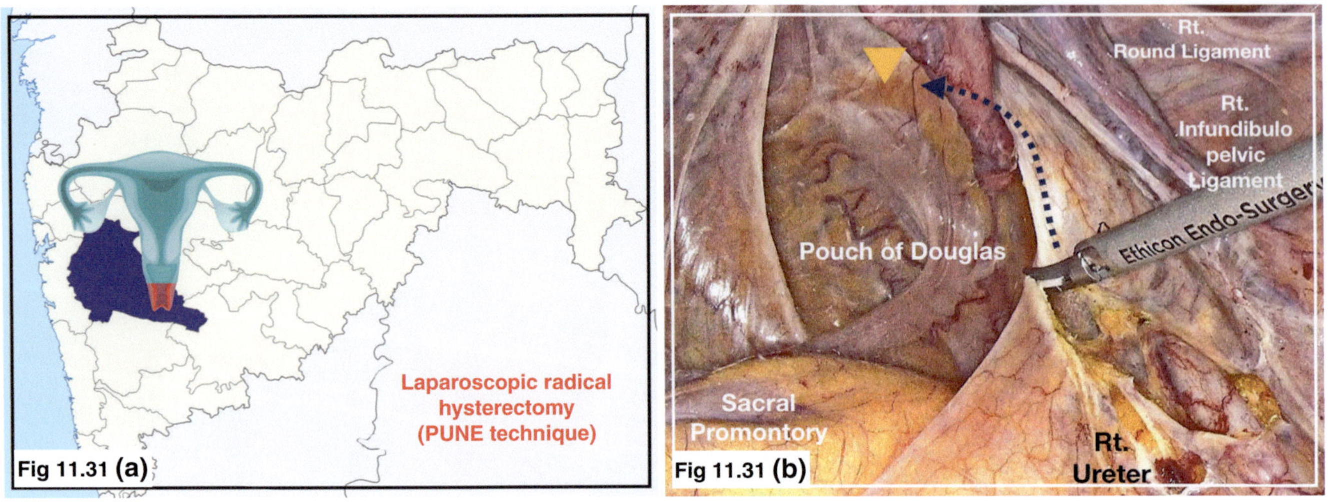

Fig. 11.31 Steps of Pune technique: (**a**) The posterior U-cut: This is the first step of the one technique comprising an incision on the peritoneum from the medial side of infundibulopelvic ligament on one side to the infundibulopelvic ligament on the other side involving the apex of both uterosacral ligaments forming a U-shaped incision. This picture shows the initial part of the posterior U-cut at the right infundibulopelvic ligament

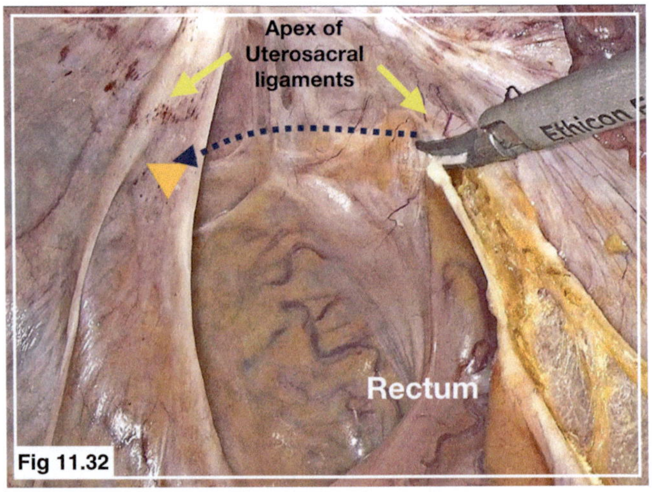

Fig. 11.32 Steps of Pune technique: (**a**) The posterior U-cut: On reaching the apex of the ipsilateral uterosacral ligament an arch-shape bent incision is extended onto the contralateral uterosacral ligament. This extension of incision is to be kept in mind to stay away from the fat. The yellow fat is the line of demarcation so as not to go beyond it. There is greater possibility of injury to the rectum here

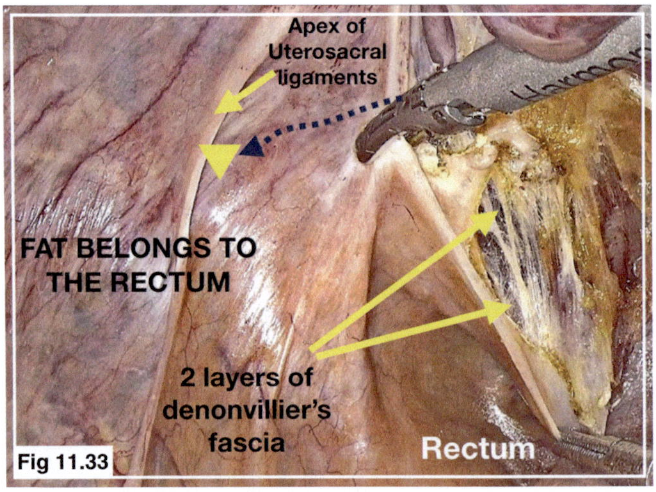

Fig. 11.33 Steps of Pune technique: (**a**) The posterior U-cut: While cutting over the pouch of Douglas, gentle traction to the rectum in a central and cranial manner keeping the uterus anteverted stretches the fat from the peritoneum layer and thus helps in better dissection. The dictum to be followed here is "fat belongs to the rectum". This reveals the two layers of Denonvilliers' fascia

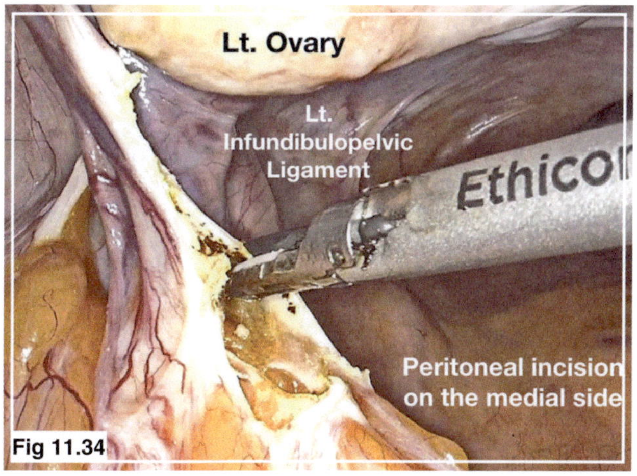

Fig. 11.34 Steps of Pune technique: (**a**) The posterior U-cut: Mirroring incision on the contralateral side is also taken. The incision from the apex of uterosacral ligaments can be extended upwards up to the medial side of the infundibulopelvic ligament but it would amount to greater risk of ureteric injuries

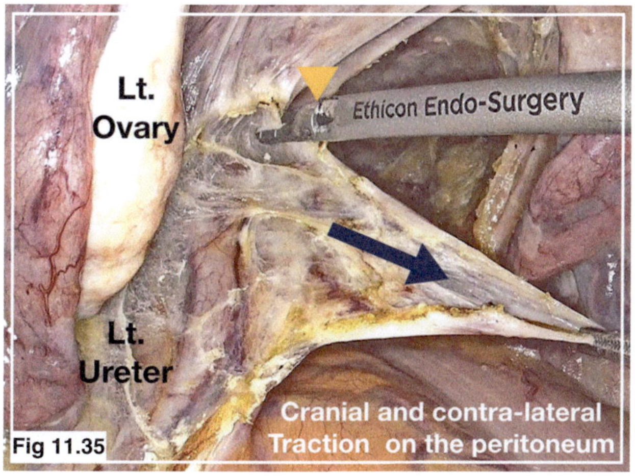

Fig. 11.35 Steps of Pune technique: (**a**) The posterior U-cut: Similar incisions on the contralateral sides help in early visualisation of the ureter. Cranial and medial traction of the posterior leaf of broad ligament opens the pararectal space and dissects easily

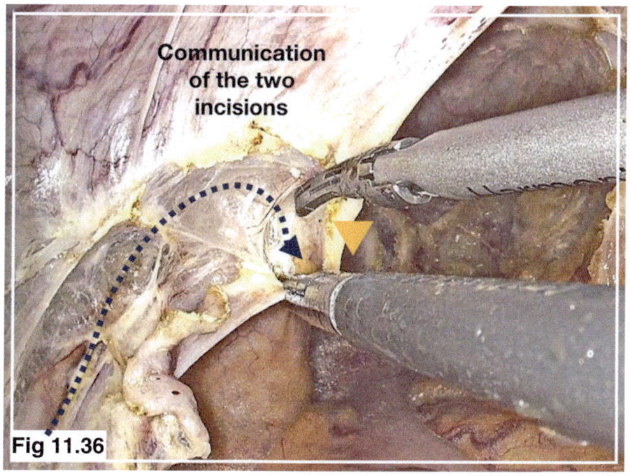

Fig. 11.36 Steps of Pune technique: (**a**) The posterior U-cut: The incision can be extended up to the apex of uterosacral ligament like in the ipsilateral side and made to communicate with the previous incision. This helps in easy mobilisation of the posterior half of the uterus

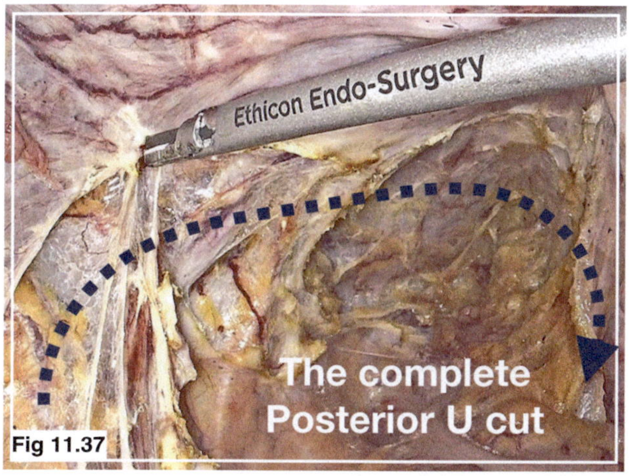

Fig. 11.37 Steps of Pune technique: (**a**) The posterior U-cut: The competed posterior U-cut or two J-shaped cuts

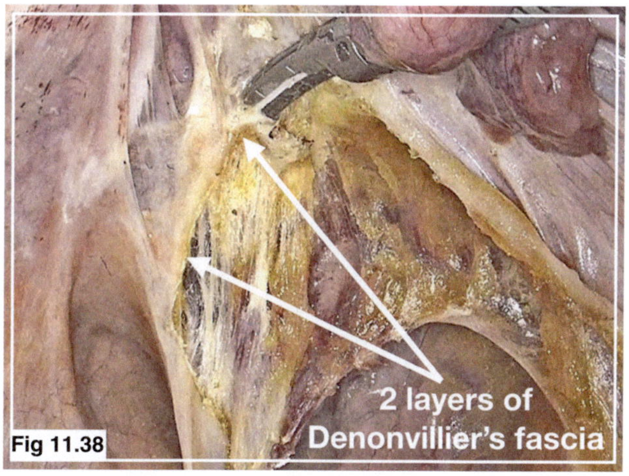

Fig. 11.38 Steps of Pune technique: (**b**) Rectovaginal space dissection: This retroperitoneal space dissection helps in completely separating the rectum from the uterus in its lower retroperitoneal (vagina) extremities or the paracolpium

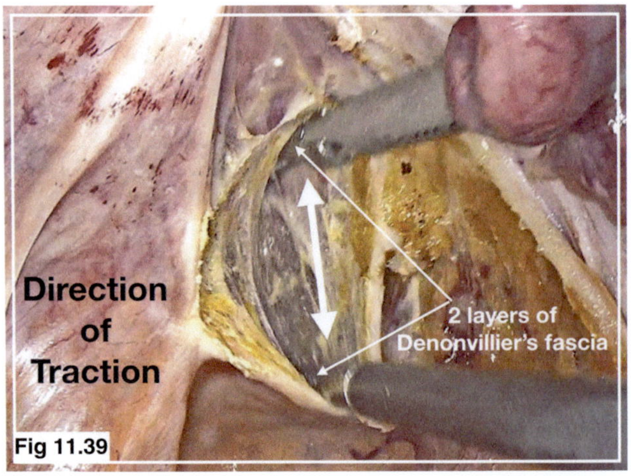

Fig. 11.39 Steps of Pune technique: (**b**) Rectovaginal space dissection: There are two layers of the Denonvilliers' fascia in the rectovaginal space. Avascular plane can be maintained by staying between these two layers at all times

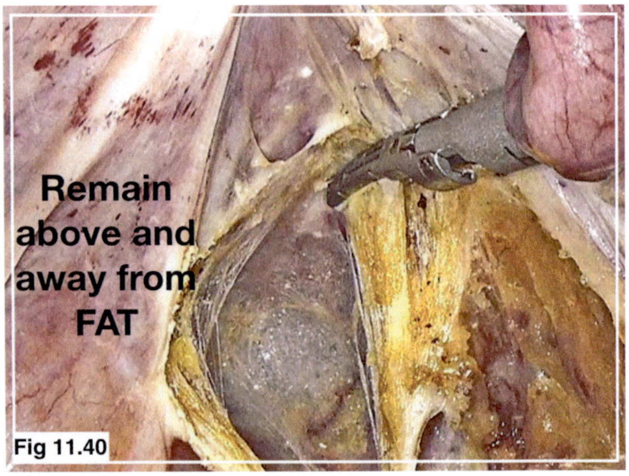

Fig. 11.40 Steps of Pune technique: (**b**) Rectovaginal space dissection: *Fat belongs to the rectum*; this dictum helps prevent injuries to the minor veins underneath the fascia

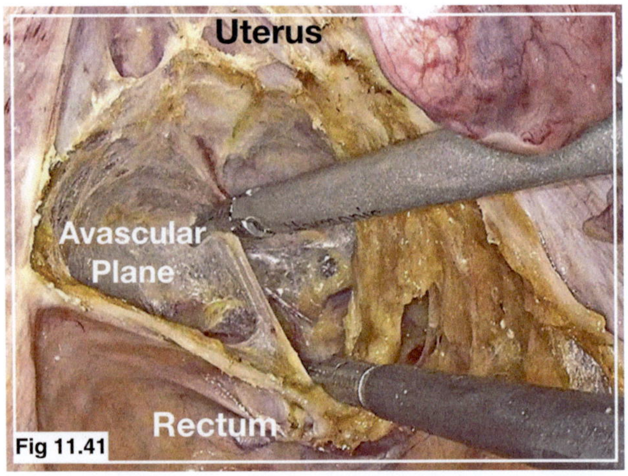

Fig. 11.41 Steps of Pune technique: (**b**) Rectovaginal space dissection: The dissection is to be carried out till the endopelvic fascia is visible underneath. At this point the rectum has been completely free from any attachments to the uterus

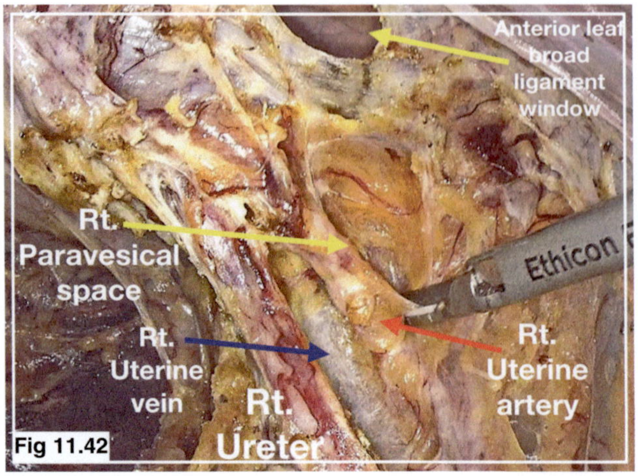

Fig. 11.42 Steps of Pune technique: (**c**) Pararectal and paravesical space dissection: As discussed in detail in prior images, the dissection of these spaces follows the same principles and steps. The uterine artery is identified and dissected free from all retroperitoneal fat. This is followed by the paravesical space dissection done parallel and above the uterine artery

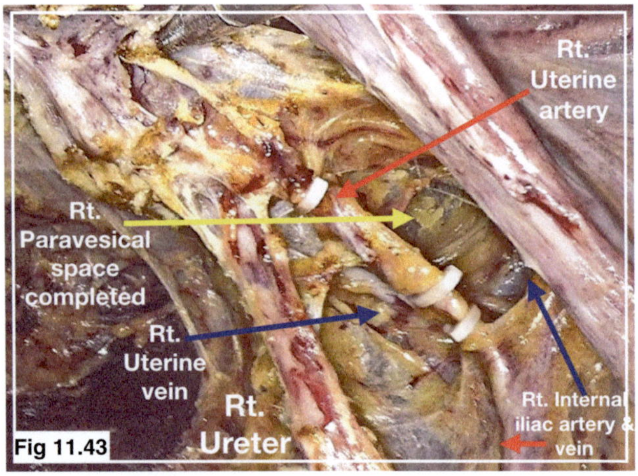

Fig. 11.43 Steps of Pune technique: (**c**) Pararectal and paravesical space dissection: The paravesical space dissection is done till the levator ani is appreciated as shiny grey reflection from the depth of the paravesical space. Clipping the major vessels, coagulating and cutting complete the pararectal space dissection

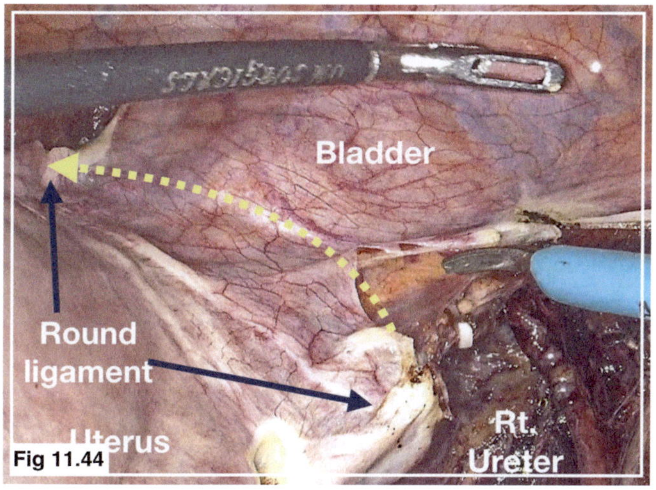

Fig. 11.44 Steps of Pune technique: (**d**) Anterior U-cut: This is called as the anterior U-cut because just like the posterior U-cut it has two fixed points. When both the round ligaments are cut in the pararectal space dissection, the anterior U-cut begins from these end points along the uterovesical fold of the peritoneum forming a U-shaped incision, hence anterior U-cut. This is done for bladder dissection

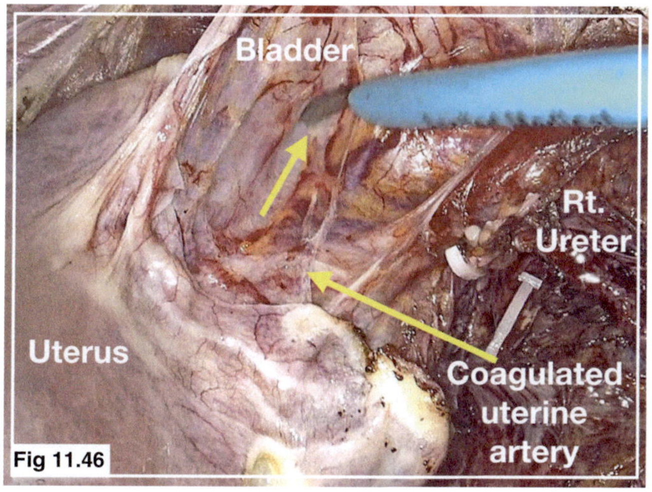

Fig. 11.46 Steps of Pune technique: (**d**) Anterior U-cut: As we dissect the bladder the uterine artery becomes more visible. Thus it is to be kept in mind that the correct plane of dissection lies anterior and above the uterine artery. All that is yellow should be pushed onto the bladder and away from the uterus. Avascular plane is an indicator that the dissection has occurred in the correct plane of fascia

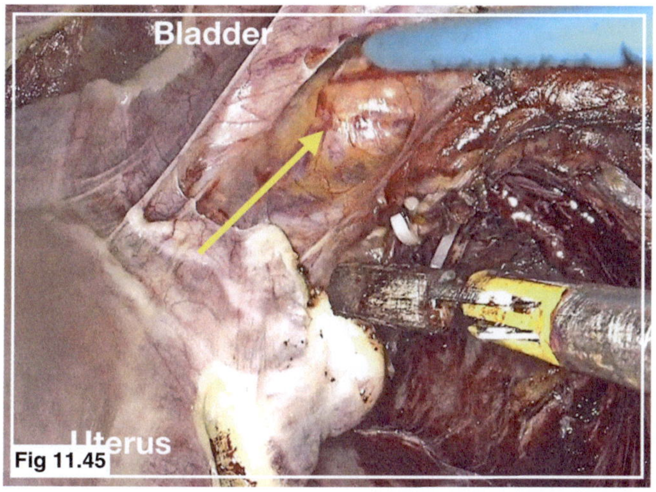

Fig. 11.45 Steps of Pune technique: (**d**) Anterior U-cut: The bladder dissection is best appreciated without the use of any energy sources. The cold scissors are the best instrument to use during bladder dissection. The dictum followed here is "fat belongs to the bladder". Thus with every small incision the fat is pushed off from the uterus and onto the bladder. The yellow arrow denotes the direction of bladder dissection

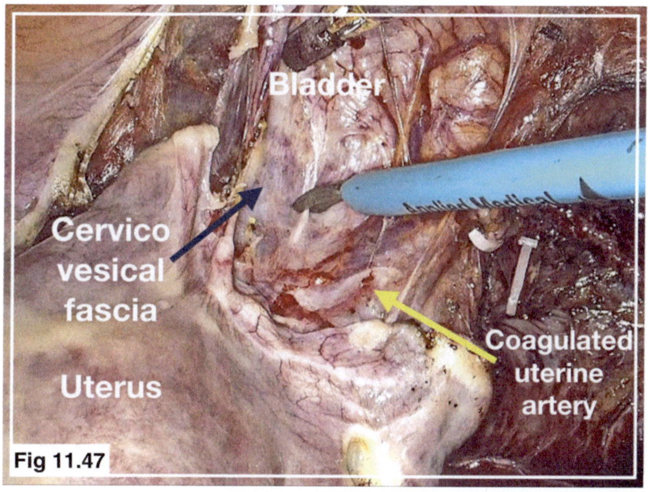

Fig. 11.47 Steps of Pune technique: (**d**) Anterior U-cut: Small bites are taken at the vascular areas and pushed away from the uterus. The energy sources can be used in case of coagulation of the minor veins on the surface of uterus. It is important to ensure that no fat is left on the uterine surface. This becomes an indicator that the dissection has been done in the correct plane. This clear plane of fascia is called the cervicovesical fascia

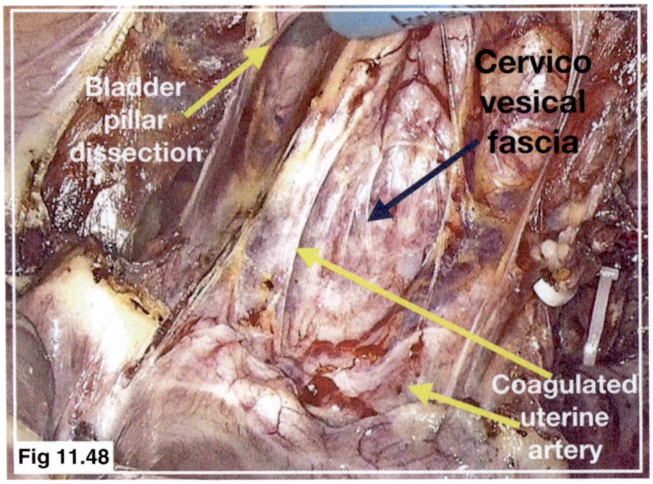

Fig. 11.48 Steps of Pune technique: (**d**) Anterior U-cut: Dissection of the bladders is most important as these areas have many vessels which are prone to injury. Secondly the bladder is raised high up in these areas as compared to the areas along the uterovesical fold. Dissection of both the bladder pillars and complete exposure of the cervicovesical fascia and both the uterine arteries denote the completion of the anterior U-cut and the bladder dissection

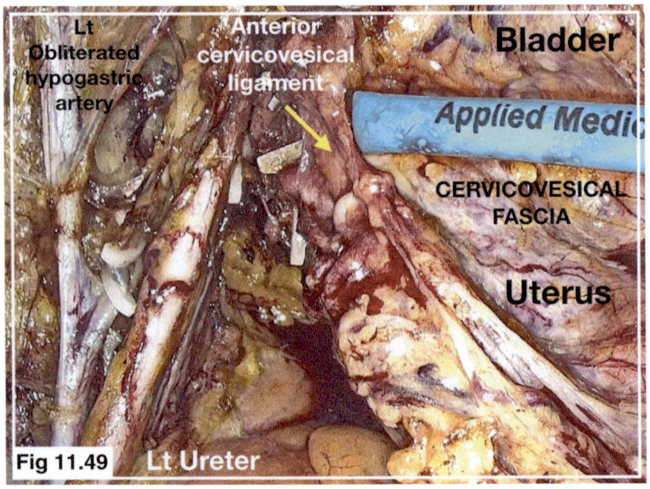

Fig. 11.49 Steps of Pune technique: (**e**) Tunnel dissection: This is also known as the Wertheim's tunnel dissection. However it is the dissection of the ligaments condensed around the cervicovesical fascia anteriorly and posteriorly. The anterior cervicovesical ligament can be identified above the scissors dissected through the Yabuki space

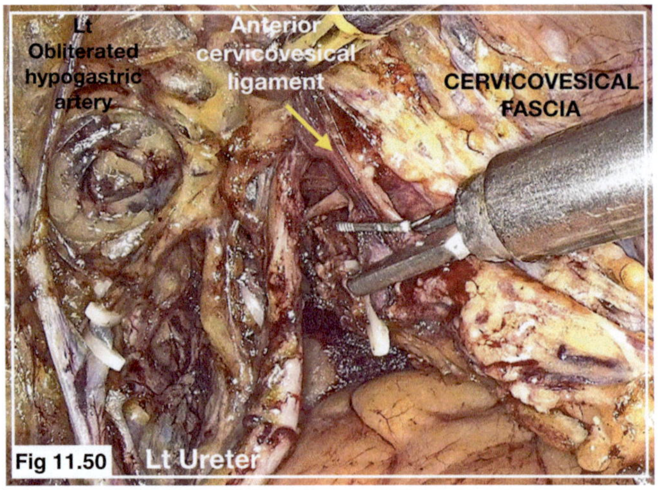

Fig. 11.50 Steps of Pune technique: (**e**) Tunnel dissection: There are unnamed veins in the cervicovesical ligament which need to be clipped before dissection to prevent bleeding into the diminutive space

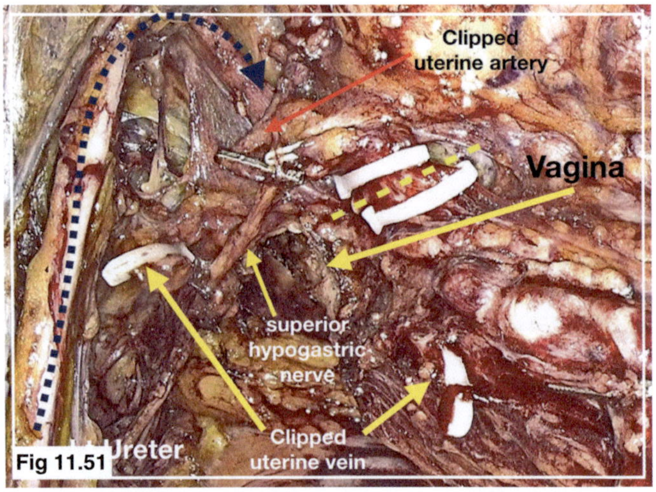

Fig. 11.51 Steps of Pune technique: (**e**) Tunnel dissection: The posterior cervicovesical ligament contains similar veins and sometime lies very close to the uterine even which needs to be clipped to prevent bleeding and free the ureter from the paracolpium and uterus. The course of the ureter can be identified with the blue arrows. The superior hypogastric nerve can be easily appreciated. The major vessels, i.e. the uterine artery and vein, can be seen clipped and cut. The yellow interrupted lines depict the final cut of the anterior cervicovesical ligament that would free the ureter from its course and the uterus

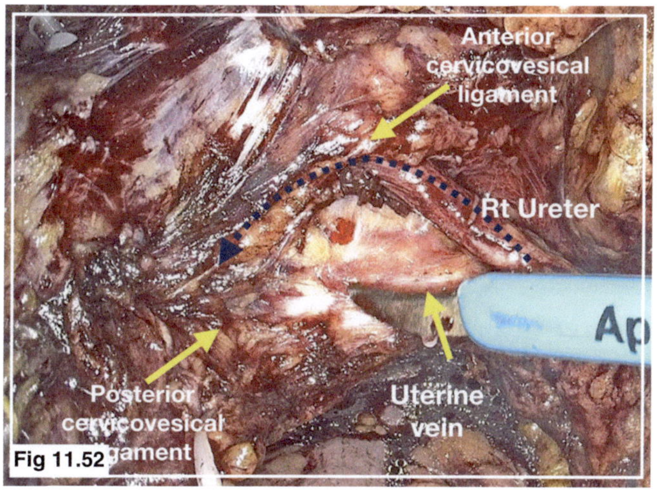

Fig. 11.52 Steps of Pune technique: (**e**) Tunnel dissection: Similar procedure is done on the right side

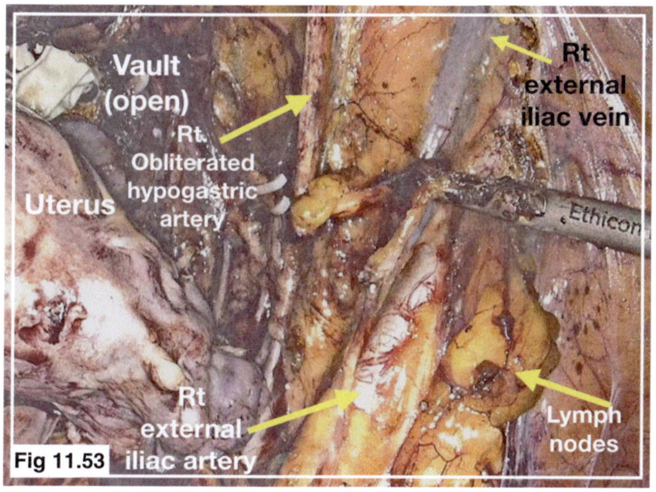

Fig. 11.53 Steps of Pune technique: (**f**) Lymph node dissection: The anterior surface of the external iliac artery does not have any branches and thus lymph node dissection is done by peeling off the fat covering the vessel and removing it en bloc along its whole length and depth

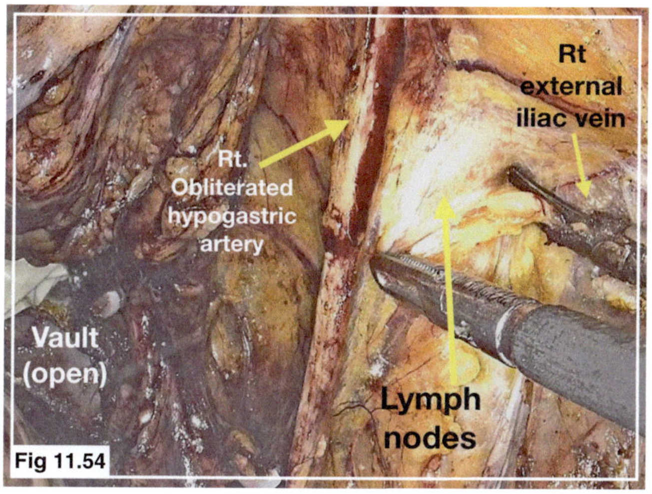

Fig. 11.54 Steps of Pune technique: (**f**) Lymph node dissection: After dissecting a significant thickness of fat it is extended upwards to the anterior abdominal wall in an attempt to remove it en bloc. The fat on the medial side of the external iliac artery is of oncological significance in gynaecology. Lateral to the external iliac vessels lie the femoral lymph nodes which have fewer significance in gynaecology

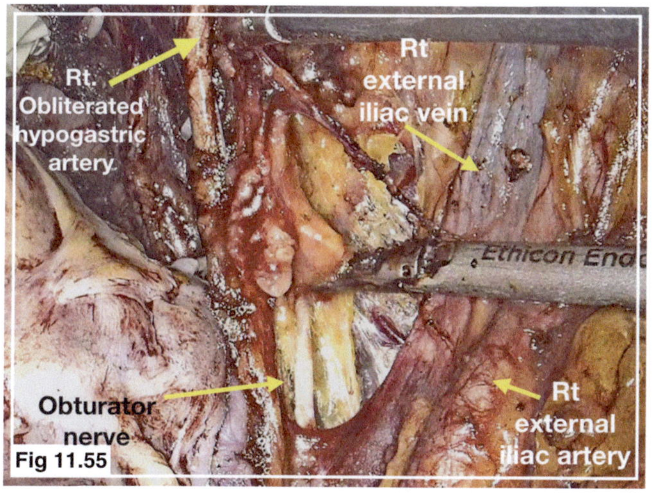

Fig. 11.55 Steps of Pune technique: (**f**) Lymph node dissection: En bloc removal of the Rt pelvic lymph node is done. The lower limit of dissection is the appearance of the obturator nerve. No attempts to be made to dissect the fat from below the obturator nerve

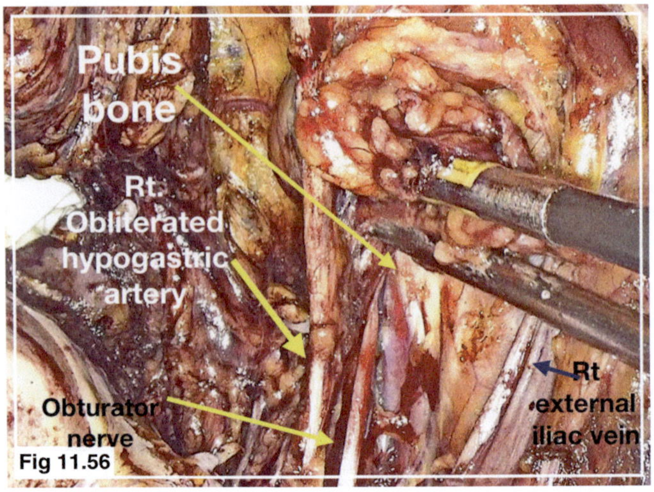

Fig. 11.56 Steps of Pune technique: (f) Lymph node dissection: Dissection is done parallel, anteriorly and at the level of obturator nerve. The obturator vessels lie underneath the nerve. Forceful strain on the nerve can lead to rupture of vessels and significant haemorrhage

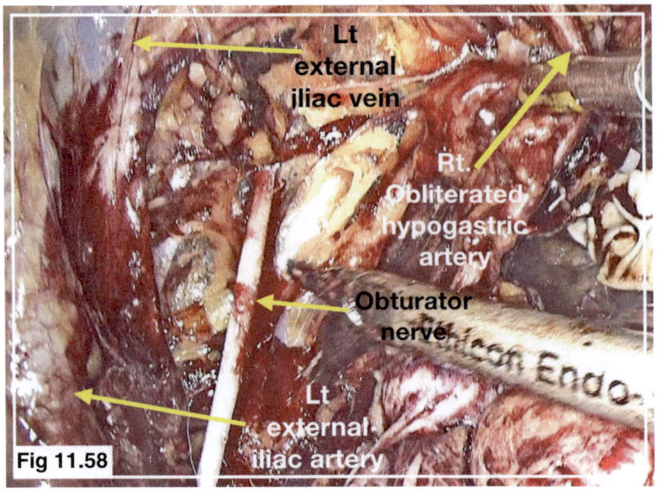

Fig. 11.58 Steps of Pune technique: (f) Lymph node dissection: Similar steps are done on the left side as well following the same principles

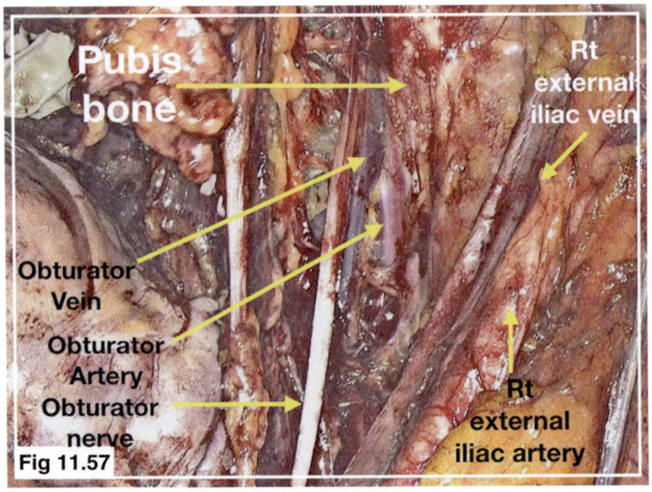

Fig. 11.57 Steps of Pune technique: (f) Lymph node dissection: *Completed picture of right pelvic lymph node dissection.* Obturator nerve, artery and vein are seen. Pubis bone is seen. Exposed external iliac artery and vein are seen. The pararectal and paravesical space appears clear free from fat

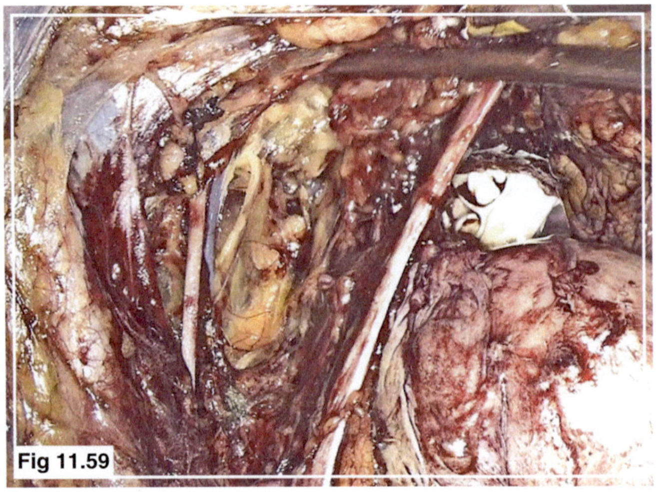

Fig. 11.59 Steps of Pune technique: (f) Lymph node dissection: Completed left-sided pelvic lymph node dissection

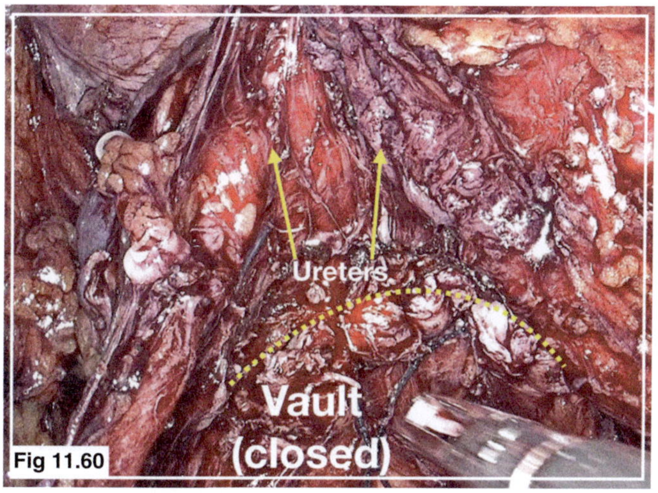

Fig. 11.60 Steps of Pune technique: The ureters are completely dissected off till their insertion into the bladder in radical hysterectomy. This is not seen in intrafascial hysterectomy where none of the retroperitoneal structures are opened

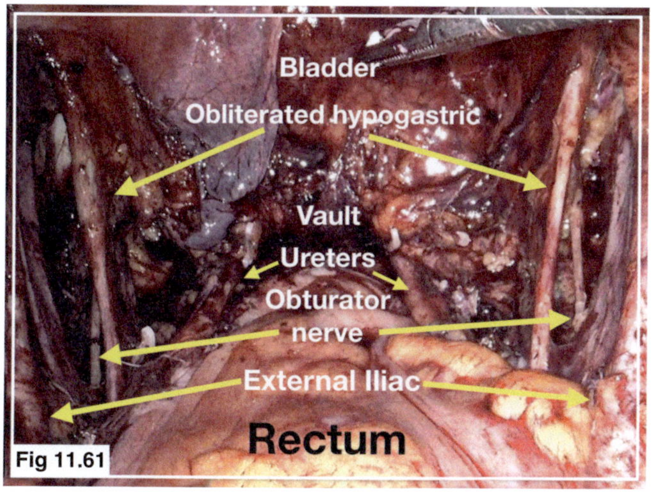

Fig. 11.61 Steps of Pune technique: Final picture of the vault: Both the ureters are seen till their insertion into the bladder, and both the external and internal iliac artery are visualised. Both obturator nerves can be seen indicating complete lymph node dissection

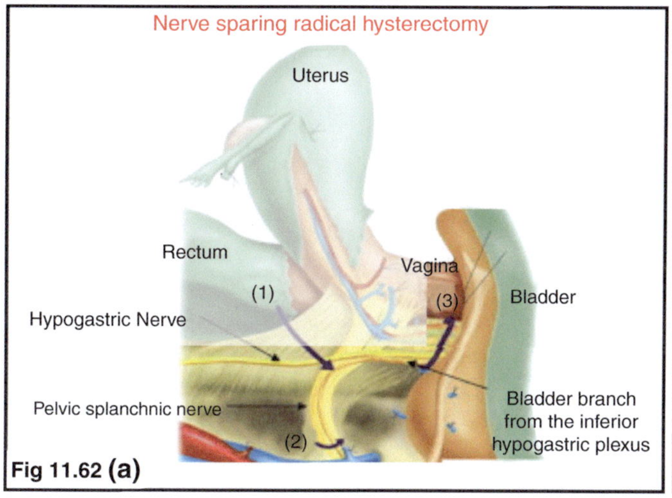

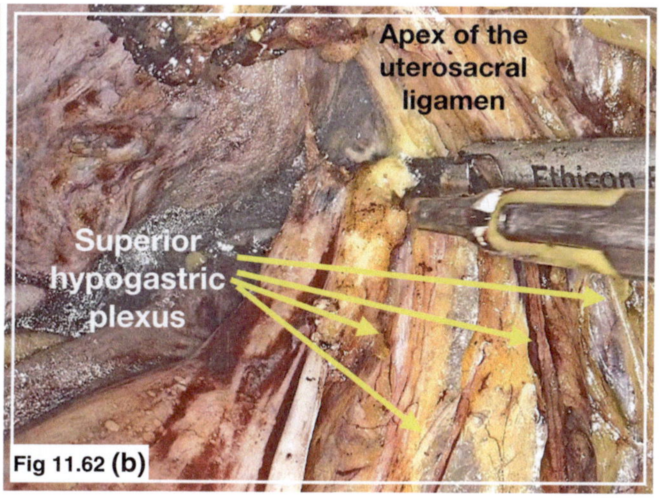

Fig. 11.62 (a, b) Steps of Pune technique: Nerve-sparing laparoscopic radical hysterectomy: Similar principles and steps are carried out as the laparoscopic radical hysterectomy. However difference lies in the identification of the uterine vein. The superior hypogastric plexus and its branches and the parasympathetic S2, 3 and 4 nerves and careful dissection around them

11.5 Nerve Sparing

Similarly only the salient steps with photos of nerve sparing. This should include:

1. Exposure of the hypogastric nerve (Figs. 11.62 and 11.63)
2. Exposure of the parasympathetic nerves (Figs. 11.64 and 11.65)
3. Exposure of the uterine vein (Fig. 11.66)
4. Clipping of the uterine vein medial to the ureter (Fig. 11.67)
5. Cutting the nerve fibres going to the uterus (Fig. 11.68)
6. Exposure of the Yabuki space (Fig. 11.69)
7. Clipping of the inferior vesicle vein in the posterior cervicovesical ligament to finally lateralise the nerve (Figs. 11.70 and 11.71)

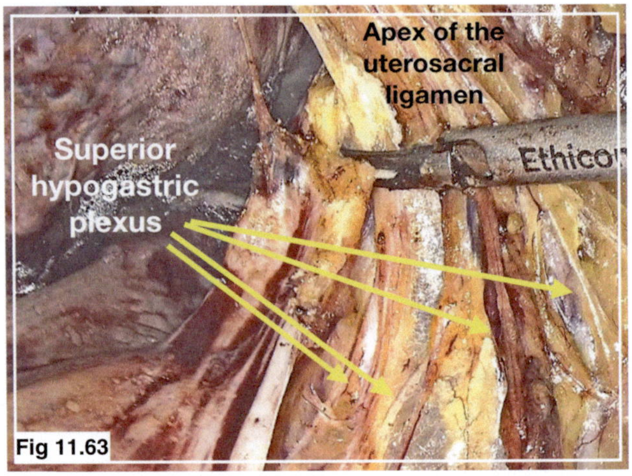

Fig. 11.63 Steps of Pune technique: Nerve-sparing laparoscopic radical hysterectomy: Exposure of the superior hypogastric nerve is done at the level of the uterosacral ligament. Many of its branches supply the uterus while the rest travel forward to supply the bladder

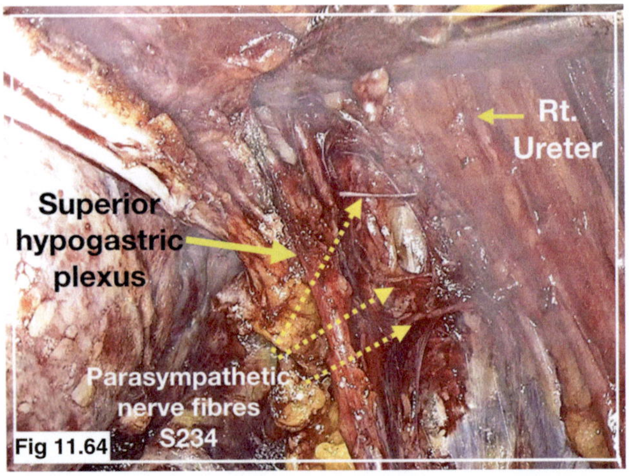

Fig. 11.64 Steps of Pune technique: Nerve-sparing laparoscopic radical hysterectomy: The parasympathetic nerves communicate with the hypogastric nerves at the level below the ureter and uterine vein

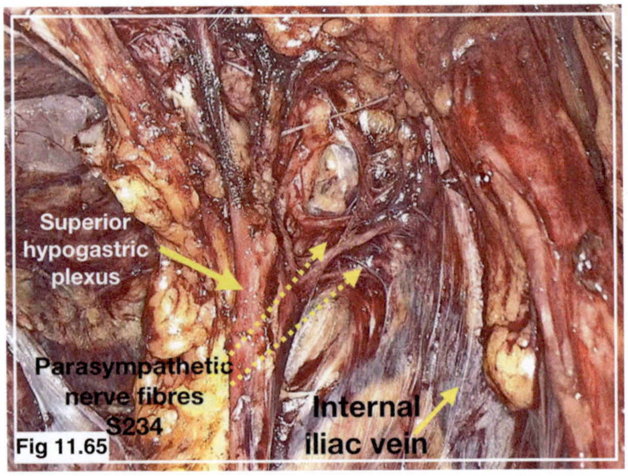

Fig. 11.65 Steps of Pune technique: Nerve-sparing laparoscopic radical hysterectomy: The parasympathetic nerves are well dissected and identified

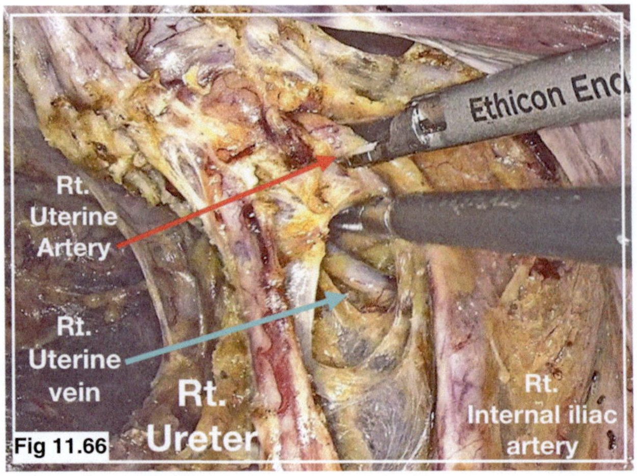

Fig. 11.66 Steps of Pune technique: Nerve-sparing laparoscopic radical hysterectomy: The uterine vein is identified early at the level below the uterine artery and traced upwards to the uterus. Identification of the length of uterine vein is important as clipping of the vein decides the nerve sparing of the procedure

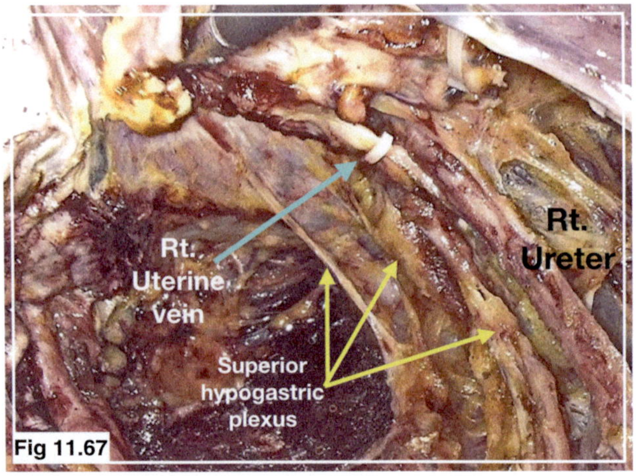

Fig. 11.67 Steps of Pune technique: Nerve-sparing laparoscopic radical hysterectomy: In nerve-sparing hysterectomy the uterine vein is clipped close to the uterus and medial to the ureter. This is so that the nerves supplying the bladder are spared and remain lateral to the clip and remain unharmed when the uterus is removed

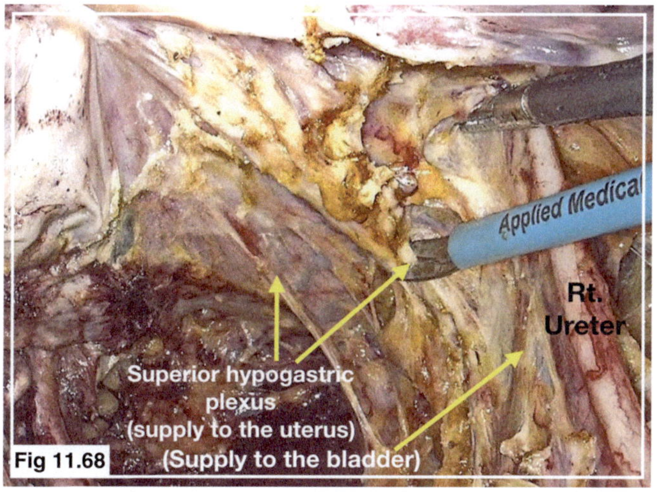

Fig. 11.68 Steps of Pune technique: Nerve-sparing laparoscopic radical hysterectomy: The nerve branches of the hypogastria nerves supplying the uterus are identified and dissected out. They are identified by tracing forward to appreciate if they innervate the uterus or travel further under the ureter

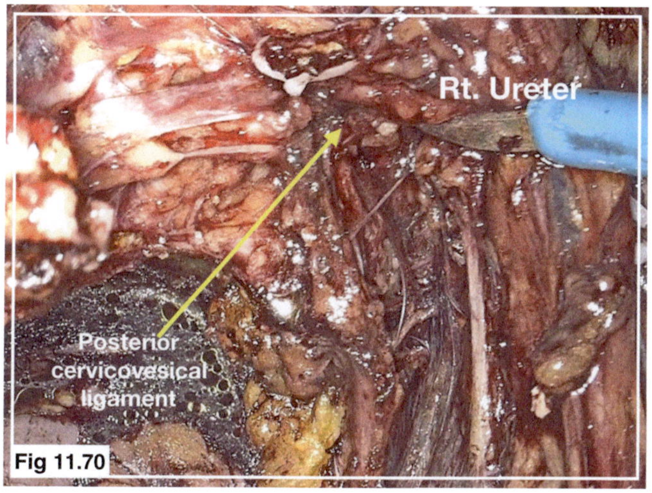

Fig. 11.70 Steps of Pune technique: Nerve-sparing laparoscopic radical hysterectomy: Finally the inferior vesicle vein and the posterior cervicovesical ligament is dissected and cut off to free the ureter posteriorly as well. This completes the nerve-sparing portion of hysterectomy. The rest of the hysterectomy is done with the same steps and principles of radical hysterectomy

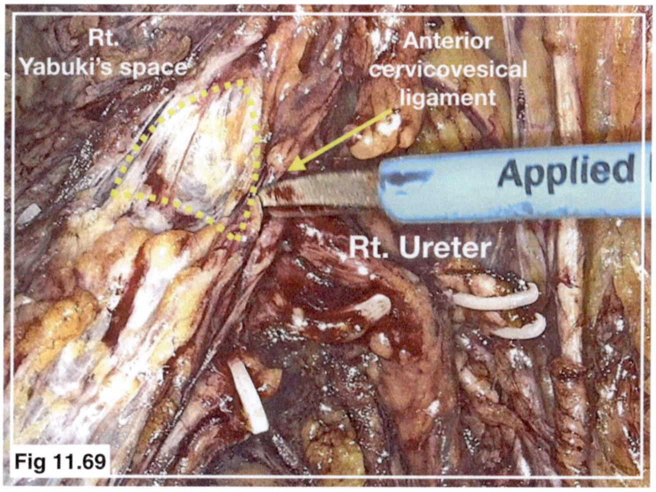

Fig. 11.69 Steps of Pune technique: Nerve-sparing laparoscopic radical hysterectomy: Opening of the Yabuki space is that last step of the nerve-sparing hysterectomy. It contains the nerve fibres which travel along the ureter and innervate the bladder. Dissection of this space is done to free the ureter and the nerves from the uterus. The scissor points at the anterior cervicovesical ligament attached to the ureter which needs to be cut and frees the ureter anteriorly

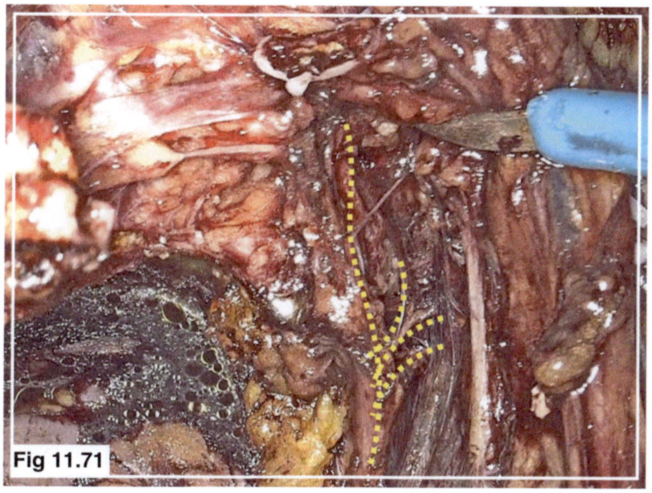

Fig. 11.71 Steps of Pune technique: Nerve-sparing laparoscopic radical hysterectomy: The yellow dotted lines denote the nerves that have been preserved which supply the bladder and the parasympathetic innervation which remains lateral to the ureter along the uterine vein. The ureter here however has been retracted laterally for a better view of the nerves

11.6 Hysterectomy Type I or Intrafascial (Figs. 11.72, 11.73, 11.74, 11.75, 11.76, 11.77, 11.78, 11.79, 11.80, 11.81, 11.82, 11.83, 11.84, 11.85, and 11.86)

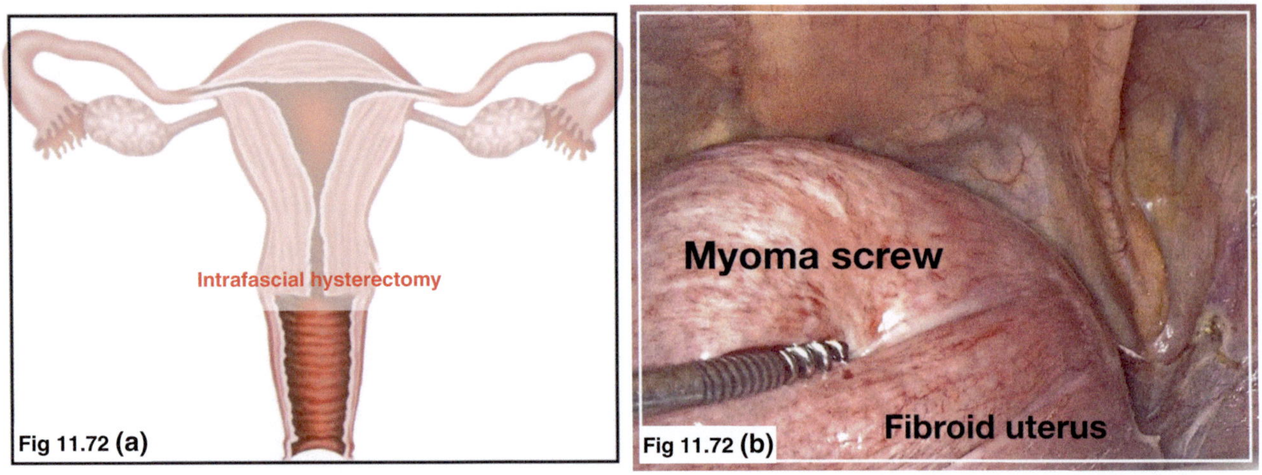

Fig. 11.72 (**a**, **b**) Type I intrafascial hysterectomy: For benign conditions myoma screw is the best instrument for manipulation of the uterus. They can be used in all gynaecological procedures except fertility-preserving surgery and endometrial carcinoma

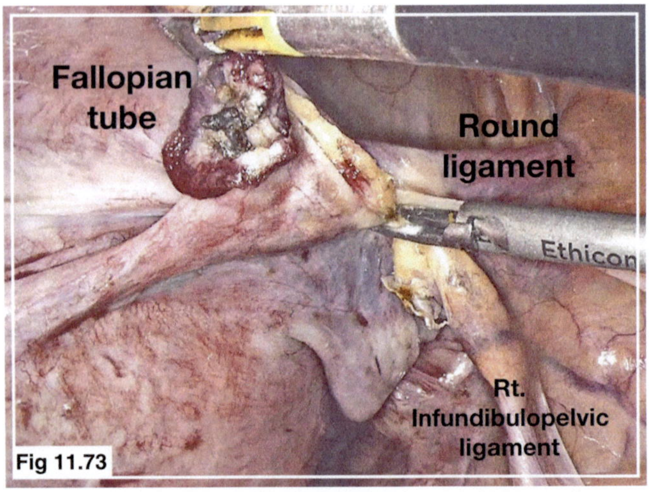

Fig. 11.73 Type I intrafascial hysterectomy: Coagulation of the cornual structures begins with the fallopian tube as it is the most flimsy and dependent structure which often obstructs vision

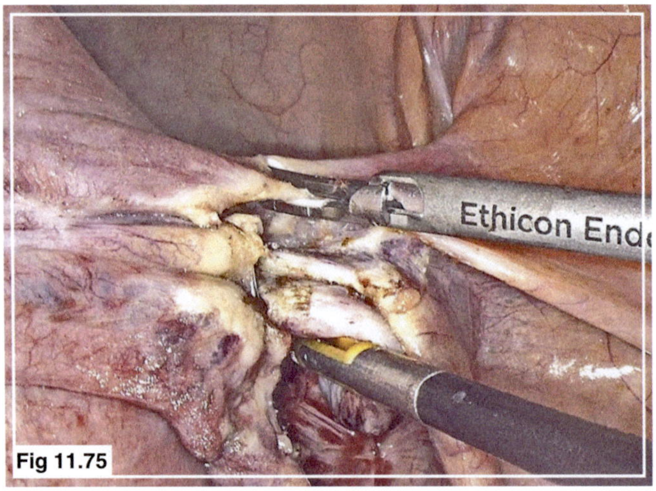

Fig. 11.75 Type I intrafascial hysterectomy: The ovarian and infundibulopelvic ligament is cut depending upon the need of oophorectomy

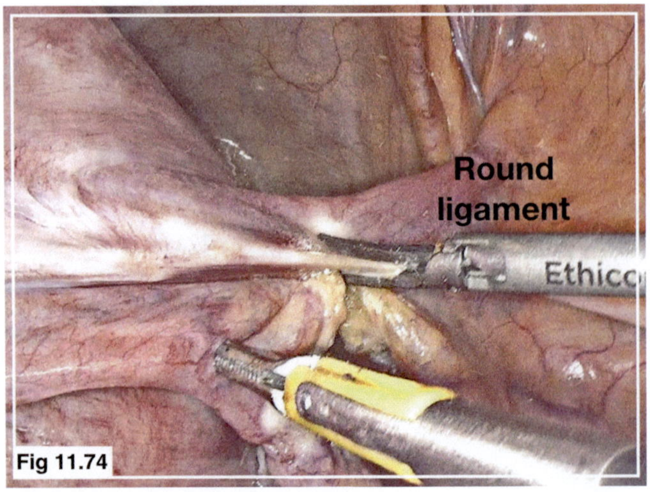

Fig. 11.74 Type I intrafascial hysterectomy: The round ligament is coagulated and cut following the fallopian tube

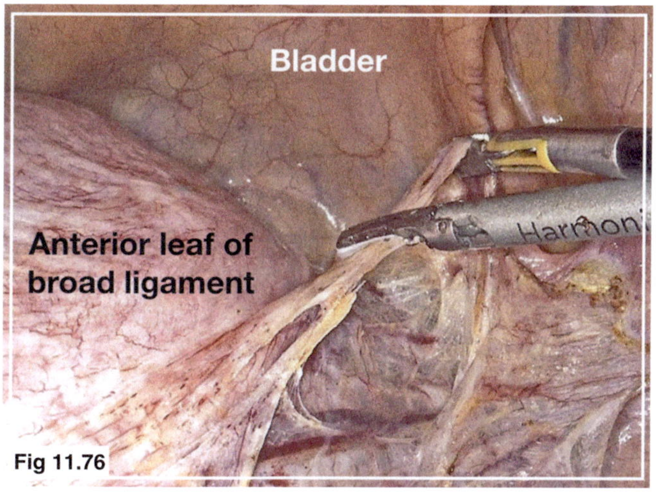

Fig. 11.76 Type I intrafascial hysterectomy: On cutting the round ligament the anterior leaf of the broad ligament becomes free and separated from the uterus. This is the starting point of the bladder dissection in benign cases. In radical hysterectomy the round ligament is cut at the junction of medial 2/3rd and lateral 1/3rd while in benign intrafascial hysterectomy the round ligament is cut close to the uterus

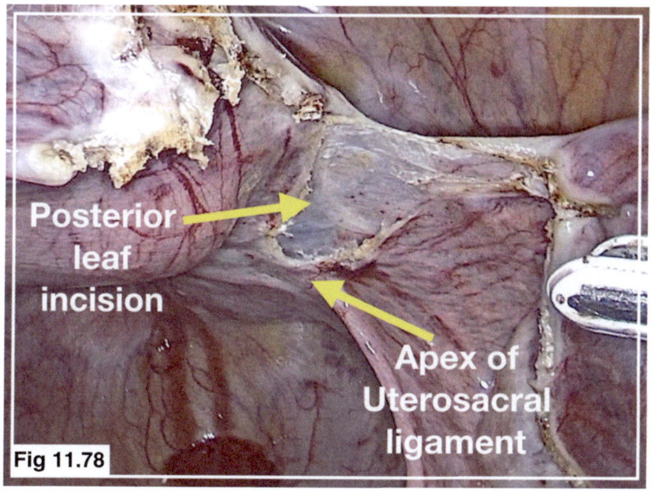

Fig. 11.78 Type I intrafascial hysterectomy: The posterior leaf of the broad ligament is dissected up to the apex of uterosacral ligament and this demarcates the extent of dissection. The dissection should not cross that level

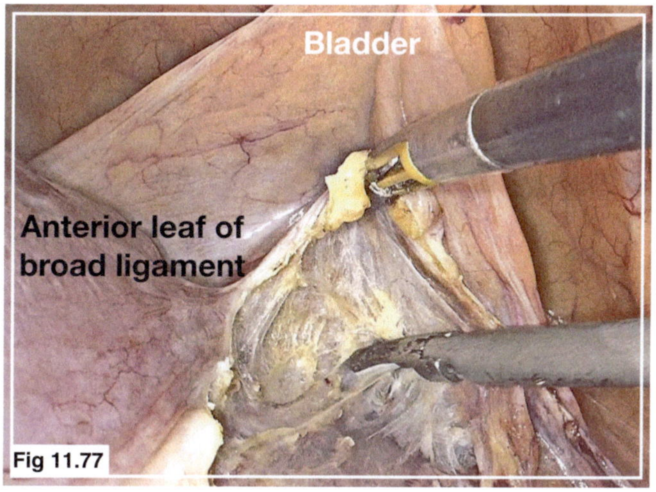

Fig. 11.77 Type I intrafascial hysterectomy: The bladder dissection is done in the same way as explained in the *Pune* technique. The cervix is palpated from the anterior surface of the uterus

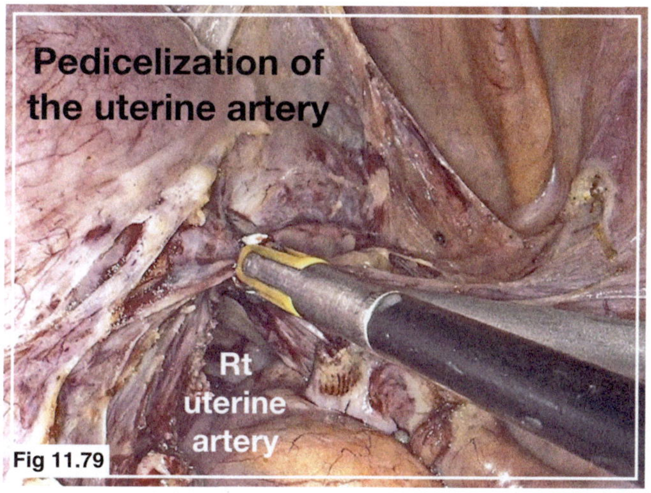

Fig. 11.79 Type I intrafascial hysterectomy: Cutting both leaves of the broad ligament exposes the uterine artery. This is also called as skeletonisation of the uterine artery. Formation of the pedicle of uterine artery is begun from near the attachment the round ligament and above the level of the cervix

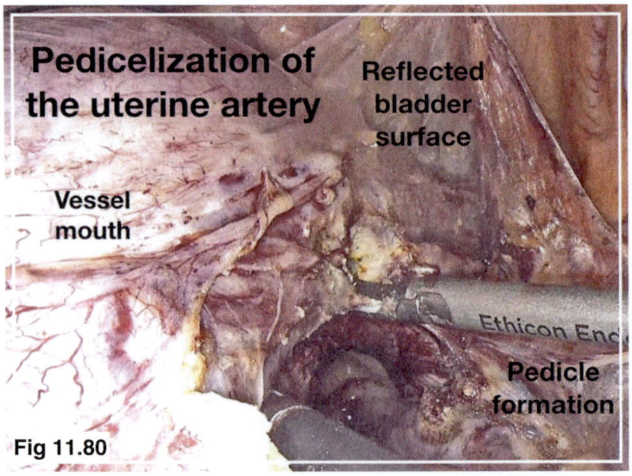

Fig. 11.80 Type I intrafascial hysterectomy: Since uterine artery is of a higher calibre, it is first cauterised with bipolar and then cut by the Harmonic scalpel. The bladder leaf is held to expose the lower uterus. The bipolar cautery should be rolled over the cervix till substantial tissue has been grasped

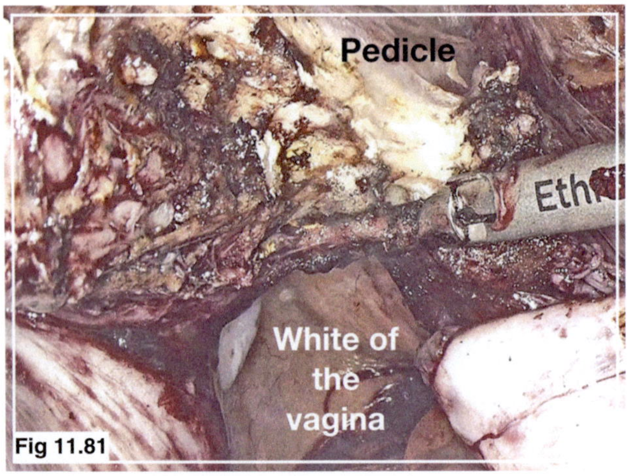

Fig. 11.81 Type I intrafascial hysterectomy: The pedicle is formed by dissecting close to the uterus travelling downwards and medially so that the pedicle falls off on the lateral side as shown in the image. The dissection is continued till the white elastic feeling of the vagina is appreciated. It is often called as the "white of the vagina". However it is relatively more elastic than the rest of the body, thus helping in distinguishing it

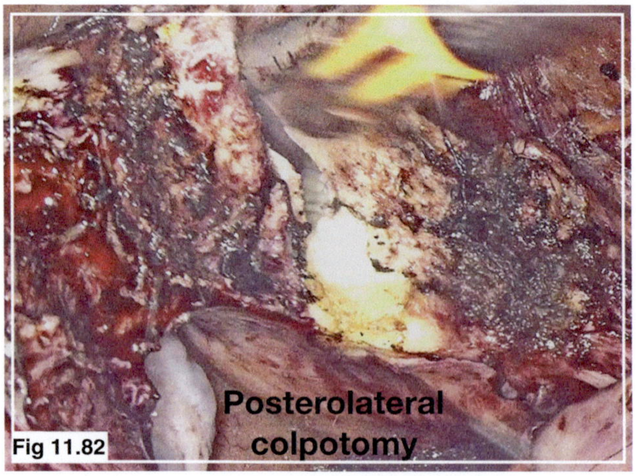

Fig. 11.82 Type I intrafascial hysterectomy: Colpotomy is the most assured step of completion of hysterectomy in the correct plane. It is preferably done on the posterolateral side as no major structures are present. It is always done at the level above the apex of uterosacral ligament

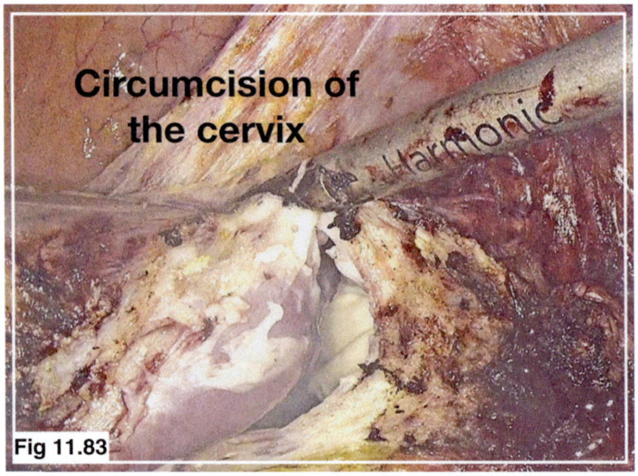

Fig. 11.83 Type I intrafascial hysterectomy: Circumcision of cervix is done to preserve significant length of the vagina

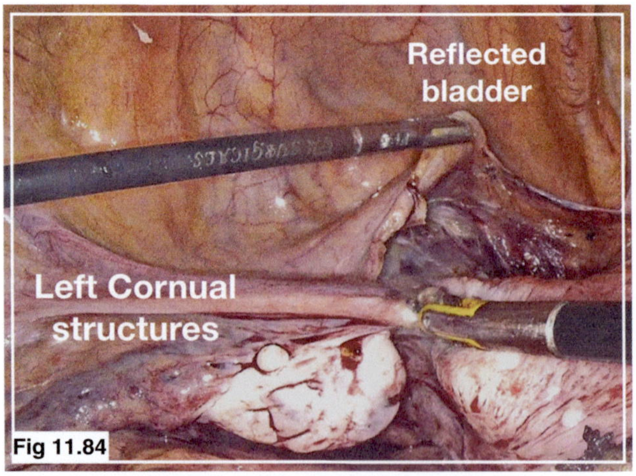

Fig. 11.84 Type I intrafascial hysterectomy: Similar steps are carried out on the contralateral side

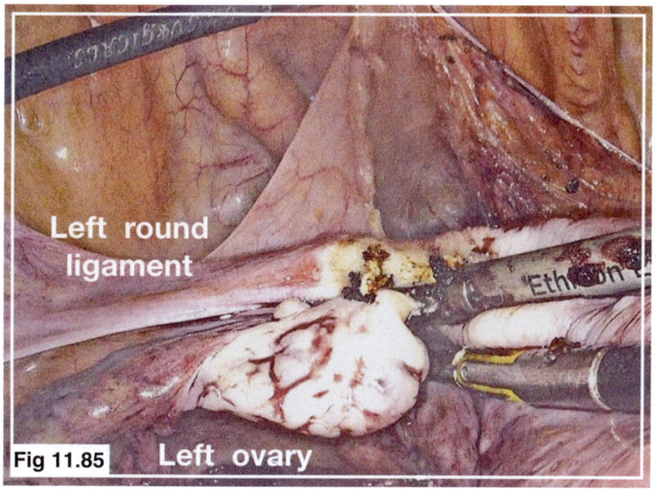

Fig. 11.85 Type I intrafascial hysterectomy: Similar steps are carried out at the cornua

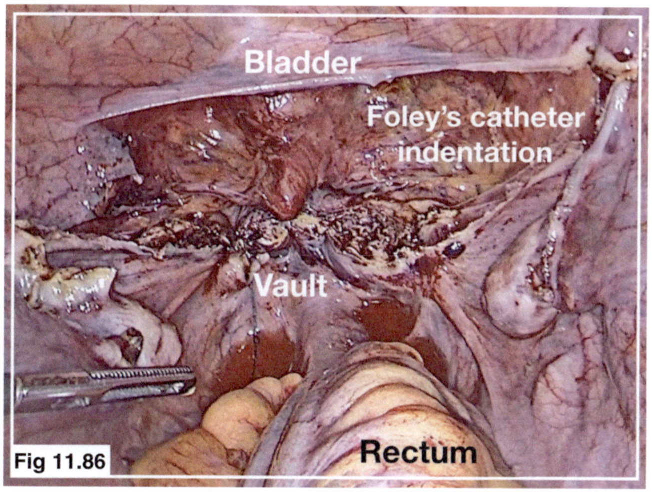

Fig. 11.86 Type I intrafascial hysterectomy: Final appearance of the vault after hysterectomy. Both ovaries are preserved, suture line is at the level of the apex of uterosacral ligaments and the uterosacral ligaments are *not* resected. Ureters are not visualised

Suggested Reading

Alkatout I, Mettler L. Laparoscopic radical hysterectomy with anterior and posterior exenteration, Gynecological perspective, Chap. 45, Hysterectomy: a comprehensive surgical approach, Springer. 2018. p. 649–659.

Ceccaroni M, Pontrelli G, Spagnolo E, et al. Parametrial dissection during laparoscopic nerve-sparing radical hysterectomy: a new approach aims to improve patients' postoperative quality of life. Am J Obstet Gynecol. 2010;202:e1–2.

Fujii S. Anatomic identification of nerve-sparing radical hysterectomy: a step-by-step procedure. Gynecol Oncol. 2008;111:S33–41.

Jamkar A, Puntambekar S. Laparoscopic anterior exenteration with Intracorporeal uretero-sigmoidostomy. J Minim Invasive Gynecol. 2015;22(4):538–9.

Mirilas P, Skandalakis J. Surgical anatomy of the retroperitoneal spaces part II: the architecture of the retroperitoneal space. Ann Surg. 2010;76:33–42.

Netter FH. Section 5 pelvis and the perineum, Atlas of Human Anatomy, Elsevier. 2015. p. 329–395.

Puntambekar S. Laparoscopic pelvic exenteration for advanced pelvic cancers: a review of 16 cases. Gynecol Oncol. 2006;102(3):513–6.

Puntambekar S. Atlas of laparoscopic surgery in gynecologic oncology, Anshan. 2007.

Puntambekar S. Laparoscopic total radical hysyterectomy by the Pune technique: our experience of 248 cases. J Minim Invasive Gynecol. 2007;14(6):682–9.

Puntambekar S. Video 5 & 7, Video atlas of Laparoscopic colorectal surgery, Jaypee. 2012.

Puntambekar S. Video 7, 8, 10 & 11, Video atlas of robotic oncosurgery, p. 19, 22, 28, 31, Jaypee. 2012.

Puntambekar S. Our experience of laparoscopic anterior exenteration in locally advanced cervical carcinoma. J Minim Invasive Gynecol. 2016;23(3):396–404.

Puntambekar S, Cuesta M. Atlas of minimally invasive surgery in oesophageal cancer, Elsevier. 2010.

Puntambekar S, Manchanda R. Surgical pelvic anatomy in gynecologic oncology. Gynecol Obstet. 2018;143(Suppl 2):86–92.

Yabuki Y, Sasaki H, Hatakeyama N, Murakami G. Discrepancies between classic anatomy and modern gynecologic surgery on pelvic connective tissue structure: harmonization of those concepts by collaborative cadaver dissection. Am J Obstet Gynecol. 2005;193:7–15.

S. Puntambekar et al., *Laparoscopic Pelvic Anatomy in Females*, https://doi.org/10.1007/978-981-13-8653-4

MIX
Papier aus verantwortungsvollen Quellen
Paper from responsible sources
FSC® C105338

If you have any concerns about our products,
you can contact us on
ProductSafety@springernature.com

In case Publisher is established outside the EU,
the EU authorized representative is:
Springer Nature Customer Service Center GmbH
Europaplatz 3, 69115 Heidelberg, Germany

Printed by Libri Plureos GmbH
in Hamburg, Germany